Sleep Apnea

Progress in Respiratory Research

Vol. 35

Series Editor *Chris T. Bolliger*, Cape Town

KARGER

Basel · Freiburg · Paris · London · New York · Bangalore · Bangkok · Singapore · Tokyo · Sydney

Sleep Apnea

Current Diagnosis and Treatment

Volume Editors *Winfried J. Randerath*, Solingen
Bernd M. Sanner, Wuppertal
Virend K. Somers, Rochester, Minn.

74 figures, 14 in color, and 19 tables, 2006

KARGER

Basel · Freiburg · Paris · London · New York ·
Bangalore · Bangkok · Singapore · Tokyo · Sydney

Prof. Dr. Winfried J. Randerath
Bethanien Hospital
Aufderhöherstrasse 169–175
DE–42699 Solingen (Germany)

Prof. Dr. Bernd M. Sanner
Bethesda Hospital
Hainstrasse 35
DE–42109 Wuppertal (Germany)

Prof. Dr. Virend K. Somers
Mayo Clinic and Mayo Foundation
200 1st Street SW
Rochester, MN 55901 (USA)

Library of Congress Cataloging-in-Publication Data

Sleep apnea / volume editors, Winfried J. Randerath Solingen, Bernd M. Sanner Wuppertal, Virend K. Somers.
p. ; cm. – (Progress in respiratory research, ISSN 1422-2140 ; v. 35)
Includes bibliographical references and indexes.
ISBN 3-8055-8049-5 (hard cover : alk. paper)
1. Sleep apnea syndromes.
[DNLM: 1. Sleep Apnea Syndromes. WF 143 S632 2006] I. Randerath, Winfried J. II. Sanner, Bernd M. III. Somers, Virend K. IV. Series.
RC737.5.S527 2006
616.2–dc22

2006004184

Disclaimer. The statements, options and data contained in this publication are solely those of the individual authors and contributors and not of the publisher and the editor(s). The appearance of advertisements in the book is not a warranty, endorsement, or approval of the products or services advertised or of their effectiveness, quality or safety. The publisher and the editor(s) disclaim responsibility for any injury to persons or property resulting from any ideas, methods, instructions or products referred to in the content or advertisements.

Drug Dosage. The authors and the publisher have exerted every effort to ensure that drug selection and dosage set forth in this text are in accord with current recommendations and practice at the time of publication. However, in view of ongoing research, changes in government regulations, and the constant flow of information relating to drug therapy and drug reactions, the reader is urged to check the package insert for each drug for any change in indications and dosage and for added warnings and precautions. This is particularly important when the recommended agent is a new and/or infrequently employed drug.

www.karger.com
Printed in Switzerland on acid-free paper by
Reinhardt Druck, Basel
ISBN 3–8055–8049–5, ISSN 1422–2140

This book is dedicated to our wives and children:

Iris, Johannes and Sophie
WR

Andrea, Jonas and Anne
BS

Phyllis, Krishen and Kiran
VKS

Contents

Foreword

Since its inception in 1963, the book series *Progress in Respiratory Research* aims at publishing cutting edge knowledge covering the widest possible area. Both clinical and basic science feature with equal prominence. Judging from sales figures and citations in the literature, the series is enjoying a rapidly increasing reputation. The last two volumes, vol 33 on 'Paediatric Pulmonary Function Testing', and vol 34 on 'Cystic Fibrosis in the 21st Century' have addressed important topics mainly relating to pediatric pulmonology. Both are outstanding books, the former just having received a 'highly commended' award by the British Medical Association!

The one area which has never been covered in the series, however, is sleep medicine. We were therefore very enthusiastic when Prof. W.J. Randerath approached us with his idea to bring out a volume entitled: Sleep Apnea: Current Diagnosis and Treatment. Together with his co-editors B.M. Sanner and V.K. Somers, he put together a comprehensive book containing all relevant topics relating to sleep apnea. True to the vision of the series *Progress in Respiratory Research*, the authors of the different chapters were chosen among the leaders in the field and from all corners of the world, giving the book the usual global appeal. Also, authors were instructed to cite the most recent literature including 2005. Combined with the usual speed of Karger Publishers to produce a book in very few months after acceptance of the final article, this results in a book presenting up-to-date knowledge, a true reflection of the series' title.

The current volume, 35 of the series, offers something for everyone interested in sleep apnea or sleep-disordered breathing and presents yet another gem in *Progress in Respiratory Research.*

To the volume editors, the chapter authors, and the editorial staff at Karger Publishers, Basel, a hearty thank you and to you, potential readers, a warm welcome!

C.T. Bolliger
Cape Town

Preface

It has been a fascinating experience to witness the development of a new discipline in science and clinical medicine. Although Charles Dickens excellently described the presentation of a patient with sleep apnea in his famous novel *The Pickwick Papers* in 1837, until 1980 there were only few scientific publications on the theme. The impressive recent evolution of sleep medicine started with the description of continuous positive airway pressure therapy by Colin Sullivan in the late 1970s. Professor Sullivan has more lately added a new and important aspect to our understanding of clinical sleep medicine by his observations on sleep-disordered breathing during pregnancy. It is therefore a great honor for us that he and some of the other most important sleep researchers enrich this book with their insights.

In the face of the rapid developments in sleep medicine, this book seeks to present the current knowledge in the pathophysiology, clinical presentation, diagnosis, and treatment of sleep apnea. As our primary focus is on breathing disturbances during sleep, it is important to differentiate these disorders from other sleep problems. Therefore, Professor Levy introduces the volume with an overview of the broad spectrum of sleep medicine.

New physiological approaches to modeling sleep are based on the observation of the fluctuations between wakefulness and sleep. Interestingly, the distribution of sleep and wakefulness follows similar laws as molecular movement. Recent research highlights respiratory instability during sleep, which also has implications for the upper airway dilator muscles.

By directly measuring the impedance of the upper airways, the mechanical changes that take place in the course of an apnea can be described precisely. Aside from these, however, the importance of inflammatory processes and oxidative stress is increasingly recognized. These mechanisms, as well as genetic and anatomic factors and compensatory processes, critically influence the structure and function of the upper airway muscles. These concepts open up new avenues of investigation for better understanding and improved therapeutic options.

The diagnosis of sleep-disordered breathing is contingent upon the history and the measurement of ventilation during sleep. Standardized tests and questionnaires have become increasingly important as objective measures of daytime sleepiness. These tests aim at better characterization and evaluation of the complexity of clinical symptoms. Despite many attempts to simplify the diagnostic process, polysomnography remains the gold standard approach to clearly define sleep apnea, to differentiate it from other sleep disorders and to introduce and supervise optimal therapy.

CPAP is the current method of choice for the treatment of sleep apnea. However, based on new pathophysiologic findings, novel therapeutic approaches are under investigation. For example, stimulation of the upper airway muscles, cardiac pacing, and surgical and pharmacological interventions have been tested. As patients often seek treatment alternatives, it seemed important to us to include the opportunities and limitations of these new approaches, and to suggest recommendations for their use. Although automatic positive airway pressure devices have broadened the therapeutic repertoire of sleep physicians, questions still remain regarding how automatic CPAP should be best used in titration and treatment.

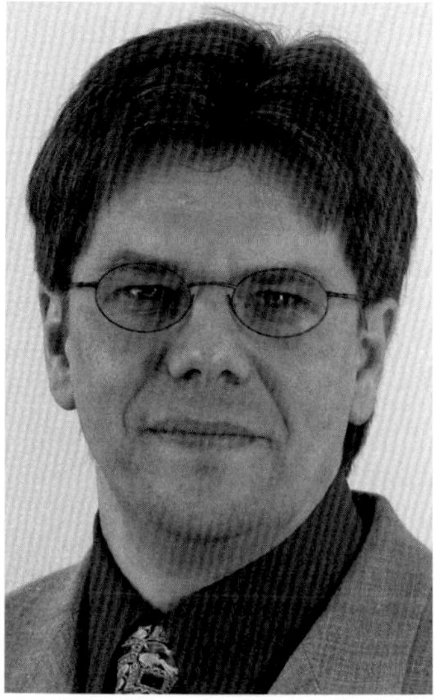

W.J. Randerath, Solingen

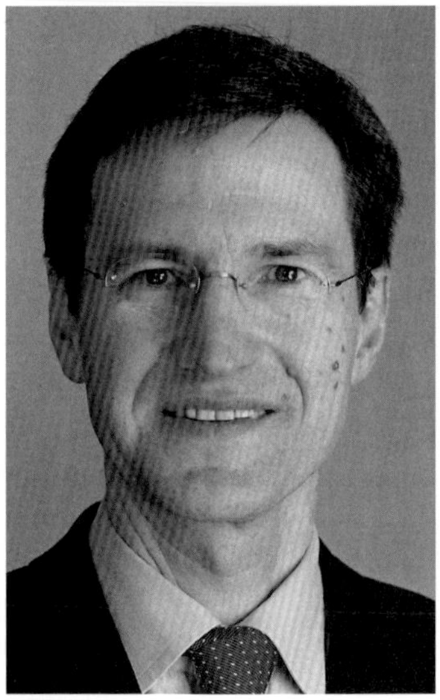

B.M. Sanner, Wuppertal

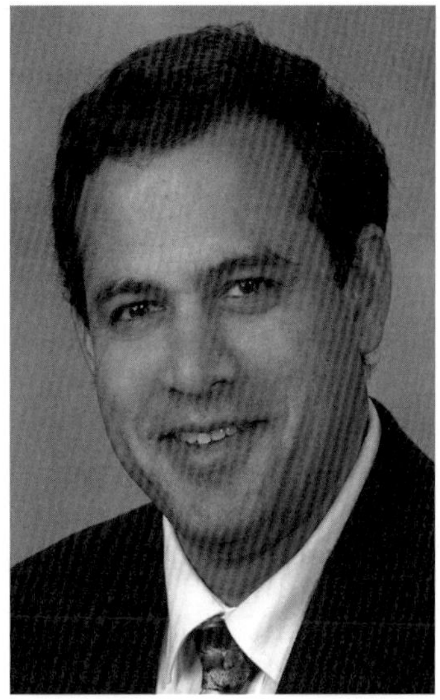

V.K. Somers, Rochester, Minn.

The general medical community has become increasingly interested in sleep disorders, because of the important influence of breathing disturbances during sleep on the cardiovascular system. Therefore, reviews of central sleep apnea and of cardiovascular complications of sleep-disordered breathing play an important role in this edition. Sleep apnea is relevant to all ages. Hence, children, the elderly and pregnancy receive special attention in dedicated chapters.

Our overall goal is to summarize the state-of-the-art knowledge on sleep-disordered breathing. We are very grateful to Prof. Bolliger and Karger Publishers for agreeing to incorporate this theme in the series *Progress in Respiratory Research*. We especially thank the expert contributors from throughout the world for sharing our mission and for excellent contributions to this volume. We do hope that this book will stimulate through discussion and research, and that it will also assist clinicians in the evaluation and management of their patients.

W.J. Randerath
B.M. Sanner
V.K. Somers

Randerath WJ, Sanner BM, Somers VK (eds): Sleep Apnea.
Prog Respir Res. Basel, Karger, 2006, vol 35, pp 1–12

Sleep Disorders and Their Classification – An Overview

Patrick Lévy[a] Véronique Viot-Blanc[b] Jean-Louis Pépin[a]

[a]Sleep Laboratory and HP2 Inserm ERI 0017, Grenoble University, Grenoble, [b]Sleep Unit, Lariboisière Hospital, Paris, France

Abstract

There are numerous sleep disorders. Many of these disorders remain poorly recognized by the general practitioners but may also be largely ignored by the respiratory physicians even though they manage patients with sleep-disordered breathing. It is nevertheless critical to be aware of the diversity of the sleep disorders. Sleep disorders represent a major challenge in terms of differential diagnosis. This is particularly relevant to excessive daytime sleepiness. On the other hand, very common conditions such as insomnia or restless legs syndrome are still neglected or ignored by the vast majority of the medical community. Thus, expanding the knowledge on both respiratory and nonrespiratory sleep disorders may contribute to improve sleep medicine quality amongst respiratory physicians. In this overview, sleep disorders have been described according to the 2nd International Classification of Sleep Disorders published in 2005, i.e. insomnia, sleep-disordered breathing, hypersomnias, parasomnias, circadian disorders and movement disorders. Lastly, excessive daytime sleepiness being a major concern for the respiratory physicians dealing with sleep, the differential diagnosis of excessive daytime sleepiness has been further detailed.

Introduction

Sleep has multiple functions including brain metabolism maintenance, rest of the cardiovascular system and glucose metabolism balance. Sleep represents one third of the human life and deeply alters many physiological regulations.

There are numerous sleep disorders. However, many behavioral changes occurring during sleep do not necessarily represent a health hazard. Moreover, the boundary between normality and disease is often difficult to establish. Snoring, for instance, obviously represents an increase in upper airway resistance. Primary snoring, however, may only be a social nuisance. On the other hand, snoring may further be associated with sleep fragmentation and sleep apnea, thus leading to excessive daytime sleepiness and cardiovascular morbidity. There are also many changes occurring with ageing without significant health impact. For instance, inspiratory flow limitation, a common feature in sleep-disordered breathing (SDB), seems to be very frequent during sleep in male adults over 40, without necessarily any symptom or health consequence.

In the present overview, we refer to the 2nd International Classification of Sleep Disorders (ICSD II) [1], published in 2005. Sleep disorders have been described in accordance with ICSD II, i.e. insomnia, SDB, hypersomnias, parasomnias, circadian disorders and movement disorders.

The ICSD II can be summarized in eight categories, as shown in table 1.

Insomnia

Definitions

Insomnia is defined as a repeated difficulty with sleep initiation, duration, consolidation, or quality that occurs

Table 1. Overall classification of sleep disorders according to ICSD II [1]

I	Insomnias
II	Sleep-related breathing disorders (SRBD)
III	Hypersomnia of central origin not due to circadian rhythm sleep disorder, SRBD or other cause of disturbed nocturnal sleep
IV	Circadian rhythm sleep disorder
V	Parasomnias
VI	Sleep-related movement disorders
VII	Isolated symptoms, apparently normal variants, unresolved issues
VIII	Other sleep disorders

despite adequate time and opportunity for sleep and results in some form of daytime impairment [1]. An adult insomniac patient usually complains of difficulty initiating or maintaining sleep. Concerns about insufficient amount of nocturnal sleep and extended periods of nocturnal wakefulness are usually present. Early awakening can also occur. Less frequently, the patient may describe a perception of poor sleep quality or nonrestorative sleep, while its length and sleep periods are perceived as adequate. Insomniac patients are usually worried and anxious about their sleep [2, 3].

Consequences of Insomnia

Insomnia usually results in daytime fatigue, irritability, decreased mood, general malaise and cognitive impairment. This includes attention, concentration and memory impairments. The cognitive impairment may result in an increased occurrence of errors, accidents, at work or at the wheel, mainly in the more severe forms. In some patients, physical symptoms are related to their insomnia, including muscle tension, gastrointestinal upset or headache. Lastly, there are few data suggesting a higher prevalence of hypertension and an increased usage of cardiovascular drugs in chronic insomnia.

Consequences on social and occupational functioning, and personal life are frequent when insomnia becomes chronic, reducing quality of life. Excessive daytime somnolence (EDS) is unusual in insomniac patients. When present, it suggests searching for a specific cause or another sleep disorder.

Causes of Insomnia

Multiple causes are possible. In some cases, insomnia represents the symptom of another condition: primary medical illness or mental disorder, other sleep disorder or use of substances or drugs. In these cases, insomnia may be qualified as secondary. In other cases, insomnia appears to be primary without identifiable causes [4]. There are however favoring factors, i.e. vulnerability triggering (environment, life events) or perpetuating insomnia (behaviors).

Insomnia is thus frequently multifactorial. The pathophysiological bases are still largely unknown and the favoring factors may change with ageing. One of the most prominent contributing factors is anxiety that can be diffuse or focused on concerns regarding the patient's insomnia and its consequences.

Objective Findings

Sleep recording is not useful unless another sleep disorder is suspected. When performed, it may or may not confirm patient sleep perception. Discordance between objective findings and sleep complaints is not unusual and does not rule out the diagnosis [5]. This is particularly true when the recording is performed in the laboratory or in unusual sleeping conditions. When sleep disturbances are present, delayed sleep onset, increased wake after sleep onset (WASO) or early awakening can be found alone or in combination. Usually, sleep onset of more than 30 min and WASO of more than 45 min are considered as pathological. Sleep structure is likely to be disturbed with slow wave sleep and REM sleep reduction whilst light sleep (stages I and II) increases in percentage. Sleep fragmentation is also common without identifiable cause in most cases [1].

Overall Treatment Principles

The multifactorial and complex determinants of insomnia represent a major challenge when treating insomniacs. A critical step is to identify the various causes and favoring or perpetuating factors and to try to implement a specific response.

To treat a mental disorder, to correct or adapt a pharmacological treatment, to restore sleep hygiene are among the first measures to envisage. These can be effective especially in case of acute or subacute insomnia. Their efficacy is much more limited when dealing with chronic insomnia.

Psychological determinants are central in chronic insomnia. Anxiety treatment is often a first-line treatment target. Pharmacological treatment, relaxation, behavioral and cognitive therapies, stimulus control may all have some degree of effectiveness. Among effective insomnia treatments, cognitive and behavioral therapies (BCT) refer to a frequent negative conditioning effect on sleep that predisposes to symptom perpetuation and aggravation [6]. It has been demonstrated that BCT are comparable to hypnotics in chronic insomnia. However, a combination or a sequential use of these treatments might be even more effective.

Modern hypnotics (zolpidem, zopiclone) that are short-time action compounds have a proven efficacy without residual sleepiness at awakening or during daytime. However, it should be reminded that most studies are short term, usually 1–3 months, and very recently 6 months for one study. Long-term studies are warranted and should be favored by the recent FDA approval for chronic hypnotic treatment.

Hypnotics' prescription needs to carefully evaluate clinical history and associated symptoms. A global care program is needed in case of chronic insomnia, including hypnotic prescription when needed. This prescription has to be adapted, limited in time and accompanied by a careful evaluation and treatment of associated favoring and perpetuating factors.

Theoretically, hypnotic treatment should be short-term aiming essentially at stopping the vicious circle perpetuating insomnia. In clinical practice, however, hypnotics are often used as long-term treatment, which can promote reduction in the therapeutic effect, increase in dosage, and make ending the drug treatment difficult. This applies particularly to classical benzodiazepines that commonly induce rebound insomnia when suddenly interrupted. It is also true for modern hypnotics that long-term use may lead to psychological dependency. This could be one of the causes of long-term treatment, although the low level of knowledge regarding sleep and insomnia among health professionals might be much more contributing. Moreover, alternative treatments are poorly available in many countries and not affordable economically for many patients, being usually not covered by health insurance. Thus the use of hypnotics although often criticized by the health authorities remains the only available solution.

Different Types of Insomnia

Adjustment or Acute Insomnia

The essential feature of adjustment insomnia is the presence of insomnia in association with an identifiable stressor. It is insomnia of relatively short duration, typically a few days to a few weeks.

Its occurrence can be related to a variety of stressors including changes or disputes in personal relationship, occupational stress, personal losses, diagnosis of a medical condition, moving to a new location, or even change in the usual sleep environment. . . . Its incidence has been reported to be up to 15–20%, with a predominance in females and elderly subjects. A previous history of anxiety or depressive symptoms or disorders is a favoring factor. This insomnia has a clearly defined acute onset and a short duration, usually less than 3 months. It will resolve when the stressor will stop or when the subject will be adapted when the stressor has become chronic. Repeated episodes may also occur. Hypnotics are usually effective in this type of insomnia, generally prescribed for a period of a few days or weeks. In this context, modern hypnotics such as zolpidem, zaleplon or zopiclone, of short duration of action, have been shown as effective and safe, without morning or daytime residual sleepiness.

Insomnia Associated with Poor Sleep Hygiene

Various habits or behaviors may be detrimental for sleep onset or quality. They represent perpetuating factors. These behaviors include: frequent, prolonged or late naps during daytime, highly variable bedtimes or rising times, time in bed much exceeding sleeping time, routine use of stimulants, alcohol, caffeine or nicotine especially in the period preceding bedtime, engagement in mentally stimulating, physically activating or emotionally upsetting activities close to bedtime, frequent use of the bed for activities other than sleep such as watching TV, snacking, studying, etc. A failure in maintaining a comfortable sleeping environment can also be noticed.

Psychophysiological Insomnia

The main characteristic is heightened arousal during daytime and a negative conditioning to sleep onset in the beginning of the night or during the night. The physiological arousal may be associated with cognitive hypervigilance, intellectual or physical hyperactivity. Mental arousal in the form of 'a racing mind' is characteristic. There is also an overconcern with the inability to sleep. A vicious cycle develops, in which the more one strives to sleep, the more agitated one becomes and the less able one is to fall asleep. This might explain why patients often report that they sleep better away from their own bedroom and usual routines. This may be learned during previous episodes of insomnia caused by other precipitating factors such as depression, pain, disturbed sleep environment or shift work. However, psychophysiological insomnia may persist long after these factors have disappeared. As in all forms of insomnia, there is a decreased feeling of well-being during daytime, with deteriorated mood and motivation, decreased attention, vigilance, energy and concentration and increased fatigue and malaise. Excessive daytime sleepiness and daytime naps are conversely rather rare. This condition is thought to be present in 1–2% of the general population and between 10 and 15% of all patients seen at sleep centers. This type of insomnia is more frequent in women and may occur during adolescence or when adult. Sleep recording may paradoxically reveal better than sleep at home, which contrasts with what is usually observed in normal individuals. When untreated, this condition may persist for decades and deteriorate progressively. There is then an increased risk of depression occurrence or aggravation. This type of insomnia is usually responsive to behavioral therapy, alone or associated with hypnotics [6].

Paradoxical Insomnia

Paradoxical insomnia is characterized by a very severe insomnia complaint, nearly every night, with very little sleep. The patient describes permanent awareness of environmental stimuli and a frequent pattern of conscious thoughts or rumination. The severity of this insomnia contrasts both with little daytime consequences and also a consistent marked mismatch between objective findings from polysomnography or actigraphy and subjective sleep estimates. Total sleep time is for instance often underestimated by 50%. This is related to the difficulty in sleep perception.

Idiopathic Insomnia

This type of insomnia is observed very early in life, during childhood. There is no precipitating factor and the condition is stable and chronic. There is usually no inter-night variability or periods of remission as seen in other forms of insomnia. There is possibly a familial component. Daytime impairment includes daytime fatigue or sleepiness, mood symptoms, or cognitive complaints such as poor attention and concentration. The sleep disturbance should not be better explained by another sleep disorder, medical or neurological disorder, mental disorder and medication use or substance abuse.

Insomnia due to Mental Disorder

Mental disorders are essentially made of mood disorders and anxiety. The insomnia typically begins with the onset of the causative mental disorder and varies in parallel. Mood disorders include major depressive disorder, dysthymic disorder, bipolar disorder and cyclothymic disorder. However, most anxiety disorders and various somatoform disorders may give rise to this condition. Difficulty falling asleep is most typical of anxiety disorders, especially in young patients. In depression and older patients, frequent awakenings during the night and early morning awakenings with difficulty returning to sleep are more typical. Insomnia usually improves when treating the causal mental disorder. However, in some individuals, insomnia may persist long after the other symptoms of their mental disorder remit. It should also be reminded that some treatments of depression or anxiety may aggravate insomnia.

Insomnia due to Drug or Substance

Sleep disruption may arise from substances that act as CNS stimulant or depressant. Among the stimulants that most commonly lead to sleep difficulties are caffeine, amphetamines and cocaine. Insomnia, however, may arise as an unintended side effect of various medications prescribed at therapeutic dosage. Insomnia may appear as a side effect of certain antidepressants, various antihypertensive agents, hypolipidemic medications, corticosteroids, antiparkinsonian drugs, theophylline, anorectic agents and some antiepileptic medications. Paradoxically, sedative drugs may generate insomnia when used chronically and interrupted. Alcohol consumption may also initially favor sleep onset but further promote sleep instability and fragmentation. Abrupt alcohol withdrawal is also possibly associated with severe insomnia.

Insomnia due to Medical Condition

All respiratory disorders, limited mobility and many neurological disorders may generate insomnia. All painful disorders may also be involved.

- Asthma, chronic respiratory failure, migraine, gastro-oesophageal reflux, prostatic hypertrophy and diabetes, dementia and neurodegenerative diseases.
- Menopause is frequently associated with insomnia.
- All painful disorders such as fibromyalgia, arthritis, primary or metastatic cancers may be involved.

Insomnia Related to Another Sleep Disorder

Insomnia may reveal another sleep disorder. Restless legs syndrome (RLS) is frequently associated with insomnia, whilst SDB and parasomnias are much more rarely revealed by insomnia.

Sleep-Disordered Breathing

Sleep breathing disorders are extensively presented in the present book. Thus there is no need for further details. However, the classification that has been suggested in 1999 by the American Academy of Sleep Medicine (AASM) [7] is of interest and has been confirmed through the ICSD II published in 2005. There are basically four different categories:

Obstructive Sleep Apnea/Hypopnea Syndrome

This includes both classical obstructive sleep syndrome (OSA) but also upper airway resistance syndrome (UARS) [8], as it has been suggested that there is no sufficient specific epidemiological, pathophysiological and clinical data to support a specific category. The definitions of SDB made by the AASM Task Force in 1999 did not include UARS as a syndrome but did define respiratory effort-related arousals (RERAs) [7]. Recently several authors have discussed about this syndrome's existence and the morbidity that might be related to RERAs [9]. ICSD II is overall in accordance with the AASM Task Force report. If baseline oxygen saturation is normal, events including an absence of oxygen desaturation, despite a clear drop in inspiratory flow, increased respiratory effort and a brief change in sleep state or arousal, are defined as RERAs. The UARS is a proposed diagnostic classification for patients with RERAs who also do not have events that would meet definitions for apneas and hypopneas [10]. However, these events are presumed to have the same pathophysiology as obstructive apneas and hypopneas (upper airway obstruction) and are believed to be as much of a risk factor for symptoms of unrefreshing sleep, daytime somnolence, and fatigue as frank apnea or hypopnea. Therefore, ICSD II recommends that they be included as part of OSA and not considered as a separate entity [1].

Regarding obstructive sleep apnea syndrome [11], there is now substantial evidence that there is a causal relationship between OSA and EDS, with cognitive impairment including increased risk of traffic accidents on the one hand [12, 13] and cardiovascular morbidity and mortality on the other [13–15]. The cardiovascular consequences seem to appear early in the disease, e.g. occurrence of atherosclerosis without other cardiovascular risk during OSA [16, 17]. This supports early treatment also because the rate of mortality is decreased with age [18].

Central Sleep Apnea Syndrome with Cheyne-Stokes Respiration

This is a condition including both central apneas and hypopneas and Cheyne-Stokes respiration (CSR) usually associated with an increase in ventilatory response to CO_2 that promotes ventilatory instability and thus sleep instability [7]. The most prevalent condition leading to central sleep apnea syndrome (CSAS)-CSR is chronic heart failure (CHF), being both a marker of severity and a factor of aggravation which affects both morbidity and mortality [19]. However, there is no doubt that treating CHF reduces CSAS-CSR. Thus, this condition might be slightly less prevalent since the systematic use of beta-blockers, as suggested by the recently published Canadian multicenter study on positive airway pressure (CANPAP) [19, 20].

Central Sleep Apnea Syndrome

This is a condition where central apneas and hypopneas occur without CSR, thus excluding CSAS-CSR. This is a rare condition, although several infectious, tumoral or inflammatory diseases affecting the brainstem may result in CSAS [7].

Obesity Hypoventilation Syndrome

This is a condition in which there is both obesity and hypercapnia [7]. There is possibly either hypoventilation or apneas or both during sleep. As the prognosis is very poor [21] and obesity more and more epidemic worldwide, this is a rapidly growing subset of SDB that needs more attention in both clinical research and care.

Hypersomnia

Hypersomnia presents with a common symptom that is EDS, and the cause of this primary symptom is not disturbed nocturnal sleep or misaligned circadian rhythm [1]. Daytime sleepiness is defined as the inability to stay awake and alert during the waking period, resulting in unintended lapses into drowsiness or sleep. This occurs more likely in boring monotonous situations and may result in large increase in daily total sleep time without significant feeling of restoration. The impact of naps may also be transitorily effective in alleviating EDS which reappears shortly thereafter. Sleepiness may also result in semiconscious behavior in the midst of a sleep episode with usually no memory of the event. It also usually significantly alters driving ability and disturbs occupational activities. This may result in potentially dangerous consequences and impaired quality of life. EDS has to be a chronic symptom and last for at least 3 months prior to diagnosis.

Narcolepsy

Narcolepsy [22, 23] is rather rare and affects 0.02–0.18% of the US and European populations regarding narcolepsy with cataplexy. A lower prevalence has been described in Israel, whereas narcolepsy is more prevalent in Japan. The onset of the disease occurs typically between the age of 15 and 25 years. Sleepiness is usually the first symptom, cataplexy often occurring within a year of onset. Hypnagogic hallucinations, sleep paralysis and disturbed nocturnal sleep often occur later in the course of the disease. Most cases of narcolepsy-cataplexy are associated with a loss of 50,000–100,000 hypothalamic neurons containing the neuropeptide hypocretin or orexin. The lack of hypocretin can be assessed by measuring cerebrospinal fluid (CSF) levels of hypocretin-1 [23, 24]. About 90% of patients with narcolepsy-cataplexy have drastically reduced levels of hypocretin-1, almost all exhibiting a specific human leukocyte antigen subtype, i.e. HLA DQB1*0602 [22–24]. It has been very recently demonstrated that these neurons are effectively lost, presumably owing to an autoimmune process resulting in hypocretin cells occurring during adolescence. This autoimmune hypothesis although never demonstrated is supported by the association with the HLA subtype. Regarding the HLA subtypes, actually both DR2/DRB1*1501 and DQB1*0602 are associated with narcolepsy in Causasians and Asians but not in African-Americans. This is supporting a genetic predisposing factor. However, environmental factors are also present. In a twin study, only 30% of monozygotic twin pairs with narcolepsy-cataplexy were reported as concordant.

The main symptom is EDS resulting in repeated episodes of naps or lapses into sleep across the daytime. Typical patients with narcolepsy with cataplexy also present with refreshing sleep episodes during daytime. They also often exhibit sudden and irresistible sleep attacks occurring in unusual situations such as eating, walking or driving [22, 23]. Nocturnal sleep is often unstable, fragmental and perceived as superficial. Sleep paralysis and hypnagogic hallucinations are also common in narcoleptic patients but may also occur occasionally in normal patients and in patients with other sleep disorders.

Cataplexy is conversely a unique characteristic of the disease. It is characterized by a sudden loss of bilateral muscle tone provoked by strong emotions that are usually positive, such as laughter, pride or surprise [22, 23]. Cataplexy can include all skeletal muscle groups or can affect specifical muscle subgroups, mostly lower or upper limb, neck or mouth. The duration of cataplexy is short, ranging from a few seconds to several minutes with usually an immediate and complete recovery [22, 23].

Sleep recording may demonstrate sleep onset in REM sleep (SOREMP) and poor sleep quality. In most cases, however, nocturnal sleep recording is nonspecific. Diagnosis is both clinical and based on the Multiple Sleep Latency Test (MSLT). This test is made of 4–5 sleep recordings during naps starting at 8 or 9 a.m. and occurring every 2 h. MSLT should follow a nocturnal polysomnography (PSG). The diagnosis is made on mean sleep latency on MSLT of less than 8 min and two or more SOREMPs. An alternative is hypocretin-1 CSF level of less than 110 pg/ml or one third of the normal values (90% of patients with narcolepsy-cataplexy) [1].

An important change in the ICSD is the recognition of narcolepsy without cataplexy. Cataplexy is either absent or doubtful or atypical [1]. The main diagnostic criteria are EDS associated with mean sleep latency less than 8 min and at least two SOREMPs on MSLT. The prevalence is unknown but may represent 10–50% of the narcoleptic population. Only 10–20% of patients with narcolepsy without cataplexy present with low CSF hypocretin-1 [24]; almost all with HLA DQB1*0602. Most probably, this subgroup represents a heterogeneous group that includes numerous etiologies [1, 23].

The differential diagnosis is critical in this late condition (see below).

Idiopathic Hypersomnia

This is a condition characterized by constant and severe excessive sleepiness with prolonged and unrefreshing naps of up to 3 or 4 h and great difficulty of waking up in the morning [25]. The major sleep episode is prolonged to at least 10 h, typically 12–14 h [1]. In the ICSD II, the term idiopathic hypersomnia has been used to include subjects with hypersomnolence without increased nocturnal sleep. The two variants have been separated.

- In case of idiopathic hypersomnia without increased nocturnal sleep time, MSLT must demonstrate mean sleep latency (SL) less than 8 min and less than two SOREMPs. This allows distinguishing from narcolepsy without cataplexy, a difficult clinical differential diagnosis [1].
- Idiopathic hypersomnia with long sleep time may be familial, and an autosomal dominant mode of inheritance has been suggested. CSF hypocretin-1 is at normal levels [1].

Principles of Treatment

In most cases, modafinil is effective in treating EDS. Methylphenidate is a possible alternative. However, in some cases, there is persistent need for naps and daily life has to be organized in taking this residual EDS into account.

In narcolepsy with cataplexy, cataplexy can be treated by antidepressant (tricyclic antidepressants, serotonin-specific reuptake inhibitors, SSRIs, and monoamine oxidase inhibitors).

Parasomnias

These diseases have been classified in the ICSD II but also in several reviews [1, 26]. Mark Mahowald, a leading expert in the field, elegantly summarized the knowledge in this field in a review recently published in the journal *Nature* [27].

Parasomnias are defined as unpleasant or undesirable behavioral phenomena that occur predominantly or exclusively during sleep. Parasomnias are not a unitary phenomenon but rather are the manifestation of a wide variety of completely different conditions, most of which are diagnosable and treatable. The common parasomnias are an example of 'dissociated sleep states', representing the simultaneous admixture of wakefulness and either NREM sleep (disorders of arousal such as sleepwalking or sleep terrors) or wakefulness and REM sleep (REM sleep behavior disorder). Parasomnias may result in striking clinical phenomena, which occur during the transition from one state to another. In addition to the phenomenon of state dissociation, in which two states of being overlap or occur simultaneously, there are probably additional underlying physiological phenomena that contribute to the appearance of complex motor behaviors during sleep. This may include activation of locomotor centers during sleep, sleep inertia (a period of confusion or disorientation during the transition from sleep to wakefulness) upon arousal and sleep state instability (oscillation between wakefulness and sleep).

NREM Sleep Parasomnias

Disorders of Arousal

The disorders of arousal are the most impressive and most common of the NREM sleep parasomnias. They share common features. They tend to arise from slow-wave sleep (stages 3 and 4 of NREM sleep) and therefore usually occur during the first third of the sleep cycle (and rarely during naps). They are common in childhood, usually decreasing in frequency with increasing age. Disorders of arousal may be triggered by febrile illness, alcohol, previous sleep deprivation, physical activity, emotional stress or medications. Such factors act, however, as triggering events in susceptible individuals. Persistence of these behaviors beyond childhood or their development in adulthood has erroneously been taken as an indication of underlying psychopathology, whilst many more recent clinical reports have demonstrated that this is not the case [27].

Confusional Arousals

These are often seen in children and are characterized by movements in bed, occasionally thrashing about or inconsolable crying. 'Sleep drunkenness' is probably a variation on this theme. The prevalence of confusional arousals in adults is approximately 4%.

Sleepwalking

Sleepwalking is prevalent in childhood (1–17%), peaking at 11–12 years of age, and is still very common in adults (nearly 4%). Sleepwalking may be either calm or agitated, with varying degrees of complexity and duration.

Sleep Terrors

The sleep terror is the most impressive disorder of arousal, frequently initiated by a loud scream associated with extreme panic, followed by prominent motor activity such as hitting the wall, running around or out of the bedroom, resulting in bodily injury or property damage. A constant feature is inconsolability, attempts at consolation being useless and often prolonging or even intensifying the confusional state. Complete amnesia for the activity is typical, but may be only partial. As with sleepwalking, sleep terrors are not rare in adults (up to 3%). Although usually benign, these behaviors may be violent, resulting in considerable injury to the victim or others or damage to the environment, with possible legal implications. Treatment options include reassurance, behavioral or pharmacological approaches, e.g. short-acting benzodiazepines.

REM Sleep Parasomnia

The most common REM sleep parasomnia [1, 26, 27] is the REM sleep behavior disorder (RBD). In patients with RBD, somatic muscle atonia, one of the defining features of REM sleep, is absent, permitting the acting out of dream mentation, often with violent or injurious results.

The presenting complaint is that of vigorous sleep behaviors usually accompanying vivid dreams. These behaviors may result in repeated injury, including ecchymoses, lacerations and fractures. Some of the self-protection measures taken by the patients (tethering themselves to the bed, using sleeping bags or pillow barricades, or sleeping on a mattress in an empty room) reveal the intensity and severity of these recurrent episodes. There are also legal issues in this disorder. RBD predominantly affects males (about 90%) and usually begins after the age of 50 years.

RBD may occur in both an acute and chronic form. The acute form is often due to undesirable side effects of prescribed medications, most commonly antidepressant medications, particularly the SSRIs.

The chronic form of RBD is usually either idiopathic or associated with neurological disorders. RBD may be associated with neurodegenerative disorders, particularly Parkinson's disease, multiple system atrophy or dementia with Lewy body disease. Interestingly, RBD may be the first manifestation of these conditions, and may precede any other manifestation of the underlying neurodegenerative process by more than 10 years. Many patients with RBD who have been followed over time, are developing neurodegenerative disorders. The striking relationship between RBD and neurodegenerative disorders has led to many neuroimaging and cerebral blood flow studies in patients with RBD. As both narcolepsy and RBD represent state boundary dyscontrol conditions, there is a higher incidence of RBD in patients with narcolepsy. Moreover, medications prescribed to treat cataplexy associated with narcolepsy (tricyclic antidepressants, SSRIs and monoamine oxidase inhibitors) can trigger or further exacerbate RBD. The benzodiazepine clonazepam is a highly effective treatment for RBD although its mechanism of action in RBD is unknown.

Circadian Rhythm Disorders

The primary symptom of circadian rhythm disorders [1, 27, 28] is the inability to sleep during the desired sleep time. Once asleep, there is no abnormality of sleep but only of the timing of sleep. The cause of all circadian rhythm disorders is an inability of the individual's biological clock to adjust to the demands of the environment. Wake-sleep schedule disorders are either primary (dysfunction of the biologic clock) or secondary (resulting from environmental effects upon the underlying clock). The secondary disorders (such as jet lag and shift work) are usually easy to identify [29, 30]. The primary disorders may be much more difficult to diagnose, as they may present as other sleep, medical or psychiatric disorders such as hypersomnia, insomnia, substance (sedative-hypnotic or stimulant) abuse or psychiatric conditions.

Treatment is based on chronotherapy and phototherapy. In addition, there are new pharmacological treatments.

In chronotherapy, the desirable total sleep time is determined by sleep logs during a 'free-running' period. The patient then delays or advances sleep onset, by a few minutes every day and sleeping only the predetermined number of hours until the sleep onset time is at the desired time.

Phototherapy (exposure to bright light) has a potent effect upon the biological clock, and exposure at specific times of the wake/sleep cycle results in a change in the underlying rhythm. The timing and duration of the phototherapy depend upon diagnosis and individual response. The patient sits at a prescribed distance from a bright light producing more than 2,500 lux. The effect of light upon human rhythms varies with intensity, wavelength, timing and duration of exposure. Once the desired sleep period time has been achieved, continued light exposure must be maintained.

Delayed Sleep-Phase Syndrome

In delayed sleep-phase syndrome (DSPS), the patient falls asleep late and rises late [28]. There is a striking inability to fall asleep at an earlier, more desirable time. This may present itself as either sleep-onset insomnia or daytime hypersomnia (particularly in the morning). DSPS is the most common of the primary circadian disorders, and may, in part, be the consequence of societal increases in nighttime activities. Combinations of chronotherapy, phototherapy and medications may be effective in 'resetting' the clock. The treatment regimen must however be maintained, or the clock will again become delayed.

Advanced Sleep-Phase Syndrome

Individuals suffering from advanced sleep-phase syndrome fall asleep early and awaken earlier than desired. They are unable to remain awake until the desired time, falling asleep in the early evening and awakening in the very early hours of the morning. This may present as hypersomnia (particularly in the evening) or sleep-maintenance insomnia. Patients complain of interruption of evening activities by their sleepiness [28]. Bright light exposure in the evening may delay the clock to a more acceptable pattern.

Other, less common, circadian dysrhythmias include a 'non-24-hour wake-sleep pattern' and 'irregular wake-sleep pattern'.

Underscoring the inherent nature of these conditions, human genetic studies have identified specific genes associated with both delayed and advanced sleep-phase syndromes [31–33].

One promising pharmacological treatment is melatonin. Melatonin is secreted by the pineal gland, and its secretion is coupled to the wake-sleep cycle. It is a valuable marker of the underlying wake-sleep period. It is likely that melatonin plays an important role in biological rhythms. There is evidence that administration of exogenous melatonin may alter the biological rhythm in certain conditions.

Restless Legs Syndrome

There are many recent excellent reviews and also several Task Force reports regarding RLS [34–37]. There is also major interest in the field since dopamine agonists have been shown as effective treatment [38, 39]. The RLS is a common disorder that encompasses an idiopathic form of genetic or unknown origin and symptomatic forms associated with many causes.

The prevalence of the syndrome has been underestimated in the past and epidemiological population-based studies show that between 3 and 10% of the population have cardinal symptoms. In several studies a female preponderance has been described. Most patients with mild symptoms do not need any pharmacological treatment. Patients who need continuous treatment are mostly older than 50 years [35]. In 1995, clinical diagnostic criteria for the RLS were established by the International Restless Legs Syndrome Study Group.The criteria for diagnosis as shown below were further published in 2003 [36] as well as a severity scale [37].

The essential criteria are:

- An urge to move the legs, usually accompanied by uncomfortable or unpleasant sensations in the legs.
- Unpleasant sensations or the urge to move begin or worsen during periods of rest or inactivity such as lying or sitting.
- Unpleasant sensations or the urge to move are partly or totally relieved by movement such as walking, bending, stretching, etc., at least for as long as the activity continues.
- Unpleasant sensations or the urge to move are worse in the evening or at night than during the day, or only occur in the evening or night.

There are supportive criteria: positive response to dopaminergic treatment, periodic limb movements (during wakefulness or sleep), positive family history of the RLS.

There are also associated features. It can begin at any age, but most patients seen in clinical practice are middle-aged or older. Most patients have a progressive clinical course, but a static clinical course is sometimes seen.

Remissions of a month or more are also reported. The leg discomfort and the need to move may result in insomnia in most cases. A neurological examination is usual in idiopathic and familial forms of the syndrome. Peripheral neuropathy or radiculopathy are sometimes carried out in the nonfamilial form of the syndrome. A low serum ferritin (<50 μg/l) may be found in the syndrome.

Periodic Limb Movements

Involuntary movements may also occur either during sleep or when awake. These movements occur periodically and are called periodic limb movements. Diagnosis of periodic limb movements during sleep is based on the definition of the American Sleep Disorders Association [38]. These movements are measured by surface electromyography from the tibialis muscle and show muscle activation in a sequence of at least four muscle contractions lasting 0.5–5 s and recurring at intervals of 5–90 s. The muscle contractions must be at least 25% of the amplitude of the voluntary leg movements. These movements can occur with or without arousals or during wakefulness. About 80% of patients with RLS have periodic limb movements during sleep. Eighty-seven percent of patients will have periodic limb movements during sleep on at least one of two nights of recording. These movements are also not specific for the diagnosis of RLS because they can occur in other disorders or as an isolated occurrence.

Individuals with the syndrome might also complain of involuntary twitching movements of the legs during wakefulness when they are sitting or lying. Actigraphy may be used to measure periodic limb movements in wakefulness during the suggested immobilization test, general motor activity during wakefulness, or periodic limb movements during the sleep period.

Symptomatic RLS

Iron deficiency is probably the most frequent cause of symptomatic RLS. The manifestation of RLS may be associated with low blood concentrations of ferritin. In most patients, iron deficiency is not detected because there is no anaemia, and low ferritin is the only pathological parameter. Another frequent association is renal failure. Moreover, the syndrome often occurs with rheumatoid arthritis, fibromyalgia, or during pregnancy. Some women exhibit the disorder for the first time or have symptoms that worsen temporarily during pregnancy. In this clinical context, a family history of the disorder is common.

Differential and Positive Diagnosis

RLS should be distinguished from neuropathy and radiculopathy. In pure peripheral neuropathy and radiculopathy, patients do not have the need to move to relieve leg discomfort and the symptoms are not usually worse at rest or at night. The RLS should also be distinguished from neuroleptic-induced akathisia induced by antipsychotic agents that block dopamine receptors.

If there is an associated peripheral neuropathy or radiculopathy, electromyography and nerve conduction studies should be performed to evaluate these disorders. Since the RLS is frequently associated with iron deficiency, all patients should have serum ferritin measured, as a sensitive means of detection of iron deficiency.

Pathophysiology

RLS pathophysiology remains largely unknown.

Dopamine

Dopaminergic A11 cell group represents a possible pathophysiological correlate of the syndrome. A11 cells are the only cells that provide dopaminergic axons to the spinal cord. Dysfunction or atrophy of these cells could explain the positive treatment response to dopaminergic drugs and the circadian component of the syndrome since these cells are located close to the hypothalamic circadian pacemaker. Although there is no firm demonstration for several methodological reasons, A11 cells remain the focus of future pathophysiological research.

Opioid System

Central pain perception could have a role in the pathophysiological mechanisms of RLS. Opioid receptor binding was measured in 12 patients with the RLS vs. controls. Binding in patients correlated with the severity of the syndrome: the more severe the disease, the greater the release of endogenous opioids within the medial pain system.

Iron

Several studies showed a relation between low ferritin concentrations and symptoms of the syndrome, especially when ferritin was measured in the CSF. There are data issued both from neuropathological studies and imaging (MRI) supporting an impairment of the transferrin receptors and cellular iron deficiency. Overall, there are changes in the iron content in RLS patients that seem critical.

Circadian Factors

There is a clear circadian rhythm of the subjective complaints of the syndrome, and similar time of night variations can be seen for periodic limb movements during sleep and during wakefulness. The changes in melatonin secretion, as a marker of the circadian rhythm, were the only changes that preceded the increase in sensory and motor symptoms in RLS patients, suggesting melatonin might worsen symptoms in the evening and during the night by inhibiting central dopamine secretion.

Genetic Factors

For the hereditary forms, at least three gene loci, located on chromosomes 12, 14, and 9 have been identified so far.

Treatment

Treatment [34, 35, 39, 40] is needed only in the moderate to severe forms of the disorder. Treatment is mainly acting on the dopaminergic system and the iron metabolism. Dopaminergic treatment with dopamine agonists, i.e. ropinirole, pramipexole, is the first choice in idiopathic RLS [39, 40]. Various other drugs, such as opioids, gabapentin, and benzodiazepines, provide alternative treatment possibilities.

Overall Treatment Recommendations

Before starting a pharmacological treatment, sleep hygiene measures should be instituted and all possibilities for treating symptomatic RLS should be considered. Iron should be supplemented if ferritin is low. According to the guidelines of the AASM [41], dopaminergic agents are the first line of treatment for the syndrome, followed by opioids, anticonvulsants, and benzodiazepines. Among anticonvulsants, gabapentin is preferable because of its superior efficacy, and among the benzodiazepines, clonazepam is preferable because of its long half-life. If symptoms begin earlier rather than later in the evening, splitting doses may be needed. However, single doses at nighttime should be tried first at the initiation of the treatment. Intermittent treatment during the day might also be helpful for activities involving long periods of sitting.

Dopaminergic Treatment

Treatment should be started with the lowest dose possible. Progressive dose increment should be carried out slowly and attention paid to possible side effects of dopaminergic agents, such as nausea, arterial hypotension, dizziness, and, sometimes, daytime sleepiness. Domperidone is usually prescribed in order to avoid nausea. Patients should also be asked for any evidence of early onset of symptoms during the day once medication has been started. If this phenomenon called 'augmentation' becomes a persistent problem, the dopaminergic agent should be lowered or discontinued, at which time the symptoms should disappear during the daytime and remit back to the nighttime hours.

Opioids

Opioids are regarded as a second-choice treatment in patients who cannot tolerate dopaminergic agents. Whenever possible, opioids should be used in sustained-release forms to avoid addiction and to benefit from a continuous efficacy in more severe cases of the RLS.

Diagnosis of Excessive Daytime Sleepiness

EDS represents a major symptom in sleep medicine. It is the main clinical symptom of OSA, narcolepsy and idiopathic hypersomnia. It may also be associated with many other medical or mental diseases. From a clinical perspective, it should also be reminded that the prevalence of EDS is high in the general population, up to 9%. Interestingly enough, in a recent paper by Bixler et al. [42], it has been shown that there is high prevalence of EDS in the young subjects (<30) and in the very old (>75). In the young, unmet sleep needs and depression seem to be the major contributing factors, while in the oldest medical illness and health problems are presumably the causes. Depression should thus be suspected especially in young subjects presenting with EDS. Actually there are several major points to keep in mind when searching for a cause of EDS:

(1) As mentioned in the AASM definition of SDB [7], EDS may have many causes. When linking PSG findings with EDS, any other major cause of EDS such as depression, other sleep disorder, use of sedative or other psychoactive drugs or simply unmet sleep needs should first be considered. This is the reason why EDS should be considered in the context of clinical diagnosis as being not better explained by one of these factors.

(2) When the clinical probability is low, it should be further established that treatment of the specific cause is effective in alleviating EDS. This does not rule out a possible placebo effect. However, in most cases, this treatment trial is valuable to secondarily support the initial diagnosis.

(3) This does not exclude a synergic effect of these various causes of EDS. The rationale is to identify the different factors and to first treat the one which is presumably the most contributing.

(4) There are clinical differences regarding EDS in the different diseases that have been reviewed in the present chapter. Sudden and irresistible sleep attacks occurring in young individuals, even in the absence of cataplexy, might strongly suggest narcolepsy. EDS in OSA or upper airway resistance is of different nature, more progressive, less intense and usually unaffected by naps. Also, from a clinical standpoint, EDS in depression usually follows the changes in mood. Thus a detailed clinical inventory of all possible causes of EDS is highly recommended even in case of supporting symptoms for SDB such as snoring or obesity, for instance.

(5) A specific clinical context is the occurrence of residual EDS in OSA treated by CPAP. Although the prevalence of this condition is much discussed, 2–4% prevalence might be estimated. There are several items that should however be checked before considering EDS as residual and treating it accordingly using modafinil. The effectiveness of CPAP in correcting sleep structure by suppressing respiratory events during sleep should be assessed. Compliance to CPAP treatment has to be verified. Mouth leaks or any other cause of sleep fragmentation such as periodic leg movements should be carefully excluded. Any other disease possibly resulting in EDS should be identified. Lastly, total sleep time should be evaluated and be not too far from estimated sleep needs. In our experience, however, most EDS causes can be identified clinically and with PSG or simplified sleep monitoring under CPAP.

(6) Lastly, EDS and vigilance assessment may be critical in specific clinical contexts such as professional drivers or other at-risk occupational activities. It has been shown that attention deficits may exist even in the absence of subjective or even objective sleepiness. This probably suggests using an extended battery of tests in order to detect these deficits [43]. Moreover, considering the impact on driving ability, this supports treating these subjects and evaluating their clinical benefit. Objective vigilance evaluation, sustained attention test, reaction time evaluation and divided-attention test are of interest in this context.

Conclusions

There are multiple sleep disorders that should be better known by the respiratory physicians even if many diagnoses are mainly performed in specialized sleep centers. Excessive daytime sleepiness is however a condition requiring extended knowledge on the various clinical contexts and clinical variations that are to be taken into account before diagnosis and treatment.

References

1 American Academy of Sleep Medicine: International Classification of Sleep Disorders, ed 2: Diagnostic and Coding Manual. Rochester, American Academy of Sleep Medicine, 2005.

2 Roehrs T, Zorick F, Roth T: Transient and short-term insomnias; in Kryger MH, Roth T, Dement WC (eds): Principles and Practice of Sleep Medicine, ed 3. Philadelphia, Saunders, 2000, pp 624–632.

3 Buysse DJ, Reynolds CF 3rd, Kupfer DJ, Thorpy MJ, Bixler E, Manfredi R, Kales A, Stepanski E, Roth T: Clinical diagnoses in 216 insomnia patients using the International Classification of Sleep Disorders (ICSD), DSM-IV and ICD-10 categories: a report from the APA/NIMH DSM-IV field trial. Sleep 1994;17:630–637.

4 Ohayon M: Epidemiology of insomnia: what we know and what we still need to learn. Sleep Med Rev 2002;6:97–111.

5 Edinger JD, Fins AL: The distribution and clinical significance of sleep time misperceptions. Sleep 1995;18:232–239.

6 Morin CM, Hauri PJ, Espie CA, Spielman AJ, Buysse DJ, Bootzin RR: Non-pharmacological treatment of chronic insomnia. Sleep 1999; 22:1134–1156.

7 The Report of an American Academy of Sleep Medicine Task Force: Sleep-related breathing disorders in adults: recommendations for syndrome definition and measurement techniques in clinical research. Sleep 1999;22:667–689.

8 Guilleminault C, Stoohs R, Clerk A, Cetel M, Maistros P: A cause of excessive daytime sleepiness. The upper airway resistance syndrome. Chest 1993;104:781–787.

9 Douglas NJ: Upper airway resistance syndrome is not a distinct syndrome. Am J Respir Crit Care Med 2000;161:1413–1416.

10 Cracowski C, Pepin JL, Wuyam B, Levy P: Characterization of obstructive non-apneic respiratory events in moderate sleep apnea syndrome. Am J Respir Crit Care Med 2001;164: 944–948.

11 Young T, Palta M, Dempsey J, Skatrud J, Weber S, Badr S: The occurrence of sleep-disordered breathing among middle-aged adults. N Engl J Med 1993;328:1230–1235.

12 Teran-Santos J, Jimenez-Gomez A, Cordero-Guevara J: The association between sleep apnea and the risk of traffic accidents. Cooperative Group Burgos-Santander. N Engl J Med 1999;340:847–851.

13 Levy P, Pepin JL, McNicholas WT: Should all sleep apnoea patients be treated? Yes. Sleep Med Rev 2002;6:17–26.

14 Marin JM, Carrizo SJ, Vicente E, Agusti AG: Long-term cardiovascular outcomes in men with obstructive sleep apnoea-hypopnoea with or without treatment with continuous positive airway pressure: an observational study. Lancet 2005;365:1046–1053.

15 Pepperell JC, Ramdassingh-Dow S, Crosthwaite N, Mullins R, Jenkinson C, Stradling JR, Davies RJ: Ambulatory blood pressure after therapeutic and subtherapeutic nasal continuous positive airway pressure for obstructive sleep apnoea: a randomised parallel trial. Lancet 2002;359:204–210.

16 Drager LF, Bortolotto LA, Lorenzi MC, Figueiredo AC, Krieger EM, Lorenzi-Filho G: Early signs of atherosclerosis in obstructive sleep apnea. Am J Respir Crit Care Med 2005;172:613–618.

17 Baguet J-P, Hammer L, Levy P, Pierre H, Launois S, Mallion J-M, Pepin J-L: The severity of oxygen desaturation is predictive of carotid wall thickening and plaque occurrence. Chest 2005;128:3407–3412.

18 Lavie P, Lavie L, Herer P: All-cause mortality in males with sleep apnoea syndrome: declining mortality rates with age. Eur Respir J 2005;25: 514–520.

19 Pepin JL, Chouri-Pontarolo N, Tamisier R, Levy P: Cheyne-Stokes respiration (CSR) with central sleep apnoea (CSA) [CSR-CSA] in chronic heart failure: proposals for a diagnostic and therapeutic strategy. Sleep Med Rev 2006;10:33–47.

20 Bradley TD, Logan AG, Kimoff RJ, Series F, Morrison D, Ferguson K, Belenkie I, Pfeifer M, Fleetham J, Hanly P, Smilovitch M, Tomlinson G, Floras JS: Continuous positive airway pressure for central sleep apnea and heart failure. N Engl J Med 2005;353:2025–2033.

21 Nowbar S, Burkart KM, Gonzales R, Fedorowicz A, Gozansky WS, Gaudio JC, Taylor MR, Zwillich CW: Obesity-associated hypoventilation in hospitalized patients: prevalence, effects, and outcome. Am J Med 2004;116:1–7.

22 Guilleminault C, Framherz S: in Kryger MH, Roth T, Dement WC (eds): Principles and Practice of Sleep Medicine, Philadelphia, Elsevier Saunders, 2005, pp 780–790.

23 Overeem S, Mignot E, Van Dijk JG, Lammers GJ: Narcolepsy: clinical features, new pathophysiologic insights and future perspectives. J Clin Neurophysiol 2001;18:78–105.

24 Mignot E, Lammers GJ, Ripley N, Okun M, Nevsimalova S, Overeem S, Vankova J, Black J, Harsh J, Bassetti C, Schrader H, Nishino S: The role of cerebrospinal fluid hypocretin measurement in the diagnosis of narcolepsy and other hypersomnias. Arch Neurol 2002; 59:1553–1562.

25 Billiard M, Dauvilliers Y: Idiopathic hypersomnia. Sleep Med Rev 2001;5:351–360.

26 Mahowald M, Schenck C: Parasomnias including the Restless Leg Syndrome. Clin Chest Med 1998;19:183–202.

27 Mahowald M, Schenck CH: Insights from studying human sleep disorders. Nature 437, 1279–1285.

28 Reid KJ, Zee PC: in Kryger MH, Roth T, Dement WC (eds): Principles and Practice of Sleep Medicine, Philadelphia, Elsevier Saunders, 2005, pp 691–701.

29 Arendt J, Stone B, Skene D: Jet Lag and sleep disruption; in Kryger MH, Roth T, Dement WC (eds): Principles and Practice of Sleep Medicine, ed3. Philadelphia, WB Saunders, 2000, pp 591–599.

30 Akerstedt T: Shift work and disturbed sleep/wakefulness. Occup Med 2003;53:89–94.

31 Archer SN, Robilliard DL, Skene DJ, Smits M, Williams A, Arendt J, von Schantz M: A length polymorphism in the circadian clock gene Per3 is linked to delayed sleep phase syndrome and extreme diurnal preference. Sleep 2003;26:413–415.

32 Xu Y, Padiath QS, Shapiro RE, Jones CR, Wu SC, Saigoh N, Saigoh K, Ptacek LJ, Fu YH: Functional consequences of a CKI-delta mutation causing familial advanced sleep phase syndrome. Nature 2005;434:640–644.

33 Toh KL, Jones CR, He Y, Eide EJ, Hinz WA, Virshup DM, Ptacek LJ, Fu YH: An hPer2 phosphorylation site mutation in familial advanced sleep phase syndrome. Science 2001;291:1040–1043.

34 Earley C: Clinical practice. Restless Leg Syndrome. N Engl J Med 2003;348:2103–2109.

35 Trenkwalder C, Paulus W, Walters AS: The restless legs syndrome. Lancet Neurology 2005;4:465–475.

36 Allen RP, Picchietti D, Hening WA, Trenkwalder C, Walters AS, Montplaisir J: Restless legs syndrome: diagnostic criteria, special considerations, and epidemiology. A report from the restless legs syndrome diagnosis and epidemiology workshop at the National Institutes of Health. Sleep Med 2003;4:101–119.

37 Walters AS, LeBrocq C, Dhar A, Hening W, Rosen R, Allen RP, Trenkwalder C: International Restless Legs Syndrome Study. Validation of the International Restless Legs Syndrome Study Group rating scale for restless legs syndrome. Sleep Med 2003;4;121–132.

38 American Sleep Disorders Association Task Force: Recording and scoring leg movements. Sleep 1993;16:748–759.

39 Allen R, Becker PM, Bogan R, et al: Ropinirole decreases periodic leg movements and improves sleep parameters in patients with restless legs syndrome. Sleep 2004;27:907–914.

40 Montplaisir J, Nicolas A, Denesle R, Gomez-Mancilla B: Restless legs syndrome improved by pramipexole: a double-blind randomized trial. Neurol 1999;52:938–943.

41 Hening W, Allen R, Earley C, Kushida C, Picchietti D, Silber M: The treatment of restless legs syndrome and periodic limb movement disorder. An American Academy of Sleep Medicine Review. Sleep 1999;22:970–999.

42 Bixler EO, Vgontzas AN, Lin H-M, Calhoun SL, Vela-Bueno A, Kales A: Excessive daytime sleepiness in a general population sample: the role of sleep apnea, age, obesity, diabetes, and depression. J Clin Endocrinol Metab 2005;90:4510–4515.

43 Mazza S, Pepin J-L, Naegele B, Plante J, Deschaux C, Levy P: Most obstructive sleep apnoea patients exhibit vigilance and attention deficits on an extended battery of tests. Eur Respir J 2005;25:75–80.

P. Lévy
EFCR
CHU Grenoble
FR–38043 Grenoble, Cedex (France)
Tel. +33 4 76 76 55 16, Fax +33 4 76 76 55 86
E-Mail PLevy@chu-grenoble.fr

Randerath WJ, Sanner BM, Somers VK (eds): Sleep Apnea.
Prog Respir Res. Basel, Karger, 2006, vol 35, pp 13–20

Physiology of Sleep and Dreaming

Thomas Penzel Karl Kesper

Sleep Laboratory, Department of Internal Medicine, Hospital of Philipps University, Marburg, Germany

Abstract

Sleep has a restorative function which is more than rest. Sleep is an active process which follows its own program with a sequence of different sleep stages and autonomous nervous system functions related to them. Slow wave sleep is mainly related to physical recreation with humoral and neuro-endocrine excretions activated. REM sleep is mainly but not exclusively related to mental recreation with associated dreaming and memory functions. The autonomous nervous system with ventilation, cardiocirculatory, vascular and temperature regulation differs between slow wave sleep and REM sleep. More regular control is found in slow wave sleep and more variability is found in REM sleep. The sleep processes follow a well-described temporal pattern with sleep cycles of a duration between 80 and 110 min. The sleep process itself is embedded in the circadian rhythm and occurs naturally during the dark phase of the day with a mean duration of 7–8 h. In order to study sleep disorders, the knowledge about physiological sleep, physiological effects of sleep deprivation, and autonomic and endocrine functions associated with it, is essential.

The key question for sleep physiology, why we sleep, is still unanswered. It is well studied that many restorative functions are linked to the sleep process. Physical recreation, endocrine and immune functions are closely linked to sleep. Mental restoration, memory consolidation, mood and behavior are also dependent on a healthy and undisturbed sleep. Our knowledge about the mechanisms of sleep-wake states is increasing even if their neuroanatomical locations still have not been found [1]. All physiological functions are embedded in the circadian day-night cycle. The sleep-wake cycle is closely linked to the circadian cycle and both influence each other. For the newborn child, the adaptation of the sleep-wake cycle to the circadian cycle takes some time and is part of the development process. With aging, the sleep period mostly occurs during the night phase and becomes as short as 8 h on average.

Sleep Structure and Sleep Stages

Sleep itself is not a steady state of unconsciousness but has an internal structure with a cyclical time course. To classify sleep, recommendations have been introduced in 1968 by a committee chaired by Rechtschaffen and Kales [2]. They introduced discrete sleep stages based on the observed electroencephalographic (EEG) waves and patterns as well as electrooculographic (EOG) patterns and mental or submental muscle tone derived by electromyography (EMG). The EEG, EOG, and EMG electrodes are attached at well standardized positions. The specific patterns of the sleep stages are described in figure 1. Sleep recording is classified into epochs of 20 or 30 s duration. At the very beginning of sleep when the person is still awake, sleepy characteristic EEG waves, alpha waves with 8–12 Hz can be observed. At the onset of sleep, on average about 10–20 min after relaxed wakefulness, muscle tone decreases and on the

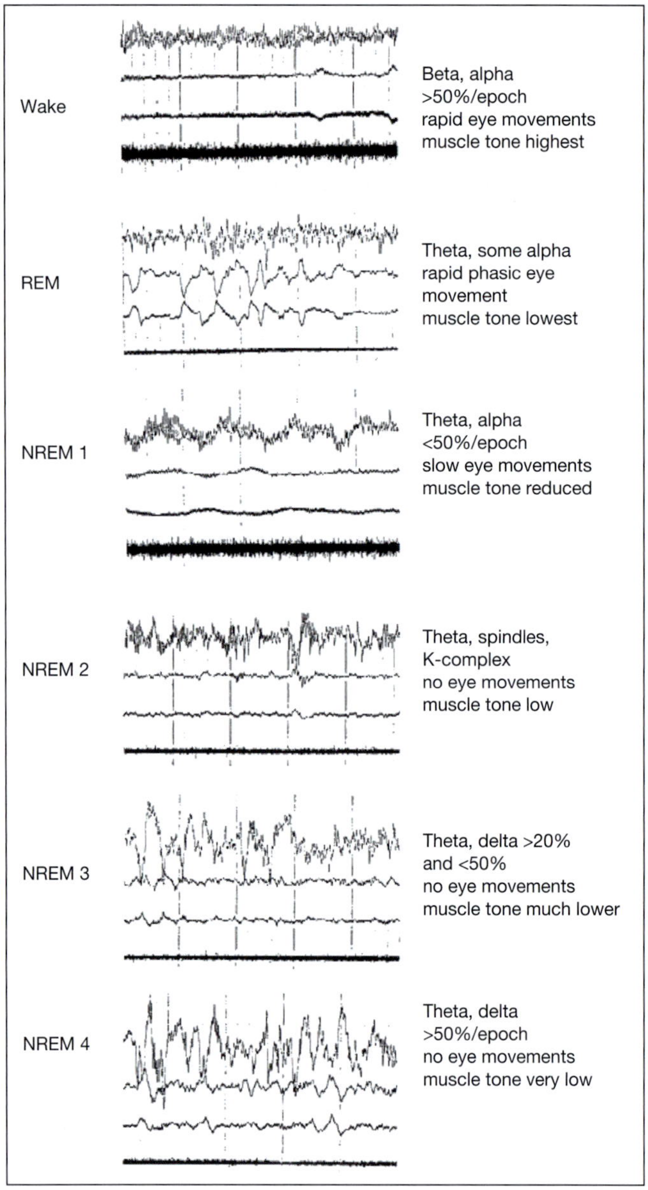

Fig. 1. The sleep stages and their characteristic features. This definition of sleep stages follows the recommendations of Rechtschaffen and Kales as used for visual sleep classification [2].

EEG the alpha waves vanish and slower frequencies, theta waves (4–7 Hz), appear. In addition, specific short patterns called vertex sharp waves can be observed. The EOG shows slow eye movements with eyes closed. This sleep stage, NREM 1, is transitional and does not last long. Often this phase is not perceived as sleep when the person is asked. After a few minutes of sleep stage 1, sleep stage NREM 2 follows. Beside the same EEG waves, the theta waves, very specific patterns are observed here. These are K complexes and sleep spindles. They belong to the classification of sleep stage 2. Both patterns are remarkably outstanding from the background EEG activity. It is assumed that sleep spindles are activities towards deeper sleep and K complexes are intermittent events reflecting an increased cerebral activity corresponding to a slowing of falling asleep. Muscle tone is slightly lower during sleep stage 2 than during sleep stage 1. Usually there are no more slow eye movements during sleep stage 2. Stages 1 and 2 together are called light sleep. When awakened from light sleep, persons still report that they did doze away but did not sleep. After another 10–20 min of stage 2, muscle tone drops further and deep sleep starts by the occurrence of slow delta waves (0.5–4 Hz) with high amplitudes (up to 150 μV) in the EEG. This slow wave sleep is artificially broken into sleep stage NREM 3 with delta waves occupying 20–50% of the time and sleep stage NREM 4 with more than 50% of delta waves which need to exceed an amplitude threshold of 75 μV. To awake a person out of deep sleep is difficult, and usually it takes a few minutes to regain full consciousness. After 20–40 min of deep sleep, a first period of paradoxical sleep follows for 5–15 min. Paradoxical sleep is called REM sleep today. The term paradoxical sleep stems from the fact that the EEG resembles wakefulness and at the same time the lowest muscle tone is observed. During REM sleep, the EEG shows mixed frequencies and low amplitude similar to wakefulness. In addition saw-tooth waves with their particular sharp patterns may occur. The very characteristic and striking pattern during REM sleep are the rapid eye movements which occur in varying density during the entire REM sleep period. Based on this, REM sleep can be split into two distinct patterns: the phasic REM sleep with eye movements present and tonic REM sleep without the rapid eye movements but similar EEG. The two patterns seem to be well correlated with different patterns observed in the signals of the autonomic system. To wake up a person out of REM sleep may be as difficult as out of deep sleep or may be very easy. In 80% of wake up experiments the person reports dreaming when taken out of REM sleep. Often vivid, colorful, and emotional dreams are reported. When waking up subjects from NREM sleep, in 20% of all cases dreams are reported. Dreams in NREM sleep are usually less colorful and less emotional. The EEG during REM sleep with mixed frequencies and small amplitude indicates high cerebral activity. This high cerebral activity has been confirmed by cerebral blood flow and positron emission tomography studies of REM sleep. With the period of REM sleep a sleep cycle is complete.

This sequence of sleep stages forms a sleep cycle with a normal duration of 80–110 min. Four to six sleep cycles are

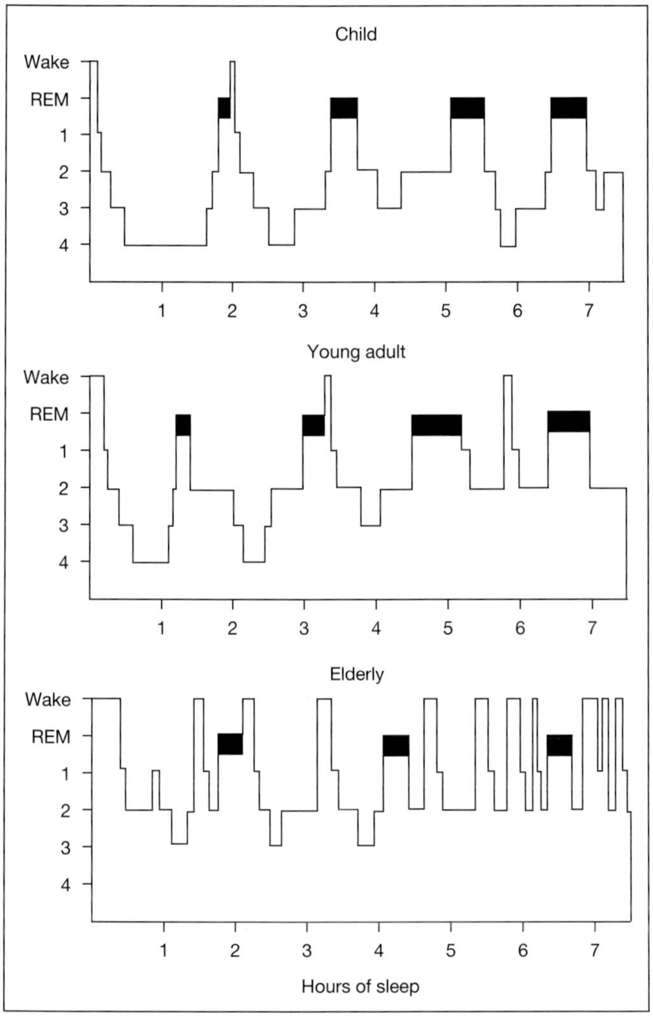

Fig. 2. The three hypnograms show the sleep structure at different ages. The normal sleep structure is shown and the effects of age are schematically drawn.

observed in a normal sleep night (fig. 2). There is a gradual change of the distribution of sleep stages within the sleep cycles over the course of the night. The first sleep cycles have more deep sleep, whereas the later ones have more REM sleep. Over the night, the total percentage of wakefulness is less than 5%, of light sleep 45–55%, of deep sleep about 20% and REM sleep 20–25%. Total duration of sleep varies between 7.5 and 8.5 h in the majority of healthy persons. Each person has an individual optimum for sleep duration. After sleep deprivation there is an increase of slow wave sleep and REM sleep during the following sleep period. The recovery from sleep deprivation is usually accomplished fast and is not carried over too many more nights.

At the transitions between sleep stages, short awakenings, incomplete awakenings and even shorter activations, so-called arousals are observed. According to the recommendations of Rechtschaffen and Kales [2], a sleep epoch is called wakefulness if the activation lasts 15 s or longer. According to additional conventions [3] on short activations, these are called arousals if they last longer than 3 s. The number of arousals in normal subjects increases with age. In normal middle-aged subjects 13–21 arousals are reported per hour of sleep [4]. In higher age groups without sleep disorders 18–27 arousals per hour have been reported [5].

The sleep structure is heavily dependent on the mental and physical workload prior to sleep time. Physical work increases deep sleep and mental work increases REM sleep percentages. Stress increases the number of awakenings and arousals.

Neuroanatomy of Sleep

The circadian system is well described and in contrast to the sleep-wake system an anatomical circadian clock has been identified. The suprachiasmatic nucleus in the anterior hypothalamus controls the timing of most circadian rhythms in mammals. In contrast, no single neural system identified so far is responsible for the generation of sleep or wakefulness [6]. Most neuroanatomical results are obtained by the observation of the effects of lesions in particular regions.

Wakefulness is maintained by multiple neural systems that extend from the brainstem reticular formation into the thalamus and through the posterior hypothalamus up to the basal forebrain. In the 1940s, Moruzzi and Magoun discovered neurons in the reticular formation which extend through the central core of the medulla, pons and midbrain of the brainstem. Neurons in the medullary and caudal pontine reticular formation are particularly important for maintaining postural muscle tone with behavioral arousal through their descending projections to the spinal cord. Neurons in the oral pontine and midbrain reticular formation are essential for sustaining cortical activation with fast EEG activity.

Sleep is promoted by neurons in the lower brainstem and upper forebrain that inhibit wake-generating neurons to dampen cortical activation and behavioral arousal [7]. Many of these neurons are located in central control regions of the parasympathetic nervous system. This includes the nucleus of the solitary tract and the anterior hypothalamus/preoptic region. These neurons receive input from the lung, heart, gut and baroreceptors. They project forward to the forebrain where they may stimulate sleep-promoting neurons. During REM sleep, the cerebral cortex is activated, whereas muscle tone along with behavioral arousal is inhibited. Many of the central activating systems including the brainstem reticular formation are active during this state. Most important are neurons within the oral pontine reticular formation [8]. The neurons that stimulate cortical activation and those that inhibit postural muscle tone are located in the pontine tegmentum. Some of these neurons project both rostrally into the forebrain and caudally into the lower brainstem and spinal cord, others to one or the other site. In the brainstem and forebrain, cholinergic neurons discharge at maximal rates during REM sleep [9]. Their discharge stimulates cortical activation and may also selectively facilitate motor inhibitory systems. The pontomesencephalic cholinergic neurons play a critical role in generating REM sleep. Gamma-aminobutyric acid (GABA)-ergic brainstem neurons also play a critical role in gating REM sleep. They inhibit the noradrenergic neurons of the locus coeruleus which must be off to permit REM sleep to occur.

The arousal system involved in wake generation utilizes a number of different neurotransmitters such as glutamate, noradrenaline, acetylcholine, dopamine, glutamic acid, histamine and orexine. Slow wave sleep occurs through the inhibition of the arousal systems. The key neurotransmitters involved in sleep generation are adenosine, GABA, acetylcholine during REM sleep, glycine and some immune modulators [10].

Functions Related to Sleep

Most physiological functions show characteristic changes with the sleep-wake regulation. Behavioral activity decreases and autonomic functions are reduced to adapt to the lower metabolic needs. The autonomic nervous system is a highly integrated system and maintains homeostasis through a control of ventilation, heart rate, arterial blood pressure, gut secretions and renal blood flow [11]. Only during REM sleep with an active brain do autonomic functions show an activated and apparently irregular behavior, while at the same time the behavioral activity remains unchanged at sleep. The changes in autonomous system regulation have been demonstrated by the recording of the sympathetic nerve activity (SNA) on the n. peroneus in healthy young humans [12]. Somers et al. [12] have shown that SNA decreases from wakefulness progressively to light sleep and further to slow wave sleep. During REM sleep, there is intermittently no SNA at all and short, very strong surges of SNA. This irregular activity of SNA corresponds to very irregular activity observed in many other autonomous nervous system variables such as respiration, heart rate and blood pressure (fig. 3).

Respiration

The ventilatory control is generated by the bulbopontine respiratory neurons, which are sensitive to central chemoreceptors and peripheral chemoreceptors. These respiratory neurons activate spinal motoneurons on which breathing muscle activity depends. This consists of the diaphragm, intercostal muscles and the muscles of the upper airways. The goal of the metabolic control of ventilation is to maintain the values of O_2, CO_2 and pH in its normal ranges. During sleep onset, the minute ventilation decreases which results in a slight increase in pCO_2. This increased value of pCO_2 is then maintained during sleep. During the transition, a variable breathing with changes in breathing frequency are observed. During this transition period, also phases of periodic breathing may occur in healthy subjects. During deeper sleep, the respiration becomes very regular with little variation in breathing rate and tidal volume. During sleep stage 2, ventilation is reduced by 13% compared to wakefulness, and it is further reduced during slow wave – up to 15% compared to wakefulness [13]. This drop in ventilation is mainly due to a reduction in tidal volume and not in breathing frequency. During REM sleep with its phasic activations of the autonomous nervous system, ventilation is still reduced compared to wakefulness but it is slightly increased compared to slow wave sleep. The activity of the intercostal muscles and the upper airway dilators are reduced by approximately 30% compared to NREM sleep, and in contrast diaphragmatic activity is increased to compensate for this effect. Thereby, upper airway resistance is higher during REM sleep, respiratory activity might become out of phase and irregular breathing can be a common consequence. Ventilation is unstable during REM sleep in terms of breathing frequency and tidal volume and this might lead to the occurrence of some apneas even in healthy subjects. The intrinsic regulation of ventilation follows different laws as has been proven by a breath-by-breath analysis [14]. Ventilation during REM sleep is very different from periodic breathing with its regularity and cannot be compared to this entirely different regulation.

Heart Rate

Heart rate drops with the onset of sleep or even before with sleepiness. Thus, heart rate follows the reduced metabolic

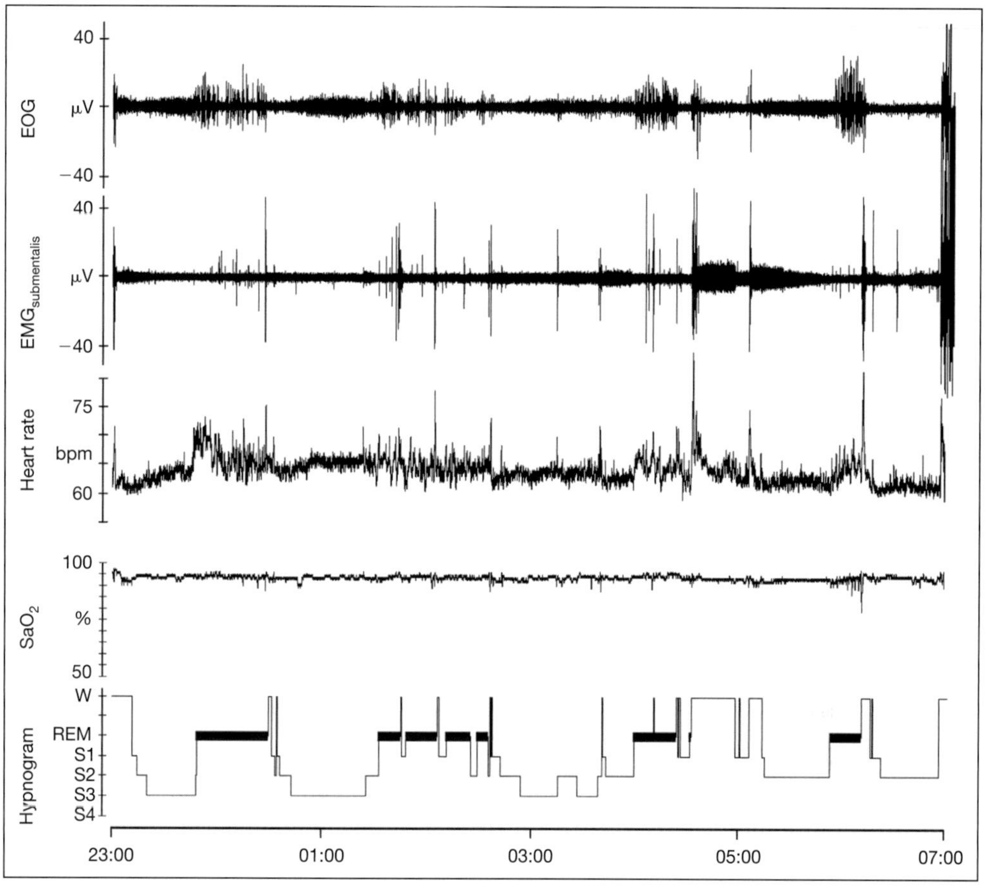

Fig. 3. Condensed plot of a polysomnographic recording showing from top to bottom EOG, EMG submentalis, heart rate, oxygen saturation (SaO_2), and the hypnogram. The EOG trace clearly indicates periods with REM sleep. The EMG shows only twitches during REM and high muscle tone during periods of wakefulness. Heart rate shows low values during sleep and high variability during REM sleep. This recording has been done in a patient under successful ventilation therapy, and therefore shows an almost normal sleep profile. The high percentage of REM sleep and deep sleep in this recording indicate the rebound effect after long sleep deprivation.

demands. Heart rate parallels much the SNA as described above [12]. Heart rate control reduces the sinus rhythm during sleep and, in addition, follows a different intrinsic regulation which has been described as irregular, similar to the time course of SNA during REM sleep. In mirroring this pattern, heart rate also increases and is followed by drops thereafter. This specific heart rate variability behavior can be quantitatively expressed as long-term correlations by non-linear signal analysis methods derived from statistical physics [15]. This long-term correlation appears to be a characteristic feature of REM sleep. Long-term correlations are also present in other autonomic variables such as ventilation during REM sleep. In NREM sleep, heart rate variability follows primarily the respiratory rhythm called sinus arrhythmia. This can be expressed as short-term correlations using the same method derived from statistical physics [15]. The respiration-linked variability of heart rate is found in the frequency range of 0.15–0.4 Hz and is called high-frequency (HF) variability. It is attributed to parasympathetic control of heart rate. The slower variability of heart rate in the range of 0.04–0.15 Hz is called low-frequency (LF) variability and reflects baroreflex sympathetic control of heart rate. Both can be set in relation to each other and the resulting index LF/HF is called sympathovagal balance. The sympathovagal balance reflects the decrease in sympathetic activation when coming to deeper sleep stages. It also reflects well the sympathetic activation during REM sleep. Many more indices derived from heart rate and heart rate variability can be used to characterize the normal sleep process and to give indications for a disturbed sleep process in multiple sleep disorders [16]. Arousals from sleep may show activation at the cortical level but may also show a sympathetic activation which is usually reflected by heart rate increases.

Blood Pressure

The arterial blood pressure reflects vascular resistance and sympathetic tone. Therefore arterial blood pressure closely follows the SNA [12]. During REM sleep, systolic blood pressure shows remarkable elevations compared to NREM sleep. In patients with hypertension or sleep disordered breathing, blood pressure during REM sleep can reach extremely high values which are the consequence of peripheral vasoconstriction and sympathetic activation.

Temperature

Prior to sleep onset, body core temperature starts to drop. At the same time, a peripheral vasodilatation leads to an increase in skin temperature which thus helps to drop body temperature. Temperature decreases further during sleep and reaches a minimum in the early phase of sleep. Thereafter temperature increases again, but more slowly than the decrease that was observed during falling asleep. The decline in metabolic rate and body temperature with sleep onset is not only a consequence of decreased motor activity and digestive activity because body temperature declines even in fasting persons in bedrest studies or in paralyzed patients. It is the effect of circadian and sleep regulation processes. Metabolic rate decreases in humans by 5–17% during sleep compared to wakefulness. Body temperature decreases already before sleep onset, thus suggesting that it plays an active part in the process of sleep onset. Indeed, a drop in body temperature with the parallel increase in peripheral skin temperature, particularly the hands, is a strong stimulus to fall asleep. In contrast a rising body temperature has an arousing effect and inhibits falling asleep. Passive heating or intense exercise in the afternoon increases slow wave sleep but has no effect on REM sleep during the following night sleep.

Thermoregulatory responses in humans are markedly inhibited during REM sleep. Shivering during sleep in cool environments is observed in light sleep and is not seen in slow wave sleep or REM sleep [17]. Sweating in warm environments which can be observed in NREM sleep declines before the onset of REM sleep and reaches minimal levels during REM sleep. The body temperature rises during REM sleep in warm environments if sweating does not help [18].

Memory and Learning

Memory functions can be related to sleep [19]. A number of experiments in the last few years could demonstrate that not only REM but also NREM sleep is important for memory functions. The theory of learning distinguishes in this context between two types of learning and associated memory. One type is declarative memory which is tested through a session of learning pairs of related terms such as glove – shoe, or tree – leaf, or water – wave, etc. This memory is needed for the learning of foreign languages. The other type is procedural memory which is tested through the learning of mirror-writing. For this task the person has to write some sentences while the writing hand is hidden and can be observed through a mirror only. The written sentence should be readable in the mirror which requires some training in writing against the usual order. Procedural memory is needed for all types of movements such as car driving, bicycle riding, skiing etc. The carefully selected experiments could show that the improvement of declarative memory can be more associated with NREM sleep, whereas the improvement of procedural memory can be more attributed to REM sleep. Further, very recent experiments have demonstrated that sleep and specifically REM sleep seems to improve problem-solving behavior in young volunteers [20]. Prior to these recent studies, memory consolidation had been attributed to REM sleep exclusively. Now it became evident, that both REM and NREM sleep take part in memory consolidation and learning processes.

Development of Sleep with Age

Sleep changes with age [1]. Very small children sleep for up to 16 h distributed over the 24 h with 50% REM sleep (called active sleep at that age). At the age of 15 years, sleep duration is only a little longer than in adults of 20 and more years. By the age of 10, REM sleep has decreased to 20–25%. Further, with increasing age the percentage of deep sleep decreases steadily (table 1), but the total sleep duration does not change much (fig. 2) [21]. The reasons for this decrease are not fully investigated. Often night sleep becomes shorter and some daytime naps add up to a similar total sleep duration. As stated above, the number of spontaneous arousals during sleep also increase with age.

Complaints about sleep quality and sleep disorders are very common in industrialized societies. Surveys do distinguish between complaints of insomnia and complaints of excessive sleepiness. The prevalence of current insomnia was 32% and of excessive sleep was 7% among 1,006 households [22]. Up to 20% of persons at the age of 40 and

Table 1. Table of sleep stages as a function of age and gender according to Redline et al. [21]

Age years	Stage 1		Stage 2		Slow wave sleep		REM sleep	
	Men	Women	Men	Women	Men	Women	Men	Women
37–54	5.8	4.6	61.4	58.5	11.2	14.2	19.5	20.9
55–60	6.3	5.0	64.5	56.2	8.2	17.0	19.1	20.2
61–70	7.1	5.0	65.2	57.3	6.7	16.7	18.4	19.3
>70	7.6	4.9	66.5	57.1	5.5	17.2	17.8	18.8

Percentages of total sleep time are listed as mean values.

older report on frequent or regular sleep problems. The complaints of insomnia and excessive sleep both increase with age.

Models for Sleep Wake Regulation

In order to explain and to predict the sleep wake process for normal and disturbed sleep, mathematical models have been developed. The most common and well-established model is the so-called two-process model, which was first presented by Daan, Beersma and Borbely in 1984. It combines chronobiological and homeostatic principles that were obtained from many previous laboratory experiments on sleep and circadian rhythms. The model has proven to explain several aspects of sleep wake regulation [23]. It has been successful in the prediction of sleep deprivation experiments and increasing sleep pressure.

Apart from this two-process model, other models based on statistical properties or Markov chain models were developed. These models were adapted to specific problems and were universally valid. However, they have not been validated by independent research groups.

According to the two-process model, the occurrence of sleep, duration of sleep, sleep intensity and the internal structure are determined by two oscillatory processes called process 'S' or sleep homeostasis and process 'C' or circadian rhythm. The timing of sleep is determined by the circadian rhythm. Process S is homeostatic and increases during wakefulness until it reaches a circadian upper threshold and sleep is initiated. The homeostatic process S has been deducted from the quantification of slow wave sleep in the sleep EEG. The larger the S is the more slow wave sleep can be observed in the sleep EEG. The circadian process C is strongly influenced by the light-dark cycle.

Both processes interact closely and can be related to neural activities. The circadian rhythm is determined by the rhythmic activity of the suprachiasmatic nuclei, being primarily responsible for changes in body temperature and endocrine secretions.

The model was able to predict sleepiness in shift work, in response to time zone transitions, in aircrew fatigue and driver fatigue risk. The model does not explain the cyclic NREM REM cycle. It is also not well suited to model cumulative effects of sleep loss over several nights. It is also obvious that different tasks may create different effects on sleepiness, and thus the increase in sleep pressure may vary with the task performed during daytime.

Today, a number of refinements have been made and have finally led to an expanded three-process model of sleep and fatigue. This refined model introduces a task-related component which contributes to sleep pressure and sleep inertia. A possible correlate for this third task-related component may be physical activity as monitored by a wrist-watch type of actigraph.

A different approach to modeling sleep is based on the observation of the alteration between wakefulness and sleep. This approach is based on the statistical properties of the regulation of sleep and wakefulness durations [24]. The distributions of sleep and wakefulness durations differ in a way that the distribution of sleep durations follows an exponential law as it is also the case with molecular movement. In contrast, the distribution of wakefulness durations follows a power law which is characteristic for systems with fractal behavior such as the branching of bronchioles. In general, exponential law and power law behavior cannot be generated by the same underlying system. Transferring this rule to the sleep wake regulation, it is very likely that different neural brain areas are responsible for the regulation of sleep and wakefulness. This difference in regulation of sleep and wakefulness durations was also found in sleep in different species [25]. There, only the exponent and the constant responsible for the decline of the distribution differed. The general characteristic remained the same throughout the species.

Circadian Rhythm

The occurrence of sleep is dependent on the circadian phase. There is an 'opening window' in the late evening, accompanied by a drop in body temperature. Then sleep is initiated best. Another, less pronounced 'opening window' for sleep is in the early afternoon. To start sleep at other times is more difficult unless a person is sleep deprived. In order to investigate the circadian rhythm systematically, a specific bedrest study protocol has been developed, which aims to minimize all external influences which can mask the intrinsic circadian rhythm. These studies are performed in isolated chambers with control of light, temperature, noise, and without any clocks. The so-called forced desynchrony protocol gives mental and physical tasks to the subjects in the circadian study laboratory at a 28-hour rhythm. This period is long enough that an adaptation to this duration does not occur. In this way the intrinsic circadian processes can be studied when averaging effects over several days.

Important zeitgeber for the circadian clock are light, ambient temperature changes, noise, nutrition, and social contacts. The classic intrinsic markers for the circadian rhythm are body core temperature and melatonin secretion. This means that these variables vary closely with the circadian rhythm. Typically subjects want to go to bed when their body temperature is reaching its minimum values. But it also means that changes in body temperature and melatonin influence the circadian rhythm.

The intrinsic circadian rhythm is a little bit longer than 24 h, on average by 15 min. The duration of REM sleep is strongly linked to the circadian sleep process, and the longest REM sleep in bedrest studies is found roughly 1–2 h after the body temperature has reached its minimum [26]. From the results of circadian research it is evident that the homeostatic sleep regulation and the circadian process interact strongly with each other and influence each other. A clear experience of this interactions can be observed at flights across several time zones during intercontinental flights.

References

1 Kryger M, Roth T, Dement WC: Principles and Practice of Sleep Medicine, ed 3. Philadelphia, Saunders, 2000.
2 Rechtschaffen A, Kales A: A Manual of Standardized Terminology, Techniques and Scoring System for Sleep Stages of Human Subjects. NIH Publication No. 204. Washington, U.S. Government Printing Office, 1968.
3 American Sleep Disorders Association: EEG arousals: scoring rules and examples. Sleep 1992;15:173–184.
4 Marthur R, Douglas NJ: Frequency of EEG arousals from nocturnal sleep in normal subjects. Sleep 1995;18:330–333.
5 Boselli M, Parrino L, Smerieri A, et al: Effect of age on EEG arousals in normal sleep. Sleep 1998;21:351–357.
6 Jones BE: Basic mechanisms of sleep-wake states; in Kryger MH, Roth T, Dement WC (eds): Principles and Practice of Sleep Medicine, ed 3. Philadelphia, Saunders, 2000, pp 134–154.
7 Jones BE: Activity, modulation and role of basal forebrain cholinergic neurons innervating the cerebral cortex. Prog Brain Res 2004;145: 157–169.
8 Saper CB, Chou TC, Scammell TE: The sleep switch: hypothalamic control of sleep and wakefulness. Trends Neurosci 2001;24:726–731.
9 Hobson JA, McCarley RW, Wyzinski PW: Sleep cycle oscillation: reciprocal discharge by two brainstem neural groups. Science 1975;189:55–58.
10 Krueger JM, Majde JA: Humoral links between sleep and the immune system: research issues. Ann N Y Acad Sci 2003;992:9–20.
11 Verrier RL, Harper RM, Hobson JA: Cardiac physiology: central and autonomic regulation; in Kryger MH, Roth T, Dement WC (eds): Principles and Practice of Sleep Medicine, ed 3. Philadelphia, Saunders, 2000, pp 179–191.
12 Somers VK, Dyken ME, Mark AL, Abboud FM: Sympathetic-nerve activity during sleep in normal subjects. N Engl J Med 1993;328: 303–307.
13 Krieger J, Maglasiu N, Sforza E, Kurtz D: Breathing during sleep in normal middle-aged subjects. Sleep 1990;13:143–154.
14 Rostig S, Kantelhardt JW, Penzel T, Cassel W, Peter JH, Vogelmeier C, Becker HF: Nonrandom variability of respiration during sleep in healthy humans. Sleep 2005;28:411–417.
15 Bunde A, Havlin S, Kantelhardt JW, Penzel T, Peter JH, Voigt K: Correlated and uncorrelated regions in heart-rate fluctuations during sleep. Phys Rev Lett 2000;85:3736–3739.
16 Penzel T, Kantelhardt JW, Grote L, Peter JH, Bunde A: Comparison of detrended fluctuation analysis and spectral analysis for heart rate variability in sleep and sleep apnea. IEEE Trans Biomed Eng 2003;50:1143–1151.
17 Palca JW, Walker JM, Berger RJ: Thermoregulation, metabolism, and stages of sleep in cold-exposed men. J Appl Physiol 1986;61: 940–947.
18 Sagot JC, Amoros C, Candas V, Libert JP: Sweating responses and body temperatures during nocturnal sleep in humans. Am J Physiol 1987;252:R462–R470.
19 Smith C: Sleep states and memory processes in humans: procedural versus declarative memory systems. Sleep Med Rev 2001;5: 491–506.
20 Wagner U, Gais S, Halder H, Verleger R, Born J: Sleep inspires insight. Nature 2004;427: 352–355.
21 Redline S, Kirchner HL, Quan SR, et al: The effect of age, sex, ethnicity, and sleep-disordered breathing on sleep architecture. Arch Intern Med 2004;164:406–418.
22 Bixler EO, Kales A, Soldatos CR, et al: Prevalence of sleep disorders in the Los Angeles metropolitan area. Am J Psychiatry 1979;236:1257–1262.
23 Borbely AA, Achermann P: Sleep homeostasis and models of sleep regulation. J Biol Rhythms 1999;14:557–568.
24 Lo CC, Amaral LAN, Havlin S, Ivanov PC, Penzel T, Peter JH, Stanley HE: Dynamics of sleep-wake transitions during sleep. Europhys Lett 2002;57:625–631.
25 Lo CC, Chou T, Penzel T, Scammell T, Strecker RE, Stanley HE, Ivanov PC: Common scale-invariant pattern of sleep-wake transitions across species. Proc Natl Acad Sci USA 2004;101:17545–17548.
26 Dijk DJ, Czeisler CA: Contribution of the circadian pacemaker and the sleep homeostat to sleep propensity, sleep structure, electroencephalographic slow waves, and sleep spindle activity in humans. J Neurosci 1995;15: 3526–3538.

T. Penzel
Department of Internal Medicine
Sleep laboratory
Division of Respiratory Disorders
Hospital of Philipps University
Baldingerstrasse 1
DE–35033 Marburg (Germany)
Tel. +49 6421 2866435
Fax +49 6421 2865450
E-Mail penzel@med.uni-marburg.de

Randerath WJ, Sanner BM, Somers VK (eds): Sleep Apnea.
Prog Respir Res. Basel, Karger, 2006, vol 35, pp 21–28

Physiology of Breathing during Sleep

Thorsten Schäfer

Department of Physiology, Ruhr University Bochum, Bochum, Germany

Abstract

Sleep-related breathing disorders are closely linked to the features of the physiology and pathophysiology of respiratory control during sleep. Sleep fosters respiratory instability due to loss of the so-called wakefulness drives, changes in the chemical drives of respiration, mainly CO_2– and hypoxic sensitivity, modifications in the neuronal control of ventilation, and increases of the respiratory arousal thresholds. The modified neuronal respiratory drive during sleep also affects the upper airway dilator muscles with respect to tonic and phasic activity. In combination with anatomical dispositions, this may lead to upper airway obstruction during sleep. Transient hyperpnea suppresses dilator muscle activity more than phrenic nerve activity, leading to a mismatch in timing during inspiration. Repeated hypoxia accounts for fatigue of the upper airway muscles which then tend to collapse more easily.

Breathing Rhythm

Breathing is maintained by rhythmically active neurons in the brainstem which are interconnected in a neuronal network and innervate the respiratory muscles. Furthermore, this rhythm can be recorded from lots of other functional systems, the cardiovascular, the upper and lower airway muscles, the somatomotoric and the autonomic nervous system. On the other hand, many exogenous and endogenous conditions can influence the breathing rhythm, leading to a complete interruption of breathing, called apnea, to partial inhibition, (bradypnea, hypopnea, hypoventilation, rapid shallow breathing) or increased breathing movements (sighs, hyperpnea, hyperventilation).

Microelectrode recordings in animals have been used to identify different types of neurons within the brainstem which are only active during precisely defined phases of the respiratory rhythm. Different types of inspiratory neurons fire during onset, the course and the end of inspiration, some are phase-spanning from inspiration to expiration, and other neurons are active during the expiratory phase [1]. The inspiratory neurons are located within a bilateral column of cells next to the nucleus ambiguous, the so-called ventral respiratory group, and more rostrally next to the solitary tract forming the dorsal respiratory group. Some other inspiratory cells have been found in the spinal cord at the levels of C1 and C2. Expiratory cells are located at the level of the pons and the caudal brainstem. Thus, respiratory-related cells form a widespread network with reciprocal inhibition, located within the pons and brainstem, rather than an explicit 'breathing center'. This network generates the breathing rhythm by timing the on- and off-switch of inspiration and expiration, but also generates a highly specific dynamic pattern of incremental and decremental neuronal output to the various respiratory muscles. During inspiration, for e.g. phrenic nerve activity is increased in a ramp-like manner to overcome the increasing elastic forces at higher lung volumes (fig. 1).

The respiratory neurons in the brain stem can hardly be identified morphologically as they resemble the other neurons within the reticular formation.

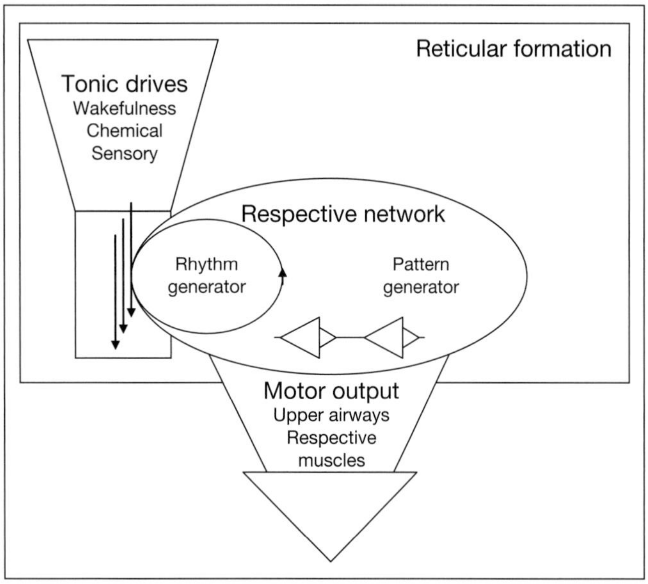

Fig. 1. The central control system of breathing. Illustration of the respiratory control system located in various sites of the brainstem. Respiratory-related cells form a network which generates the rhythm of inspiration and expiration and a complex dynamic pattern of motor output to the airways, respiratory muscles and other systems. The activity of this network depends upon the tonic drive of the surrounding reticular formation, which is influenced by chemical (hypoxia, hypercapnia) and sensory afferents, as well as wakefulness drives from higher cortical areas.

The phasic activity of the respiratory network is dependent upon a tonic drive arising from the surrounding reticular formation. Suppression of this tonic drive leads to inhibition of respiratory activity, which results in a decreased respiratory rate and/or decreased tidal volume. The tonic reticular drive is influenced by all kinds of sensory inputs, including specific chemical information on O_2 and CO_2 partial pressures and the pH in the arterial blood and the brain extracellular fluid. In addition, brain activity including motor tasks leads to increased reticular activity and thus drives to the respiratory network.

Sleep leads to a modification of the activity of the reticular formation. Consequently, the breathing rhythm is influenced by sleep in a characteristic manner which differs between light and deep NREM sleep and REM sleep.

Breathing Rhythm during NREM Sleep

Compared to quiet wakefulness the frequency and amplitude of breathing are slightly lower during light and deep NREM sleep. In a study in 18 young healthy adults [Szczyrba and Schäfer, unpubl.] breathing frequency fell from 17 to $16\,min^{-1}$ and $15.5\,min^{-1}$. At the same time, tidal volume decreased by 10–15% from 560 to 490 and 480 ml, respectively. Thus, ventilation decreased by approximately 12% from wakefulness to light sleep and by 16% from wakefulness to deep NREM sleep. Energy expenditure, however, decreased by only 4% to light sleep and 8% to deep NREM sleep. Consequently, the CO_2 partial pressure rose from 38.9 to 41.6 and 43.0 mm Hg, respectively. The variability of the inspiratory time, expiratory time, respiratory rate, and tidal volume decreases significantly from quiet wakefulness to light and deep NREM sleep.

These sleep-related changes are the results of a decreased tonic drive of the respiratory network and an increased upper airway resistance. Quantitative analysis of neuron activity during sleep shows that neurons with a greater proportion of tonic activity are predominantly affected by sleep. Experimental excitation of silenced cells using excitatory neurotransmitters re-establishes the phasic respiratory activity [2], which indicates that a 'subthreshold' rhythm still persists. On the other hand, neurons, which are more strongly related to the respiratory rhythm, do not show greater changes in their activity during NREM sleep compared to wakefulness. Thus, NREM sleep decreases tonic input to the respiratory network, which silences cells with stronger non-respiratory inputs. There are other state-related changes in telencephalic and mesencephalic respiratory neuronal activity, but the functional significance is not known.

Several tonic excitatory inputs to the respiratory neuronal network besides the reticular formation have been identified: (1) the behavioral control on the respiratory system including both involuntary activation by sneezing and coughing and voluntary activation as during vocalization, breath holding and hyperpnea, the activity of which is strongly reduced during sleep; (2) serotonergic and norepinephrine-containing excitatory brainstem nuclei, which are most active during wakefulness, less in NREM sleep and almost absent during REM sleep; (3) orexin-containing hypothalamic neurons, targeting wakefulness-related nuclei. They are candidates for the cellular representation of the so-called wakefulness drive of ventilation [3].

Recently, several genes were identified which cause variation in daytime and nighttime respiratory rates [4]. The heritability was found to be moderate during the daytime, but to sharply increase during sleep, which suggests that respiratory rate is under more genetic control during sleep than during wakefulness, when many behavioral and environmental influences affect the control system of breathing. This genetic influence may be due to sleep-related impact on candidate genes coding for the adenosine receptor and serotonin receptor subtypes which are involved in the control of breathing.

Breathing Rhythm during REM Sleep

In REM sleep, breathing becomes more irregular, the mean frequency of breathing slightly increases, whereas tidal volume decreases. In summary, minute ventilation is reduced. Metabolic rate increases in REM sleep, which coincides with a large increase in cerebral perfusion. During phasic events in REM sleep tidal volume is significantly reduced. This leads to short periods of rapid shallow breathing positively related to the occurrence of rapid eye movements [5]. The mean arterial CO_2 partial pressures, however, are lower in REM sleep than during NREM sleep. Already, the initial description of REM sleep noted the changes in the breathing rhythm. The excitatory drives arise from central efferents, which influence inspiratory as well as expiratory cells. These excitations persist even after removal of mechanical feedback, e.g. from airways or stretch receptors, which means that they originate from endogenous sources. Early studies support the idea that the variability of breathing during REM sleep may be related to dream content, others have argued that the irregularity during REM sleep is a side effect of neuronal REM sleep processes. Nevertheless, these two ideas are not mutually exclusive.

Another characteristic of REM sleep is the markedly reduced muscle tone. This is also true for the intercostal and accessory respiratory muscles, but not for the diaphragm. This leads to a strong impairment of breathing movements in patients with ineffective diaphragmatic breathing, who depend upon the effectiveness of the other respiratory muscles. Neurophysiologic experiments led to the identification of a discrete area in the dorsomedial pontine tegmentum containing cholinergic neurons that are activated during REM sleep. Injection of acetylcholine agonists at the vicinity of these cells trigger REM-like muscle atonia.

Pathophysiology of Breathing Rhythmicity during Sleep

There is a sleep-related physiologic reduction in tidal volume and minute ventilation during NREM sleep caused by the loss of tonic activation of the respiratory network and by increased airway resistance. During REM sleep endogenous mechanisms lead to phasic inhibitions of tidal volume, the muscle atonia also involves upper airways, intercostal and accessory respiratory muscles. In healthy subjects these sleep-related changes are adequately compensated. Blood gases remain within normal limits. In patients with a handicapped respiratory system, e.g. in neurologic or neuro-muscular disease or in obstructive lung disease, compensatory efforts are less or not effective. This results in an impaired gas exchange and often in disordered sleep.

Control of Ventilation

The majority of sleep-related breathing disorders are related either to physiological changes of the control system of ventilation during sleep or to pathophysiological conditions arising from these special features. There are several feedback loops in the control system of ventilation which include mechanical information from the lungs and the airways as well as chemical information from peripheral chemoreceptors and central chemosensitivity. In addition, there are interactions between the neuronal respiratory network and mechanical, chemical or 'unspecific' afferents, which may cause instability of breathing during sleep. These instabilities most likely occur during sleep onset or during the transition from one sleep state to another [6].

Neuronal Mechanisms

Within the respiratory control system there are mechanisms which may lead to increased instability during sleep. One of these is the feature of short-term potentiation of respiratory neurons [7]. During wakefulness, transient excitation of respiratory neurons leads to a prolonged afterdischarge of these neurons. After a short augmentation, tidal volumes gradually decrease to pre-stimulus values rather than being reduced to zero, i.e. cessation of breathing. During sleep, however, this afterdischarge is reduced. Brief augmentations of tidal volume may lead to apneas not prevented by short-term potentiation of respiratory neurons. A second mechanism is an obvious hysteresis in the control of inspiratory onset. Especially during sleep there is a higher threshold to re-establish the respiratory rhythm than to stop it [8]. This control system inertia facilitates the occurrence of apneas during sleep. Third, the lung inflation reflex is activated during sleep by increasing tidal volumes above 1–1.5 liters. This may cause inhibition of inspiration after sighs [9]. Short periods of hyperpnea, e.g. due to phasic activations during REM sleep, can lower the CO_2 partial pressure below the apnea threshold [10]. This leads to a loss of the strong CO_2-dependent respiratory drive during normoxia. Sleep unmasks this highly sensitive hypocapnia-induced apnea threshold and apnea is initiated if the arterial PCO_2 slightly falls below eupnoeic values [11]. During wakefulness the wakefulness drives can prevent apneas under these conditions. During sleep, however, single or periodic apneas may occur.

Chemical Control of Breathing

Hypercapnia, hypoxia and metabolic acidosis are potent respiratory stimuli. Their impact on ventilation, however, differs between states of wakefulness and sleep.

Hypoxia stimulates breathing via peripheral chemoreceptors located in the carotid and – with a threshold at much lower PO_2 values – in the aortic bodies. They sense arterial oxygen concentration and send afferent impulses in a nonlinear fashion to the dorsal medulla oblongata via the glossopharyngeal nerve. The threshold of this feedback loop, however, is low. Only when the PaO_2 falls below 60 mm Hg ventilation increases. Further drop of the PaO_2 below 30–40 mm Hg leads to central nervous depression which also inhibits the respiratory network and leads to suppression of breathing. The carotid bodies are responsible for the majority of the hypoxic afferences to the respiratory network and supply 40–15% of total drive to ventilation at rest [12]. Denervation causes an acute fall in minute ventilation with an increase in $PaCO_2$ by 5–10 mm Hg. After accommodation, normocapnia is re-established, but the hypoxic ventilatory response remains attenuated.

Peripheral chemoreceptors also sense the $PaCO_2$ and arterial pH and elicit a brisk increase in ventilation when the $PaCO_2$ rises or the pH drops. These changes, however, tend to adapt after minutes to hours. After experimental denervation of the carotid bodies a strong CO_2- and pH-dependent respiratory drive persists, which comes from central chemosensitive areas. At first, areas on the ventral medullary surface were identified as the site of respiratory chemosensitivity. Small changes in the PCO_2 and/or pH of the extracellular fluid cause marked changes in ventilation, mainly by changing tidal volume. Experimental elimination of these areas by various methods led to a loss of central CO_2 sensitivity of respiration during anesthesia and different states of sleep and wakefulness [13]. Besides these chemosensitive areas other widespread sites of CO_2 chemosensitivity have been found, which in part may function only during certain states of sleep and wakefulness [14, 15]. The connection with the respiratory network and the sleep-related changes in excitability to CO_2 at physiological levels, however, remain to be determined for most putative chemosensor sites.

In general, chemical control of ventilation is blunted during sleep compared to wakefulness. Nevertheless, the feedback loops involving chemical information are still functioning and appear to prevent major changes in blood gases during sleep, either by driving respiration or by evoking arousal responses, which may lead to changes in sleep states. In children suffering from congenital central hypoventilation syndrome (CCHS) the consequences of CO_2 insensitivity can be observed: during wakefulness spontaneous ventilation is maintained, the variability of the arterial CO_2 partial pressure is increased. There are periods of hyperventilation followed by hypoventilation. The CCHS patients exhibit deficient hypercapnic and hypoxic ventilatory responses and chronic respiratory insufficiency in the absence of lung, cardiac, or neuromuscular disease, and fail to show breathlessness to hypercapnia, some arouse from sleep to high CO_2. Functional magnetic resonance imaging (fMRI) in CCHS and healthy control subjects was used to determine brain areas controlling different aspects of breathing [16]. The fMRI response deficits revealed neural processes for the hypercapnic ventilatory and arousal response that included disruption of the connection of cerebellar deep nuclei to rostral motor control sites; posterior thalamic, midbrain and dorsal pontine areas, which are involved in arousal; failure to recruit limbic sites to sense discomfort of hypercapnic breathlessness; and failure of limbic and cerebellar sites to regulate autonomic outflow. These data illustrate that there are complex systems beyond the primary chemical chemosensor sites that are involved in an appropriate response to hypercapnia and hypoxia [17].

With sleep onset, there is a dramatic decrease in ventilation in CCHS patients, sometimes with central apneas, and the $PaCO_2$ increases to values above 60–80 mm Hg during NREM stage 4. During REM sleep, the endogenous drive of respiration may lead to an improvement of ventilation [18]. These observations again support the idea of different modes of the ventilatory control system during NREM vs. REM sleep.

Hypoxic and hypercapnic ventilatory drives can be assessed by hypoxic and CO_2 response tests, which have been performed during wakefulness and during sleep.

Hypoxic and Hypercapnic Ventilatory Responses

There are two principles to test ventilatory responses to changes of oxygen and carbon dioxide partial pressures: In the steady state method, experimental changes of inspired air are in a stepwise manner. First, baseline values are recorded. Then, the fraction of inspired O_2 or CO_2 is slightly changed. It takes about 7–20 min until there is a new steady state. These stepwise changes are repeated several times. The advantage of this method is the more physiological range of blood gas changes. On the other hand, waiting for the new steady states takes up much time. The other method is the rebreathing technique. The hypercapnic ventilatory response (according to Read) starts with breathing from a bag which contains 7% CO_2 in O_2. This leads to a rapid increase of the $PaCO_2$ above mean venous PCO_2 at rest. By rebreathing from the bag, the PCO_2 progressively increases to 60–70 mm Hg within 3–5 min. This shortness of time is a major advantage of the rebreathing method, the blood gas changes, however, are far beyond the physiological range.

Hypoxic Ventilatory Response during Sleep

In general, the hypoxic ventilatory response drops during sleep, reaching the lowest level during REM sleep in both men and women [19]. Men, however, have a much stronger hypoxic drive during wakefulness, which is significantly reduced during NREM sleep and further during REM sleep. In contrast, there is no difference of the hypoxic drive in women between wakefulness and NREM sleep. The underlying mechanisms, whether central or peripheral, are still unclear.

The hypoxic response in neonates shows that there are different strategies to get away from hypoxic threat: Newborns pursue a conservative approach by lowering metabolism and reducing ventilation. A similar strategy can be found in the diving reflex, which results in apnea, bradycardia, vasoconstriction, and an increase in catecholamine release. These actions are likely to conserve oxygen for the brain and the heart and to lengthen the tolerance towards hypoxia [20]. Alternatively, there is the struggle for more oxygen by increasing the ventilatory response to hypoxia, the cardiac output and the oxygen concentration, trying to optimize the use of limited oxygen resources in adult humans. Third, hypoxic arousal may help to escape from the dangerous situation by waking up. The hypoxic arousal threshold varies considerably between sleep states and between men and women. It appears to be at lower oxygen saturation levels during REM sleep compared to NREM sleep.

Hypercapnic Ventilatory Response during Sleep

The hypercapnic ventilatory response (HCVR) in adult humans varies markedly during sleep. Rebreathing tests during well-defined, EEG-documented sleep states showed that the HCVR was significantly reduced in all stages of sleep compared with wakefulness, falling to less than 50% during NREM sleep and less than 30% during REM sleep [21] (fig. 2c). Furthermore, there is a circadian rhythm of the HCVR, measured in awake subjects, with an amplitude of 30% of the mean HCVR with lowest slopes of the response curve in the early morning hours [22, 23]. Continuously repeated CO_2 challenges by moderate increases of the inspired CO_2 fraction to 2.5 and 4.0% for 7 min each throughout the whole night revealed a marked variation of slopes and apnea points of the HCVRs with respect to tidal volume and ventilation, but not of the frequency of breathing [24] (fig. 2a, b). The mean of the lowest slopes in 10 subjects was 0.31 ± 0.13 liters/min/mm Hg, the mean of the highest slopes 1.45 ± 0.35 liters/ min/mm Hg per night. Lowest slopes occurred in the early morning hours between 3 and 6:30 a.m. There was a reduced tidal volume response during REM sleep, which was not completely offset by the increased frequency response. This may be one of the reasons for the lower overall HCVR during REM sleep. Despite the large scatter of the slopes of the HCVR, baseline ventilation and resting PCO_2 remained constant due to offsetting shifts of the apnea points. The slopes of the HCVR during REM sleep were significantly lower than during wakefulness or NREM sleep [21, 25], but, at the same time, the CO_2 response curves were shifted to the left. Therefore, it can be concluded that the chemical control of breathing is maintained during sleep, but that there are periods during which ventilation varies independently of the chemical drives, due to endogenous features of REM sleep, loss of the 'wakefulness drives' and other factors.

Studies in obstructive sleep apnea (OSA) patients indicate that chemoreflex control of breathing may vary over night due to the repetitive episodes of hypoxia, hypercapnia and arousal. In contrast to non-OSA, patients with apnea-hypopnea indices (AHI) greater than 30 showed a significant over night increase in chemoreflex sensitivities by approximately 30%, which tends to further destabilize breathing during sleep [26].

With respect to the pathophysiological relevance, the variation in the HCVR as measured by end-tidal or arterial PCO_2 and ventilation could be a 'peripheral' phenomenon, because the PCO_2 at the sensor sites in the central chemosensitive areas is the main stimulus, which is dependent upon local blood flow. There are considerable sleep-related changes in brain blood flow, which may explain variations in 'peripheral' CO_2 sensitivity. The increase in brain blood flow during REM sleep could explain the blunted HCVR in this sleep

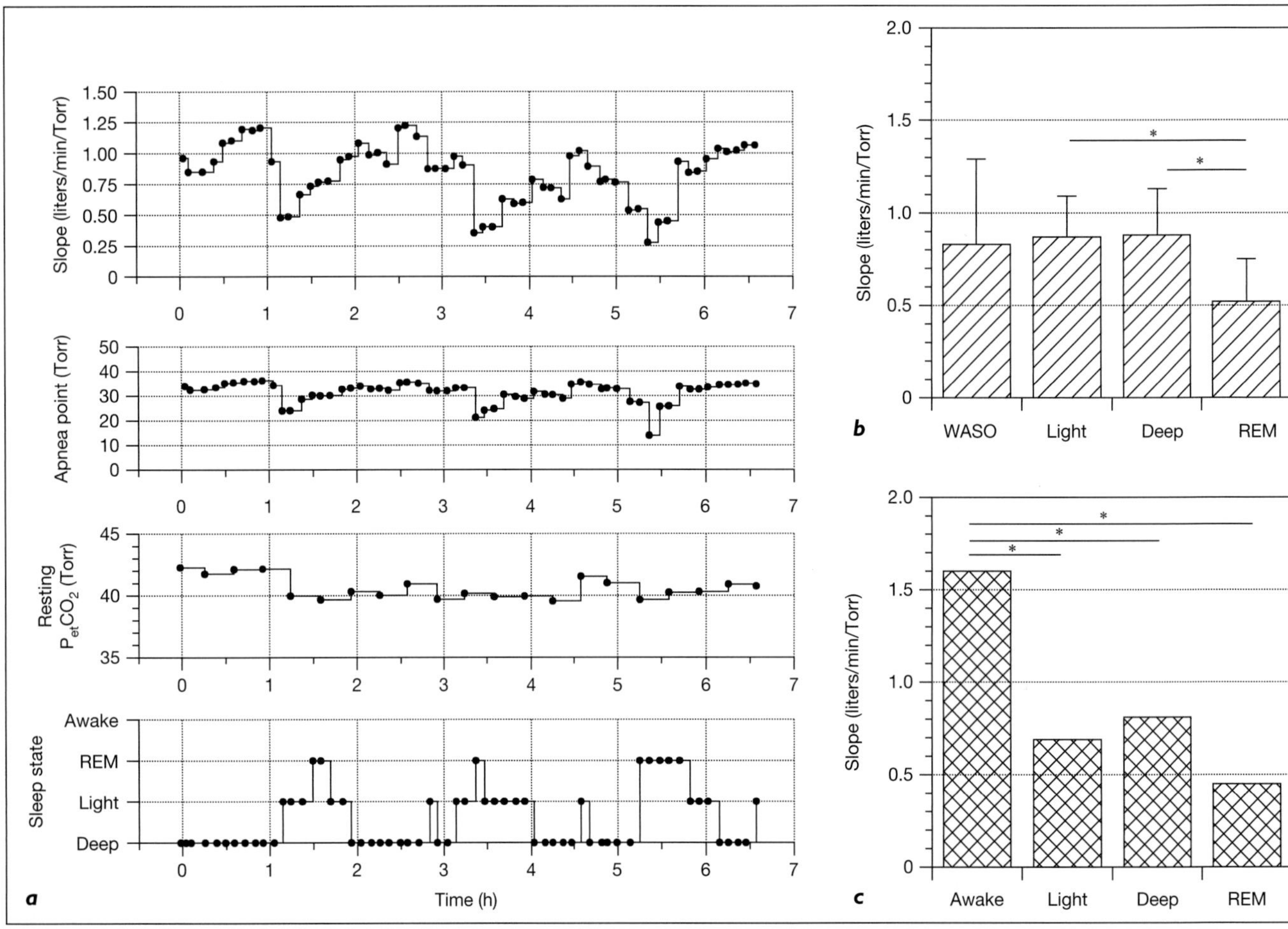

Fig. 2. Hypercapnic ventilatory responses during wakefulness and sleep. ***a*** Variability of the hypercapnic ventilatory response (HCVR) during the night in a healthy male subject determined by 60 stepwise changes of the inspiratory CO_2 fraction. Decreases in the slope of the HCVR coincide with REM sleep. Note that apnea points shift to the left during REM sleep. Therefore, ventilation does not decrease at normocapnic conditions despite the flattening of the CO_2 response curve. ***b*** Summary of the sleep state-related slopes of 10 subjects. The HCVR was significantly lower during REM sleep than during light and deep sleep [25]. WASO means 'wakefulness after sleep onset', with slopes not different from light and deep sleep. ***c*** In contrast, slopes during wakefulness before sleep onset are steeper, as shown by Douglas et al. [21].

state. Experiments in waking and sleeping goats showed that there was a strong relationship between mean venous PCO_2 drawn from the jugular vein, and the phrenic EMG, independent from sleep states [27].

Upper Airway Muscles

In order to maintain airway caliber there is a tonic and phasic activation of upper airway muscles, including the genioglossus and the sternohyoid muscles. There is an increase in upper airway muscle tone during inspiration, followed by a decrease during expiration. This activation is sensitive to CO_2: hypercapnia increases the phasic activation of airway muscles. During sleep, however, this response to CO_2 appears to be blunted [28]. Furthermore, the CO_2-dependent drive to the respiratory muscles, including the diaphragm and the intercostals, is much higher than to the airway muscles. Under certain circumstances this fact may foster the occurrence of mixed and obstructive apneas, especially following short periods of hyperventilation, when the PCO_2 falls below the apnea threshold. Rising PCO_2 levels will at first reactivate phrenic activity, and later, at higher levels of PCO_2, airway muscles will be recruited. Recently, low concentrations of CO_2 added to conventional continuous positive airway pressure

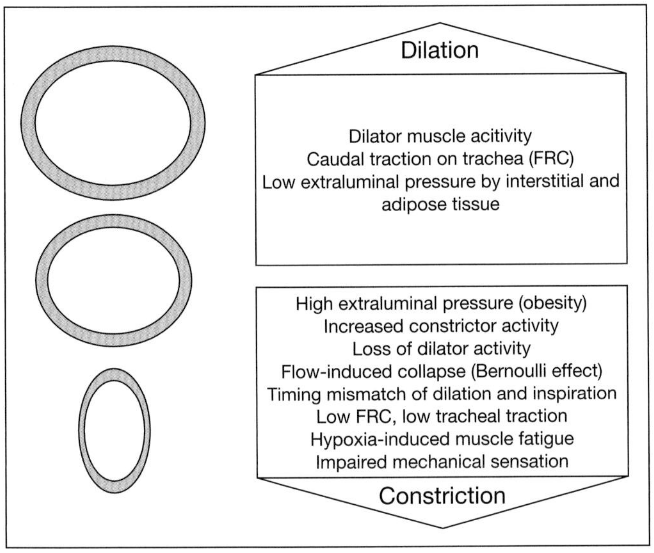

Fig. 3. Factors influencing upper airway patency.

(CPAP) therapy have been shown to improve treatment of mixed and central sleep apneas in patients with poorly controlled mixed sleep-disordered breathing despite CPAP therapy [29].

In addition, upper airway muscle activity is also dependent on other factors (fig. 3), such as distortions of the upper airways, the pattern of inspiratory flow, the air temperature, and the functional residual capacity. The neuromechanical activation of the upper airways appears to be dependent upon sensory afferents to the central nervous system. Studies in patients with obstructive sleep apnea showed that they had a blunted vibration sensation and a diminished two-point discrimination in the upper airways [30].

The tonic activation of upper airway muscles appears to be more or less independent of the control of ventilation and more related to the general muscle tone. There is a sleep-related decrease in tonic activity in the tensor veli palatini, which correlates with the increase in upper airway resistance [31]. Similar decreases in tonic activity were found in the genioglossus, the geniohyoid and the posterior cricoarytenoid. A large increase in total airway resistance during NREM sleep has been shown [32], whereas the elastic properties of the lung are not altered.

During wakefulness, upper airway resistance was similar between the oral and nasal breathing routes. However, during sleep in a supine position, upper airway resistance was much higher while breathing orally than nasally [33].

In animal experiments, intermittent hypoxia, a frequent condition in patients with obstructive sleep apnea, triggers muscle fiber composition changes in the geniohyoid muscle toward the fast-twitch types, which may account for the fatigue of the upper airway muscles [34]. These changes could already be observed after 10 h of exposure. There is increasing evidence that episodic hypoxia, the consequence of periodic airway collapse, is responsible for the maintenance and progression of obstructive sleep apneas through impairment of the neural control of upper airway patency by altering upper airway muscle contractile function. This vicious cycle seems to perpetuate the condition of periodic airway obstruction and recurrent hypoxia [35].

References

1 Richter DW: Neural regulation of respiration: rhythmogenesis and afferent control; in Greger R, Windhorst U (eds): Comprehensive Human Physiology. Berlin, 1996, vol 2, pp 2079–2095.
2 Foutz AS, Boudinot E, Morin-Surun MP, Champagnat J, Gonsalves SF, Denavit-Saubié M: Excitability of 'silent' respiratory neurons during sleep-waking states: an iontophoretic study in undrugged chronic cats. Brain Res 1987;404:10–20.
3 Peyron C, Tighe DK, van den Pol AN, de Lecea L, Heller HC, Sutcliffe JG, Kilduff TS: Neurons containing hypocretin (orexin) project to multiple neuronal systems. J Neurosci 1998;18:9996–10015.
4 de Geus EJ, Posthuma D, Kupper N, van den BM, Willemsen G, Beem AL, Slagboom PE, Boomsma DI: A whole-genome scan for 24-hour respiration rate: a major locus at 10q26 influences respiration during sleep. Am J Hum Genet 2005;76:100–111.
5 Schäfer T, Schläfke ME: Respiratory changes associated with rapid eye movements in normo- and hypercapnia during sleep. J Appl Physiol 1998;85:2213–2219.
6 Dempsey JA, Smith CA, Harms CA, Chow CM, Saupe KW: Sleep-induced breathing instability: state of the art review. Sleep 1996; 19:236–247.
7 Badr MS, Skatrud JB, Dempsey JA: Determinants of poststimulus potentiation in humans during NREM sleep. J Appl Physiol 1992;73:1958–1971.
8 Leevers AM, Simon PM, Xi L, Dempsey JA: Apnoea following normocapnic mechanical ventilation in awake mammals: a demonstration of control system inertia. J Physiol 1993;472:749–768.
9 Iber C, Simon P, Skatrud JB, Mahowald MW, Dempsey JA, Reicks M, McArthur C: The Breuer-Hering reflex in humans: effects of pulmonary denervation and hypocapnia. Am J Respir Crit Care Med 1995;152:217–224.
10 Skatrud JB, Dempsey JA: Interaction of sleep state and chemical stimuli in sustaining rhythmic ventilation. J Appl Physiol 1983;55: 813–822.
11 Dempsey JA, Smith CA, Przybylowski T, Chenuel B, Xie A, Nakayama H, Skatrud JB: The ventilatory responsiveness to CO(2) below eupnoea as a determinant of ventilatory stability in sleep. J Physiol 2004; 560:1–11.
12 Pan LG, Forster HV, Martino P, Strecker PJ, Beales J, Serra A, Lowry TF, Forster MM, Forster AL: Important role of carotid afferents in control of breathing. J Appl Physiol 1998;85: 1299–1306.
13 Schläfke ME: Central chemosensitivity: a respiratory drive. Rev Physiol Biochem Pharmacol 1981;90:172–244.
14 Nattie E: Multiple sites for central chemoreception: their roles in response sensitivity and in sleep and wakefulness. Respir Physiol 2000;122:223–235.

15 Krimsky WR, Leiter JC: Physiology of breathing and respiratory control during sleep. Semin Respir Crit Care Med 2005;26:5–12.
16 Harper RM, Macey PM, Woo MA, Macey KE, Keens TG, Gozal D, Alger JR: Hypercapnic exposure in congenital central hypoventilation syndrome reveals CNS respiratory control mechanisms. J Neurophysiol 2005;93:1647–1658.
17 Macey PM, Woo MA, Macey KE, Keens TG, Saeed MM, Alger JR, Harper RM: Hypoxia reveals posterior thalamic, cerebellar, midbrain, and limbic deficits in congenital central hypoventilation syndrome. J Appl Physiol 2005;98:958–969.
18 Schläfke ME, Schäfer C, Schäfer T: Das Undine-Syndrom als kongenitales zentrales Hypoventilationssyndrom (CCHS). Somnologie 1999;3:128–133.
19 Douglas NJ, White DP, Weil JV, Pickett CK, Martin RJ, Hudgel DW, Zwillich CW: Hypoxic ventilatory response decreases during sleep in normal men. Am Rev Respir Dis 1982;125:286–289.
20 Foster GE, Sheel AW: The human diving response, its function, and its control. Scand J Med Sci Sports 2005;15:3–12.
21 Douglas NJ, White DP, Weil JV, Pickett CK, Zwillich CW: Hypercapnic ventilatory response in sleeping adults. Am Rev Respir Dis 1982;126:758–762.
22 Raschke F, Möller KH: Untersuchungen zur Tagesrhythmik der Chemosensitivität und deren Beitrag zu nächtlichen Atmungsregulationsstörungen. Pneumologie 1989;43:568–571.
23 Spengler CM, Czeisler CA, Shea SA: An endogenous circadian rhythm of respiratory control in humans. J Physiol Lond 2000;526: 683–694.
24 Schäfer T, Schläfke ME: Variability of CO_2-sensitivity during sleep. Adv Exp Med Biol 2001;499:459–463.
25 Schäfer T: Variability of vigilance and ventilation. Studies on the control of respiration during sleep. Respir Physiol 1998;114:37–48.
26 Mahamed S, Hanly PJ, Gabor J, Beecroft J, Duffin J: Overnight changes of chemoreflex control in obstructive sleep apnoea patients. Respir Physiol Neurobiol 2005;146:279–290.
27 Parisi RA, Edelman NH, Santiago TV: Central respiratory carbon dioxide chemosensitivity does not decrease during sleep. Am Rev Respir Dis 1992;145:832–836.
28 Pillar G, Malhotra A, Fogel RB, Beauregard J, Slamowitz DI, Shea SA, White DP: Upper airway muscle responsiveness to rising PCO(2) during NREM sleep. J Appl Physiol 2000;89: 1275–1282.
29 Thomas RJ, Daly RW, Weiss JW: Low-concentration carbon dioxide is an effective adjunct to positive airway pressure in the treatment of refractory mixed central and obstructive sleep-disordered breathing. Sleep 2005;28: 69–77.
30 Kimoff J, Sforza E, Champagne V, Ofiara L, Gendron D: Upper airway sensation in snoring and obstructive sleep apnea. Am J Respir Crit Care Med 2001;164:250–255.
31 Tangel DJ, Mezzanotte WS, White DP: Influence of sleep on tensor palatini EMG and upper airway resistance in normal men. J Appl Physiol 1991;70:2574–2581.
32 Lopes JM, Tabachnik E, Muller NL, Levison H, Bryan AC: Total airway resistance and respiratory muscle activity during sleep. J Appl Physiol 1983;54:773–777.
33 Fitzpatrick MF, McLean H, Urton AM, Tan A, O'Donnell D, Driver HS: Effect of nasal or oral breathing route on upper airway resistance during sleep. Eur Respir J 2003;22: 827–832.
34 Pae EK, Wu J, Nguyen D, Monti R, Harper RM: Geniohyoid muscle properties and myosin heavy chain composition are altered after short-term intermittent hypoxic exposure. J Appl Physiol 2005;98:889–894.
35 Bradford A, McGuire M, O'Halloran KD: Does episodic hypoxia affect upper airway dilator muscle function? Implications for the pathophysiology of obstructive sleep apnoea. Respir Physiol Neurobiol 2005;147: 223–234.

Thorsten Schäfer, MD, PD
Department of Physiology
Ruhr University Bochum
DE–44780 Bochum (Germany)
Tel. +49 234 32 24889
Fax +49 234 32 14250
E-Mail Thorsten.Schaefer@rub.de

Randerath WJ, Sanner BM, Somers VK (eds): Sleep Apnea.
Prog Respir Res. Basel, Karger, 2006, vol 35, pp 29–36

Physiology of the Cardiovascular, Endocrine and Renal Systems during Sleep

J.G. Peter I. Fietze

Department of Cardiology, Pneumology and Angiology, Center for Sleep Medicine,
Charité – Universitätsmedizin Berlin, Berlin, Germany

Abstract

In humans, the period for optimal mental and physical performance is found during the light period of the day whereas the dark period provides optimal regenerational capacities. A variety of biological parameters follow a circadian rhythm of approximately 24 h according to the earth's rotational period. Other parameters exclusively underlie the ultradian influence of state, i.e. wake state vs. sleep state, or the rhythmic sleep process with cyclically returning stages of NREM 1–4 sleep and REM sleep. Long-term blood pressure and ECG recordings show a circadian pattern of blood pressure and heart rate. At night, blood pressure physiologically decreases by 10–15% which is referred to as dipping. Non-dipping is prognostically adversarial. In addition, the mean heart rate drops at night. Blood pressure and heart rate are modulated according to the sleep stages. At the transition from wake to sleep, blood pressure and heart rate decrease in trend reaching the lowest values during deep sleep. During REM sleep, blood pressure and heart rate exhibit pronounced changes, thereby generating a nightly recurring stress test for the cardiovascular system. Circadian and ultradian rhythms influence endocrine parameters as well as hydromineral balance and renal function. Cortisol secretion exhibits a characteristic circadian rhythm pattern. Adversely, renin secretion for example is strongly related to sleep stage control.

Cardiovascular Function

Introduction

Control of cardiovascular parameters is a vital function during wake and sleep. Maintaining blood pressure within normal limits ensures sufficient oxygen and energy supply as well as transport of metabolic products to the organs. The autonomous nervous system regulates blood pressure via heart rate and total peripheral resistance. Cardiovascular function follows a circadian rhythm which is closely related to the states of sleep and wake. In addition, the role of the sleep stages (NREM 1–4) and REM on cardiovascular function must be emphasized. Whilst in a relaxed wake state circulatory function remains largely constant, in sleep characteristic changes are lawfully present. NREM sleep is characterized by a downregulation of cardiovascular activity whereas REM sleep displays a high variability.

Cardiovascular parameters are closely interrelated by feedback loops which ensure a homeostatic control and adequate response to physiological needs. In this chapter, we introduce basic mechanisms of cardiovascular regulation and relate them to circadian and sleep-dependent changes.

Basic Mechanisms

Blood Pressure

Arterial blood pressure is the key control for the cardiovascular system. It is constantly maintained within a certain range allowing tissues to regulate blood flow according to their metabolic requirements. Arterial blood pressure is adjusted by cardiac output and total peripheral resistance. Furthermore, cardiac output is calculated as the product of stroke volume and heart rate. In the latter lies a neural regulatory moment as heart rate is under control of the autonomic nervous system (ANS). This is of particular interest as autonomic modulation is sleep stage dependent and varies strongly – especially in REM sleep. Stroke volume is modulated by cardiac preload. Total peripheral resistance is determined by arteriole tone which in part underlies local regulatory mechanisms [1]. Additionally, systemic sympathetic activation via adrenalin and local sympathetic nervous control via noradrenalin vasomotor pathways are crucial for the amount of total peripheral resistance.

Heart Rate

Heart rate is a key target of cardiovascular regulation mechanisms and feedback loops. Herein, the final common pathway is the efferent autonomic response to the heart by vagal and sympathetic activity. These mechanisms include: Firstly, respiratory sinus arrhythmia due to central nervous interactions and as a consequence of increased venous return in inspiration. Secondly, this leads to increased cardiac preload with consecutive heart rate increase due to stretch receptors in the right atrium – the Bainbridge reflex [2]. Thirdly, baroreceptors in the aortic arch and carotid sinus respond to blood pressure fluctuations – the baroreflex. Regarding REM sleep, emotional activity is of central interest as it goes hand in hand with dream activity. Thereby, it modulates autonomic outflow and thus heart rate via the limbic system and the insular cortex.

Sympathetic Nerve Activity

A method to experimentally measure sympathetic nerve activity (SNA) is the direct recording of muscle sympathetic nerve activity (MSNA) by microneurography in the perineal nerve of the lower legs. Elevated sympathetic activity is of central interest as it modulates total peripheral resistance and heart rate and correlates well with sleep stages and also with pathological conditions such as obesity, hypertension, heart failure, diabetes and sleep apnea.

Heart Rate Variability

The fluctuations in the interval between normal heartbeats are referred to as heart rate variability. As fluctuations are mediated autonomically, indices of heart rate variability provide insights into autonomic modulation of the heart. For this purpose, parameters of time domain analysis and spectral analysis are employed.

Time domain indices are directly calculated from heart beat intervals. Calculated from 24-hour Holter ECG recordings, they provide information on circadian rhythmicity and the general presence of vagal modulation of the sinuatrial node. Low modulation is referred to as decreased heart rate variability and hints at low vagal modulation. This heart rate rigidity is either due to high sympathetic tone or due to denervation for example in the transplanted heart or in autonomic polyneuropathies. In population studies, decreased heart rate variability has had a predictive value for higher mortality among healthy adults.

Frequency domain analysis is mathematically more complex and provides spectral information on heart rate variability – the so-called spectral power. Spectral cutouts represent different autonomic influences. High frequency (HF) spectral power is mediated parasympathetically to the heart via the vagus nerve. It reflects for instance vagally transmitted respiratory-related changes. Low frequency (LF) spectral power is modulated by sympathetic and to a minor degree parasympathetic influences. The latter can be reduced mathematically. Besides, very low frequency (VLF) and ultra low frequency (ULF) power reflect slower modulations of heart rate such as renin-angiotensin system oscillations and circadian rhythms [3].

LF spectral power has been defined as sympathetic tone. This has been challenged for two reasons:

Firstly, the assumption of a general sympathetic tone has been disproved. Regional differences in sympathetic tone have been demonstrated. The assumption of a general tone does not adequately reflect the function of the autonomic nervous system as it operates in a complex way on different levels. As a consequence, the term cardiac sympathetic tone has been introduced.

Secondly, major limitations of this concept have been brought up by experimental evidence mainly showing that LF power under some circumstances does not represent sympathetic modulation of heart rate but also includes distorting parasympathetic components [4]. Despite the criticism, in most conditions limits can be neglected, so that cardiac sympathetic tone is nicely reflected by LF power spectra during wake and sleep.

Sympathovagal balance, i.e. a ratio of sympathetic and vagal power, is another feature of spectral analysis of heart rate variability. It reflects autonomic changes of cardiac control, e.g. in different sleep stages.

Baroreflex

The baroreflex responds to blood pressure fluctuations in the carotid sinus and the aortic arch where baroreceptors are located. Herein, the baroreflex serves as a blood pressure buffer system. The receptor signal is afferently transmitted to autonomic centers in the medulla oblongata. Vagal efferent fibers increase cardiac vagal tone in response to blood pressure increases. Sympathetic efferent fibers alter cardiac sympathetic tone and total peripheral resistance. The latter is achieved through vasomotor response in splanchnic beds and more importantly through skeletal muscle vasomotor response.

The intensity of baroreflex response is referred to as baroreceptor gain. The means of expressing baroreceptor-mediated changes is baroreceptor sensitivity (BRS). It displays the resulting difference in heart rate per blood pressure change in milliseconds per mm of mercury. BRS is not constant but changes with central and peripheral autonomic modulation. Baroreceptor feedback adapts to new conditions by resetting of blood pressure setpoints, e.g. in hypertension. Baroreceptor function decreases with age as well as in a variety of pathologic conditions such as hypertension, congestive heart failure, postmyocardial infarction, metabolic syndrome, insulin resistance and in sleep apnea. Positive pressure ventilation with a CPAP (continuous positive airway pressure) device in healthy subjects shows an increase in vagal baroreflex modulation but underlying mechanisms are only partially understood [5]. BRS can be assessed directly e.g. through pharmacological manipulation. Another method is spontaneous BRS which utilizes spontaneous fluctuations in the baroreflex feedback loop. It is based on a mathematic approach to calculate BRS from heart rate and blood pressure variability. In this case, blood pressure variability is a means of expressing beat-to-beat changes in blood pressure and requires invasive or noninvasive continuous blood pressure monitoring.

Blood Pressure Variability

Increased blood pressure variability from a 24-hour ambulatory blood pressure monitoring (ABPM) has been linked to organ damage [6]. Due to a lack of data, the relevance of blood pressure variability remains a point of discussion. Evidence hints at a high blood pressure variability as an adverse prognostic marker.

Circadian Control

Circadian variations in cardiovascular parameters are known from large amounts of pooled 24-hour blood pressure monitoring and ECG data. They represent a mixture of real circadian changes and sleep-dependent changes. From a chronobiological point of view, this difference does not account for practical aspects as most people sleep at night and are awake during the day. Regarding 24-hour blood pressure and ECG measurements, this means a quasi circadian pattern that satisfies clinical requirements. Thus, normal values for nocturnal blood pressure could be defined in the absence of sleep monitoring. A dipping of blood pressure of at least 10% of the systolic and 15% of the diastolic mean daily values during the period from 10 p.m. to 7 a.m. is expected to be physiological. Another clinical definition refers to maximal systolic and diastolic blood pressure values for the same nightly time span. A value below 120/70 mmHg is considered normotensive. Autonomic modulation of cardiac control in spectral analysis of heart rate variability and baroreflex function changes according to the circadian rhythm.

Sleep Stage Control

Apart from circadian variations, the different sleep stages provoke profound differences in autonomic cardiac control and cardiovascular function. This is most pronounced comparing NREM with REM sleep.

NREM Sleep

After the transition from quiet wake to sleep, the sleep process progresses from NREM 1 and 2 – light sleep – to NREM 3 and 4 – slow-wave sleep or deep sleep – as described in 'Physiology of Sleep and Dreaming'.

Blood pressure and heart rate drop from stages NREM 1 to NREM 4. This has been shown to correlate with a reduction in SNA [7]. Increased heart rate variability and decreased blood pressure variability in NREM are indicative for cardiac health and autonomic stability.

NREM sleep presents with heightened baroreceptor gain compared to wake. Cardiac autonomic modulation shows decreased sympathetic and increased vagal components. However, vagal components increase only in the first three of five sleep cycles during NREM sleep. This means that NREM sleep in the first half of the night does not equal NREM sleep in the second half, suggesting an additional component of ultradian or circadian control [8].

Due to slow and regular breathing, the stable autonomic state provides a good basis for normal respiratory sinus arrhythmia which is indicative for cardiac health. Nevertheless, in 50% the EEG phenomenon of K complexes – which is a hallmark of light NREM sleep – is accompanied by bursts of muscle SNA. These are accompanied by transient low-scale blood pressure increases [9]. Not all K complexes display the phenomenon and overall sympathetic activity in NREM sleep is reduced and stable in comparison to quiet wakefulness. Still, this shows the active nature of the sleep process even in stages NREM 1 and 2.

REM Sleep

REM sleep periods are initiated at 80- to 110-min intervals at the end of a sleep cycle. The hallmarks of REM sleep are rapid eye movements which further divide REM sleep into phasic episodes with REMs and tonic episodes without REMs. Compared to NREM sleep, REM sleep is accompanied by higher brain activity reflected in elevated cerebral blood flow and brain metabolism. For the cardiovascular system and its regulatory mechanisms this implicates a lower level of central regulation. Linked to fluctuating autonomic activity REM-sleep-related brain activity includes structures of the limbic system. Additionally, central responses to peripheral feedback loop regulatory control are diminished. As a consequence, blood pressure and heart rate display pronounced variability that disrupts cardiorespiratory homeostasis. This 'stress test' for the cardiovascular system has been found to be associated with a high incidence of cardiovascular events during the early hours of the morning when REM sleep density increases.

Blood Pressure and REM Sleep. In REM sleep, mean arterial blood pressure is higher than in deep sleep and averages NREM 2. Strikingly, the blood pressure oscillations are higher than during NREM sleep.

Blood Flow and REM Sleep. Coronary artery blood flow during sleep has been studied in different animal models. Higher sympathetic activity in REM increases the metabolic demand of the myocardium due to increasing heart rate and total peripheral resistance. This results in vasodilation and an increase in coronary blood flow in healthy subjects. In the pathological condition of experimental coronary artery stenosis, coronary blood flow decreases in response to heart rate accelerations during REM sleep probably due to the reduced diastolic perfusion time [10]. This underlines the pathophysiological implications of REM sleep in coronary artery disease.

Heart Rate and REM Sleep. In REM sleep, heart rate fluctuates physiologically, displaying phases of tachycardia and heart rate surges as well as phases of bradycardia even to the point of heart rhythm pauses. Heart rate surges increase the mean arterial blood pressure which in turn downregulates the heart rate via baroreceptor pathways. Surges are abolished by bilateral stellectomy in Baboons, proving a sympathetic causal relation. As a consequence, parasympathetic influence is negligible concerning the origin of the surges.

Sudden decelerations in heart rhythm occur predominantly during tonic REM sleep. They are independent from blood pressure increases and related baroreflex function as well as respiratory interaction. In cats, experimentally conducted beta-blockade did not alter decelerations whereas muscarinic blockade abolished the phenomenon, suggesting vagus nerve dependence. As a different phenomenon, vagally mediated short-term heart rhythm pauses occur responding to blood pressure increases as shown in canines and young adults [11]. These baroreceptor-mediated pauses appear at the transition from slow wave sleep to REM sleep, being more closely related to phasic than tonic REM. Preceding REMs by some seconds, central nervous system activity increases vagal nerve tone which then slows sinus node activity.

Heart Rate Variability and REM Sleep. Compared to NREM sleep, heart rate variability power spectra demonstrate increased sympathetic components and unchanged vagal components. On average, they are similar to those during quiet wakefulness. This shift in autonomic modulation precedes REM onset by several minutes. It thereby parallels similar changes of autonomic peripheral activity that have been shown by peripheral arterial tonometry (PAT). PAT is a technique that measures sympathetic vasomotor control in the fingertip. Total peripheral resistance also increases in REM sleep due to sympathetic activation.

Baroreflex and REM Sleep. Baroreceptor gain in REM sleep is reduced compared to NREM but higher than in wake. Baroreflex seems to alter its buffering capability during sleep with higher capability towards the morning hours, counteracting the increased length of REM periods.

Implications for Epidemiology and Pathophysiology

Autonomic activation associated with REM sleep including surges in sympathetic activity can be seen as a natural 'stress test' for the cardiovascular system occurring night by night. In individuals with coronary atherosclerosis, it predisposes for myocardial ischemia and its consequences. This is supported by epidemiologic data showing nonuniform nighttime distribution of cardiac mortality increasing in the morning hours with high REM density.

Different from cardiac mortality, the peak of total cardiac events was found to be around midnight in another study [12]. Baroreflex function presents with lower gain in the first sleep cycle and increasing gain in the following cycles. This might in part explain the findings of total cardiac events [13, 14].

Respiratory function is closely interconnected with cardiac function, especially heart rate due to increased venous return during inspiration. Thus, in REM sleep diminished breathing control leads to irregular fluctuations and instability in cardiorespiratory feedback loops, predisposing for tachycardic and bradycardic episodes, independent from sympathetic surges. As a consequence, respiratory instability adds on existing deficits of blood pressure control during REM sleep.

Enhanced SNA at REM onset and during REM sleep predisposes for cardiac arrythmias due to profibrillatory catecholaminergic properties. Concerning breathing control, the diaphragm is not inhibited whereas accessory and upper airway muscles reduce activity. Irregular breathing can cause oxygen desaturation, particularly in patients with cardiac or pulmonary disease.

Endocrine Function

Introduction

Endocrine systems and sleep physiology underlie complex, bidirectional interactions. In this chapter, we will focus on the influence of sleep and circadian rhythm on several hormone systems, including hormones of the hypothalamic pituitary axis as well as appetite regulation and carbohydrate metabolism.

In general, sleep and the circadian system modulate endocrine functions following two different patterns. One is the influence of sleep or certain sleep stages on hormone release. This is an ultradian process as the changing frequency is higher than once per 24 h. Another is the influence of the circadian rhythm. Most commonly, a mixture of both types is found with one type predominating.

Most endocrine functions follow a more or less pronounced circadian rhythm. As sleep normally takes place during nighttime, it can be difficult to distinguish influences of sleep from circadian influences. To elucidate underlying mechanisms, experimental settings with nighttime sleep restriction and daytime sleep periods have been introduced. A classical example of a predominantly circadian system is the hypothalamo-pituitary-adrenocortical (HPA) axis which determines cortisol release. A classic example of sleep-triggered hormone release is found in growth hormone.

Hypothalamo-Pituitary-Adrenocortical Axis

The HPA system is an important mediator of the response to psychological and physical load. Activation of this system includes hypothalamic excretion of corticotropin-releasing hormone followed by pituitary adrenocorticotropic hormone (ACTH) release and finally the secretion of cortisol from the adrenals.

Plasma levels of ACTH and cortisol demonstrate an association with the circadian rhythm. Predisposing for sleep initiation and sleep maintenance, a cortisol decrease is found towards the late evening and night hours with a minimum at around 2–3 a.m. called cortisol nadir. A short-term cortisol inhibition is reported to derive from the onset of the sleep period. Towards the morning hours, cortisol levels rise steadily preparing the organism for the wake state with peak levels around awakening. The rise of cortisol levels is linked to the anticipated time of waking as shown by means of plasma ACTH levels in figure 1. The actual waking is followed by an extra pulse of ACTH secretion. In case the anticipated time of waking is preceded by actual waking, the following ACTH pulse is more pronounced as a means of compensation [15].

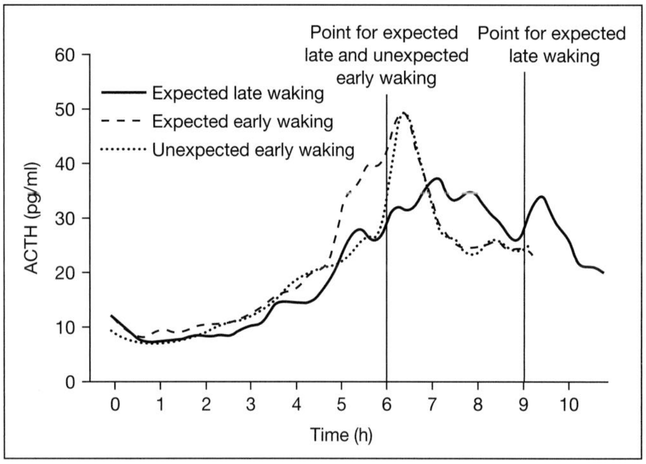

Fig. 1. Morning ACTH plasma levels dependent on anticipated time of waking. Modified with permission from Born et al. [15].

HPA feedback inhibition is attenuated in the sleep state but becomes sensitive again in light sleep and wake state. Cortisol pulses occur as an unspecific reaction to arousal stimuli during sleep. However, total cortisol release is not reported to differ between sleep deprivation, fragmented and undisturbed sleep [16].

Growth Hormone

Growth hormone (GH) is released by the anterior pituitary in a pulsatile fashion and has major anabolic properties. In children, growth hormone deficiency causes growth deficiency. It has direct effects on body cells but mostly exerts its anabolic function by stimulating insulin-like growth factor-1 (ILGF-1) production in the liver and other organs.

Being anabolic, GH is secreted with a slightly elevated baseline during a phase when behavioral rest usually occurs.

This is the dark phase of the day. Additionally, and even more strongly, it is linked to the state when behavioral rest usually occurs, which is sleep. It demonstrates associations with the circadian rhythm as well as the ultradian sleep process showing a marked increase in the first half of the night. They can be explained by the stimulating mechanisms which foster GH secretion. On the one hand, there are two stimulating factors: growth hormone-releasing hormone (GHRH) and ghrelin. On the other hand, somatostatin inhibits GH secretion and GH itself is part of a negative feedback loop to stop its secretion. The minor circadian influences on GH secretion are due to lower inhibitory somatostatin tone and higher stimulating ghrelin tone at nighttime which both occur independent of the actual presence of sleep. However, the major determinant of GH secretion is the actual state of sleep – especially slow wave sleep (SWS) – regardless of whether it occurs during nighttime or daytime. Sleep onset reliably produces a GH pulse. Interestingly, both the onset of SWS and the peak of GH levels are initiated by activity of the same GHRH neuron populations in the hypothalamus displaying a direct neurostructural link between SWS and GH secretion. The sleep GH coupling is still true for shift workers who lack their nocturnal sleep episode and recover during daytime sleep. In contrast, an overall sleep deprivation decreases GH secretion. Thus, in children chronic sleep disturbances and sleep-related syndromes like obstructive sleep apnea (OSA) can cause diminished growth.

Gonadal Hormones

Gonadotropin hormones, i.e. luteinizing hormone (LH) and follicle-stimulating hormone (FSH), control the production of gonadal steroid levels. In women, the menstrual cycle is gated by an infradian monthly rhythm of both gonadotropin hormones, whereas in men LH is the key player in the production of testosterone which is pivotal for erectile function and libido.

Prior to puberty, gonadotropins are secreted in a pulsatile fashion displaying acceleration in pulse frequency with the onset of sleep. As one of the main characteristics of puberty, the amplitude of gonadotropin release increases during sleep. Thus, sleep disorders in children can delay puberty. In early adulthood, daytime pulse amplitude increases as well, diminishing the sleep-wake-dependent rhythm. Despite this, testosterone levels in healthy sleeping adult men exhibit a robust diurnal rhythm, requiring control mechanisms other than LH. In adult women gonadotropin circadian activity depends on the menstrual cycle [17].

Appetite Regulation and Glucose Metabolism

Both the appetite-diminishing hormone leptin and appetite-enhancing hormone ghrelin are elevated in normal sleep. So the balance of both hormones is responsible for a good sleep not disrupted by appetite attacks. Attention has been drawn to the fact that recurrent partial sleep restriction in young healthy adults decreases the plasma levels of leptin and increases ghrelin levels [18]. Additionally, decreased glucose tolerance and insulin sensitivity have been demonstrated. Thus, chronic sleep loss may represent a risk factor for weight gain, insulin resistance and type 2 diabetes.

Conclusion

Sleep has a stabilizing effect on a variety of endocrine functions. Chronic sleep loss – both behavioral and sleep disorders related – impairs functioning in several organ systems and predisposes for the development of pathological conditions such as obesity, diabetes and in children retarded growth.

Renal Function

Introduction

Renal function includes water and electrolyte balance, excretion of metabolites, acid-base balance, blood pressure control and haematopoiesis.

Renal function, especially hydromineral balance during wake and sleep is under the control of the central nervous system, of sympathetic outflow and of endocrine mechanisms such as the renin-angiotensin-aldosterone system (RAAS), the natriuretic peptides and arginine vasopressin (AVP) and other hormones. Within normal blood pressure limits, the kidneys autoregulate their own blood flow.

In a normal sleep-wake cycle, urine flow and electrolyte excretion are higher during the day than during the night. Herein, the state – i.e. sleep or wake – plays the decisive role whereas circadian rhythm influences are of minor importance. This follows the need for undisturbed sleep without awakening for nycturia. Thus, overnight urine excretion during sleep is physiologically limited by bladder volume. Diminished urine output is achieved by increased activity of the RAAS and changes in autonomic activity during sleep, especially a decreased sympathetic tone [19].

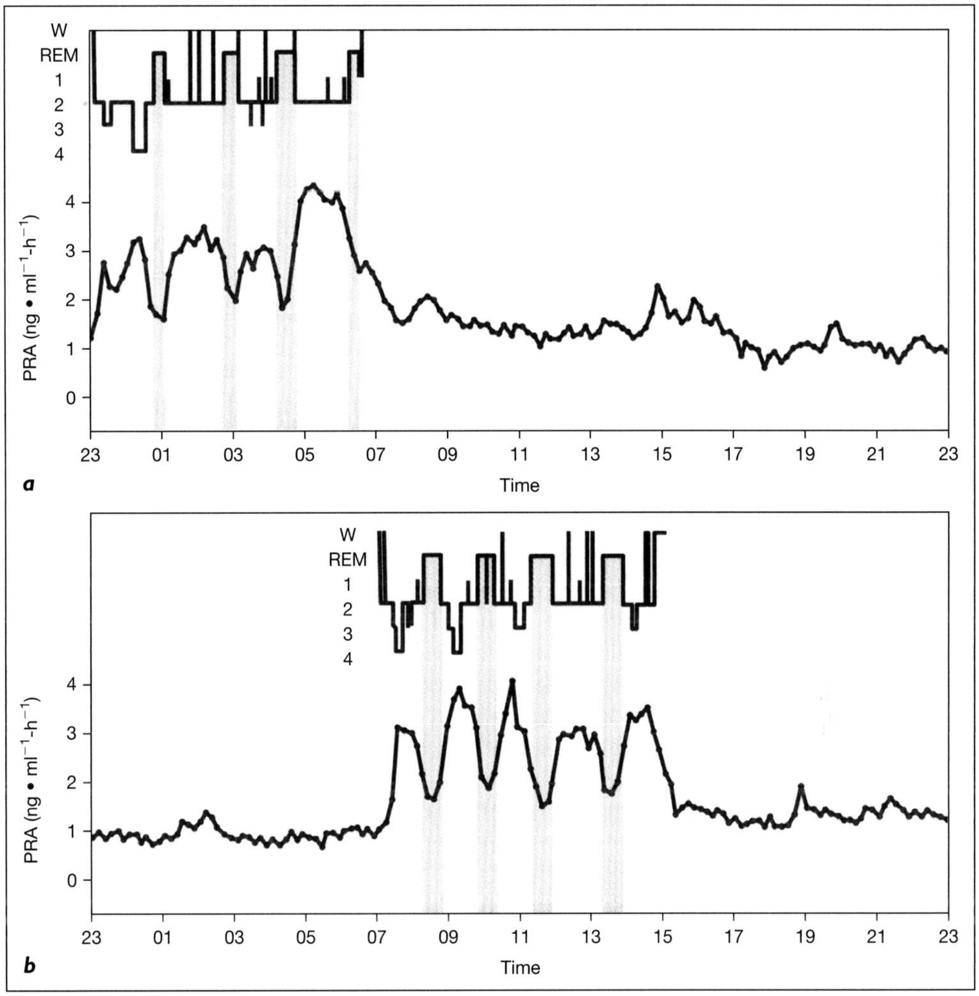

Fig. 2. The 24-hour profiles of plasma renin activity sampled at 10-minute intervals in a healthy subject. ***a*** Nocturnal sleep from 23:00 to 7:00. ***b*** Daytime sleep from 7:00 to 15:00 h after a night of total sleep deprivation. The temporal distribution of stages wake (W); REM 1, 2, 3 and 4 are shown above the hormonal values. The oscillations of plasma renin activity are synchronized to the NREM-REM cycle during sleep. From Brandenberger G, Follenius M, Goichot B, et al: Twenty-four-hour profiles of plasma renin activity in relation to the sleep-wake cycle. J Hypertens 1994;12:277–283.

Renin-Angiotensin-Aldosterone System

The RAAS represents the renal humoral pressor system which reduces renal water and electrolyte loss to maintain blood pressure. Renin is secreted by the juxtaglomerular cells of the kidneys as a response to dropping blood pressure. Renin secretion is also influenced by the autonomic nervous system. A decrease in sympathetic activity increases renin secretion. Renin triggers the conversion from angiotensinogen to angiotensin I and further from angiotensin I to the vasoactive angiotensin II by the angiotensin-converting enzyme (ACE). In addition to its inherent vasoconstricting pressor properties, angiotensin II fosters the release of aldosterone from the adrenal cortex which has antidiuretic effects and thus acts conform to the pressure-maintaining process. Plasma renin levels are not interconnected with the circadian rhythm itself but very much so with the process of sleep and the difference between NREM and REM sleep. At the onset of sleep, renin levels increase parallel to slow wave activity with its reduced blood pressure and sympathetic activity. In REM sleep, when blood pressure is highly variable and sympathetic activity rises to levels similar to wakefulness, renin levels drop significantly to rise again with the termination of REM sleep at the beginning of the next sleep cycle as shown in figure 2.

Atrial Natriuretic Peptide and Brain Natriuretic Peptide

Atrial natriuretic peptide (ANP) is secreted by the right atrium in response to sodium concentration and to dilation caused by an increase in cardiac venous preload. ANP has natriuretic, diuretic and vasorelaxant properties. Circadian rhythm influences on ANP secretion are controversially discussed. Diurnal influences might also play a role [19]. A short-term increase has been described for the initiation phase of sleep when a lying body position facilitates venous return from the lower body parts. This effect is transitory so that the generally lowered urinary output during sleep is not afflicted [20]. Nevertheless, ANP increases play a pivotal role for the pathogenesis of nycturia in OSA when respiratory effort during obstruction of the upper airways leads to intrathoracic pressure swings followed by right heart volume overload and ANP increase [21].

Brain natriuretic peptide (BNP) has similar properties as ANP. In contrast to ANP, BNP is not secreted by the right atrium but by the right ventricle in response to right heart pressure and volume overload causing ventricular dilation. Circadian and ultradian influences on BNP release have not been found. BNP does not increase in OSA [22].

Arginine Vasopressin = Antidiuretic Hormone

AVP does not display relevant circadian or sleep dependent interactions but a light increase in the second half of the night is reported.

Conclusion

Under normal conditions, urine production does not disturb sleep. Nycturia resulting from pathological conditions interrupts sleep continuity and may affect restorative function.

References

1 Podszus T, Greenberg H, Scharf SM: Influence of sleep state and sleep-disordered breathing on cardiovascular function; in Saunders NA, Sullivan CE (eds): Sleep and Breathing, ed 2. New York, Marcel Dekker, 1994, pp 257–310.

2 Barbieri R, Triedman JK, Saul JP: Heart rate control and mechanical cardiopulmonary coupling to assess central volume: a systems analysis. Am J Physiol 2002;283:R1210–R1220.

3 Stein PK, Kleiger RE: Insights from the study of heart rate variability. Annu Rev Med 1999;50:249–261.

4 Franzini C: Cardiovascular physiology: the peripheral circulation; in Kryger MH, Roth T, Dement WC (eds): Principles and Practice of Sleep Medicine, ed 4. Philadelphia, Saunders, 2005, pp 203–212.

5 Fietze I, Romberg D, Glos M, et al: Effects of positive-pressure ventilation on the spontaneous baroreflex in healthy subjects. J Appl Physiol 2004;96:1155–1160.

6 Sega R, Corrao G, Bombelli M, et al: Blood pressure variability and organ damage in a general population: results from the PAMELA study (Pressioni Arteriose Monitorate E Loro Associazioni). Hypertension 2002;39: 710–714.

7 Somers VK, Dyken ME, Mark AL, Abboud FM: Sympathetic-nerve activity during sleep in normal subjects. N Engl J Med 1993;328: 303–307.

8 Ako M, Kawara T, Uchida S, et al: Correlation between electroencephalography and heart rate variability during sleep. Psychiatry Clin Neurosci 2003;57:59–65.

9 Tank J, Diedrich A, Hale N, et al: Relationship between blood pressure, sleep K-complexes, and muscle sympathetic nerve activity in humans. Am J Physiol 2003;285: R208–R214.

10 Verrier RL, Harper RM, Hobson JA: Cardiovascular physiology: central and autonomic regulation; in Kryger MH, Roth T, Dement WC (eds): Principles and Practice of Sleep Medicine, ed 4. Philadelphia, Saunders, 2005, pp 192–202.

11 Guilleminault C, Pool P, Motta J, Gillis AM: Sinus arrest during REM sleep in young adults. N Engl J Med 1984;311:1006–1010.

12 Lavery CE, Mittleman MA, Cohen MC, Muller JE, Verrier RL: Nonuniform nighttime distribution of acute cardiac events: a possible effect of sleep states. Circulation 1997;96: 3321–3327.

13 Iellamo F, Placidi F, Marciani MG, et al: Baroreflex buffering of sympathetic activation during sleep: evidence from autonomic assessment of sleep macroarchitecture and microarchitecture. Hypertension 2004;43:814–819.

14 Legramante JM, Galante A: Sleep and hypertension: a challenge for the autonomic regulation of the cardiovascular system. Circulation 2005;112:786–788.

15 Born J, Hansen K, Marshall L, Molle M, Fehm HL: Timing the end of nocturnal sleep. Nature 1999;397:29–30.

16 Spath-Schwalbe E, Gofferje M, Kern W, Born J, Fehm HL: Sleep disruption alters nocturnal ACTH and cortisol secretory patterns. Biol Psychiatry 1991;29:575–584.

17 Van Cauter E: Endocrine physiology; in Kryger MH, Roth T, Dement WC (eds): Principles and Practice of Sleep Medicine, ed 4. Philadelphia, Saunders, 2005, pp 266–282.

18 Spiegel K, Knutson K, Leproult R, Tasali E, Van CE: Sleep loss: a novel risk factor for insulin resistance and type 2 diabetes. J Appl Physiol 2005;99:2008–2019.

19 Brandenberger G, Charloux A, Gronfier C, Otzenberger H: Ultradian rhythms in hydromineral hormones. Horm Res 1998;49:131–135.

20 Ehlenz K, Peter JH: Volumenregulation und Hochdruckgenese beim OSAS; in Peter JH, Penzel T, Cassel W, von Wichert P (eds): Schlaf-Atmung-Kreislauf. Berlin, Springer, 1993, pp 135–141.

21 Krieger J, Laks L, Wilcox I, et al: Atrial natriuretic peptide release during sleep in patients with obstructive sleep apnoea before and during treatment with nasal continuous positive airway pressure. Clin Sci (Lond) 1989;77: 407–411.

22 Svatikova A, Shamsuzzaman AS, Wolk R, Phillips BG, Olson LJ, Somers VK: Plasma brain natriuretic peptide in obstructive sleep apnea. Am J Cardiol 2004;94:529–532.

J.G. Peter, MD
Department of Cardiology, Pneumology and Angiology, Center for Sleep Medicine
Charité – Universitätsmedizin Berlin
Campus Mitte
DE–10117 Berlin (Germany)
Tel. +49 30 450513122
Fax +49 30 450513906
E-Mail jan_giso.peter@charite.de, ingo.fietze@charite.de

Randerath WJ, Sanner BM, Somers VK (eds): Sleep Apnea.
Prog Respir Res. Basel, Karger, 2006, vol 35, pp 37–42

History and Questionnaires

Karl-Heinz Rühle

Department of Pneumology, Allergology and Sleep Medicine, Klinik Ambrock, Witten-Herdecke University, Hagen, Germany

Abstract

Questionnaires to assess medical history, sleepiness and quality of life (QOL) are valuable tools to define the functional impact of the sleep-related breathing events in patients with obstructive sleep apnea syndrome (OSAS). If the answers of standardized history questionnaires are systematically evaluated, groups of different risk can be identified. Severity of symptoms together with anthropometric data predict with high sensitivity the probability of an increased apnea/hypopnea index. Sleepiness is a typical symptom of OSAS and can be characterized by subjective ratings, including the Stanford Sleepiness Scale and Epworth Sleepiness Scale. The Epworth Sleepiness Scale is most often applied in clinical routines because of its practicability. QOL is significantly impaired in OSAS patients. Evaluative instruments like the Medical Outcomes Study Short Form 36 (SF-36) measure multidimensional health components. The general questionnaires such as the SF-36 and Nottingham Health Profile were constructed to compare QOL of patients with different diseases with QOL of healthy subjects (discriminative property) and are not sensitive enough to changes. The Sleep Apnea Quality of Life Index and Quebec Sleep Questionnaire were developed to assess the specific effects of sleep apnea on QOL and within-subject changes after treatment. The choice of the instrument depends on whether sleepiness, impairment or treatment effects should be measured.

History

As a consequence of fragmented sleep in obstructive sleep apnea syndrome (OSAS), sleepiness is the most important daytime symptom in these patients, leading to impaired quality of life (QOL). Additionally, systemic hypertension may develop, and cardiovascular disease and increased mortality have been associated with OSAS. The sleep history is critical for the recognition of persons with potentially treatable sleep disorders. It is therefore necessary to know which questions are best for identifying increased apnea activity.

Several different sleep apnea clinical prediction rules have been developed, using patients' and bed partners' reports of symptoms relating to snoring, apneas, choking and/or gasping and anthropomorphic data such as the body mass index (BMI), waist and neck circumference. Other important clinical information concerning symptom severity, comorbidities, and QOL should be registered. In a study to predict relevant sleep apnea activity with an apnea/hypopnea index (AHI) >15 with high sensitivity, four terms were identified: apneas observed by bed partners, hypertension, BMI and age [1]. Snoring and daytime sleepiness did not discriminate between patients with and without sleep-related breathing disorder (SRBD) due to selection biases because all patients were referred to the clinic with such symptoms. When a low cutoff probability was selected, 33 of 36 patients were correctly classified. The resulting sensitivity was 92%, while the specificity was only 51%.

The validity of symptom questions to predict sleep apnea activity (AHI > 20) was assessed using a self-administered sleep questionnaire [2]. Sixteen questions were clustered into clinically meaningful dimensions like performance ability, snoring intensity, fallen asleep while driving and frequent awakenings. When the severity of the symptoms was taken into account, the odds demonstrating apnea activity increased progressively. Mild snoring, for instance, had an odds ratio of 2.1, very severe snoring 21.1 compared with those who never snore. In addition to 3 selected questions, data on BMI and gender improved the prediction ability by 10%.

The Berlin questionnaire includes self-reported questions and focuses on a screening approach in a primary care population and a limited set of risk factors [3]. The questions include weight, snoring loudness, frequency, disturbing other people, breathing pauses, tiredness after sleeping or during waketime, falling asleep while driving and high blood pressure. Three domains were defined, namely snoring behavior, waketime sleepiness and a history of obesity or hypertension. Persistent or frequent symptoms in 2 of the 3 domains were considered as high risk. In the high risk group, the sensitivity and specificity for a respiratory disturbance index (RDI) > 5 measured with a portable monitoring was 86 and 77%, respectively.

Patients with OSAS seem to be well informed about their symptoms because there is a modest to good agreement between patients' and bed partners' answers on identical questionnaires [4]. Nevertheless, an interview of the bed partner is recommended to assess the reliability of the patient report.

Questionnaires on their own are only of limited value as a clinical screening tool because they only modestly predict apnea activity. By using more stringent criteria in order to ascertain patients with OSAS, more patients with the disease are excluded (more false negatives), and if weaker criteria are used more unaffected persons are included (more false positives). In order to gather a sampling frame for ambulatory monitoring, it is more important to get a high sensitivity than specificity because no patient should be missed who could benefit from continuous positive airway pressure (CPAP) or other treatment. Thus, if any risk is suspected, the judgment of a physician is needed to decide about further evaluation, especially using objective measurements like polysomnography.

Table 1. The Stanford Sleepiness Scale

Tick only the *one* of the seven options presented that best describes the degree of your momentary sleepiness or alertness.

Degree of sleepiness	Scale rating
Feeling active, vital, alert, or wide awake	1
Functioning at high levels, but not at peak; able to concentrate	2
Awake, but relaxed; responsive but not fully alert	3
Somewhat foggy, let down	4
Foggy; losing interest in remaining awake; slowed down	5
Sleepy, woozy, fighting sleep; prefer to lie down	6
No longer fighting sleep, sleep onset soon; having dream-like thoughts	7
Asleep	×

For reference values, see Herscovitch and Broughton [28].

Daytime Sleepiness

Stanford Sleepiness Scale

Subjective sleepiness can be estimated with the Stanford Sleepiness Scale (SSS) which reflects the actual state of sleepiness at the time when the questionnaire is administered (table 1). This 7-point scale features verbal descriptions of the different stages of sleepiness. It indicates sleep deprivation or sleep fragmentation and is a useful tool to reflect treatment efficiency of CPAP. The effect of this treatment on sleepiness was studied by applying the SSS before and during CPAP therapy [5]. Without CPAP, the baseline value was 3.5 ± 1.3 after 30 days. Under CPAP, the score decreased by about 0.8 ± 1.0 and increased by the same amount immediately after the first night without CPAP. Generally the SSS is used in clinical studies but in clinical routines the SSS could not be established.

Epworth Sleepiness Scale

This questionnaire was constructed with the intention to describe the probability of falling asleep in 8 specific situations with varying soporific situations (table 2). In contrast to the multiple sleep latency test, different situations concerning sleepiness of the daily life are considered. The advantage of the Epworth Sleepiness Scale (ESS) consists in representing the average sleep propensity [6–10]. The ESS is applied mostly because of its simplicity and practicability in routine especially to describe sleepiness of patients with sleep apnea syndrome (OSAS) [11]. The mean ± SD of ESS scores in 30 normal men and women was 5.9 ± 2.2.

Quality of Life

SRBD considerably reduce the QOL, that should improve with an adequate therapy. Forty percent of all studies of the last years reported no symptoms or QOL outcomes. It is well recognized that the AHI correlates poorly with these outcomes, so alone it is not an appropriate measure. Since QOL is what matters most to patients with sleep apnea, clinical

Table 2. The Epworth Sleepiness Scale

How likely are you to doze off or fall asleep in the following situations, in contrast to feeling just tired? This refers to your usual way of life in recent times. Even if you have not done some of these things recently try to work out how they would have affected you. Use the following scale to choose the most appropriate number for each situation:

Situation	Chance of dozing
Sitting and reading	
Watching TV	
Sitting inactive in a public place (e.g. a theatre or a meeting)	
As a passenger in a car for an hour without a break	
Lying down to rest in the afternoon when circumstances permit	
Sitting and talking to someone	
Sitting quietly after a lunch without alcohol	
In a car, while stopped for a few minutes in traffic	

0 = No chance of dozing; 1 = slight chance of dozing; 2 = moderate chance of dozing; 3 = high chance of dozing.

To check your sleepiness score, total the points. Check your total score to see how sleepy you are.

trials should include it as an important outcome measure. In addition to the registration of the polysomnographic data, it is therefore recommended to apply to all patients at least one of the following instruments to measure QOL prior to and during therapy. In the following, the questionnaires most frequently used internationally will be reviewed.

General Health Status Questionnaires

General indices such as the Medical Outcomes Study Short Form 36 (SF-36), Nottingham Health Profile (NHP), Sickness Impact Profile (SIP), Munich Life Quality Dimension List (MLDL) are in common use and have been applied in many diseases. The advantage of these and other well established questionnaires consists in the possibility to compare consequences of sleep apnea and its treatment with other diseases like asthma or chronic obstructive lung disease. However, the disadvantage of these indices is that they do not cover important consequences of sleep apnea. Many questionnaires are construed to distinguish between conditions with a better QOL from those with a worse QOL at a single date (discriminative property). In many cases they are insensitive to important changes experienced with treatment, because they were not specifically designed to measure changes following a therapeutic intervention.

Medical Outcomes Study Short Form 36

The SF-36 includes 8 domains: physical and social functioning, role function (physical and emotional), mental health, vitality, pain, and general perceptions of health. Normative data for adults are available [12]. In all dimensions, considerable differences between the normal population and patients with OSAS were detected. In a longitudinal study, the impact of OSAS and CPAP therapy on the overall QOL was determined. In a study of consecutive patients, all qualities of life factors expressed as a percentage of normative data were reduced (physical and emotional health, social functioning, physical functioning, 75%; vitality, 41%; role functioning: physical, 54%, emotional, 61%, and social, 66%; general health, 88%, and mental health, 76%). After 8 weeks of CPAP therapy, vitality (75%), social functioning (90%), and mental health (96%) markedly improved. The magnitude of improvement was related to the degree of QOL impairment before treatment, it was not closely related with the RDI and arousal indices. Adherence to therapy was only weakly correlated with changes of QOL.

In a study in patients with OSAS comparing CPAP and autotitrating positive airway pressure, compliance and treatment response were measured [13]. Compliance, ESS score, SF-36, side effects and treatment pressures were compared. There were no differences between treatment modes in overall compliance, ESS scores relative to baseline and between modes, SF-36 scores significantly improved in physical role and vitality domains relative to baseline; however, differences between the two modes were not detected.

In patients with chronic heart failure (CHF) QOL is also severely affected. In about 50% of these patients with severe CHF, Cheyne-Stokes Respiration or OSAS are observed. The resulting fragmentation of sleep leads to excessive daytime sleepiness with lower QOL than in patients without SRBD and CHF [14]. Bodily pain, physical functioning and social functioning are largely impaired in patients with SRBD.

Nottingham Health Profile

The NHP includes 38 items. The score of 100 is correlated to an extremely reduced QOL, 0 to a very good one. It contains subscales for energy, pain, emotional reactions, sleep quality, social isolation and physical mobility [15]. In almost all dimensions except emotional perception, significant differences relative to a control group of healthy people were discovered [16].

Before and during daily CPAP, the correlation between changes of daytime function and CPAP adherence was examined. Only a few measures like symptoms, sleepiness and QOL, measured with the NHP predicted weakly the time of

CPAP use [17]. However, providing an intensive additional education program which increased CPAP use did not influence significantly the QOL measured with the NHP [18]. The questionnaire was also validated in French. In a large population of more than 3,000 patients with OSAS under long-term CPAP therapy, the NHP was applied. Even during therapy some scores were increased: The worst value was found for energy (33.6), followed by physical mobility (21.4). Social isolation (9.9) seems to be a problem for females [19]. The reduced QOL of patients under CPAP may be due to the associated conditions as obesity and cardiovascular diseases.

Sickness Impact Profile

This 136-item questionnaire depicts behavioral changes and shows sensitivity to treatment effects. It includes several categories, i.e. social interaction, locomotion, sleep and rest, nutrition, usual daily work, household, mobility, body movement, communication, leisure, intellectual functioning, interaction with family, emotions, feelings and personal hygiene. From these dimensions a global scale can be derived. Using the SIP as outcome measure, the global score improved under CPAP from a pretreatment value of 17.2 ± 13.6 to 5.4 ± 6.3 under CPAP [5].

Munich Life Quality Dimension List

The MLDL includes 19 items which can be assigned to 4 categories, namely physical and psychical conditions, social life and everyday life. The questions concern the degree of satisfaction, degree of importance, desire for change and belief in changes. Untreated patients with OSAS differed significantly from control subjects. If they were treated for 3 months or longer, their QOL attained similar values as the controls [20]. In a study with 40 controls and 41 OSAS patients, 3 questionnaires were compared. The calculation of the effect size revealed the strongest effect of therapy in the subscale vitality of the SF-36 with 0.93. With the MLDL, good effect sizes were found in the domains physical satisfaction (0.70) and psychical satisfaction. Its feasibility and simple use make the MLDL a more useful instrument to cover QOL in clinical routine [21].

Specific Questionnaires Concerning Sleep

Functional Outcome of Sleep Questionnaire

The Functional Outcome of Sleep Questionnaire (FOSQ) was developed to estimate the functional impact of diseases with sleep disturbances on the activities of everyday living [22]. The ESS and SSS describe sleepiness in different dimensions but not how patients are constrained in their daily activities. By means of the FOSQ, efficiency of daily routine should be estimated. Instruments like the SIP or SF-36 comprise a large area of functions, therefore they are appropriate for comparing different diseases. By responding especially to sleepiness, the FOSQ can better characterize data of specific diseases like OSAS. As a result, better graduations are possible. The FOSQ is a paper and pencil test. It includes 30 questions and lasts 15 min. Five factors were identified: level of activity, vigilance, intimacy and sexual impact. The results of the FOSQ were compared with SF-36 and SIP data in OSAS patients. As there is only a moderate correlation, one can conclude that additional characteristics of OSAS are covered by the FOSQ. The FOSQ was adapted by several working groups in different languages, e.g. Spanish and German, and is available for scientific issues.

Before answering the questionnaire, the patient is informed about the difference between sleepiness and fatigue after physical endurance. The patient should differentiate between 4 degrees of severity in each question, that means: no, some, considerable and extreme problems in the actual situation. Points between 4 and 0 are given per question, respectively. The sum score is calculated in percentage of the maximal possible score. In healthy persons, the single value of the subscales ranges from 3.5 to 3.9 [23]. The evaluation is done by composing a global sum score of all 5 factors. If one or several questions are not answered, the mean value is calculated by the diminished number of questions.

Controls and patients with OSAS in comparison showed both significant differences in the global score (90 ± 9 vs. 68 ± 21) and the 5 subscales [22]. In a comparison of CPAP with sham CPAP in a group of 45 patients with moderate and severe OSAS, the SF-36 and FOSQ were applied to examine the efficiency of therapy. Vigilance and general fitness in the FOSQ scales increased significantly. Therefore, in addition to minimizing the symptoms the positive impact of improved sleep on fitness during daytime could also be proved.

In a study in patients with mild OSAS (AHI 12.9 ± 6.3, range 5–30), the effect of CPAP in a randomized placebo-controlled study was examined [23]. The data of the FOSQ showed that 72% of the patients had a reduced QOL before CPAP treatment. A tablet as placebo was used, and the patients were told that it had been developed to improve their breathing during the night. Three of 5 domains improved during placebo treatment. Except for vigilance, no significant difference was found between placebo and CPAP. These results demonstrate that patients are susceptible to placebo treatment effects. Treatment results measured with the FOSQ and other questionnaires are subjective data and should be compared with a control group.

OSAS-Specific Questionnaires

Calgary Sleep Apnea Quality of Life Index

Generic health measures, for instance the above-mentioned NHP and the SF-36 do not detect more subtle effects of the disease on QOL. Also, they were not constructed to evaluate within-subject change after treatment. Additional questionnaires are needed to assess the specific effects of sleep apnea on QOL.

The Sleep Apnea Quality of Life Index (SAQLI) was developed as an evaluative instrument to measure within-subject change in response to a therapeutic intervention [24]. It contains 35 questions with 4 domains: daily functioning, social interactions, emotional functioning, and symptoms. Treatment-related symptoms were added in a further domain to take the possible negative impact of treatment into consideration. The questionnaire was thoroughly developed by reviewing the literature, meetings with experts, discussions with patients with OSAS and their partners, as well as interviews. From all these results, a list of 133 items with importance to patients with OSAS was constructed. For each item, the product of frequency and importance was calculated. The best items were selected in the Calgary SAQLI and organized into 5 domains: The highest scores were associated with alertness, concentration, the feeling of tiredness and significant problems in relationships.

The SAQLI should be administered by a trained interviewer, using response cards with a seven-level Likert scale. The SAQLI showed a good reliability on testing and retesting at 2 weeks; a good construct validity because the within-subject change in SAQLI scores correlated significantly with the SF-36; a very high responsiveness index of 1.9 and an effect size in the range of 1.1, which was much greater compared with the domains of the SF-36 [25].

The questionnaire was used to examine effects of an education program [26]. In a comparative study, the standard program consisted of a 10-min CPAP education program, and handing out a brochure on OSAS and CPAP treatment. The patients were subsequently followed up by physicians and nurses at the CPAP clinic at 1 month and 3 months. In addition to receiving the same information as in the basic support group, patients in the augmented support group were given extra information on OSAS and CPAP by physicians via videotape and an additional 15-min education session. At weeks 1 and 2, the patients were reviewed by physicians. Telephone support was added on days 1 and 2, and at weeks 1, 2, 3, 4, 8, and 12. Objective CPAP adherence and compliance improvement of ESS score were not significantly different between the two groups. However, the group with augmented support reported a significantly greater improvement of QOL with an increase in the total SAQLI score from 9.1 $\pm$ 2.5 to 21.9 $\pm$ 5.2 at 4 and 12 weeks.

Quebec Sleep Questionnaire

The SAQLI is time-consuming because patients are asked in an interview to select from a list of items the most important symptoms they have experienced. Therefore, a self-administered standardized QOL questionnaire was developed (Quebec Sleep Questionnaire, QSQ). The QSQ can be administered without supervision and even mailed to patients [27]. The ease and convenience of standardized items of the QSQ exceeds the benefits of individualized items of the SAQLI. The QSQ is a 32-item OSAS-specific questionnaire. The questions were selected by their impact score, defined as the product of frequency and importance. It is used to describe baseline and changes in domain scores (daytime sleepiness, diurnal symptoms, nocturnal symptoms, emotions and social interactions). Each domain includes 4–7 items and each item is scored on a 7-point scale. The QSQ is available in English and French. The minimal clinically important difference, namely the smallest difference perceived by the patient, was calculated for a better interpretability of the scores before and during the CPAP treatment.

To compare the sensitivity of different questionnaires, the standardized response mean (magnitude of change/standard deviation of change) was calculated. The QSQ was more responsive to treatment-induced changes than the FOSQ, a property that is required for clinical trials and in routine.

Conclusions

We conclude that apart from the objective registration of respiratory disturbances during sleep, the description of QOL is needed, because the domains of QOL remain unexplored by the nocturnal recordings in the sleep laboratory. There exist only minor correlations between sleepiness, QOL and frequency and duration of the disorder. For scientific purposes, to describe the broad range of impairment in OSAS generic QOL scales like the SF-36 or NHP should be used. But even in clinical routine, QOL should be registered. As an evaluative instrument to measure therapeutic effects, a disease-specific self-administered questionnaire like the QSQ is preferable because it is sensitive to treatment-induced changes. If there is no relevant improvement of QOL after several weeks on CPAP, a thorough check-up of the diagnosis and the treatment modality should be performed.

References

1 Crocker B, Olson LG, Saunders NA, Hensley NJ, McKeon JL, Allen KM, Gyulay SG: Estimation of the probability of disturbed breathing during sleep before a sleep study. Am J Respir Crit Care Med 1990;142:14–18.

2 Kump K, Whalen C, Tishler PV, Browner I, Ferrette V, et al: Assessment of the validity and utility of a sleep-symptom questionnaire. Am J Respir Crit Care Med 1994;150:735–741.

3 Netzer NC, Stoohs RA, Netzer CM, Clark K, Strohl KP: Using the Berlin Questionnaire to identify patients at risk for the sleep apnea syndrome. Ann Intern Med 1999;131:485–491.

4 Virkkula P, Bachour A, Hytönen M, Malmberg H, Salmi T, Maasilta P: Patient- and bed partner-reported symptoms, smoking, and nasal resistance in sleep-disordered breathing. Chest 2005;128:2176–2182.

5 Kribbs NB, Pack AI, Kline LR, Getsy JE, Schuett JS, Henry JN, Maislin G, Dinges DF: Effects of one night without nasal CPAP treatment on sleep and sleepiness in patients with obstructive sleep apnea. Am Rev Respir Dis 1993;147:1162–1168.

6 Johns MW: A new method for measuring daytime sleepiness: the Epworth Sleepiness Scale. Sleep 1991;14:540–545.

7 Johns MW: Reliability and factor analysis of the Epworth Sleepiness Scale. Sleep 1992;15: 376–381.

8 Johns MW: Daytime sleepiness, snoring, and obstructive sleep apnea. The Epworth Sleepiness Scale. Chest 1993;103:30–36.

9 Johns MW: Sleepiness in different situations measured by the Epworth Sleepiness Scale. Sleep 1994;17:703–710.

10 Johns MW: Sensitivity and specificity of the multiple sleep latency test (MSLT), the maintenance of wakefulness test and the Epworth Sleepiness Scale: failure of the MSLT as a gold standard. J Sleep Res 2000;9:5–11.

11 Rühle KH, Feier Ch, Galetke W, Büttner A, Nilius G: Analysis of the 8 items of the Epworth Sleepiness Scale. Somnologie 2005;9: 154–158.

12 Jenkinson C, Coulter A, Wright L: Short form 36 (SF-36) health survey questionnaire: normative data for adults of working age. BMJ 1993;306:1437–1440.

13 Hukins C: Comparative study of autotitrating and fixed-pressure CPAP in the home: a randomized, single-blind crossover trial. Sleep 2004;27:1512–1517.

14 Skobel E, Norra C, Sinha A, Breuer C, Hanrath P, Stellbrink C: Impact of sleep-related breathing disorders on health-related quality of life in patients with chronic heart failure. Eur J Heart Fail 2005;7:505–511.

15 Engleman HM, Douglas NJ: Sleep. 4: sleepiness, cognitive function, and quality of life in obstructive sleep apnoea/hypopnoea syndrome. Thorax 2004;59:618–622.

16 Fornas C, Ballester E, Arteta E, Ricou C, Diaz A, Fernandez A, Alonso J, Montserrat JM: Measurement of general health status in obstructive sleep apnea hypopnea patients. Sleep 1995;18:876–879.

17 Kingshott RN, Vennelle M, Hoy CJ, Engleman HM: Predictors of improvements in daytime function outcomes with CPAP therapy. Am J Respir Crit Care Med 2000;161: 866–871.

18 Hoy CJ, Vennelle M, Kingshott RN, Engleman HM, Douglas NJ: Can intensive support improve continuous positive pressure use in patients with the sleep apnea/hypopnea syndrome? Am J Respir Crit Care Med 1999;159: 1096–1100.

19 Meslier N, Lebrun T, Grillier-Lanoir, Rolland N, Henderick C, Saily JC, Racineux JL: A French survey of 3225 patients treated with CPAP for obstructive sleep apnoea: benefits, tolerance, compliance and quality of life. Eur Respir J 1998;12:185–192.

20 Bolitschek J, Schmeiser-Rieder A, Schobersberger R, Rosenberger A, Kunze M, Aigner K: Impact of nasal continuous positive airway pressure treatment on quality of life in patients with obstructive sleep apnea. Eur Respir J 1998;11:890–894.

21 Büttner A, Rühle KH: Quality of life before and during nCPAP. Comparison of different questionnaires – SWLS, MLDL and SF-36. Pneumology 2004;58:651–659.

22 Weaver TE, Laizner AM, Evans LK, Maislin G, Chugh DK, Lyon K, Smith PL, Schwartz AR, Redline S, Pack AI, Dinges DF: An instrument to measure functional outcomes for disorders of excessive sleepiness. Sleep 1997;20:835–843.

23 Barnes M, Houston D, Worsnop CJ, Neill AM, Mykytyn IJ, Kay A, Trinder J, Saunders NA, Douglas McEvoy R, Pierce RJ: A randomized controlled trial of continuous positive airway pressure in mild obstructive sleep apnea. Am J Respir Crit Care Med 2002;165:773–780.

24 Flemons WW, Reimer MA: Development of a disease-specific health-related quality of life questionnaire for sleep apnea. Am J Respir Crit Care Med 1998;158:494–503.

25 Lacasse Y, Godbout C, Series F: Independent validation of the Sleep Apnoea Quality of Life Index. Thorax 2002;57:483–488.

26 Hui DSC, Chan JKW, Choy DKL, Ko FWS, Li TST, Leung RCC, Lai CKW: Effects of augmented continuous positive airway pressure education and support on compliance and outcome in a Chinese population. Chest 2000;117:1410–1416.

27 Lacasse Y, Bureau MP, Series F: A new standardised and self-administered quality of life questionnaire specific to obstructive sleep apnoea. Thorax 2004;59:494–499.

28 Herscovitch J, Broughton R: Sensitivity of the Stanford Sleepiness Scale to the effects of cumulative partial sleep deprivation and recovery oversleeping. Sleep 1981;4:83–91.

Prof. K.H. Rühle
Klinik Ambrock, Ambrockerweg 60
DE–58091 Hagen (Germany)
Tel. +49 2331 974 201
Fax +49 2331 974 209
E-Mail klinik-ambrock.pneumo@t-online.de

Randerath WJ, Sanner BM, Somers VK (eds): Sleep Apnea.
Prog Respir Res. Basel, Karger, 2006, vol 35, pp 43–46

Objectifying Sleepiness

Holger Hein

Praxis für Innere Medizin, Pneumologie, Allergologie und Schlafmedizin, Reinbek, Germany

Abstract

Objectifying sleepiness should encompass a number of tests: (1) Subjective self-assessment with the aid of standardized questionnaires (e.g. Epworth Sleepiness Scale, Stanford Sleepiness Scale); (2) Determination of reaction times or the time taken to solve standardized tasks (e.g. Trail Making Test, Mackworth Clock Test, Psychomotor Vigilance Test, Vienna Test System); (3) EEG-based measurements of sleep latency and/or ability to remain awake under standard conditions (Multiple Sleep Latency Test, Maintenance of Wakefulness Test). The place of tests of sympathetic activity like pupillometry needs to be determined. The time requirement and costs of 'real' driving simulators are high, therefore this procedure is hardly suitable for use in the clinical practice setting.

Sleepiness is a form of attention deficit associated with a reduction in reaction and vigilance. Vigilance and cognitive performance are complex processes. The former is dependent upon the time of the day, quality of sleep and the oxygen supply to the brain. If sleep is fragmented, it loses its regenerative function, and vigilance and cognition are disordered.

Sleep-related breathing disorders occur as a result of repeated constriction of the pharynx or as a result of a central disturbance of breathing regulation [1]. According to the model proposed by Bebee and Gozal [2], respiratory events lead to a drop in oxygen saturation, or hypercapnea on the one hand and, as a result of arousals, to sleep fragmentation on the other. The percentage of REM and slow-wave sleep decreases, sleep loses its restorative function, and cognitive process and vigilance are disturbed [2, 3]. Daytime sleepiness [4] or insomnia [5] and impaired vigilance occur. These cardinal symptoms are of central importance for the diagnosis and evaluation of the severity of sleep-related respiratory disorders, and should therefore be accurately measured and identified. It is interesting that only about one quarter of all those affected report sleepiness to be a leading symptom, with almost a half of the patients suffering mainly from a lack of energy and drive, and about one quarter complaining of exhaustion [6]. Since the symptoms develop and progress only gradually, some patients are hardly aware of the abovementioned problems. Daytime sleepiness can have a considerable impact on the patient's fitness to drive. A meta-analysis revealed that, in comparison with controls, persons with the obstructive sleep apnea syndrome have a 2.5- to 3-fold higher rate of accidents [7]. An interesting observation is the fact that women with sleep-related respiratory disorders have a lower accident risk than men suffering from the same problem. The number of nocturnal respiratory disorders that are expressed by means of the apnea/hypopnea index, which identifies the average number of nocturnal events (disturbances per hour of sleep), is not indicative of the extent of sleepiness [3] or the incidence of accidents [8]. For this reason, the demonstration of a sleep-related respiratory disorder alone does not permit an evaluation of a person's fitness to drive. Patients with sleep-related respiratory disorders do, however, have a reduced quality of life as a result of sleep fragmentation. Measurements employing quality of life scales in severe sleep-related respiratory disorders show a significant reduction in the parameters vitality, physical functioning, general health and social functioning [9]. Furthermore, patients with sleep-related respiratory disorders demonstrate a reduction in the amount of grey matter in the brain [10], together with cognitive performance problems in comparison with control subjects [2].

The clinical evaluation of sleepiness reveals two striking points in patients with sleep-related respiratory disorders: (1) the sleep disorder is chronic and (2) is improved only insignificantly by prolonging sleep time. As a rule, the patient himself is aware of his sleepiness problem. Yawning, heavy eyelids (ptosis), lethargy, difficulty in concentrating, and delayed reaction to stimuli are typical signs. The following tests are often used for the clinical evaluation of sleepiness and vigilance deficits:

Questionnaires

Sleep quality questionnaires can provide good evidence for nonrestorative sleep. In cooperative patients, standardized questionnaire-based sleepiness scales reliably reflect the patient's sleepiness. As a measure of momentary sleepiness, the 7-stage Stanford Sleepiness Scale has proven useful [11]. As a measure of the patient's ability to remain awake or propensity to doze off in typical daily situations, the Epworth Sleepiness Scale is often employed [12]. Both sleepiness scales are discussed in the paper by Rühle [this vol., p. 37].

Paper and Pencil Tests

Classical psychophysiological tests measure the time taken to solve concentration tasks as, e.g. connecting a series of numbers with an alphabetic series of letters. The trail making test A and B in particular has proved useful, and well-validated normative figures are available. Part A consists of encircled numbers from 1 to 25 randomly spread on a sheet of paper. The object of the test is to connect the numbers in order, in as little time as possible. Part B requires the subject to connect numbers and letters in an alternating pattern as fast as possible (reference value: 66–85 s). Part B requires more thought processing and attention of the subject.

Electronically-Based Reaction Time and Vigilance Tests

Other procedures electronically determine the reaction time to randomly presented, unchanging stimuli. In the case of the psychomotor vigilance test, reaction times to the sudden appearance of an ascending series of numbers is measured. A red light flashes on the display of the device at random intervals throughout the 10-min duration of the test. Subjects have to press a button as soon as possible as an answer while the red light is flashing. In each individual, results are expressed as mean reaction time and, also, as the slope of the relationship between the inverse of the reaction time vs. time. This slope is used as a measurement of reaction fatigue. A negative slope indicates an increase of the reaction time over time (i.e. more reaction fatigue). The 10% slowest and fastest reactions, as well as the number of all the events not recognized within 500 ms, are recorded. Reference figures are available and have been published [13].

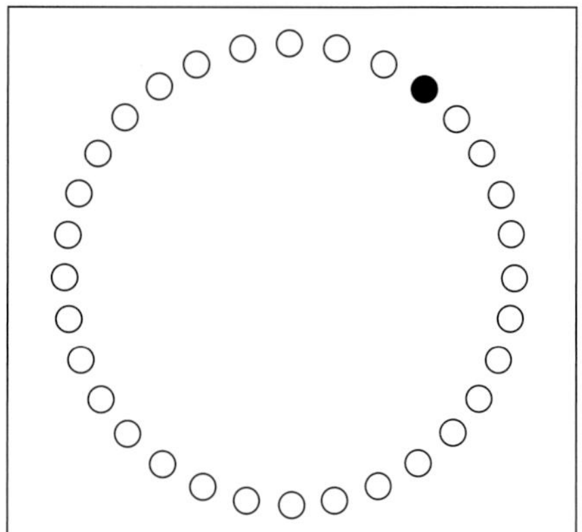

Fig. 1. The Mackworth Clock.

Another scientifically proven examination is the Mackworth Clock Test. It was originally developed to evaluate vigilance in British Air Force radar technicians during World War II. It is used to establish the increase in misses and the increase in reaction time. Subjects watching a white light, which jumps one step further every second on a clock with 32 intercepts. Whenever the light jumps two steps instead of one, the subjects has to report it (fig. 1). Research showed that within the first 30 min the decrement in the hit rate is most pronounced. After that the decrement levels off and stays at an almost constant value. This test is currently under further examination by the SIESTA (**S**ystem for **I**ntegrating Polygraphic Recordings and **D**escribing **S**leep Archi**t**ecture and Its V**a**lidation) group and a task force of the Deutsche Gesellschaft für Schlafforschung und Schlafmedizin.

The Vienna Test System consists of several performance test. Tests of general ability are included, e.g. Continuous Attention (DAUF [Daueraufmerksamkeits-Test zur Quantifizierung der Aufmerksamkeitsleistungen]), Reaction Time Analysis, Signal Detection, Vienna Determination Test, Vienna Reaction Test, Vigilance (VIGIL), Work Performance Series (ALS). The Continuous Attention test, for instance, is an assessment of the long-term selective attention and concentration ability, general performance and commitment. Rows of triangles are shown on the screen pointing either up or down. Whenever a predefined number of triangles points down, the respondent is required to press the reaction. The VIGIL test is an application of the Mackworth Clock Test. The Work Performance Series (ALS) is an assessment of concentration, psychic saturation and fatigability in mental tasks under time pressure. The computerized administration of the ALS includes a standardized instruction and a practice phase, as well as a test phase of 20 min, during which the respondent is required to add as fast as possible two numbers at a time. They are displayed on top of each other on the screen. The respondent enters the results of the arithmetical problems via the keys of the panel. For the short-term memory tasks, the lower number moves up and is covered each time the respondent enters a result. Thus the respondent needs to memorize the lower number before entering the result in order to be able to carry out the next task [14].

Computer-Based Driving Simulator Tests

Computer-based driving simulator tests, such as the Steer-Clear [15] measure the frequency of tracking errors. During 30 min, the subject looks on a computer screen, where a car runs through a long, linear road. At random intervals and unexpectedly an object appears on the road. The subject has to press the space bar of a computer keybord to avoid hitting. The number of hits is recorded by the computer every minute. Other authors used commercially available driving simulators. Subjects performed, e.g. over 20 min, a divided attention driving simulation test. The object of the test is to steer an image of a car bonnet down the centre of a winding road as accurately as possible (measuring the ability to track) using a standard computer game steering wheel. The error rate of these off-road events correlated with the number of road accidents involving those investigated, but only slightly, with an odds ratio of 1.004. Patients who have not had an accident are readily identified, but only 10% of those who have been involved in an accident are identified [16].

Driving Simulators

Measurements obtained in 'real' driving simulators require the coordination of complex actions. They show good correlation with the incidence of actual road traffic accidents, and changes in vigilance under treatment can also be well documented [17]. Since, however, the time requirement and costs of the measuring equipment are very high, this procedure is hardly suitable for use in the clinical practice setting.

Pupillometry

In recent years, measurement of the pupil diameter in the darkness has attracted considerable interest. In the presence of sleepiness, the diameter of the pupil varies considerably over a measuring period of 11 min, while in the alert person, it remains constant at roughly 7 mm during measurement in the dark. The pupillary unrest index correlates well with other sleepiness tests. However, only those values measured before noon are of significance for discriminating between alertness and sleepiness [18].

Electrophysiological Measurements of Brain Activity

The gold standard – also for diagnosis – is the determination of sleep latency based on the electrophysiological curves reflecting brain activity. The recording of EEGs in channels C3/C4 enables the accurate determination of the sleep onset time points. Under standardized conditions in a low-stimulus environment, the Multiple Sleep Latency Test (MSLT) [19] and the Maintenance of Wakefulness Test (MWT) [20] are employed. In the case of the MSLT, the rapidity of sleep onset in a subject lying in bed in a darkened room is measured over a period of 20 min every 2 h, four to five times during the day. The subjects are instructed to try to go to sleep. Since, however, the ability to remain awake predominates during the daytime, the MWT was developed as an exactly reversed test. Here the subject, seated for 40 min in a comfortable armchair in a darkened room, is requested to remain awake for as long as possible. Measurements are made four times during the day at intervals of 2 h. Here, too, the sleep latency is determined electrophysiologically, applying the criteria of Rechtschaffen and Kales [21]. The measurements must be constantly monitored so as to exclude the influence of such aids as light, reading, listening to music, etc. Normative values derived from meta-analyses are available, and vary according to age between 9 and 13 min (MSLT) and 29–38 min (MWT) [22]. A disadvantage is the dependence on a laboratory, special equipment and the need to obtain measurements throughout the whole of the day. The results, however, are objective, and also recognized for use in diagnosis. Interestingly, the MWT correlates well with driving simulator performance [23].

If the results of various tests are ambiguous, the so-called practice test remains as a general evaluation option. If, e.g. the likelihood of a significant reduction of fitness to drive as a result of a disease possibly associated with excessive sleepiness is to be determined, a driving test in normal road traffic can provide the necessary information about attention deficits. This test, of course, requires the use of a driving school car permitting the tester to take over if necessary.

In summary, the testing of sleepiness should encompass a number of tests:

1 Subjective self-assessment with the aid of standardized questionnaires (e.g. Epworth Sleepiness Scale, Stanford Sleepiness Scale).
2 Determination of reaction times or the time taken to solve standardized tasks (e.g. Trail Making Test, Mackworth Clock Test, Vienna Test System).
3 EEG-based measurements of sleep latency and ability to remain awake under standard conditions (MSLT, MWT).

References

1 American Academy of Sleep Medicine: International Classification of Sleep Disorders, ed 2: Diagnostic and coding manual. Westchester, American Academy of Sleep Medicine, 2005.

2 Beebe DW, Gozal D: Obstructive sleep apnea and the prefrontal cortex: towards a comprehensive model linking nocturnal upper airway obstruction to daytime cognitive and behavioral deficits. J Sleep Res 2002;11:1–16.

3 Colt HG, Haas H, Rich GB: Hypoxemia vs. sleep fragmentation as cause of excessive daytime sleepines in OSA. Chest 1991;100: 1542–1548.

4 Barbé F, Pericás J, Munoz A, Findley L, Anto JM, Agusti AGN: Automobile accidents in patients with sleep apnea syndrome. Am J Respir Crit Care Med 1998;158:18–22.

5 Guilleminault C, Elridge FL, Dement WC: Insomnia with sleep apnea: a new syndrome. Science 1973;181:856–858.

6 Chervin RD: Sleepiness, fatigue, tiredness, and lack of energy in obstructive sleep apnea. Chest 2000;118:372–379.

7 Sassani A, Findley LJ, Kryger M, Goldlust E, George C, Davidson TM: Reducing motor-vehicle collisions, costs, and fatalities by treating obstructive sleep apnea syndrome. Sleep 2004;27:453–458.

8 Young T, Blustein J, Finn L, Palta M: Sleep-disordered breathing and motor vehicle accidents in a population-based sample of employed adults. Sleep 1997;20:608–613.

9 Baldwin CM, Griffith KA, Nieto FJ, O'Connor GT, Walsleben JA, Redline S: The association of sleep-disordered breathing and sleep symptoms with quality of life in the sleep heart health study. Sleep 2001;24:96–105.

10 Macey PM, Henderson LA, Macey KE, Alger JR, Frysinger RC, Woo MA, Harper RK, Yan-Go FL, Harper RM: Brain morphology associated with obstructive sleep apnea. Am J Respir Crit Care Med 2002;166:1382–1387.

11 Hoddes E, Zarcone VP, Smythe H: Quantification of sleepiness: a new approach. Psychophysiology 1973;10:431–436.

12 Johns, MW: A new method for measuring daytime sleepiness: the Epworth sleepiness scale. Sleep 1991;14:540–545.

13 Dinges DF, Pack F, Williams K, Gillen KA, Powell JW, Ott GE, Aptowicz C, Pack AI: Cumulative sleepiness, mood disturbance, and psychomotor vigilance performance decrements during a week of sleep restricted to 4–5 hours per night. Sleep 1997;20:267–277.

14 Wiener Testsystem. Mödling, Dr. G. Schuhfried.

15 Findley L, Unverzagt M, Guchu R, Fabrizio M, Buckner J, Suratt P: Vigilance and automobile accidents in patients with sleep apnea or narcolepsy. Chest 1995;108:619–624.

16 Turkington PM, Sircar M, Allgar V, Elliott MW: Relationship between obstructive sleep apnoea, driving simulator performance, and risk of road traffic accidents. Thorax 2001;56: 800–805.

17 Orth M, Leidag M, Kotterba S, Widdig W, de Zeeuw J, Walther JW, Duchna HW, Schafer D, Schlafke ME, Malin JP, Schultze-Werninghaus G, Rasche K: Estimation of accident risk in obstructive sleep apnea syndrome (OSAS) by driving simulation. Pneumologie 2002;56: 13–18.

18 Wilhelm B, Rühle KH, Widmaier D, Lüdtke H, Wilhelm H: Objektiverung von Schweregrad und Therapierfolg beim obstruktiven Schlafapnoesyndrom mit dem pupillographischen Schläfrigkeitstest. Somnologie 1998;2: 51–57.

19 Carskadon M, Dement WC, Mitler MM, Roth R, Westbrook PR, Keenan S: Guidelines for the multiple sleep latency test (MSLT): a standard measure of sleepiness. Sleep 1986;9: 519–524.

20 Sangal R, Thomas L, Mitler M: Disorders of excessive sleepiness: treatment improves ability to stay awake but does not reduce sleepiness. Chest 1992;102:699–703.

21 Rechtschaffen A, Kales A: A Manual of Standardized Terminology, Techniques, and Scoring Systems for Sleep Stages of Human Subjects. Washington, US Government Printing Office, 1968.

22 Arand D, Bonnet M, Hurwitz T, Mitler M, Rosa R, Sangal RB: The clinical use of the MSLT and MWT. Sleep 2005;28:123–144.

23 Banks S, Catcheside P, Lack LC, Grunstein RR, McEvoy D: The maintenance of wakefulness test and driving simulator performance. Sleep 2005;28:1381–1385.

Holger Hein, MD
Bahnhofstr. 9
DE–21465 Reinbek (Germany)
Tel. +49 40 722 8393, Fax +49 40 722 8466
E-Mail dr.holger.hein@web.de

Randerath WJ, Sanner BM, Somers VK (eds): Sleep Apnea.
Prog Respir Res. Basel, Karger, 2006, vol 35, pp 47–50

Portable Monitoring Systems

Holger Hein

Praxis für Innere Medizin, Pneumologie, Allergologie und Schlafmedizin, Reinbek, Germany

Abstract

Portable monitoring systems may be useful for the diagnosis of moderate to severe obstructive sleep-related respiratory disorders, in the case of an attended measurement. Attended polysomnography is considered to be the gold standard. Three different levels of portable monitoring systems are in use: unattended polysomnography, polygraphy with the recording of at least 3 cardiorespiratory parameters and body posture, recording of oxygen saturation and one other parameter. Since no high-evidence studies are available, unattended polysomnography is not generally recommended either for the detection or the exclusion of sleep-related breathing disorders. An exception is attended polygraphy (level 3: recording of at least cardiorespiratory parameters and body posture) in the case of detecting sleep-related respiratory disorders with an apnea-hypopnea index >15/h. Careful manual evaluation of the recorded curves and the absence of concomitant diseases (e.g. COPD, cardiac insufficiency) are a precondition. Neither unattended ambulatory polygraphy (recording of at least three cardiorespiratory parameters and body posture) nor attended or unattended recording of oxygen saturation and one further parameter are suitable for the exclusion or confirmation of a sleep-related respiratory disorder with an apnea-hypopnea index <15/h. All portable monitoring systems are not suitable for split-night studies. Interpretation of the recorded values requires a good knowledge of the patient's history and symptoms. Portable monitoring systems should be applied only by properly trained staff. For follow-up examinations of patients with sleep-related respiratory disorders there are no high-evidence studies available. For the detection of central sleep-related respiratory disorders and hypoventilation syndromes there are also no high-evidence studies available.

Therapy-requiring sleep-related respiratory disorders in childhood have a reported incidence of approximately 2% [1], and in adulthood of some 2% of women and 4% of men aged between 30 and 60 years [2]. Sleep-related breathing disorders manifest in three different forms [3]:

- obstructive sleep apnea syndrome,
- central sleep apnea syndrome,
- sleep-hypoventilation syndrome.

In the case of obstructive sleep apnea syndrome, repeated constrictions of the pharynx lead to:

- vibrations of the walls of the pharynx, audible as snoring;
- partial occlusion manifesting as hypopnea or breathing-related arousal;
- complete obstruction (apnea).

The diagnosis of obstructive sleep apnea syndrome is established whenever respiratory events occur more frequently than 15/h of sleep, or if more than 5 events/h are observed and clinical symptoms indicative of nonrefreshing sleep are present [3, 4]. In the case of the central sleep apnea syndrome, at least ten cessations of breathing per hour of sleep are recorded, each of which lasting for at least 10 s and characterized by an absence of ventilatory effort [3, 4]. In the sleep-hypoventilation syndromes, primary disorders of breathing regulation or secondary sequelae of diseases of the lungs, thorax or respiratory muscles result in lengthy nocturnal desaturations or nocturnal increases in $PaCO_2 > 10$ mm Hg as compared with the values measured in the wake, recumbent patient [3, 4].

To diagnose the above-mentioned diseases, it is necessary to record, continuously and throughout the night, the respiratory movements, respiratory flow, oxygen saturation of the blood, and where indicated the carbon dioxide concentration in the blood, snoring, ECG, sleep stages and body posture under simultaneous video monitoring. In the event of specific medical questions, further functions are additionally continuously recorded. All these measurements require prior biocalibration. The measuring sensors must be accurately placed and must remain in position for the entire measurement. For this reason placement of the sensors and implementation of the measurement must be carried out by qualified staff, who must be present throughout the entire night to monitor possible sensor displacement and to make necessary corrections. Since the signs of nonrefreshing sleep are also of central importance for the diagnosis and symptom-oriented assessment of severity, they must be accurately recorded and described.

Ideally, ambulatory measurements should enable the entire spectrum of the above-mentioned disorders to be identified. In order to achieve this, measurements of respiration, sleep and cardiovascular function are important. Many of the above-mentioned parameters can, however, be recorded only with considerable technical effort. This therefore limits the information yield of ambulatory measurements. The term portable monitoring encompasses a wide range of devices that can record as many signals as does attended polysomnography, or only one signal, such as oximetry [5]. On the other hand, less effort is required to obtain ambulatory measurements, which also enable the investigation of large groups of persons at acceptable cost [6].

A task force of experts from different fields of sleep medicine summarized 2003 and 2004 recommendations for the use of portable monitoring in the investigation of suspected sleep apnea in adults. These recommendations are a thorough evidence-based review of available publications. The results were published by the American Academy of Sleep Medicine, the American Thoracic Society and the American College of Chest Physicians [5, 6]. Four levels are distinguishable in the diagnosis and differential diagnosis of sleep-related breathing disorders: level 1, attended polysomnography; level 2, unattended polysomnography; level 3, polygraphy with the recording of at least 3 cardiorespiratory parameters and body posture; level 4, recording of oxygen saturation and one other parameter.

Attended polysomnography (level 1) is considered to be the gold standard [7–9]. The information yield of the other approaches is therefore measured against the results of polysomnography performed in the sleep laboratory.

For all the diagnostic approaches listed above, the proviso applies that the results obtained must be evaluated only in the light of a knowledge of the patient's history and current complaints. The curves recorded must be checked manually, validated and evaluated. The recording methods employed have a considerable influence on the quality of the curves obtained and thus on the validity of the results. The best signal for the determination of respiratory flow is provided by a pneumotachograph. With the portable monitoring systems, however, this method is not employed; in most cases, a thermistor is used, but its signal provides only qualitative data. The course of the nasal pressure, in contrast, provides a quantitative assessment of respiratory flow and also permits identification of a pathophysiologically and clinically relevant flow limitation [10]. The number of apneas and hypopneas detected is greatly influenced by the definition of respiratory flow reduction [11]. In comparison with normal respiration, flow reductions of 30–80% have been described for hypopneas. Occasionally, the definition of hypopnea requires a subsequent decrease in oxygen saturation of 2%, in some cases of 3%, and in others of 4% [9]. It would therefore appear to make good sense to use the standard of a 3% desaturation supported by the American Academy of Sleep Medicine as a basis for the evaluation [4]. Hypopneas resulting merely in arousals but not desaturations cannot be identified by level 3 or level 4 ambulatory monitoring systems, since no EEG signals are obtained.

The sole validated method for measuring respiratory movements is induction plethysmography. However, it is only rarely employed in portable monitoring systems. In most cases, strain gauges with built-in piezo crystals – rarely, pressure tubes – are employed.

The measured values obtained for oxygen saturation largely depend on the method used and the subsequent processing of the signals. Some devices provide the directly measured value for each pulse beat, while others provide mean values for time periods varying between 3 and 12 s; yet, others give mean values for several pulse beats. Information on the minimum oxygen saturation, the number and extent of saturation decreases, and the detection of artifacts is of critical importance. Owing to the S-shaped course of the oxygen-binding curve, the evaluation of desaturations in patients with prior reduced basal oxygen saturation (e.g. COPD) is not only very difficult, but also of particular importance. Studies on the sensitivity and specificity of ambulatory monitoring in these groups have not been carried out. Snoring signals are recorded in some systems with a microphone, while in others they are derived from the nasal pressure curves. Studies to validate the signals have not been carried out to date.

Of decisive importance for the evaluation of the usefulness of portable monitoring systems is the agreement of the results with those of the diagnostic gold standard, i.e. with polysomnography. The determination of a Pearson correlation coefficient is of limited usefulness, since only an association, but not an agreement, is thereby described. The determination of the difference in measured values using the method described by Bland and Altman is superior [12]. Since the likelihood of identifying or excluding a disease depends not only on sensitivity and specificity but also on the prevalence of the disease, the ratios of sensitivity and of frequency of false-positive and false-negative test results are used to calculate a likelihood ratio for a positive test. A likelihood ratio of 1.0 signifies that the gold standard and the compared test are equally likely to identify the disease. In an analogous manner, the specificity can be used to determine the likelihood that a sleep-related respiratory disorder can be excluded by portable monitoring systems [9, 13]. In a systematic review of English-language studies, these likelihood ratios were calculated. In that review, as well as in the recommendations of the American Thoracic Society [5], the following conclusions were drawn:

1 Level 2 examinations (unattended polysomnography): Since no high-evidence studies are available, this method is not recommended, either for the detection or the exclusion of sleep-related breathing disorders.
2 Level 3 examinations, staff-monitored in the laboratory (polygraphy with recording of at least cardiorespiratory parameters and body posture): These are suitable for detecting sleep-related respiratory disorders with an apnea-hypopnea index (AHI) >15/h. This applies under the following provisos:
   - careful manual evaluation of the recorded curves,
   - the evaluator must be able to assess the device employed, and in particular the limitations of the sensor system used,
   - the evaluator should have a good knowlodge of sleep medicine,
   - the patients should be free of such concomitant diseases as COPD and cardiac insufficiency,
   - since sleep is not measured, the respiratory disturbance index (RDI) may be smaller than the AHI measured by polysomnography,
   - it must be ensured that patients experiencing non-refreshing sleep and with an RDI <15/h will be submitted to further investigations by polysomnography in the sleep laboratory,
   - any CPAP titration that might be necessary must be done under polysomnography control,
   - level 3 examinations are not suitable for split-night studies.
3 Level 3 examinations, unattended (ambulatory polygraph with recording of at least three cardiorespiratory parameters and body posture): This is not suitable for the exclusion or confirmation of a sleep-related respiratory disorder with an AHI< or >15/h.
4 Level 4 examinations, attended or unattended (recording of oxygen saturation and one further parameter): This is not suitable for the exclusion or confirmation of a sleep-related respiratory disorder with an AHI< or >15/h.

A critical health-economic comparison of costs associated with the use of polysomnography or portable monitoring systems for the diagnosis and treatment of sleep-related respiratory disorders revealed an advantage of 13.431 USD/QALY for polysomnography. According to this cost-utility analysis of a hypothetical cohort of persons suspected of having obstructive sleep apnea, the use of portable monitoring systems may result in the establishment of an incorrect diagnosis and inappropriate treatment, and thus cause the above-mentioned costs. Using polysomnography as the gold standard, a level 3 home study would misclassify 5.2% of all patients. A diagnosis based solely on clinical data would be incorrect for 15% of all [14].

A promising new method for the detection of sleep apnea is whole-body impedance cardiography (ICGWB). These signals could be a by-product of 24-hour ECG measurements. Obstructive apneas, central apneas and hypopneas all cause characteristic patterns in the ICGWB tracing. A study which compared simultaneous whole-night ICGWB with standard polysomnographic recordings revealed a sensitivity of 89% and a specificity of 80% [15] for patients with an AHI >15/h. It seems that ICGWB signal includes valuable physiological information that can be effectively used for the detection of sleep apnea episodes. The method is promising in cases where the multichannel polysomnography is not applicable or when ICGWB is used for hemodynamic monitoring in seriously ill and postoperative patients.

The question whether follow-up examinations of patients with sleep-related respiratory disorders are possible with level 3 recordings was seldom an issue. One study analyzed the use of ambulatory monitoring devices for the home management of patients with severe sleep apnea (AHI 41 ± 17.5/h). The authors concluded that they were able to diagnose and treat these patients in an entirely outpatient setting [16]. High-evidence studies are not available, and there are also no studies of patients with less severe diseases.

In summary, portable monitoring systems may be useful only for the diagnosis or exclusion of severe obstructive sleep-related respiratory disorders. Patients with a symptom of unrefreshing sleep should be further evaluated by polysomnography. For the detection of central sleep-related respiratory disorders and hypoventilation syndromes there are no high-evidence studies available. All portable monitoring systems are not suitable for split-night studies. Interpretation of the recorded values requires a good knowledge of the patient's history and symptoms. Portable monitoring systems should be applied only by properly trained staff.

References

1 Section on Pediatric Pulmonology, Subcommittee on Obstructive Sleep Apnea Syndrome. American Academy of Pediatrics: Clinical practice guideline: diagnosis and management of childhood obstructive sleep apnea syndrome. Pediatrics 2002;109:704–712.

2 Young T, Palta M, Dempsey J, Skatrud J, Weber S, Badr S: The occurrence of sleep-disordered breathing among middle-aged adults. N Engl J Med 1993;328:1230–1235.

3 American Academy of Sleep Medicine: International Classification of Sleep Disorders, ed 2: Diagnostic and Coding Manual. Westchester, American Academy of Sleep Medicine, 2005.

4 American Academy of Sleep Medicine Task Force: Sleep-related breathing disorders in adults: recommendations for syndrome definition and measurement techniques in clinical research. Sleep 1999;22:667–689.

5 ATS/ACCP/AASM Taskforce Steering Committee: Executive summary on the systematic review and practice parameters for portable monitoring in the investigation of suspected sleep apnea in adults. Am J Respir Crit Care Med 2004;169:1160–1163.

6 Chesson AL Jr, Berry RB, Pack A; American Academy of Sleep Medicine; American Thoracic Society; American College of Chest Physicians: Practice parameters for the use of portable monitoring devices in the investigation of suspected obstructive sleep apnea in adults. Sleep 2003;26:907–913.

7 Penzel T, Hajak G, Hoffmann RM, Lund R, Podszus T, Pollmächer T, Schäfer T, Schulz H, Sonnenschein W, Spieweg I: Empfehlungen zur Durchführung und Auswertung polygraphischer Ableitungen im diagnostischen Schlaflabor. Ztschr EEG EMG 1993;24:65–70.

8 Chesson AL Jr, Ferber RA, Fry JM, Grigg-Damberger M, Hartse KM, Hurwitz TD, Johnson S, Kader GA, Littner M, Rosen G, Sangal RB, Schmidt-Nowara W, Sher A: The indications for polysomnography and related procedures. Sleep 1997;20:423–487.

9 Flemons WW, Littner MR, Rowley JA, Gay P, Anderson WM, Hudgel DW, McEvoy RD, Loube DI: Home diagnosis of sleep apnea: a systematic review of the literature. An evidence review cosponsored by the American Academy of Sleep Medicine, the American College of Chest Physicians, and the American Thoracic Society. Chest 2003;124:1535–1542.

10 Norman RG, Ahmed MM, Walsleben JA, Rapoport DM: Detection of respiratory events during NPSG: nasal cannula/pressure sensor versus thermistor. Sleep 1997;20:1175–1184.

11 Redline S, Sanders M: Hypopnea, a floating metric: implications for prevalence, morbid ity estimates and case finding. Sleep 1997;20: 1209–1217.

12 Bland JM, Altman DG: Statistical methods for assessing agreement between two methods of clinical measurement. Lancet 1986;1:307–310.

13 Flemons WW, Littner MR: Measuring agreement between diagnostic devices. Chest 2003;124:1535–1542.

14 Chervin RD, Murman DL, Malow BA, Totten V: Cost-utility of three approaches to the diagnosis of sleep apnea: polysomnography, home testing, and empirical therapy. Ann Intern Med 1999;130:496–505.

15 Saarelainen S, Himanen SL, Hasan J, Virkkala J, Koobi T: Whole-body impedance recording a practical method for the diagnosis of sleep apnoea. Clin Physiol Funct Imaging 2003; 23:110–113.

16 Coppola MP, Lawee M: Management of obstructive sleep apnea syndrome in the home. The role of portable sleep apnea recording. Chest 1993;104:19–25.

Holger Hein, MD
Bahnhofstr. 9
DE–21465 Reinbek (Germany)
Tel. +49 40 722 8393, Fax +49 40 722 8466
E-Mail dr.holger.hein@web.de

Randerath WJ, Sanner BM, Somers VK (eds): Sleep Apnea.
Prog Respir Res. Basel, Karger, 2006, vol 35, pp 51–60

Polysomnography

Thomas Penzel   Sebastian Canisius

Department of Internal Medicine, Sleep Laboratory, Hospital of Philipps University, Marburg, Germany

Abstract

The method for the definite diagnosis of disordered breathing during sleep is cardiorespiratory polysomnography. It was introduced in the 1980s and is now the accepted standard. Cardiorespiratory polysomnography includes the recording of sleep signals, respiratory effort, muscle movement and cardiovascular signals. For these signals, different electrodes and sensors are available with some being better than others but also more expensive. Evaluation of polysomnography is based on a number of rules all focusing on visual evaluation of the traces. For sleep, the visual evaluation according to the recommendations of Rechtschaffen and Kales is the gold standard. For respiration and movement there are recommendations compiled by committees of the American Academy of Sleep Medicine. Computer-based polysomnography supports the sleep expert primarily in the monitoring, recording, and archiving tasks. In addition, it tries to help with automated analysis of sleep, respiration, and movement. These methods have not replaced visual evaluation methods until now because the results of automatic scoring do not meet the results of visual scoring in a satisfying manner. Currently, the definitions for visual sleep stage scoring are reassessed. The revised definitions will improve the basis for the development of computer-based algorithms by being more procedural. Then an automatic analysis can achieve better validity compared to visual expert evaluation.

The sleep EEG recording is the core part with the longest tradition of cardiorespiratory polysomnography [1]. Cardiorespiratory polysomnography consists of a set of established signals recorded on a polygraph. Based on cardiorespiratory polysomnography, most common sleep disorders can be diagnosed [2]. The success of treatment studies can be evaluated successfully. Cardiorespiratory polysomnography is performed in a sleep laboratory attended by trained personnel using a polygraph. The polygraph is mostly a digital system and has five distinct tasks related to polysomnography:

(1) Amplification and monitoring of signals from different electrodes, transducers, and sensors during sleep for continuous signal acquisition, detection of unexpected events and continuous quality control. The monitoring mode displays signals in adequate time and amplitude resolution and must allow notes to be added to the data displayed online.

(2) Recording of signals together with notes and comments on the digital media with appropriate resolution for later accessibility (with previous equipment, recordings were made on paper).

(3) Visualization of recorded data for review and classification purposes, support of classification task (e.g. visual marking of events and scoring of sleep stages) in order to draw diagnostic conclusions.

(4) In order to support the evaluation of data, many computer-based polygraphs provide software to analyze the sleep recordings with programs to determine sleep stages, arousals, respiratory, cardiac, and movement-related events.

(5) The polygraph should support procedures for archiving recorded sleep data as well as archiving summarizing

Table 1. Signals required for cardiorespiratory polysomnography: mandatory and optional signals are indicated

Function	Signal	Mandatory/ optional	Method
Sleep	EEG (2 leads)	M	Electrophysiological electrodes
	EOG (2 leads)	M	Electrophysiological electrodes
	EMG submentalis (1 lead)	M	Electrophysiological electrodes
Respiration	Oronasal airflow	M	Thermistor, thermocouple probe, differential pressure
	Ribcage and abdominal movement (2 leads)	M	Piezo sensors, impedance or inductance plethysmography
	Snoring noise	O	Microphone, pressure swings, foil sensors
	Oxygen saturation	M	Pulse oximetry
	Esophageal pressure	O	Pressure sensors
	Blood gases, end-tidal pCO_2	O	Transcutaneous O_2 and CO_2 partial pressure sensors, ultrared absorption spectroscopy (URAS)
	Mask pressure on ventilation	O	Pressure transducer
Cardiovascular	ECG, heart rate	M	Electrophysiological electrodes
	Arterial blood pressure	O	Pressure transducers, indirect techniques
Movement	EMG tibialis (2 leads for the legs)	M	Electrophysiological electrodes
Position, movement	Body position	M	Switches, mechanical
Brain, neurology	EEG (multiple leads)	O	Electrophysiological electrodes
Gastrointestinal system	Esophageal pH	O	pH sensor
Circadian system	Core body temperature	O	Thermistor, thermocouple probe
Behavior	Video, audio	M	Camera, microphone

reports. This can be done with the help of a database for patients investigated in the sleep laboratory.

Cardiorespiratory polysomnography requires a minimum of 12 physiological signals [4]. These signals are indicated in table 1 as mandatory (fig. 1). The specific selection of optional signals recorded in a sleep study depends on the physiological function of interest. Audiovisual recording is part of polysomnography using a video camera and a room microphone in the sleep lab. Notes on patient behavior are taken by the attending personnel throughout night.

Sleep Recording

To recognize the sleep stages with the help of cardiorespiratory polysomnography, the recording always requires electrophysiological signals for the visualization. The minimum set of signals has been described in full detail in the recommendations of Rechtschaffen and Kales [6]. The minimum requires one EEG lead with electrodes placed either at C3-A2 or C4-A1 according to the 10–20 system for placement of electroencephalography electrodes on the skull. It is well established to have at least one second EEG lead in order to have an alternative signal if one lead loses its quality during the night. For better sleep evaluation, three leads are preferable, reflecting frontal, central and occipital EEG activity. Two EOG leads are always needed. Often they are abbreviated as ROC (right outer cantus) and LOC (left outer cantus). The electrodes are arranged in such a way that the eyeball movements result in signals going in opposite deflections whereas head movement and EEG artifacts result in signals going in the same deflection. One EMG lead is required on the chin. The chin muscles

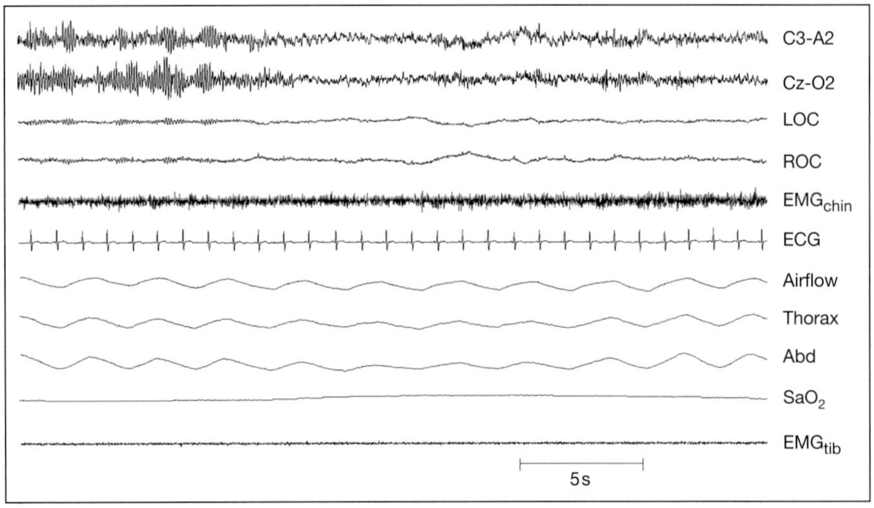

Fig. 1. An example of signals recorded in a sleep laboratory exactly as required by the standards for cardiorespiratory polysomnography. The example presents 30 s, which corresponds to one epoch. Looking at the EEG, it is visible that the epoch contains just the beginning of falling asleep. On the left side alpha waves are still visible and then theta waves follow. The eye movements start with slow eye movements. Respiration is regular.

present a perfect signal to record muscle tone in general. Based on these signals, a visual sleep scoring can be done. The rules for sleep scoring are also given by the recommendations of Rechtschaffen and Kales [6]. According to this manual, it is possible to distinguish the sleep stages wake, REM sleep, and NREM sleep stages 1–4. NREM sleep stages 1 and 2 are summarized as 'light sleep' and stages 3 and 4 are summarized as 'deep sleep' or 'slow-wave sleep' due to the dominance of slow delta waves in the EEG. This sleep scoring is performed for time episodes of either 20 or 30 s duration which are called 'epochs'. An 8-hour sleep consists of 960 30-second epochs to be classified visually. The visual sleep stage scoring according to the rules of Rechtschaffen and Kales [6] is regarded as the gold standard for sleep classification. Besides the scoring of sleep stages, interruptions of sleep, or central nervous activations, so-called arousals from sleep are evaluated and counted [7]. An arousal is an increase in EEG frequencies for at least 3 s and less than 15 s. It may occur during any sleep stage. During REM sleep there is an additional increase in EMG muscle tone. A certain number of arousals often associated with changes in body position is found during normal sleep. An excessive number of arousals does disturb sleep considerably and needs to be documented.

Respiratory Signal Recording

To detect sleep-related breathing disorders, it is necessary to record oronasal airflow, respiratory movements with two independent signals at the ribcage and the abdomen, and the effect of respiration reflected by blood gases (fig. 2). The most convenient way to record blood gases is pulse oximetry. The gold standard to record respiration is the quantitative recording of airflow using a pneumotachograph with a closed face mask [8]. This airflow measurement is combined with the quantitative recording of respiratory effort using intrathoracic pressure changes with an esophageal pressure transducer [9]. Both these methods have the trade-off of not being very comfortable for the patient and in addition they may disturb sleep. Therefore, usually less intrusive and less accurate methods are used for the recording of respiration. Among the less intrusive methods, pressure transducers appear to be best for airflow and inductive plethysmography for respiratory effort. The pressure transducers measure air pressure with nasal prongs. Between absolute flow values and pressure there is a quadratic relationship which can be considered using dedicated amplifiers or post-acquisition correction by algorithms. Inductive plethysmography is the best noninvasive method for respiratory effort because the principle is based on frequency changes in a coil around the body. The change in signal is proportional to the enclosed area which is much closer to actual changes in lung volume than other methods. Most other respiratory belts use piezo elements which only assess changes in length or circumference of the chest and the abdomen. In addition, the small piezo sensors pick up changes only at a small part of the respiratory belt and therefore these signals often have small amplitudes and are confounded with artifacts (e.g. body movements, cardiogenic movements).

The respiratory signals are used to detect events of sleep-related breathing disorders such as apneas and hypopneas. If the respiratory flow is reduced to less than 50% of

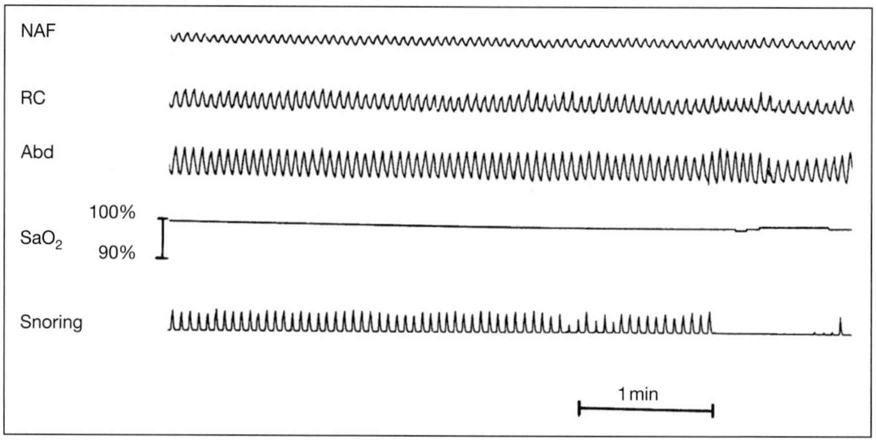

Fig. 2. The recording example demonstrates the respiratory signals in a compressed visualization for better classification of sleep-related breathing disorders. The example shows normal respiration during sleep with snoring during most of the time (NAF = nasal airflow, RC = ribcage, Abd = abdominal movements). Inductive plethysmography has been used for respiratory movement recording.

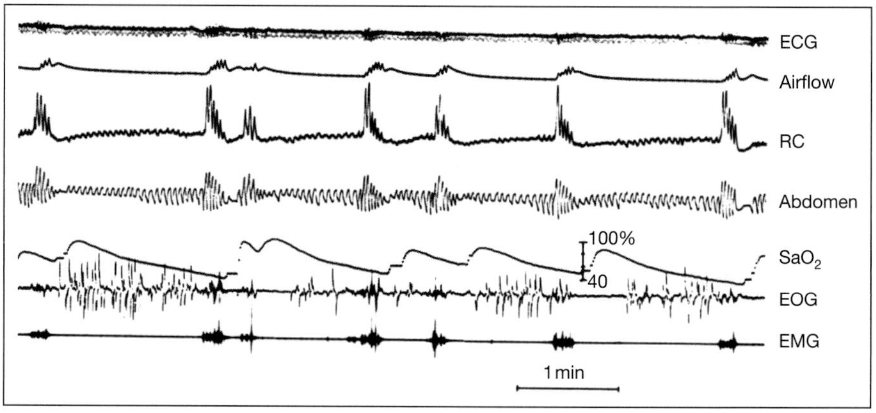

Fig. 3. The recording example shows a sequence of obstructive sleep apnea events in an even more compressed recording. This period depicts REM sleep as can be seen from the eye movements. It is very typical for sleep apnea events during REM sleep to observe long events with severe oxygen desaturation followed by short events with less desaturation in an irregular sequence. The recording method and the signal labels are the same as in figure 2.

normal flow, then the event is classified as hypoventilation or hypopnea. If the flow is zero then the event is classified as an apnea. After that, the events are sub-classified into either obstructive, mixed or central events. Obstructive events exhibit respiratory cessation of airflow with ongoing respiratory effort. This ongoing respiratory effort can be recognized by respiratory movements in opposite directions at the chest and the abdomen belt. Central events exhibit respiratory cessation of airflow with no respiratory effort in either belt. If cessations of airflow have some initial seconds without and some subsequent seconds with respiratory effort movements then the event is called a mixed apnea or hypopnea (fig. 3).

A tracheal microphone or as a less favorable alternative a room microphone to pick up snoring noise serves as an indirect way to detect partial upper airway obstruction during sleep. A complete obstruction cannot be detected because then no sound is produced. Simple piezo microphones are sufficient to pick up snoring noise. For subsequent interpretation, the microphone recordings are only interpreted in terms of relative loudness and therefore the recording of this signal does not need to preserve sound signal characteristics.

The recording of blood gases is usually limited to pulse oximetry. Pulse oximetry can detect changes in oxygen saturation by evaluating the light extinction of hemoglobin either using transmission or reflection of red and infrared light. The time course of oxygen saturation allows the easiest detection of apnea and hypopnea events. Unfortunately, results vary depending on the manufacturer of the pulse oximeter and the device settings [11]. In a considerable number of patients, the interpretation of oxygen saturation is limited. Due to the oxygen-binding curve oxygen saturation may not show clear drops with apnea or hypopnea events in a patient with a healthy lung and a very high blood gas baseline. In patients with additional lung diseases (e.g. chronic obstructive pulmonary disease or alveolar hypoventilation), the baseline oxygen saturation may be low even when awake. In these patients, it is difficult to detect apnea-related desaturation events based on the time course of oxygen saturation.

A better interpretation of the blood gases situation is obtained by the investigation of CO_2 in patients with chronic obstructive pulmonary disease or with alveolar hypoventilation during sleep. The recording of CO_2 is done using a capnography based on the ultra-red absorption spectroscopy (URAS). The derived readings are end-tidal CO_2 values. The disadvantage of this method is impairment of patient sleep comfort due to the need for a mask or a small tube inserted in the exhaled air. Another disadvantage is that CO_2 cannot be analyzed during the course of an apnea because there is no airflow. Only after the end of an apnea when breathing is resumed can end-tidal CO_2 be determined.

In small children with disordered breathing during sleep, the monitoring of blood gases is very useful. The recording of blood gases is best done with transcutaneous pO_2 and pCO_2 partial pressure electrodes. The technique uses heated electrodes on the skin and the electrodes have to be attached carefully because placement and sensor temperature are important modifiers for signal quality. If the sensor is placed correctly then the time course of the signal is reliable and it usually exhibits a constant offset compared to partial pressure pO_2 and pCO_2 values taken by a blood sample. Since the electrodes are heated at 43°C, their position needs to be changed every 90 min or alternatively two electrodes are applied and the heating is switched between the two. Due to these practical limitations, this technique is rarely used in adults.

Patients with sleep-related breathing disorders are most often treated with a ventilation therapy applied by a nasal mask. If a cardiorespiratory polysomnography is conducted as a ventilation therapy control study in a patient using CPAP, BiPAP or similar devices, it is most feasible to record the applied air pressure at the nasal mask continuously. The fluctuations observed in the air pressure signals can serve as a very good alternative to a thermistor or thermocouple respiration signal. In addition, if the pressure transducer has a rapid pressure response which allows the detection of high frequency pressure fluctuations, then these can be evaluated in terms of snoring persisting under ventilation therapy.

Cardiorespiratory Signal Recording

Usually one lead of ECG is recorded during cardiorespiratory polysomnography. This can be used to derive heart rate and may give hints on the presence of arrhythmias. ECG and heart rate are also used to investigate sleep-related transient tachycardia or bradycardia. Some arrhythmias may be associated with specific sleep stages, e.g. REM sleep. Heart rate changes are very characteristic for sleep apnea. Along with each apnea event, a relative bradycardia followed by a relative tachycardia is observed. This pattern has been described as a cyclical variation of heart rate [12]. Changes in heart rate also occur with arousal from sleep. Central nervous activations cause an increase in heart rate.

Even if there are guidelines for regular 12-lead ECG and Holter ECG recordings there are no established evaluation guidelines for the recording of ECG during sleep. It is possible to refer to general long-term ECG analysis if sampling rate and leads are chosen according to those criteria. This would require the recording of at least two leads of ECG.

The recording of blood pressure has major importance for sleep recordings because elevated blood pressure presents the direct link to cardiovascular consequences of sleep disorders. Several studies proved that obstructive sleep apnea is an independent risk factor to develop daytime hypertension with an increased morbidity and mortality. Blood pressure shows immediate rises with events of apnea and shows impressive changes associated with sleep stages.

Unfortunately, most measurement methods either disturb sleep or are invasive. Therefore, no method has been established as a gold standard for sleep so far. The method used most is blood pressure readings using periodic arm cuff inflations. These arm cuff inflations disturb sleep quite often. As a consequence, the blood pressure readings more often present readings for nocturnal awakening than for continuous sleep. Also, the arm cuff readings cannot keep track of such rapid blood pressure changes as are observed in sleep apnea and during arousals. The finger photoplethysmography method provides a continuous blood pressure signal derived from one (e.g. Finapres) or two inflated finger cuffs (e.g. Portapres). The signal proved to have high reliability but the finger cuffs create some discomfort because the venous return of blood flow is reduced and this may disturb sleep as well. The gold standard for blood pressure is the invasive arterial line pressure recording. This requires intensive care-like settings and is used in few and very specific sleep laboratory studies only.

Movement Recording

For limb movement recording, the gold standard is to record the EMG at the m. tibialis with two ECG electrodes placed 5 cm apart on the skin of the lower leg where the m. tibialis is found [5, 13]. It is recommended to record both legs with two bipolar EMG leads. The required minimum is one EMG leg recording.

Body Position Recording

The recording of body position is essential because body position may modify many sleep disorders. In a number of patients sleep-related breathing disorders occur in one body position only. Therefore, it is useful to keep track of this modifier and present the results in the sleep lab report. Simple sensors code the angle of the body into a continuous voltage. Other transducers use miniature contacts to convert an angle into a voltage or a digital code. Switch or contact based sensors are usually able to code not only the angle but also upright or supine position. This is very useful in order to have an indirect indication for patient behavior based on a biosignal besides observation.

Optional Signal Recording

Optional signals are selected according to the disorders to be diagnosed in a particular patient. Mostly, additional EEG leads are used. Additional EEG leads are useful to see the spatial distribution of sleep-related EEG patterns. The additional EEG leads are indispensable in the case of sleep-related epilepsy or other neurological disorders with associated sleep disturbance.

In patients with complaints of gastroesophageal reflux during the night, it is useful to record esophageal pH to verify whether gastric acid reflux events occur during the night and whether they are related to nocturnal awakening. A reflux event is defined as a drop in esophageal pH <4 for at least 30 s duration. It is common to find nocturnal reflux events in patients with such complaints. Few patients without complaints of esophageal reflux experience such events during the night. The majority of the nocturnal gastroesophageal reflux events are observed during awakening from sleep or are associated with an arousal event during sleep. Very few events are found during undisturbed sleep without any arousal. The potential danger of nocturnal reflux events is that the natural esophageal clearance during sleep is much slower due to the reduced motor activity of the esophagus and due to lying in a horizontal position.

If disorders of the circadian rhythm are investigated, the recording of core body temperature can give insights on the actual circadian phase of the patient [14]. Core body temperature is closely linked to the circadian system and its recording will allow the evaluation of jet lag and delayed or advanced sleep phase problems. The normal difference between maximum and minimum body temperature in the diurnal rhythm is close to 0.5°C. Rectal or ear temperature probes are most appropriate. Body temperature depends much on physical activity, postural changes, psychological excitement, type of food, and environmental conditions. Therefore, a scientifically correct and undisturbed recording of body temperature requires a standardized setting usually not available in a clinical routine sleep laboratory. High quality body temperature recording requires a 'constant routine' protocol with a well-defined reduction of all external zeitgebers. This means a constant low level of light, a protein-reduced food given at fixed intervals during the day and night, isolation from external light and external sound sources, lying in bed for at least 26 h without any activities beside questionnaires and psychophysiological tests.

In addition to the physiological signals, a sleep laboratory should provide the possibility for audiovisual recording of the sleeping subject. Video recording is useful to document sleep apnea events, movement disorders, epileptic seizures or REM sleep behavior disorders with uncontrolled movements during sleep. Usually, patients are not aware of the events occurring during sleep. Talking during sleep can be recorded using an audio channel in this way. The presentation of these recorded events to the patient the next morning can be very helpful to explain the disorder and to educate the patient about the need to use the recommended therapy. This education generally improves compliance with therapy.

Digital Polysomnography

The digital recording of polysomnography follows the requirements concerning sensors and signals as specified above. In addition, some more issues need to be taken into consideration due to the digital recording and storage of signals [15]. A digital polysomnography system must fulfill minimal criteria on quality of digitized signals to obtain a good presentation on computer screens and to enable a solid analysis by subsequent processing. The requirements for sampling rate and minimal sampling rate are given in table 2. When a particular sampling rate is chosen, the appropriate anti-aliasing filter has to be set in addition to the correct electrophysiological filter settings. The digital range of the A/D converter should provide a range of 12 bits or better 16 bits to provide good amplitude resolution.

If signals are presented to a sleep expert on a computer screen, this should follow the guidelines for interpretation by

Table 2. Minimal requirements for digital recording of sleep data

Signal	Quantification per bit	Sampling rate	Filter settings
EEG	0.5 μV (1.0)	200 Hz (100)	0.3–40 Hz
EOG	0.5 μV (1.0)	200 Hz (100)	0.3–40 Hz
EMG	0.5 μV	200 Hz	10–75 Hz
ECG	10 μV	250 Hz (100)	0.3–100 Hz
Blood pressure	1 mm Hg	100 Hz (25)	0.0–40 Hz
Esophageal pressure	1 mm Hg	100 Hz (25)	0.0–40 Hz
Respiration	Arbitrary	25 Hz	–
SpO_2	1%	4 Hz (1)	–
pO_2, pCO_2	0.1 mm Hg	4 Hz (1)	–
Temperature	0.05°C	4 Hz (1)	–

Minimal values are given in parentheses. Common filter settings are specified. A low frequency of 0.0 Hz indicates that the amplifier must preserve the DC component. A '–' indicates that the DC component is most interesting and that the frequency content is not of interest. Internal anti-aliasing should be respected for the acquisition.

Rechtschaffen and Kales [6]. Sleep interpretation can be done in either 20- or 30-second epochs. A sleep spindle has a frequency range of 12–16 Hz and beta waves have frequencies between 16 and 25 Hz. This is usually impossible to distinguish on a computer screen with standard resolution. Therefore, it is recommended to use at least 1,600 × 1,400 pixels resolution for computer monitors installed for sleep EEG monitoring and evaluation.

Computer-Based Sleep Analysis

Almost all currently available sleep recording systems are computer based, usually PCs, and provide help for automatic or at least partial automatic analysis of the sleep recording [16]. Some parts of the signal analysis are straightforward in terms of algorithms whereas others are much more complicated and their results are often not satisfying for the sleep physician.

Automated sleep analysis primarily focuses on the sleep EEG signal. Several analysis algorithms restrict themselves to the analysis of one EEG only. The definition of sleep stages according to the recommendations of Rechtschaffen and Kales [6] require the interpretation of EOG and EMG in addition. Therefore, some but not all sleep analysis software also evaluate EOG and few programs evaluate EMG. The adding of EOG analysis in terms of slow and rapid eye movements improves automatic sleep analysis considerably.

Sleep analysis has to follow a sequence of steps listed here. The analysis of the sleep EEG first requires the removal of artifacts. Artifacts can occur due to many causes. Electrode cable movements are a common cause. Changes in electrode impedance cause waves which can be misinterpreted. Then there may be ECG, EOG and EMG artifacts in the EEG signal. As far as possible these influences have to be removed. The analysis of background sleep EEG activity can follow as a first step to detect sleep stages. The analysis of background activity will quantify the amount of alpha-, beta-, theta- and delta-waves. The analysis of these waves can be any kind of spectral analysis, e.g. Fourier transform, filter banks, or time-domain wave analysis. Overall, the result of this part is usually power in the defined frequency band. The next step is the detection of distinct patterns in the sleep EEG. Such sleep patterns are the K complex, the sleep spindle and the vertex wave. The recognition of these patterns is important, because the occurrence of sleep spindles and K complexes is essential for the definition of sleep stage 2 according to the Rechtschaffen and Kales [6] recommendations. Besides, the number of sleep spindles increases with some specific sleep medications (e.g. benzodiazepines) and therefore their occurrence is of high interest in the later sleep report. After having identified waves and patterns at a high time resolution (a resolution of 1 second appears to be appropriate), the next step is to map these high time and component resolution results to the low time and stage resolution sleep classification as defined by Rechtschaffen and Kales [6]. This means a reduction to five sleep stages (stages 1–4, REM) and a reduction to 30-second epochs. In order to achieve this reduction, many different methods have been applied and tested against each other. No optimum method has been identified. The methods are based on either rules, neural networks, or fuzzy logic approaches [16]. All methods try to mimic the visual classification of Rechtschaffen and Kales [6]. The accuracy of the automatic sleep staging is measured against the visual sleep staging and may come as close as 90% in some studies. Algorithms based on sleep EEG alone do have difficulties to distinguish wake, sleep stage 1, and REM sleep. Many algorithms do have difficulties to distinguish sleep stages 3 and 4 since this is just a gradual difference in the amount of delta waves which meet the amplitude criteria. The biggest advantage of automatic sleep analysis is that it can provide objective and quantitative measures of spectral power in well-defined frequency bands. This way, it is possible to observe small influences on sleep EEG which may not be reflected by rough visual sleep stages evaluation. A good and important example for this is the added information described as sleep spindle density (fig. 4).

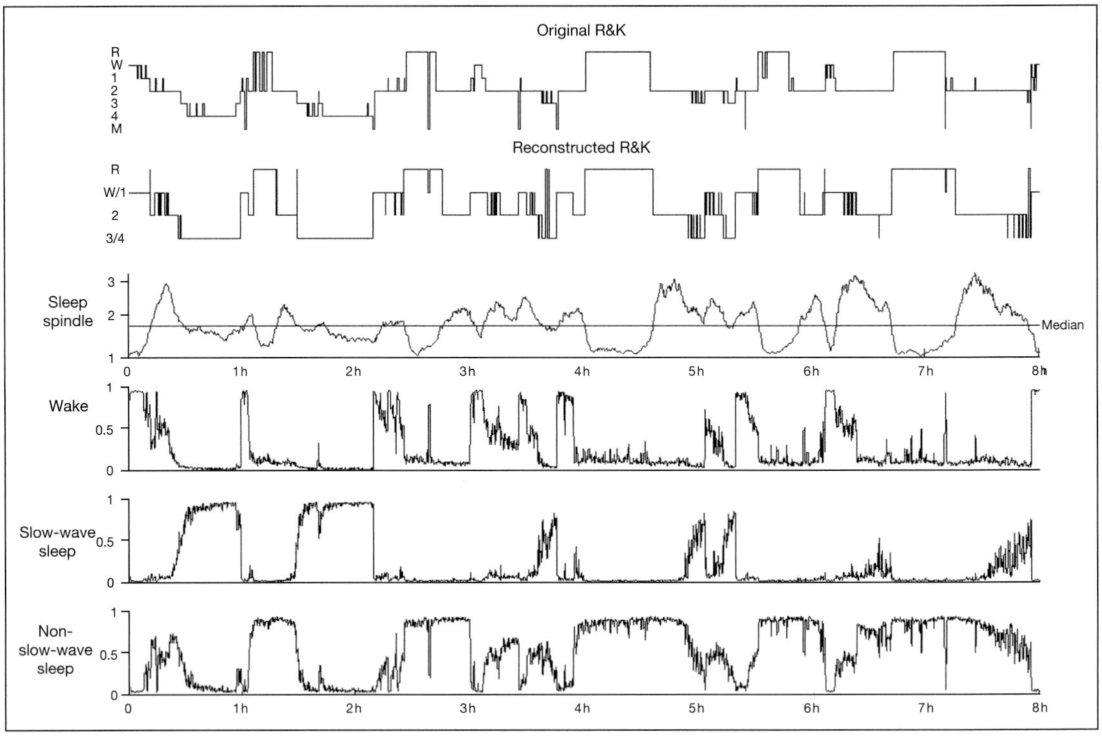

Fig. 4. The automatic sleep evaluation of one night shows the visual sleep staging according to Rechtschaffen and Kales [6] (original R&K) and the automatically determined sleep staging (reconstructed R&K). Below there are continuous parameters calculated from the sleep EEG. These are measures for sleep spindles, for wakefulness or arousal, for slow-wave sleep, and finally the residuum calculates as 1.0 – wake – slow-wave sleep. This residuum is called non-slow-wave sleep in this analysis.

The analysis of respiration is essential for the recognition of sleep-related breathing disorders. The main issue is to identify events of sleep apnea, hypopnea and to distinguish the different categories, such as obstructive, mixed and central apnea. In addition, the oxygen desaturation events need to be counted and evaluated. Recognition and removal of artifacts is the first step in the analysis of respiratory signals. For respiration, the type of analysis depends much on the type of signals, because signal characteristics vary very much with the type of sensors used. Esophageal pressure, inductive plethysmography, impedance plethysmography and piezo belt sensors produce completely different signals. Therefore, the respiratory signal analysis is usually optimized for a specific sensor. After this specification the analysis itself is straightforward. The analysis has to recognize each breath and calculate its amplitude. Based on amplitude criteria, it is possible to define an apnea (amplitude drops to zero) and to define hypopnea (amplitude drops below 50% of normal value) [8]. The minimum event duration is 10 s. The recognized respiratory events are checked by a trained sleep expert in order to adjust amplitude criteria in a specific recording, to reject movement artifacts, changes in posture, and signal quality. The result of the analysis is the total number of apnea and hypopnea events, split according to sleep stages and body positions. As an index of severity the apnea/hypopnea index (AHI) is calculated as the number of apnea and hypopnea events per hour of total sleep time. For oxygen saturation, a similar index is calculated as the oxygen desaturation index (ODI). In addition, baseline oxygen saturation, mean value during sleep, and the time spent with oxygen below 90%, 80%, 70% and so on is calculated. This additional information allows to determine the respiratory implications of apnea and hypopnea events over the course of the night.

Based on a one-lead ECG recording only little analysis is possible. The key task is a very reliable R-wave detection with proper identification of artifacts and ectopic beats. After that, the analysis of the ECG is limited to the calculation of heart rate [17]. Based on the heart rate, periods with low and high heart rate are detected and counted. The thresholds can be set by the user of the analysis system in order to adjust for age and for some concomitant disorders, such as diabetes. In patients with sleep apnea, an additional analysis which identifies the cyclical variation of heart rate associated with sleep-related breathing disorders is very useful. The cyclical variation of heart rate consists of relative bradycardia during each apnea, followed by relative tachycardia during each compensatory hyperventilation. Time-frequency presentations of heart rate variability over the course of the night are very useful to identify this characteristic pattern.

Blood pressure in normal subjects shows a drop in systolic, mean and diastolic values during the night. This is known as the nocturnal blood pressure dip. Analysis to recognize this dip in blood pressure has been implemented in ambulatory blood pressure recording software. No currently available sleep analysis system has such a blood pressure analysis implemented.

The analysis of nocturnal movements in terms of periodic leg movements is straightforward and very reliable since the definitions for scoring of leg movements are unambiguous [13]. Leg movements of at least 0.5 s duration have to be detected from the EMG tibialis. Trains of leg movements with at least 4 events separated by 4–90 s are called periodic leg movements.

The analysis of muscle tone in order to support sleep staging is difficult and no reliable method has been established. Only relative changes in the amplitude of the EMG can be evaluated and the EMG amplitude is often confounded by ambient noise or by ECG artifacts or other movement artifacts. Degrading electrode impedance over the time course of the night has a strong effect on EMG signal quality and this effect is difficult to recognize using automatic analysis.

Data Format Specifications

Digital polysomnography systems store the recorded raw data on the computer disk using a proprietary data format. The exchange of data between sleep laboratories is desirable and can be easily performed using a writable CD-ROM as the exchange media. In addition, data format specifications need to be followed.

A raw data interchange format has gained high acceptability between the sleep laboratories. This data format has been developed within an European Community founded project on sleep in 1989 and therefore it is called European Data Format – EDF [18]. Most systems allow a conversion of their proprietary data format to this exchangeable data format. Some few sleep analyzing systems also allow to import the EDF files. Supportive software for the Matlab and Labview programming environment and free viewing software for the EDF format are available at a web site (http://www.hsr.nl/edf/index.htm).

Limitations of Polysomnography

Evaluation studies have tested the reliability of the gold standard for sleep stage scoring and for respiratory event scoring and for periodic leg movement scoring. Reliability studies can test the reliability of one human scorer for repeated scorings (intra-rater reliability) and the reliability of a human scorer against another human scorer (inter-rater reliability). Experienced scorers with long training are able to produce very similar scorings even after long breaks between a repetition. In these cases, inter-rater reliability is usually above 90% and may reach 96% matching previous results [19]. Often inter-rater scoring is much lower. Only if experienced scorers do work closely together and train each other frequently might they then reach an inter-rater reliability similar to the intra-rater reliability. If they only had one common training session, or eventually none, just using the same published Rechtschaffen and Kales [6] criteria then inter-rater reliability has a mean value of 76% (range 65–85%) in healthy subjects and is lower in patients with sleep-related breathing disorders with a mean value of 71% (range 65–78%) if sleep stages are compared on an epoch by-epoch basis [20]. The highest agreement is found for REM sleep followed by wake, slow-wave sleep (stages 3 and 4) and sleep stage 2 and it is worst for sleep stage 1 [21]. The agreement between scorers also decreases the older the subject being investigated is [21]. Comparative studies therefore underline the need to develop computer-based quantitative sleep analysis with clear and validated criteria.

Since the visual classification of sleep stages according to the recommendations of Rechtschaffen and Kales [6] has its limitations and has a considerable subjective component, any computer-based algorithm to mimic these rules can only come as close as an experienced sleep expert can [16]. A new automatic sleep-staging algorithm is often trained by one sleep expert and therefore comes close to this person but not to other sleep experts [19]. Therefore, the training of an automatic sleep analysis algorithm is crucial for later approval by many sleep experts [21].

Due to the considerable differences between visual sleep scoring and automated sleep analysis, none of the current methods has been accepted as an alternative for visual sleep analysis.

The limited agreement of automatic methods for the detection of sleep stages and sleep-related breathing disorders is also due to the fact that the current definitions of sleep stages and apnea/hypopnea have inherent limitations. In order to overcome these limitations, research has to be performed by applying automated methods and by proving that their results are better suited to solve the medical problems in the patients with sleep disorders. Sleep medicine as a relatively young discipline is still in the process of refining current definitions and therefore there is great potential to improve definitions. Sleep disorders occur at night. But their consequences, sleepiness and not being refreshed, are experienced during the day. Better definitions are found if better correlations between daytime functions and nighttime or sleep features are discovered. The current values derived from Rechtschaffen and Kales [6] sleep stages from counting arousals, apnea and hypopnea events, and periodic leg movements have their limitations exactly here. There are some correlations, but they are not really high. Therefore, any method which improves this correlation will draw major attention in sleep research and sleep medicine.

Reliability in apnea and hypopnea scoring is similar to sleep scoring because the definitions for apnea and hypopnea are fuzzy due to having 'normal breathing' as the reference of amplitude criteria [22]. The scoring of apnea and hypopnea events can be taken as the respiratory events without considering anything else. Then the intraclass correlation coefficient (ICC) according to kappa statistics is moderate, ICC = 0.74 when using the AHI as a measure for comparison. If associated EEG arousals are used for the identification of apnea and hypopnea events, the ICC increases slightly to 0.77. If the apnea and hypopnea events were scored dependent on associated oxygen desaturation events then reliability was highest with an ICC >0.90.

Studies dedicated to the reliability in the scoring of leg movements is much better because the definition of leg movements is rather simple. There the correlation between two scorings are as high as r = 0.98. This confirms at the same time the high reliability for automatic identification of leg movements if an appropriate method is used.

References

1 Block AJ, Cohn MA, Conway WA, Hudgel DW, Powles ACP, Sanders MH, Smith PL: Indications and standards for cardiopulmonary sleep studies. Sleep 1985;8:371–379.

2 Ross SD, Sheinhait IA, Harrison KJ, Kvasz M, Connelly JE, Shea SA, Allen IE: Systematic Review and Meta-analysis of the Literature Regarding the Diagnosis of Sleep Apnea. Sleep 2000;23:519–532.

3 American Thoracic Society (ATS): Indications and standards for cardiopulmonary sleep studies. Am Rev Respir Dis 1989;139:559–568.

4 Penzel T, Hajak G, Hofmann RM, Lund R, Podszus T, Pollmächer T, Schäfer T, Schulz H, Sonnenschein W, Spieweg I: Empfehlungen zur Durchführung und Auswertung polygraphischer Ableitungen im diagnostischen Schlaflabor. Z EEG-EMG 1993;24:65–70.

5 Chesson AL, Wise M, Davila D, Johnson S, Littner M, McDowell Anderson W, Hartse K, Rafecas J: Practice parameters for the treatment of restless legs syndrome and periodic limb movement disorder. Sleep 1999;22:961–968.

6 Rechtschaffen A, Kales A: A Manual of Standardized Terminology, Techniques and Scoring System for Sleep Stages of Human Subjects. NIH Publ No 204. Washington, US Government Printing Office, 1968.

7 American Sleep Disorders Association: EEG arousals: scoring rules and examples. Sleep 1992;15:173–184.

8 American Academy of Sleep Medicine Task Force: Sleep-related breathing disorders in adults: recommendations for syndrome definition and measurement techniques in clinical research. Sleep 1999;22:667–689.

9 Kushida CA, Giacomini A, Lee MK, Guilleminault C, Dement WC: Technical protocol for the use of esophageal manometry in the diagnosis of sleep-related breathing disorders. Sleep Med 2002;3:163–173.

10 Norman RG, Ahmed MM, Walsleben JA, Rapoport DM: Detection of respiratory events during NPSG: nasal cannula/pressure sensor versus thermistor. Sleep 1997;20:1175–1184.

11 Davila DG, Richards KC, Marshall BL, O'Sullivan PS, Gregory TG, Hernandez VJ, Rice SI: Oximeter performance. Chest 2002; 122:1654–1660.

12 Guilleminault C, Connolly S, Winkle R, Melvin K, Tilkian A: Cyclical variation of the heart rate in sleep apnoea syndrome. Lancet 1984;i:126–131.

13 Atlas Task Force of the American Sleep Disorders Association: Recording and scoring of leg movements. Sleep 1993;16:748–759.

14 Kryger M, Roth T, Dement WC: Principles and Practice of Sleep Medicine, ed 3. Philadelphia, Saunders, 2000.

15 Penzel T, Peter JH: Diagnostik von Schlafstörungen und von schlafmedizinischen Erkrankungen – eine Übersicht. Biomed Tech 2003;48:47–54.

16 Penzel T, Conrad R: Computer based sleep analysis. Sleep Med Rev 2000;4:131–148.

17 Task force of the European Society of Cardiology and the North American Society of Pacing and Electrophysiology: Heart rate variability. Standards of measurement, physiological interpretation, and clinical use. Circulation 1996;93:1043–1065.

18 Kemp B, Värri A, Rosa AC, Nielsen KD, Gade J: A simple format for exchange of digitized polygraphic recordings. Electroencephalogr Clin Neurophysiol 1992;82:391–393.

19 Ferri R, Ferri P, Colognola RM, Petrella MA, Musumeci SA, Bergonzi P: Comparison between the results of an automatic and a visual scoring of sleep EEG recordings. Sleep 1989;12:354–362.

20 Norman RG, Pal I, Stewart C, Walsleben JA, Rapoport DM: Interobserver agreement among sleep scorers from different centers in a large dataset. Sleep 2000;23:901–908.

21 Danker-Hopfe H, Kunz D, Gruber G, Klösch G, Lorenzo JL, Himanen SL, Kemp B, Penzel T, Röschke J, Dorn H, Schlögl A, Trenker E, Dorffner G: Interrater reliability between scorers from eight European sleep laboratories in subjects with different sleep disorders. J Sleep Res 2004;13:63–69.

22 Whitney CW, Gottlieb DJ, Redline S, Norman RG, Dodge RR, Shahar E, Surovec S, Nieto FJ: Reliability of scoring respiratory disturbance indices and sleep staging. Sleep 1998; 21:749–757.

T. Penzel, PhD
Department of Internal Medicine, Division of Respiratory Disorders, Sleep Laboratory
Hospital of Philipps University
Baldingerstrasse 1
DE–35033 Marburg (Germany)
Tel. +49 6421 2866435
Fax +49 6421 2865450
E-Mail penzel@med.uni-marburg.de

Randerath WJ, Sanner BM, Somers VK (eds): Sleep Apnea.
Prog Respir Res. Basel, Karger, 2006, vol 35, pp 61–68

Nasal, Lung and Cardiovascular Function Tests

Wolfgang Galetke

Institute for Pneumology at the University Witten/Herdecke, Clinic for Pneumology and Allergology, Center of Sleep Medicine and Respiratory Care, Bethanien Hospital, Solingen, Germany

Abstract

The obstructive sleep apnea syndrome (OSAS) is frequently interrelated to the upper airway, the lung and the cardiovascular system both with regard to pathophysiological aspects and diagnostic tools. Nasal resistance and upper airway muscle activity both contribute to the appearance of apneic events. Impulse oscillometry and esophageal manometry, on the other hand, are diagnostic instruments not included in standard polysomnography, but may help differentiating different patterns of respiratory events. Lung function testing may identify OSAS patients with worse prognosis because of additional hypercapnia or chronic obstructive lung disease. Autonomic nerve activation during apneic events is thought to be the link between obstructive sleep apnea and the development of cardiovascular diseases. Therefore, assessment of autonomic system function plays an important role in OSAS patients. The aim of this chapter is to summarize the most relevant nasal, lung, and cardiovascular function tests and to discuss their indications and limitations. Finally, the assessment of sleep-related erections in the context of sleep apnea will be discussed.

Rhinomanometry

Increased nasal resistance results in an increase in negative oropharyngeal pressure during inspiration and may therefore contribute to upper airway collapse. However, there are conflicting data regarding the relationship between nasal resistance and the occurrence of sleep-disordered breathing. McNicholas et al. [1] and Lavie et al. [2] demonstrated that nasal obstruction due to allergic rhinitis was associated with obstructive sleep apnea (OSA). In another study, experimentally induced nasal obstruction was able to induce episodes of apneic breathing in normal subjects [3]. Lofaso et al. [4] showed that in a stepwise multiple regression analysis nasal resistance was one of the independent risk factors for OSA. On the other hand, other studies failed to show any difference in nasal resistance between OSA patients and normal subjects. Interestingly, in one study, the patients with sleep-disordered breathing switched from nasal to oronasal breathing during sleep more frequently. Since oronasal breathing has been postulated to increase work of breathing these studies suggest that although the degree of nasal resistance is not predictive of OSA, the presence of increased nasal resistance may lead to a switch from nasal to oronasal breathing, thereby increasing the work of breathing and further compromising the upper airway.

Rhinomanometry is probably the test most frequently performed to assess nasal airway resistance [5]. It measures both nasal flow and resistance, and can be divided into passive and active procedures as well as into anterior and posterior rhinomanometry according to the location of the transducer used to measure posterior pharyngeal pressure. Since active rhinomanometry is quicker to perform, it is recommended for most purposes [6]. Anterior rhinomanometry may be influenced by nasal cycles, by deformation of the nares and by the instrument inserted to the nares. Posterior rhinomanometry, on the other hand, is more

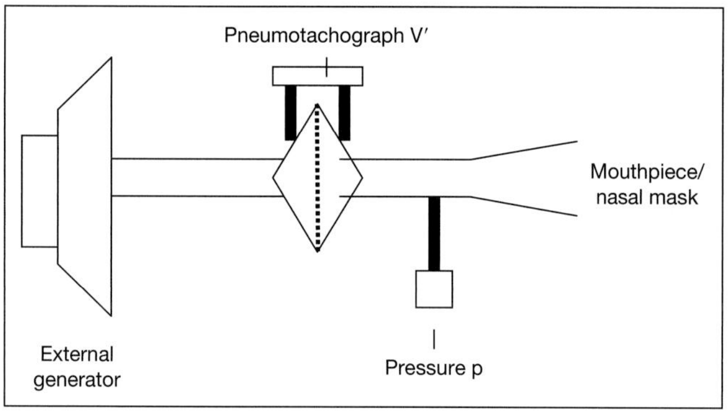

Fig. 1. Schematic arrangement of the forced oscillation technique. To enable spontaneous breathing, a shunt pathway open to the atmosphere placed in parallel to the external generator is necessary. V′ = Airflow.

expensive and requires more patient cooperation. However, both anterior active and posterior active rhinomanometry can be successfully performed in calculating nasal resistance, although well-established normal values do not exist. Other methods like acoustic rhinometry or nasal peak flow are less able to reflect nasal airway resistance.

Forced Oscillation Technique and Impulse Oscillometry

The forced oscillation technique (FOT) is a noninvasive method to investigate respiratory mechanics. Described in simplified terms, FOT or impulse oscillometry uses external signals (i.e. forced oscillations) produced by an external generator and superimposed on spontaneous breathing of the patient via a nasal mask or a mouthpiece; a pneumotachograph and a pressure-transducer register both the respiratory system flow and pressure, and the superimposed forced oscillation signals (fig. 1). After discriminating between these signals the so-called 'impedance' (Z) can be calculated, which is the relationship between pressure (P) and flow (V′): $Z = P/V'$.

Therefore, impedance can be conceived as a generalization of resistance that consists of a real part (resistance R) and an imaginary part (reactance X). In other words, the resistance R describes the dissipative mechanical properties of the respiratory system, whereas the reactance X is more related to the elastic properties [7, 8]. The main advantages of impulse oscillometry are that only minimal cooperation and no respiratory maneuvers are needed, so that it can be applied in children or even during sleep. The portable device allows to investigate even patients confined to bed.

Clinical applications of impulse oscillometry include the evaluation of chronic obstructive pulmonary diseases, restrictive lung diseases and nasal provocation tests with histamine [9] or allergens [10].

In sleep apnea patients FOT allows to detect respiratory events [11], and may help distinguish between obstructive and central apneas/hypopneas (fig. 2). Navajas et al. [12] demonstrated that in upper airway obstructions respiratory resistance measured by FOT was strongly correlated with esophageal pressure swings indicating that FOT can be used as an alternative to esophageal balloon in the diagnosis of OSA. Moreover, as new devices were developed to apply continuous positive airway pressure and forced oscillation simultaneously, FOT now serves as the basis for automatic continuous positive airway pressure (APAP) in the long-term treatment of the obstructive sleep apnea syndrome.

Lung Function Testing

Obstructive sleep apnea syndrome (OSAS) and chronic obstructive pulmonary disease (COPD) are both frequent diseases. Chaouat et al. [13] have suggested that the prevalence of COPD in patients with OSAS exceeds the prevalence of COPD in the general population, and other studies estimated the prevalence of COPD in OSAS patients to be 10–20% [14]. Conversely, a high prevalence of OSAS in COPD patients has also been reported. In view of these facts, is there a need to carry out lung function testing in all OSAS patients?

Hoffstein et al. [15] investigated 1296 patients without any lung disease and demonstrated no correlation between apnea/hypopnea index and pulmonary function parameters including flow-volume curve, body plethysmography and diffusing capacity. Data from 5,954 participants of the Sleep Heart Health Study suggested that when COPD and OSAS occur in the same individual, they occur by chance and not on the basis of a common pathophysiological link [16]. On the other hand, pulmonary function tests in OSA patients appear to be a useful tool regarding two aspects. Firstly, in one study there was a high correlation between OSAS severity and two lung function parameters, i.e. specific respiratory conductance (sGrs) and daytime arterial oxygen saturation (SaO_2). The authors concluded that a statistical model based on these parameters may effectively exclude OSAS in individual obese patients [17]. Secondly, and more importantly, Chaouat et al. [18] observed that the presence of an associated obstructive lung disease was a significant and independent predictor of death in OSA

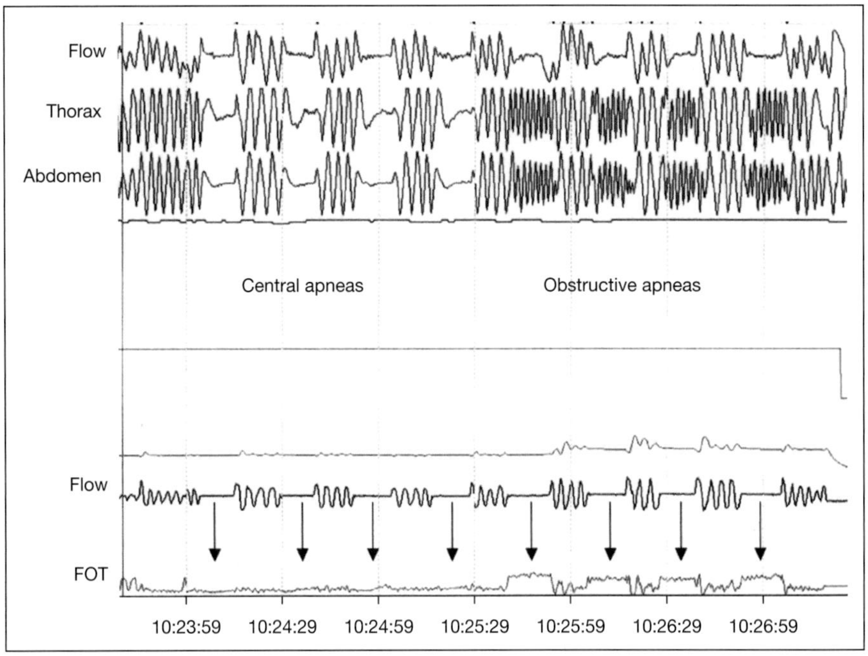

Fig. 2. Distinction between central and obstructive apneas using forced oscillation technique (FOT). During obstructive respiratory events a clear increase in the FOT signal (arrows) can be recognized, while this is missing during central respiratory events.

patients. These patients with a so-called 'overlap syndrome' have lower daytime PaO_2 and higher $PaCO_2$ and they have higher resting and exercising pulmonary artery mean pressure than OSA patients without COPD.

Even in the absence of COPD OSAS patients with massive obesity frequently have daytime hypercapnia which is related to the severity of obesity and the obesity-related impairment in lung function [19].

In conclusion, pulmonary function tests cannot effectively predict the presence of obstructive sleep apnea syndrome, but may detect associated COPD or daytime hypercapnia, which have a major importance for treatment and prognosis in OSA patients.

Esophageal Manometry

Because detection of apneas or hypopneas using thermistors or nasal cannulas may overlook respiratory events, esophageal pressure recording is regarded as a 'gold standard' in sleep medicine. However, it is an invasive method and some patients undergoing full polysomnography do not accept the esophageal catheter.

There are two different types of catheters usually employed in recording esophageal pressure. The first catheter consists of a small, air-filled balloon at its distal end transmitting esophageal pressure changes to a pressure transducer located at the proximal end of the catheter. Because these catheters were developed for pulmonary function testing, particularly measuring pulmonary compliance, many patients do not tolerate this kind of catheter for the whole night resulting in sleep fragmentation during polysomnography. Therefore newer, thin catheters have been introduced using a miniature transducer at the distal end, which are more expensive but better tolerated by the patients. Apart from patients' problems there are some technical difficulties in recording esophageal pressure signals. Artefacts due to cardiac or aortic oscillations may be eliminated by changing the transducer's position. Positive pressure swings are frequently related to swallowing, coughing or esophageal spasms.

During increased upper airway resistance, classically esophageal pressure becomes more and more negative until an arousal occurs (fig. 3).

There are two clinical applications in which esophageal pressure recording is particularly helpful: Firstly to differentiate between obstructive and central respiratory events [20], and, secondly, in the diagnosis of upper airway resistance syndrome. The upper airway resistance syndrome (UARS) is a form of sleep-disordered breathing characterized by repetitive increases in resistance to airflow within the upper airway leading to brief arousals and daytime hypersomnolence [21].

Blood Pressure and Pulse Transit Time

There is concurrent evidence in several studies confirming the relationship between OSA and hypertension independent of confounding factors such as obesity, age or

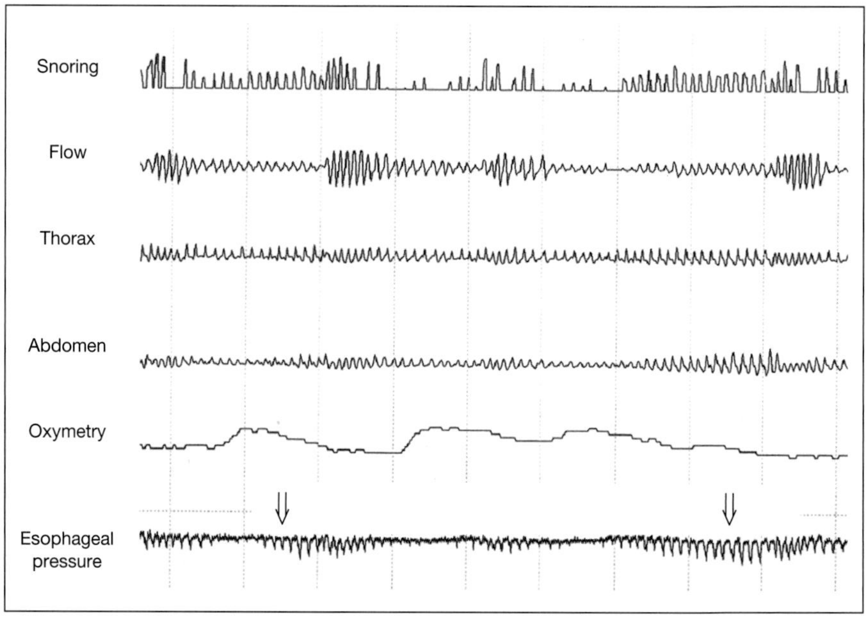

Fig. 3. Esophageal pressure in sleep apnea. During obstructive events esophageal pressure becomes more and more negative (arrows).

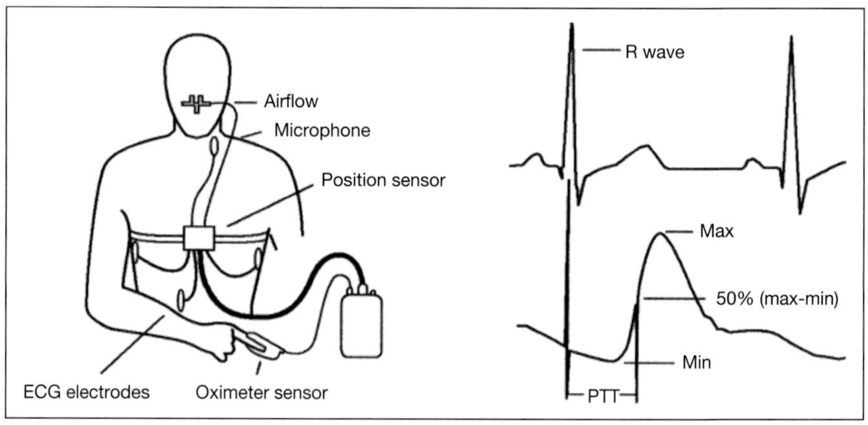

Fig. 4. Schematic arrangement of a PTT device including oximetric photoplethysmography for pulse transit time, electrocardiograph (ECG), thermistors to measure inspiratory flow, a body position sensor, and a microphone to detect snoring. The diagram demonstrates the calculation of pulse transit time using the R wave from the electrocardiogram as the starting point and the arrival of the arterial pulse wave as the end point. Adopted from Smith et al. [27].

smoking. In the cross-sectional analyses of 6,120 participants in the Sleep Heart Health Study OSA was associated with systolic/diastolic hypertension particularly in those younger than 60 years, while elevation of diastolic blood pressure seems to occur early in the course of OSA [22]. Even normotensive OSA patients develop diastolic blood pressure elevation at an earlier stage during exercise compared to normal subjects.

Noninvasive 24-hour blood pressure monitoring is a useful ambulatory procedure for detecting the typical pattern of circadian variation of blood pressure in OSA patients with increased diastolic blood pressure both day and night and increased systolic blood pressure at night ('non-dipping'). Beat-to-beat photoplethysmographic blood pressure monitoring devices are able to demonstrate the short-term variability of blood pressure, which is greater in apneic snorers and correlates with the severity of sleep apnea and sleep fragmentation [23]. When the recordings of blood pressure devices are interpreted, it should be taken into account that the cuff inflations may cause appreciable arousal from sleep and therefore lead to an increase in blood pressure [24].

Pulse transit time (PTT) is the time interval that the arterial pulse pressure wave takes to travel from the aortic valve to the periphery and is usually recorded as the time between the opening of the aortic valve ('R wave' on the electrocardiogram) and the arrival of the corresponding pulse wave at a finger. The latter is detected by a finger photoplethysmograph determining either 25 or 50% (depending on which equipment is used) of the height of the maximum value as the arrival point of the pulse wave. The device calculating PTT this way is small and portable (fig. 4). PTT depends on the degree of stiffness and tension of the arterial wall which is directly proportional to blood pressure. Therefore, as blood pressure increases, arterial wall becomes stiffer leading to an acceleration of the pulse wave and a decrease of PTT. Conversely, when blood pressure falls, a decrease of the vascular tone causes an increase of PTT.

Because inspiratory fall of systolic blood pressure is proportional to the degree of inspiratory effort, PTT can provide a quantitative measure of inspiratory effort in patients with obstructive sleep apnea [25]. There was a good correlation between the magnitude of negative pleural pressure, as measured with esophageal manometry, and the amplitude of PTT oscillations (ΔPTT) during upper airway obstructive events. An alternative way of using PTT to demonstrate an index of respiratory effort is to calculate the mean ΔPTT over the whole night, which is less useful for diagnostic purposes but can be used to assess therapeutic efficiency. Argod et al. [26] were able to demonstrate a good sensitivity, specificity and negative predictive value of PTT in differentiating between obstructive and central apneas and hypopneas by using an increase in ΔPTT to detect obstructive episodes and a decrease in ΔPTT for central events. PTT is also capable of detecting 'autonomic arousals' as a result of a respiratory event by exhibiting a transient dip in the baseline value that reflects the brief burst of sympathetic activity which in turn produces a surge in blood pressure.

PTT has some remarkable flaws that may limit its clinical usefulness. It has to be regarded as only semi-quantitative and cannot differentiate between patterns of obstructive events without an additional signal such as nasal pressure [27]. There is a tendency of undersampling PTT signals because PTT recording is only possible with each cardiac cycle. In addition, artefacts due to interference with the photoplethysmographic finger signals or chest wall movements may lead to a misinterpretation of the PTT signals. Finally, the impact of variations in cardiac contraction like left-ventricular dysfunction or cardiac arrhythmias such as atrial fibrillation on ΔPTT is unclear and needs further investigations.

Heart Rate Variability

The analysis of heart rate variability (HRV) is a useful tool evaluating autonomic nervous system function. Based on digital, high-frequency, 24-hour, multichannel electrocardiogram recordings the variations in heart rate can be assessed by different methods. While time domain methods reflect on the heart rate at any point in time or the intervals between successive normal QRS complexes, frequency domain methods provide information of variance distribution as a function of frequency by using spectral analyses [28]. Studies on spectral analyses of HRV have demonstrated the existence of three major periodic components: Firstly the high frequency (HF) oscillation (0.15–0.4 Hz), which is centered around breathing frequency, and which is mainly under vagal control and therefore represents parasympathetic activity. Secondly, a low-frequency (LF) oscillation (0.04 to 0.15 Hz), which is believed to reflect baroreflex dynamics, and, finally, a very-low-frequency (VLF) component (0.01–0.04 Hz) relating to thermoregulation [29]. While in some studies the LF component is considered as a marker of sympathetic modulation, other authors appraise it including parasympathetic and sympathetic influences.

In sleep apnea patients there is a decrease in time domain HRV, an increase of normalized LF variability and LF-to-HF ratio variability and a decrease of normalized HF variability during the night. LF and HF components of HRV demonstrate a typical pattern during an apneic phase with an increase in the HF component throughout the apnea followed by a sudden decrease with resumption of ventilation and, conversely, a peak of the LF component with resumption of ventilation and a decrease during obstructive respiratory efforts, reflecting the increased sympathetic activity at the end of an obstructive apnea [30].

Peripheral Arterial Tonometry

Peripheral arterial tonometry (PAT) is used to monitor vasoconstriction on the finger continuously and non-invasively as a marker of sympathetic nerve activation to the peripheral vasculature. The PAT device consists of a finger pneumo-optic plethysmograph, which generates its own pressure field at a fixed level of pressure irrespective of the size of the finger, thus avoiding distal venous pooling and distension (fig. 5). The optical density changes associated with pulsatile blood volume changes are measured at opposing lateral sides at the middle of the distal phalanx of a finger [31]. To register simultaneously the PAT signal, heart rate and oxygen saturation, a pulse oximeter placed on another finger completes the PAT device.

In patients with obstructive sleep apnea syndrome, Schnall et al. [32] demonstrated a transient attenuation in the pulse wave with each apneic event, thus indicating peripheral vasoconstriction particularly at the end of an obstructive apnea. The reduction in PAT amplitude is dependent on the degree of airway obstruction, such that greater airflow obstruction produces greater reduction in PAT amplitude. Even in the absence of detectable EEG arousals short periods

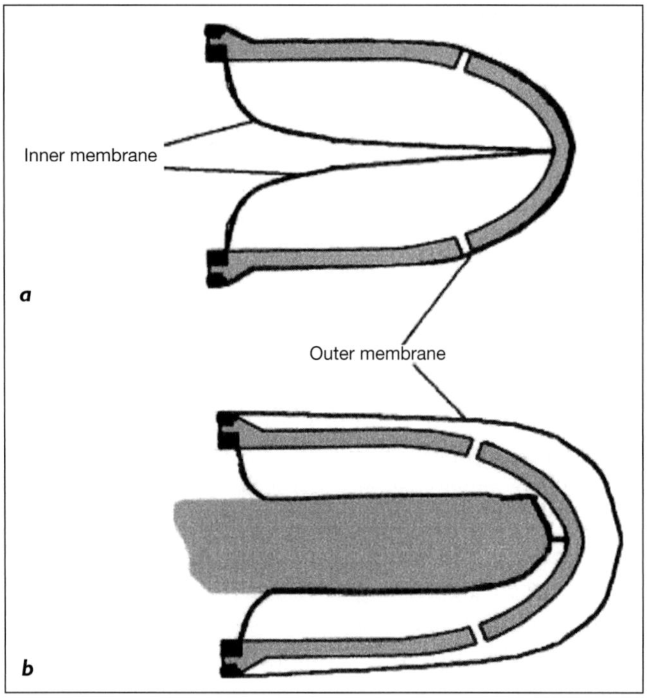

Fig. 5. Structural principle of a PAT device. It consists of an inner and an outer membrane on either side of a rigid plastic thimble. Approximately 10 ml of air is placed between the inner membrane and the plastic thimble (***a***). When a finger is inserted, a proportionate amount of air is shifted from the inner to the outer compartment of the probe thus applying pressure to the air within the probe (***b***). Adopted from Bar et al. [31].

of airflow obstruction can be detected by an attenuation in the PAT signal.

The PAT signal is not able to substitute assessment of blood pressure but provides a good recognition of apneas and subcortical arousals and gives additional information on sympathetic activation in patients with sleep apnea.

Muscle Sympathetic Nerve Activity

Muscle sympathetic nerve activity (MSNA) is another tool assessing sympathetic neural mechanisms in sleep apnea. Usually the peroneal microneurography is used for this purpose [33]. The microneurographic recordings are made with tungsten microelectrodes that are moved manually or with a pair of forceps percutaneously into the peripheral nerve. A suitable recording site for MSNA is obtained when spontaneous pulse-synchronous bursts with a greater than 2:1 to 3:1 signal-to-noise ratio are observed and nerve traffic directed to skin is excluded by the absence of responses to arousal stimuli or skin manipulations. The signals obtained in this way are multiunit action potentials from C fiber-containing nerve fascicles that are thought to reflect postganglionic vasoconstrictor nerve traffic [33]. Data are usually expressed as bursts per minute and as the total amplitude of the bursts per minute.

In patients with sleep apnea syndrome Somers et al. [34] could prove a high level of sympathetic nerve activity even when awake with a further increase of activity during sleep. This increase was typically marked at the end of an apneic episode. As MSNA and heart rate decrease during chemoreflex deactivation by 100% oxygen tonic activation of excitatory chemoreflex afferents is thought to contribute to the chronically increased efferent sympathetic activity to muscle circulation in patients with OSA. Effective CPAP therapy is able to decrease the sympathetic nerve activity.

Assessment of Muscle Function

The upper airway is surrounded by skeletal muscles that contribute mainly to maintaining airway patency. These upper airway dilator muscles can be divided into inspiratory phasic upper airway muscles, with the genioglossus being the one best studied, and tonic or postural muscles which, such as the tensor palatine, maintain a relatively constant level of activity throughout the respiratory cycle [35]. As the inspiratory phasic muscles become active before the onset of diaphragmatic contraction or inspiratory flow, these muscles are thought to prepare the pharyngeal airway for the negative pressure during inspiration [35]. Furthermore, in patients with OSA even during wakefulness there is an augmented activity of the pharyngeal dilator muscles, like the genioglossus muscle, which is thought to represent a compensatory mechanism for the more collapsible upper airway. This increased upper airway dilator muscle activity is lost at sleep thus contributing to pharyngeal collapse. Therefore, assessment of upper airway muscle function may contribute to understanding the pathophysiology of sleep-related breathing disorders.

Electromyography (EMG) is the method of choice to record the activity of upper airway muscles. According to the anatomic location different techniques in placing the electrodes are recommended. Genioglossus muscle EMG is measured with intramuscular hooked-wire electrodes directly inserted into the muscle. A peroral approach can be used to place the electrode wires into muscles in the oral cavity and soft palate, while a retractable needle catheter advanced through a fiberoptic scope is required to reach upper airway muscles that are not easily accessible through a peroral approach. Finally, the cricothyroid and thyroarytenoid muscles can be assessed by a transcutaneous method [35]. To verify the correct position of the electrodes, the subjects have to perform voluntary maneuvers associated with activation of the particular muscle.

Given the complex anatomy of the upper airways EMGs are technically difficult. Furthermore, the EMG of a single upper airway muscle is not necessarily representative of others and does not reflect interactions with the simultaneous activation of other upper airway muscles to influence airway patency [35]. The inability to calibrate the recordings makes comparison of EMG results of a specific muscle between different days or between subjects difficult. Thus clinical indications for upper airway muscle EMG are rare, and this method should be reserved for scientific questions.

The diaphragm is innervated exclusively by the phrenic nerve. The method of phrenic nerve stimulation (PNS) has been used to investigate upper airway dynamics in awake patients with OSA demonstrating that a flow limitation can be induced by an application of the twitch stimulus at end expiration. There are four PNS techniques, two of them, needle stimulation and implanted wire stimulation, being invasive. Needle stimulation is not recommended because of the risk of phrenic nerve damage [35]. Transcutaneous electrical PNS and magnetic stimulation have been studied more often and have only few side effects [35].

Recently, diaphragmatic electromyogram was demonstrated to effectively reflect the short-term changes in esophageal pressure during obstructive events indicating that this could be an alternative procedure to differentiate respiratory events in conditions where esophageal pressure is not available or not tolerated [36].

Nocturnal Penile Tumescence

The assessment of sleep-related erections is diagnostically useful in the evaluation of impotence. In this context, the measurement of nocturnal penile tumescence (NPT) is usually employed. Since sleep apnea is often associated with impotence or erectile dysfunction the combination of polysomnography and NPT is recommended in this case [37].

Traditional NPT evaluation contains the measurement of penile circumference by placing two strain gauges around the base of the penis and at the coronal sulcus. The strain gauges are mercury-filled and passed by a small electrical current so that penile expansion produces via elongation and thinning of the gauges an increased resistance of the mercury. The registered changes in electrical current are proportional to the changes in penile tumescence [38]. Newer devices will be provided measuring penile tumescence and rigidity continuously. In these devices the strain gauges tighten every 15 or 30 seconds and, if tumescence is recognized, an assessment of rigidity will performed every 30 s [39].

Furthermore, a visual inspection of an erection to detect penile anatomic problems is recommended in the diagnostic evaluation of sleep-related erections [38]. The lack of well-established normal values and difficulties in the technical procedures may complicate the interpretation of NPT in the clinical routine.

References

1 McNicholas W, Tarlo S, Cole P, Zamel N, Rutherford R, Griffin D, Phillipson EA: Obstructive apneas during sleep inpatients with seasonal allergic rhinitis. Am Rev Respir Dis 1982;126:625–628.

2 Lavie P, Gertner R, Zomer J, Podoshin L: Breathing disorders in sleep associated with microarousals in patients with allergic rhinitis. Acta Otolaryngol 1981;92:529–533.

3 White D, Cadieux R, Lomard R, Bixler EO, Kales A, Zwillich CW: The effects of nasal anesthesia on breathing during sleep. Am Rev Respir Dis 1985;132:972–975.

4 Lofaso F, Coste A, d'Ortho MP, Zerah-Lancner, Delclaux C, Goldenberg F, Harf A: Nasal obstruction as a risk factor for sleep apnoea syndrome. Eur Respir J 2000;16:639–643.

5 Rappai M, Collop N, Kemp S, deShazo R: The nose and sleep-disordered breathing. Chest 2003;124:2309–2323.

6 Clement P: Committee report on standardization of rhinomanometry. Rhinology 1984;22: 151–155.

7 Smith HJ, Reinhold P, Goldman MD: Forced oscillation technique and impulse oscillometry. Eur Respir Mon 2005;31:72–105.

8 Oostveen E, MacLeod D, Lorino H, Farré R, Hantos Z, Desager K, Marchal F: The forced oscillation technique in clinical practice: methodology, recommendations and future developments. Eur Respir J 2003;22: 1026–1041.

9 Randerath W, Smith HJ, Knarr D, Rühle KH: Comparison of anterior rhinomanometry and forced oscillation impulse technique in nasal provocation test with histamine. Pneumologie 1998;52:97–103.

10 Galetke W, Randerath W, David M, Rühle KH: Comparison between anterior rhinomanometry and impulse-oscillometric rhinometry found within nasal allergen provocation. Pneumologie 2001;55:420–424.

11 Badia JR, Farré R, Montserrat JM, Ballester E, Hernandez L, Rotger M, Rodriguez-Roisin R, Navajas D: Forced oscillation technique for the evaluation of severe sleep apnoea/hypopnoea syndrome: a pilot study. Eur Respir J 1998;11:1128–1134.

12 Navajas D, Farré R, Rotger M, Badia R, Puig-de-Morales M, Montserrat JM: Assessment of airflow obstruction during CPAP by means

of forced oscillation in patients with sleep apnea. Am J Respir Crit Care Med 1998;157: 1526–1530.
13 Chaouat A, Weitzenblum E, Krieger J, Ifoundza T, Oswald M, Kessler R: Association of chronic obstructive pulmonary disease and sleep apnea syndrome. Am J Respir Crit Care Med 1995;151:82–86.
14 Fletcher EC: Chronic lung disease in the sleep apnea syndrome. Lung 1990;168(suppl): 751–761.
15 Hoffstein V, Oliver Z: Pulmonary function and sleep apnea. Sleep Breath 2003;7:159–165.
16 Sanders MH, Newman AB, Haggerty CL, Redline S, Lebowitz M, Samet J, O'Connor GT, Punjabi NM, Shahar E: Sleep and sleep-disordered breathing in adults with predominantly mild obstructive airway disease. Am J Respir Crit Care Med 2003;167:7–14.
17 Zerah-Lancner F, Lofaso F, D'Ortho MP, Delclaux C, Goldenberg F, Coste A, Housset B, Harf A: Predictive value of pulmonary function parameters for sleep apnea syndrome. Am J Respir Crit Care Med 2000;162:2208–2212.
18 Chaouat A, Weitzenblum E, Krieger J, Sforza E, Hammad H, Oswald M, Kessler R: Prognostic value of lung function and pulmonary haemodynamics in OSA patients treated with CPAP. Eur Respir J 1999;13:1091–1096.
19 Laaban JP, Chailleux E: Daytime hypercapnia in adult patients with obstructive sleep apnea syndrome in France, before initiating nocturnal nasal continuous positive airway pressure. Chest 2005;127:710–715.
20 Hirshkowitz M, Kryger MH: Monitoring techniques for evaluating suspected sleep-disordered breathing; in Kryger MH, Roth T, Dement WC (eds): Principles and Practise of Sleep Medicine. Philadelphia, Saunders, 2000, pp 1378–1393.
21 Guilleminault C, Stoohs R, Clerk A, Cetel M, Maistros P: A cause of daytime sleepiness: the upper airway resistance syndrome. Chest 1993;104:781–787.
22 Haas DC, Foster GL, Nieto FJ, Redline S, Resnick HE, Robbins JA, Young T, Pickering TG: Age-dependent associations between sleep-disordered breathing and hypertension. Circulation 2005;111:614–621.
23 Leroy M, Surell CV, Pilliere R, Hagenmuller MP, Aegerter P, Raffestin B, Foucher A: Short-term variability of blood pressure during sleep in snorers with or without apnea. Hypertension 1996;28:937–943.
24 Davies RJ, Jenkins NE, Stradling JR: Effect of measuring ambulatory blood pressure on sleep and on blood pressure during sleep. BMJ 1994;308:820–823.
25 Pitson DJ, Sandell A, van den Hout R, Stradling JR: Use of pulse transit time as a measure of inspiratory effort in patients with obstructive sleep apnoea. Eur Respir J 1995;8: 1669–1674.
26 Argod J, Pépin JL, Lévy P: Differentiating obstructive and central sleep respiratory events through pulse transit time. Am J Respir Crit Care Med 1998;158:1778–1783.
27 Smith RP, Argod J, Pépin JL, Lévy P: Pulse transit time: an appraisal of potential clinical applications. Thorax 1999;54:452–458.
28 Task Force of the European Society of Cardiology and the North American Society of Pacing and Electrophysiology: Heart rate variability: standards of measurement, physiological interpretation, and its clinical use. Circulation 1996;93:1043–1065.
29 Parati G, Saul JP, Di Rienzo M, Mancia G: Spectral analysis of blood pressure and heart rate variability in evaluating cardiovascular regulation: a critical appraisal. Hypertension 1995;25:1276–1286.
30 Spicuzza L, Bernardi L, Calciati A, Di Maria GU: Autonomic modulation of heart rate during obstructive versus central apneas in patients with sleep-disordered breathing. Am J Respir Crit Care Med 2003;167:902–910.
31 Bar A, Pillar G, Dvir I, Sheffy J, Schnall RP, Lavie P: Evaluation of a portable device based on peripheral arterial tone for unattended home sleep studies. Chest 2003;123:695–703.
32 Schnall RP, Shlitner A, Sheffy J, Kedar R, Lavie P: Periodic, profound peripheral vasoconstriction: a new marker of obstructive sleep apnea. Sleep 1999;22:939–946.
33 Vallbo AB, Hagbarth KE, Torebjörk HE, Wallin BG: Somatosensory, proprioceptive, and sympathetic activity in human peripheral nerves. Physiol Rev 1979;59:919–957.
34 Somers VK, Dyken ME, Clary MP, Abboud FM: Sympathetic neural mechanisms in obstructive sleep apnea. J Clin Invest 1995;96:1897–1904.
35 ATS/ERS: Statement on respiratory muscle testing. Am J Respir Crit Care Med 2002;166:518–624.
36 Stoohs RA, Blum HC, Knaack L, Butsch-von-der-Heydt B, Guilleminault C: Comparison of pleural pressure and transcutaneous diaphragmatic electromyogram in obstructive sleep apnea syndrome. Sleep 2005;28:321–329.
37 Seftel AD, Strohl KP, Bayard D, Kress J, Netzer NC: Erectile dysfunction and symptoms of sleep disorders. Sleep 2002;25:637–640.
38 Ware JC, Hirshkowitz M: Assessment of sleep-related erections; in Kryger MH, Roth T, Dement WC (eds): Principles and Practice of Sleep Medicine. Philadelphia, Saunders, 2000, pp 1394–1402.
39 Licht MR, Lewis RW, Wollan PC, Harris CD: Comparison of RigiScan and sleep laboratory nocturnal penile tumescence in the diagnosis of organic impotence. J Urol 1995;154: 1740–1743.

Wolfgang Galetke, MD
Institute for Pneumology at the University Witten/Herdecke, Clinic for Pneumology and Allergology
Center of Sleep Medicine and Respiratory Care, Bethanien Hospital
Aufderhöherstrasse 169–175
DE–42699 Solingen (Germany)
Tel. +49 212 63 6000
Fax +49 212 63 6005
E-Mail galetke@klinik-bethanien.de

Randerath WJ, Sanner BM, Somers VK (eds): Sleep Apnea.
Prog Respir Res. Basel, Karger, 2006, vol 35, pp 69–78

Upper Airway Imaging in Sleep Apnea Syndrome

Rita Pinto Basto Daniel O. Rodenstein

Pneumology Unit, Cliniques universitaires Saint-Luc, Université Catholique de Louvain, Brussels, Belgium

Abstract

Obstructive sleep apnea is due to repetitive obstructions of the collapsible pharyngeal airway during sleep. It is therefore natural to search for local anatomical abnormalities to unveil the possible causes of the disease, and to look for potential curative interventions. Up to now, imaging of the upper airway has contributed more to the understanding of the pathophysiology of obstructive sleep apnea than to the identification of individual and solvable problems. The upper airway can be examined in multiple ways beginning with simple clinical observation. Clinical examination can provide the first visual information and can be useful to discard severe craniofacial abnormalities. Predictive morphometric scores have been based on simple clinical measurements, but their clinical utility requires further validation. Computed tomography and magnetic resonance imaging have provided extensive static and dynamic information on the process of obstruction of upper airway. Endoscopy with the Mueller maneuver has also been applied to the study of sleep-related breathing disorders but its predictive value is dubious. Cephalometry has pointed to different anatomical indicators of increased risk for sleep apnea and may be of help in the evaluation of patients submitted to maxillomandibular advancement or treated with oral appliances. Upper airway imaging is a valuable research tool and has provided insight into the pathophysiology of obstructive sleep apnea, thus permitting to improve the medical approach to this syndrome. However, it seems, at present, to have no role in the routine assessment of the patient with sleep-related breathing disorder.

Obstructive sleep apnea syndrome (OSAS) is a highly prevalent disease leading to severe medical consequences if left untreated. The search for a simple diagnostic method has led to the application of different imaging modalities in the study of the upper airway. Imaging of upper airway, however, has not entirely fulfilled its promises as a diagnostic tool. It has, by contrast, played a major role in the comprehension of the pathophysiology of OSAS. It allowed to access a dynamic and complex structure as the pharynx, permitting to understand its morphological and functional involvement in OSAS.

Different imaging methods have been used to study the upper airway from the simple medical observation to the modern radiological modalities with capability of three-dimensional reconstruction and dynamic imaging. These methods are used in the research and clinical fields presenting different advantages and disadvantages that condition their applicability.

We will summarize the main imaging methods of exploring the upper airway, their advantages and disadvantages and their contribution to the insight into physiopathology of OSAS. We will also try to present some conclusions about the clinical usefulness of these medical tools.

Upper Airway Anatomy

To appreciate the role of upper airway imaging in the assessment of OSAS, it is first important to understand the upper airway anatomy and function. The upper airway is a complex and highly dynamic structure that participates in very different and independent but interrelated actions like swallowing, breathing, coughing, sneezing, vomiting, yawning, singing and speaking. These actions require movements that have to be performed in a confined space and involve as well synergistic as antagonist mechanisms, which requires a very delicate and coordinated control. The relationships between the different structures of the upper airway in order to fulfil such different performances are not yet fully understood.

The acts of phonation, deglution or breathing render a static anatomic description inadequate and also limit the usefulness of the currently available static imaging methods. Although a static anatomic description is possible and necessary, dynamic imaging representing the physiological modifications during breathing and sleeping belongs at present to the research field. In order to simplify the understanding and description of the upper airway anatomy, it is useful to schematically consider it as comprising different compartments. The main anatomic elements of the upper airway are the nose and nasal fossae, the mouth and soft palate and the pharynx. These anatomic segments are constituted by some bony structures (cranial base, hyoid bone, mandible and maxilla) that are connected mainly by soft tissue and several muscles. Many of the muscles that form the upper airway, namely the pharyngeal ones, form a continuum and their theoretical limits overlap frequently.

In the nasal cavity, the inspired air is conducted through the nasal fossae where the turbinates impose a turbulent flow that facilitates its humidification and heating. The air is delivered, water saturated and at around 34°C temperature, to the nasopharynx – the posterior communication of the nasal fossae with the pharynx above the hard and soft palate.

Breathing can also be performed through the mouth when this virtual cavity becomes real by the action of the digastric muscle and the temporomandibular joint. This cavity encloses the tongue which is a complex structure formed by several muscles that either insert in other structures (extrinsic muscles – genioglossus muscle, the major tongue muscle, styloglossus, hyoglossus and palatoglossus muscles) or are completely imbibed on the tongue (intrinsic muscles – superior longitudinal, inferior longitudinal, verticalis and transversus). These muscles interact providing an amazing mobility to the tongue that has been compared to an elephant trunk [1]. In fact, the tongue may move side to side inside the mouth, protrude out of the mouth and orient its extremity in several directions and it can also wind around itself. The tongue is an example of a muscular hydrostat; like an octopus arm or an elephant trunk, it contains muscles, but has no internal skeletal support and achieves its movement as if it had an incompressible fluid compartment upon which the muscles would act, much as an earthworm does.

The tongue is attached to the hyoid bone. This is a floating bone the position of which is dependent upon the action of different muscles. It is attached to the mandible by the mylohyoid and geniohyoid muscles, has caudal connections via sternohyoid and omohyoid muscles, and also has cephalic connections to the base of the skull via the stylohyoid muscle. The participation of these muscles in the mechanics of breathing in humans remains unclear.

Behind the mouth there is another important structure – the soft palate – which allows the communication between the mouth and the pharynx. The soft palate is a membranous and muscular structure that comprises different striated muscle groups: the levator palatini which elevates the soft palate, promoting oral breathing; the palatoglossus, which forms the anterior tonsillar pillar, has an opposite action approaching the soft palate downwards and forwards towards the base of the tongue, and thus promotes nasal airflow; the palatopharyngeus muscle which forms the posterior tonsillar pillar and moves the palate downwards, and the tensor palatini muscle which tightens the palate in the coronal plane augmenting the tension of the palate aponeurosis to which the other muscles are attached. The posterior and inferior border of the soft palate presents in its median part the musculus uvulae, which may be involved in nasopharyngeal closure.

All these palatal muscles have demonstrated electromyographic activity during inspiration [2, 3] with the exception of the tensor palatini that seems to have no role in the respiratory cycle [4].

The pharynx is a muscular tube that extends from the cranial base to the larynx rostrally, and to the upper esophageal sphincter dorsally. It is placed in the median line in front of the cervical spine, behind the nasal fossae, mouth cavity and hyoid bone and between the neck vascular structures. The pharynx may be subdivided into three anatomic segments: (1) nasopharynx (the region between the nasal fossae and the posterior border of the hard palate); (2) oropharynx (the region behind the mouth cavity that can be subdivided into the retropalatal and retroglossal regions), and (3) hypopharynx (the region from the base of the tongue to the larynx).

In OSAS, the collapse of the upper airway occurs at the level of the oropharynx and/or hypopharynx. This segment lacks rigid support, and its patency is dependent upon the balance between anatomic characteristics and physiological factors, both during wakefulness or sleep.

The soft palate (when it comes in apposition to the tongue) and the tongue are the main constituents of the anterior wall of the oropharynx; its posterior wall, located in front of the cervical spine, is a muscular wall composed by the superior, middle and inferior constrictor pharyngeal muscles. The lateral walls of the oropharynx are complex structures with numerous muscles including the constrictor pharyngeal muscles of the posterior wall, lymphatic tissue, vascular elements, autonomic structures, different soft tissue structures and fat pads which have been studied extensively (see below [5, 6]).

Pathophysiology: The Upper Airways in OSAS

The pathophysiology of OSAS involves complex mechanisms that are yet to be completely unveiled. Ventilation proceeds from the nose and/or mouth to the lungs through an open upper airway, driven by the negative intrathoracic pressure. In fact, the stability and patency of the upper airway are essential and dependent upon the action of oropharyngeal dilator and abductor muscles.

The collapse of the upper airway takes place when the force generated by the upper airway muscles does not counteract the negative airway pressure produced by the inspiratory activity of the diaphragm and intercostal muscles. The neuromuscular control of ventilation has a natural protection against this phenomenon: inspiratory muscles are activated downwards in a progressive and controlled form, introducing a 150- to 200-ms delay between the alae nasi muscles and diaphragm contractions. In this way, pharyngeal muscles will be already contracted and stiffened when submitted to the airway negative pressure. A peak of muscular pharyngeal activity precedes the muscular thoracic activity. If there is any incoordination in the intensity or timing of pharyngeal muscular activity with respect to the thoracic one, the upper airway may collapse. In addition, negative pressure inside the pharynx results in activation of pharyngeal muscles, a second protective mechanism against collapse.

Activity of the upper airway muscles is also modulated by other stimuli that have been extensively studied. Among them are chemical stimuli, vagal input, inspired air temperature, blood pressure, sex-specific hormones, baroreceptor activity and sleep-wake states [2, 7]. Investigations in humans in wakefulness have demonstrated linear increments in diaphragmatic and genioglossal electromyogram (EMG) during both normoxic hypercapnia and isocapnic hypoxia. The combined effects of various stimuli result in a final integrated activation of the upper airway muscles.

All the muscles that control the tongue, palate and hyoid appear to be involved in the maintenance of upper airway patency, but the literature presents different views on the relative importance of these muscles [3, 4]. This issue is reviewed in detail in another chapter.

During sleep, besides recumbence and gravitational forces, there are various factors contributing to narrow the upper airway. As any structure formed essentially by striated skeletal muscle, the upper airway will present, in sleep, a generalized hypotonia. The electromyographic activity of all the upper airway muscles has shown tonic and phasic decreases during NREM sleep. During NREM sleep upper airway mechanoreceptors are also much less active and there is a delayed and decreased response to negative airway pressure [2].

In OSAS upper airway muscles present structural and functional alterations. In an effort to maintain upper airway patency palatal muscles have increased activity in wakefulness through a neuromuscular compensation mechanism. Probably reflecting this increased activity a number of morphological abnormalities have been described in upper airway muscles. A change of muscle fibers (more fast-twitch type IIA instead of type IIB fibers), increased levels of aerobic metabolism in addition to signs characteristic of neurogenic lesions (fiber hypertrophy and atrophy), attributed to the snoring trauma to the pharyngeal tissues, have all been described [8].

This histological documentation of sensory neuropathic changes may justify the decreased sensitivity in the response to negative pressure of OSAS patient's upper airway. In fact, upper airway muscles of patients with OSAS do respond to negative pressure, however, the magnitude of such response is less in patients with OSAS than in normal subjects. This impaired ability in the reflex response to negative pressure may also be attributed to the mucosal edema thought to arise from airway trauma secondary to snoring. CPAP therapy can revert mucosal edema. Recent studies have shown that reducing surface tensions forces in pharyngeal mucosa by the instillation of surfactant led to a reduction in mucosal folding and liquid bridging stabilizing the pharyngeal airway [9].

During sleep in patients with OSAS, the occurrence of apneas or hypopneas are most common in stages 1 and 2 of NREM and in REM sleep. Pharynx collapsibility increases with sleep fragmentation and with mouth opening during sleep [2, 3].

We can conclude that OSAS arises from an intricate relation between anatomic and functional factors. In order to define OSAS, the presence of an anatomic predisposition like alterations in the upper airway soft tissue (fat deposition) or in craniofacial structures cannot be dissociated from the reorganization of neural events that occur during sleep. Imaging of upper airways has contributed to our understanding of the physiopathology of sleep apnea [10, 11].

We will review the main imaging methods to study the upper airway, and summarize their contributions to assessment of physiology and their clinical usefulness. We will review the role of clinical examination, cephalometry, computed tomography (CT) scanning, magnetic resonance imaging (MRI), endoscopy and ultrasound in the study of the patient with OSAS.

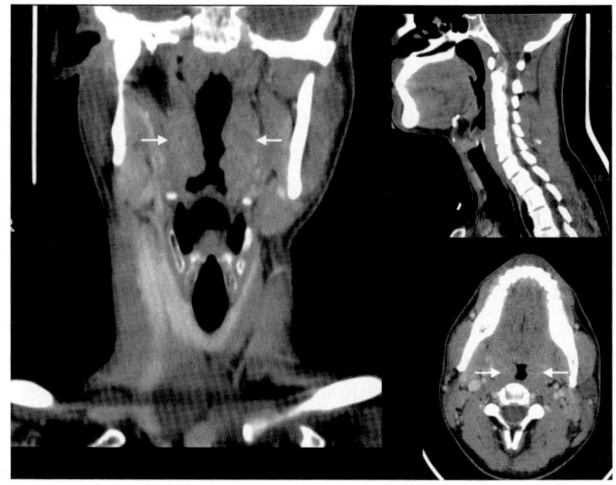
a b c

Fig. 1. Lateral pharyngeal walls enlargement (arrows) due to lymphoid tissue hyperplasia, with reduction in the transverse diameter of the pharynx. ***a*** Coronal reconstructed view. ***b*** Sagittal reconstructed view. ***c*** Axial view. Courtesy of Prof. E. Coche, Imaging Department, Cliniques Universitaires Saint-Luc.

Clinical Examination

The first 'image' that we can have from a patient suspected of sleep-related disordered breathing is given by simple visual inspection. Taking into account that movement alters the upper airway anatomy, different dynamic maneuvers should be performed.

Although the inspection of the face and neck and also mouth and pharynx has poor predictive value, it can provide identification of risk factors for the development of sleep apnea [12]. A consensual standard ENT evaluation has been proposed to evaluate the sleep-disordered breathing patient [13].

The patient should be observed in the seated and supine positions. Any obvious malformations (retrognathia, micrognathia) should be noted. Mandibular retroposition is associated with posterior displacement of the tongue base narrowing the upper airway. The maneuver of dental occlusion easily explores the presence of overjet – when the mandibula extrudes forward as compared with mandible. Nasal patency should be assessed even with simple procedures as a sniff test. The collapse of nasal valves may be suggestive of nasal obstruction. Anterior rhinoscopy will help to diagnose valve anomalies, septum deviation, and hypertrophic turbinate or nasal polyposis. The inspection of the oropharynx should include the size and consistency of the tongue, the size, length and consistency of the soft palate and of the uvula. Grading the relationship between the tongue and the oral cavity (Mallampati score) has been proven useful as an indicator of difficult endotracheal intubations and may also be used in the evaluation of the sleep apnea patient. Tonsillar hypertrophy should also be graded, especially in children.

This methodical evaluation through readily available means has permitted to identify some main risk factors for sleep apnea. The lateral narrowing of the upper airway in OSAS patients is due to two main anatomic reasons – fat deposition in the soft tissue structures surrounding the upper airway and facial bone structure. In some rare cases, tumors or enlarged tonsils may also result in lateral pharyngeal walls enlargement with narrowing of the pharynx (fig. 1). Neck circumference is a well-known risk factor for OSAS and may be a marker of regional fat distribution within the neck. Body mass index and neck circumference have been shown to independently correlate with the apnea/hypopnea index (AHI). It has been shown that the association of impaired nasal flow and a small oral airway is also a risk factor for OSAS. These can be assessed using the Mallampati score for the oral cavity and a simple sniff test for nasal obstruction [14].

Facial bone structure abnormalities, such as retrognathia, have already been mentioned and they are an example of the importance of genetic factors in the determination of the size and conformation of upper airway bony and soft tissue structures. The Pierre Robin and Treacher Collins syndromes are examples of mandibular and palatal abnormalities seen in infancy that almost invariably result in OSAS. Macroglossia is a common feature in Down syndrome and also can be associated with systemic diseases such as amyloidosis, hypothyroidism, acromegaly and nutritional deficiencies.

Although these main findings have been consistent with a higher risk of sleep-disordered breathing they do not permit the differentiation between subjects with or without OSAS.

Deegan and McNicholas [15] concluded in 215 patients evaluated for the suspicion of OSAS that no individual clinical feature is predictive of obstructive sleep apnea. The combination of features such as gender, age, snoring, observed apneas, hypersomnolence, alcohol consumption and BMI have been useful to exclude OSAS but they cannot correctly identify it.

More recently patient morphometric characteristics have been included in the analysis of predictive features for OSAS. Kushida et al. [16] described a clinical model that incorporates the quantification of both craniofacial bony and soft tissue structures as well as the BMI and neck circumference. According to the results this morphometric model has a high sensitivity (97.6%) and specificity (100%) and also presents better power to distinguish patients with OSAS than other models, which only have used BMI or neck circumference alone. The measurements proposed by this model are performed with a caliper in the oral cavity including assessment of palatal height, intermolar distance and measurement of overjet. The proposed mathematical formula includes quantification of craniofacial dysmorphism on one side and obesity on the other side and according to the authors has allowed the correct identification of 245 patients with OSAS from a group of 300 subjects. Further validation of this model is necessary to prove its clinical usefulness.

Ethnicity influence on the craniofacial characteristics has also been examined. A recent report from Lam et al. [17] prospectively studied 239 patients (164 Asian and 75 white subjects) with clinical suspicion of OSAS to determine whether the craniofacial profile predicts the presence of OSAS. They chose simple and easy-to-perform clinical measurements such as the neck circumference, the thyromental distance, the thyromental angle and the Mallampati oropharyngeal score. These measurements are thought to represent features of both obesity and abnormal craniofacial skeletal structure. Mallampati score and thyromental distance are correlated with difficult endotracheal intubation and OSAS. The authors first describe thyromental angle, which reflects the central obesity and the length of the anterior cranial base. They found that Asian patients had higher Mallampati scores, shorter thyromental distances and larger thyromental angles, and tended to have more severe OSAS than white subjects. The application of these measurements into the routine physical examination may be of value, although they have not been tested in other ethnic groups.

Cephalometry

Cephalometry is a radiological technique that has been extensively used in the fields of orthodontics and anthropology for the study of craniofacial characteristics. Its extension to the area of sleep-related breathing-related disorders has been a natural process since it provides some insight on the bony and soft tissue characteristics of the upper airway. Cephalometry procedure consists of a standardized lateral radiograph of the head and neck on which several anatomic points are identified. The distance between these points and the angles between the lines connecting them are measured. Although cephalometry is widely available, inexpensive and reproducible it requires a well-standardized performance. It can be performed in a sitting or standing position and requires a fixed head position, with the gaze in a horizontal plan. The cephalometry should be done at end-expiration. Interpretative skills should also be standardized. The main disadvantage of this technique concerns the fact that it provides only a two-dimensional analysis of a three-dimensional structure and in this way it limits the information provided about antero-posterior structures and lateral soft tissue structures of the upper airway. Moreover, it yields a single static image of an essentially dynamic structure, and the image represents the pharynx in the upright posture, whereas sleep apnea usually manifests itself in the supine position. Nevertheless, cephalometry has been used to study sleep apnea patients and has demonstrated significant differences, when compared with normal reference values. Table 1 shows a review of the main findings of cephalometry in the published literature.

Cephalometry has pointed to the following anatomical indicators of an increased risk for sleep apnea: narrow posterior airway space, enlargement of the tongue and soft palate, inferiorly positioned hyoid bone, retroposition of the mandible and small nasion-sella-basion angle. Obesity has also been implicated as a major risk factor for OSAS. However, it has been more commonly reported that craniofacial abnormalities are more important as a risk factor in nonobese than in obese OSAS patients [23].

A qualitative analysis and meta-analysis of the published literature about craniofacial structure and OSAS has found only one cephalometric measurement with clinical significance and diagnostic accuracy for OSAS: mandibular body length [26]. Although this conclusion may question the performance of cephalometry as a diagnostic tool, it has even been used to develop a craniofacial index score to differentiate patients with OSAS from habitual snorers [27]. Pracharktam et al. [28] have proposed a craniofacial index

Table 1. Review of the main findings of cephalometry in the published literature

Study	Population	Main findings	Other conclusions
Jamieson et al. [18]	155 OSAS patients 41 control subjects	Low position of the hyoid bone, retroposition of the mandible, acute nasion-sella-basion angle	
Lyberg et al. [19]	25 OSAS patients 10 control subjects	Greater length of soft palate, greater area of soft palate, low position of the hyoid bone, mandibular retrognathia	
Maltais et al. [20]	40 OSAS patients 12 snorers 34 control subjects matched by age	Low position of hyoid bone (for OSAS patients), greater length of soft palate (for snorers and OSAS patients)	Low position of hyoid bone correlates significantly with age
Lowe et al. [21]	80 OSAS patients 25 control subjects + CT scan	Larger soft palate, larger tongue, retroposition of the mandible, higher total upper and lower face height, elongated maxilla and mandibular incisors and mandibular molars	Tongue and soft palate volumes are positively correlated with BMI
Tangugsorn et al. [22]	100 OSAS patients 36 controls	Greater length and area of soft palate, larger sagittal area of tongue with an upright position, retroposition of the mandible, shorter dimension of cranial base, larger cranio-cervical angle, decreased sagittal dimension of nasopharynx, velopharynx and residual oropharynx area	
Nelson et al. [23]	72 nonobese snorers 70 obese snorers	Predictors of apnea: Nonobese: increased tongue length, smaller size of the middle cranial fossa, age Obese: low position of hyoid bone, increased tongue length	In OSAS patients interaction between lower hyoid position and increased tongue length may contribute to the obstruction of hypopharynx
Brander et al. [24]	42 nonobese OSAS patients 31 obese OSAS patients wide range of AHI (1–131 events/h sleep)	Both groups: larger hyoid-posterior pharyngeal wall distance, shorter uvular protrusion-posterior pharyngeal wall, skeletal craniofacial structure was similar between obese and nonobese, changes in upper airway caliber with posture were similar between groups	significant correlations between measurements incorporating upper airway size at different levels
Pépin et al. [25]	96 OSAS patients 35 snorers + CT scan	Identification in awake patients of hooking of the soft palate as a risk factor for OSAS	Hooking: angulation of 30° or greater between the distal part of the uvula and the longitudinal axis of the soft palate

constructed with cephalometric and anthropometric measurements, including age, BMI, hyoid mandibular plane distance and tongue length, to classify heterogeneous groups of patients with OSAS into subgroups with varying degrees of anatomic risk for the disease.

The concept that an anatomic abnormality with etiologic relevance in OSAS could be identified on cephalometry has led to its use in some therapeutic approaches. In fact, cephalometry has been used to evaluate bony structure before facial surgery (mandibular advancement) and to evaluate the efficacy of oral appliances. Cephalometric measurements have also been advocated for the pre-operative evaluation of patients submitted to uvulopalatopharyngoplasty (UPPP). Although the surgical outcome is not accurately predicted, some authors contend that the presence of moderate OSAS, a mandibular-hyoid distance <20 mm and the absence of retrognathia could be predictors of improvement after UPPP [29].

It should be noted that very few studies on cephalometry have been performed in recent years.

Computed Tomography and Magnetic Resonance Imaging of Upper Airways

Computed tomography (CT) and magnetic resonance imaging (MRI) have contributed in a greater extent to the understanding of the pathophysiology of OSAS. CT scan is widely available and allows pharyngeal measurements through axial slices at several levels, permitting the accurate assessment of upper airway cross-sectional area. Scans are performed on awake patients in supine position. The potential for three-dimensional reconstruction of axial CT images (fig. 1) provides for a volumetric evaluation of the pharynx. Ultrafast CT allows for higher spatial and temporal resolution with the possibility of dynamic imaging.

CT scan permits excellent airway and bony image resolution, however, when compared to MR images, it lacks soft-tissue contrast, particularly for adipose tissue. MRI also has the advantage of multiplanar images with no radiation. This characteristic provides the possibility to perform studies during wakefulness and induced sleep. Furthermore, this technique has already been considered the most useful tool to study OSAS patients because it permits measurement of cross-sectional area and volume of upper airway, three-dimensional reconstructions, multiplanar images and provides excellent resolution of soft tissue identifying not only the fat, but also the water content of tissues. However, its high cost limits its widespread use.

As assessed by CT scan [10, 11] and MRI [5], patients with OSAS have smaller upper airways than normal subjects even during the wake state.

The size of upper airway structures (tongue, soft palate, parapharyngeal fat pads, lateral pharyngeal walls and mandible) has been extensively studied and is thought to be an important determinant of upper airway caliber in OSAS. Cephalometric studies have proved that craniofacial abnormalities contribute to the smaller size of the upper airway. Imaging studies by CT scan and MRI have elucidated the differences in the soft tissue structures of the OSAS patients. In fact, these studies have demonstrated an increased cross-sectional area and volume of the soft palate, tongue, parapharyngeal fat pads and lateral pharyngeal walls in patients with sleep apnea [5, 30, 31].

The level of minimum cross-sectional area of the upper airway has been systematically searched and although the retropalatal area has been most frequently identified, other structures, such as an enlarged tongue or thickened lateral pharyngeal walls, have been pointed as contributors to the obstruction of the upper airway. Probably the interaction between these structures is responsible for the upper airway narrowing seen in OSAS patients. Pépin et al. [28] demonstrated, using CT and cephalometry, that the presence of soft palate hooking in awake patients with OSAS who had long soft palates, a wide oropharynx, and a wide hypopharynx had a 100% specificity for the identification of OSAS patients. However, this sign had a low sensitivity and was a transient phenomenon.

Obesity is believed to predispose to OSAS, which is mainly associated with neck adipose tissue deposition. MRI studies have permitted to identify that adipose tissue is deposited adjacent and laterally to the pharyngeal airway in patients with OSAS when compared with obese control subjects and that the volume of that tissue is related to the presence and degree of OSAS. Even in nonobese patients excess fat deposition has been described [32]. Fat pads are located especially anterolateral to the upper airway in nonobese OSAS patients when compared with controls with the same body weight assessed using BMI and neck circumference.

Schwab et al. [5], using MRI images, found that thickness of the lateral pharyngeal muscular walls rather than enlargement of the parapharyngeal fat pads played the critical role in determining airway caliber. However, the factors that control the thickness of the lateral walls of the pharynx were not determined.

Besides the size also the shape of the apneic airway is different from the normal airway [33]. The upper airway in apneic patients has an anteroposterior elliptical shape in contrast with normal subjects that present also an elliptical shape but with the major axis oriented in the coronal plane. This reduced lateral diameter of the upper airway is reported to predispose to apnea during sleep.

A recent study by Schwab et al. [30], using state-of-the-art volumetric MRI methods, concluded that the volume of the upper airway soft tissue structures was significantly greater in subjects with sleep apnea than in normal subjects. Therefore, they contend that volumetric MRI should become the standard equipment to objectively quantify the enlargement of the upper airway soft tissue structures in OSAS patients. According to the authors there is an increased risk of developing sleep apnea if an increased volume of the lateral pharyngeal walls, tongue and total soft tissue is found. It is also admitted that other factors besides obesity (in addition to age, sex, craniofacial size and ethnicity), namely genetic factors, may be important in mediating the enlargement of the soft tissue structures. It is proposed that volumetric MRI is the ideal modality to phenotype the pharynx and elucidate genetic traits in OSAS patients.

Noninvasive MRI has also been useful to evaluate the efficacy of nasal continuous positive airway pressure therapy (nCPAP), a very effective option for OSAS treatment. Ryan et al. [34] have reported that chronic CPAP therapy modifies the upper airway morphology in wakefulness: it increases pharyngeal volume and minimal pharyngeal cross sectional area and decreases tongue volume. These changes are achieved through the resolution of upper airway edema, which is thought to be secondary to the trauma of repeated obstruction of upper airway in OSAS patients. In this study the majority of the increase in pharyngeal volume occurred in the oropharynx. Other authors [35] showed that progressive increases in CPAP pressure (up to 15 cm H_2O) alter the lateral dimension of the pharynx, with an increase in this diameter due to a thinning of the lateral pharyngeal wall.

Imaging studies have not yet been able to identify the morphological predictors of the surgical success of UPPP. UPPP improves AHI in OSAS patients but has a low success rate and its determinants are still poorly understood. However, using CT scan, it was possible to identify an increase width of the soft palate after surgery. It allowed also to establish the site of pharyngeal narrowing postoperatively in those patients in whom surgery failed. Persistence of oropharyngeal narrowing after UPPP was linked to an increase in thickness of the soft palate combined with a change in palatal position in relation to the base of the tongue [36].

Recently, Sanner et al. [37] extended the use of MRI to the evaluation of the efficacy of mandibular advancement devices. Airway patency during the Mueller maneuver (see below) while wearing the device was reported to predict the outcome of this treatment in OSAS patients.

Static imaging methods are performed to study the anatomic level of obstruction, but in order to have a comprehensive view on the pathophysiology of OSAS, dynamic studies are essential.

The upper airway anatomy changes that occur throughout inspiration and expiration have been compared in normal persons and in patients with sleep apnea using cine-CT. These studies have measured the upper airway dimension during different phases of the respiratory cycle [38]. At the beginning of inspiration there is a small increase in upper airway area probably due to an increased activity of the upper airway dilator muscles. During most of the inspiration upper airway is kept relatively constant as a result of the balance between negative intraluminal pressure and the action of the upper airway dilator muscles. In the phase of early expiration upper airway reaches its greatest size presumably because of positive intraluminal pressure. At the end of expiration, the upper airway narrows significantly because its caliber cannot longer be kept open by the phasic action of the upper airway dilator muscles. These data suggested that, at end expiration, the pharynx is particularly vulnerable to collapse, making collapse not only an inspiratory, but also an expiratory phenomenon. The notion that sleep implies decreased tonic activity of the dilator muscles and decrease pharyngeal cross-sectional area below normal helps to understand why apnea appears during sleep.

Recently, ultrafast MRI that produces one imaging per 0.8 s has been used in the understanding of the dynamic changes that take place in the upper airway. Ciscar et al. [31], using this technique found that the velopharyngeal airway was smaller in OSAS patients, when compared to controls, only during part of the respiratory cycle. The variation of the velopharyngeal area was also larger in apneic patients, particularly during sleep, suggesting an increased compliance in this region of the upper airway.

CT and MRI imaging have been valuable instruments in the comprehensive understanding of the dynamic phenomena of the upper airway during the wake state and during sleep in OSAS patients. However, none of these techniques may be considered a routine clinical tool.

CT scan can also be used to visualize brain structures. In the context of sleep apnea this capability is useful to evaluate the sella turcica when acromegaly is suspected as a cause for sleep apnea.

Endoscopy

Endoscopic examination of the pharynx is easily performed with a flexible fiberoptic endoscope passed through the nose. It allows to directly visualize the behavior of the retropalatal area, retroglossal area, the larynx and the trachea during breathing in wakefulness or sleep. Although it is an invasive imaging method and requires nasal anesthesia, nasopharyngoscopy is a widely available dynamic exam that has already been included in the standard ENT evaluation.

Nasopharyngoscopy is commonly accompanied by the Mueller maneuver. This maneuver consists of a voluntary inspiration against a closed mouth and obstructed nares. It is thought to simulate the upper airway collapse that occurs during an apnea. In case of a narrowed pharynx the examiner can visualize a collapse and describe it.

The Mueller maneuver has several limitations that have to be taken into account. The degree of collapse is always a subjective measure by the examiner, even when using grading scores. Moreover, the negative pressure generated during the maneuver is variable and is highly dependent on the effort generated by the patient. The degree of this inspiratory effort is seldom assessed during the Mueller maneuver. The use of a manometer can obviate this problem but will limit the accessibility of the technique and is not routinely recommended [13]. The assumption that the physiological changes noted during the maneuver mimic those on sleep breathing remains to be proven.

Nevertheless, bearing in mind these considerations, it has been suggested that Mueller maneuver can add important information in identifying possible sites of obstruction and predict the outcome for patients submitted to UPPP. It was reported that patients with predominantly retroglossal obstruction are not ideal candidates for UPPP whereas identifying an obstruction at the retropalatal level would predict a better outcome for UPPP [39]. However, even when the velopharynx appears normal the diagnosis of OSAS cannot be excluded. Selection of patients for a surgical approach cannot rely only on the results of this technique. The value of nasopharyngoscopy and Mueller maneuver in predicting the outcome of UPPP is yet to be proven.

Other Imaging Studies

Fluoroscopy/Ultrasound

Fluoroscopy can provide a dynamic evaluation of the upper airways during wakefulness and sleep, but it implies a high level of radiation exposure, which limits its applicability. Moreover, as cephalometry, it does not provide any information relative to the soft tissues surrounding the upper airways.

At present, ultrasound technique has not yet been applied to the study of the upper airways in the context of sleep-related breathing disorders. Several years ago, Kwok et al. [40] devised a bi-directional ultrasound technique able to image the base of the tongue. However, ultrasound has not found any useful clinical application up to now.

Clinical Point of View

The imaging of the upper airway has contributed to the understanding of the physiopathology of OSAS. In fact, with the initial aim of accurately differentiating OSAS patients from normal subjects, these different techniques ended up opening a new window to the knowledge of upper airway anatomy and physiology.

Despite the greater understanding of sleep apnea physiopathology that imaging methods have allowed, they are not useful as a routine clinical tool. No imaging technique permits a diagnosis of sleep apnea in an individual patient nor predicts the surgical outcome of OSAS patients.

The upper airway is, by definition, an area of complexity and dynamic behavior and sleep state induces specific changes in the physiology of upper airway. It has already been stated that the ideal upper airway imaging method for OSAS patients should be inexpensive, non-invasive, permitting supine imaging and not exposing the patient to radiation [11]. In addition, such a method should also be capable of performing dynamic state-dependent imaging and allow for three-dimensional volumetric reconstructions of the upper airway and soft tissues. Although MRI imaging has some of this requisites, it is not widely available.

Both static and dynamic imaging methods have been used to study the causes of the differences in size and shape of the apneic upper airway. They have highlighted the importance of facial bone structure, fat deposition, obesity and gender in the determination of pharyngeal conformation in OSAS patients. Many studies tried to define the clinical predictors of OSAS, which would be important screening methods, useful to improve the utilization of sleep laboratory facilities and to reduce the number of unnecessary sleep studies. However, many of the prediction formulas presented are laborious to apply routinely, and have yet to be validated.

Clinical examination may be considered as the only 'imaging' method that should be applied to every individual suspected of OSAS. Surgical approaches for treatment, and mandibular appliances, may justify the performance of cephalometry, CT scan or MRI studies. In patients being considered for CPAP, no specific imaging study appears necessary.

References

1 Rodenstein DO: Anatomia y Fisiologia de la via aérea superior; in Jimenez JFM (eds): Apneas e Hipopneas durante el sueno – visión actual. Aula Médica Ediciones, Madrid, 2001, pp 13–20.
2 Deegan PC, McNicholas WT: Pathophysiology of obstructive sleep apnoea. Eur Respir J 1995;8:1161–1178.
3 Douglas NJ: Obstructive sleep apnoea/hypopnoea syndrome; in Arnold (ed): Clinicians' Guide to Sleep Medicine. Arnold, London, 2002, pp 23–100.
4 Malhotra A, Pillar G, Fogel RB, Beauregard J, Edwards JK, Slamowitz DI, Shea SA, White DP: Genioglossal but not palatal muscle activity relates closely to pharyngeal pressure. Am J Respir Crit Care Med 2000;162:1058–1062.
5 Schwab RJ, Gupta KB, Gefter WB, Metzger LJ, Hoffman EA, Pack AI: Upper airway and soft tissue anatomy in normal subjects and patients with sleep-disordered breathing: significance of the lateral pharyngeal walls. Am J Respir Crit Care Med 1995;152:1673–1689.
6 Schwartz AR, O'Donnell CP, Baron J, Schubert N, Alam D, Samadi SD, Smith PL: The hypotonic upper airway in obstructive sleep apnoea: role of structures and neuromuscular activity. Am J Respir Crit Care Med 1998;157:1051–1057.
7 Stanchina ML, Malhotra A, Fogel RB, Ayas N, Edwards JK, Schory K, White DP: Genioglossus muscle responsiveness to chemical and mechanical stimuli during non-rapid eye movement sleep. Am J Respir Crit Care Med 2002;165:945–949.
8 Friberg D, Ansved T, Borg K, Carlsson-Nordlander B, Larson H, Svanborg E: Histological indications of a progressive snorers disease in an upper airway muscle. Am J Respir Crit Care Med 1998;157:586–593.
9 Morrell MJ, Arabi Y, Zahn BR, Meyer KC, Skatrud JB, Badr SM: Effect of surfactant on pharyngeal mechanics in sleeping humans: implications for sleep apnoea. Eur Respir J 2002;20:451–457.
10 Smurra MV, Rodenstein DO: Upper airway imaging in sleep apnoea syndrome: clinical applications. Monaldi Arch Chest Dis 1998; 53:520–523.
11 Schwab RJ: Imaging for the snoring and sleep apnoea patient. Dent Clin North Am 2001;45: 759–796.
12 Schellenberg JB, Maislin G, Schwab RJ: Physical findings and the risk for obstructive sleep apnoea: the importance of oropharyngeal structures. Am J Respir Crit Care Med 2000;162:740–748.
13 Rombaux Ph, Bertrand B, Boudewyns A, Deron Ph, Goffart Y, Leysen J, Liistro G, Marien S, Moerman M, Remacle M: Standard ENT clinical evaluation of the sleep-disordered breathing patient: a consensus report. Acta Otorhinolaryngo Belg 2002;56:127–137.
14 Liistro G, Rombaux Ph, Belge C, Dury M, Aubert G, Rodenstein DO: High Mallampati score and nasal obstruction are associated risk factors for obstructive sleep apnoea. Eur Respir J 2003;21:248–252.
15 Deegan PC, McNicholas WT: Predictive value of clinical features for the obstructive sleep apnoea syndrome. Eur Respir J 1996;9: 117–124.
16 Kushida CA, Efron B, Guilleminault C: A predictive morphometric model for the obstructive sleep apnoea syndrome. Ann Intern Med 1997;127:581–587.
17 Lam B, Ip MSM, Tench E, Ryan CF: Craniofacial profile in Asian and white subjects with obstructive sleep apnea. Thorax 2005;60:504–510.
18 Jamieson A, Guilleminault C, Partinen M, Quera-Salva MA: Obstructive sleep apnoeic patients have craniomandibular abnormalities. Sleep 1986;9:469–477.
19 Lyberg T, Krogstad O, Djupestand G: Cephalometric analysis in patients with obstructive sleep apnoea syndrome: skeletal and soft tissue morphology (I, II). J Laryngol Otol 1989;103:287–297.
20 Maltais F, Carrier G, Cormier Y, Séries F: Cephalometric measurements in snorers, nonsnorers and patients with sleep apnoea. Thorax 1991;46:419–423.
21 Lowe AA, Fleetham JA, Adachi S, Ryan CF: Cephalometric and computed tomographic predictors of obstructive sleep apnoea severity. Am J Orthod Dentofacial Orthop 1995; 107:589–595.
22 Tangugsorn V, Skatredt O, Krogstad O, Lyberg T: Obstructive sleep apnoea: a cephalometric study – uvulo-glossopharyngeal and cervicocraniofacial morphology (I, II). Eur J Orthod 1995;17:45–67.
23 Nelson S, Hans M: Contribution of craniofacial risk factors in increasing apnoeic activity among obese and non-obese habitual snorers. Chest 1997;111:154–162.
24 Brander PE, Mortimore IL, Douglas NJ: Effect of obesity and erect/supine posture on lateral cephalometry: relationship to sleep-disorder breathing. Eur Respir J 1999;13: 398–402.
25 Pépin JL, Veale D, Ferrety GR, Mayer P, Lévy P: Obstructive sleep apnoea syndrome/ hooked apperance of the soft palate in awake patients – cephalometric and CT findings. Radiology 1999;210:163–170.
26 Miles PG, Vig PS, Weyant RJ, Forrest TD, Rockette HE: Craniofacial structure and obstructive sleep apnoea syndrome – a qualitative analysis and meta-analysis of the literature. Am J Orthod Dentofacial Orthop 1996; 109:163–172.
27 Hans MG, Nelson S, Pracharktam N, Baek S, Strohl K, Redline S: Subgrouping persons with snoring and/or apnoea by using anthro pometric and cephalometricial measures. Sleep Breath 2001;5:79–91.
28 Pracharktam N, Nelson S, Hans MG, Broadbent BH, Redline S, Rosenberg C, Strohl KP: Cephalometric assessment in obstructive sleep apnea. Am J Orthod Dentofacial Orthop 1996;109:410–419.
29 Millman RP, Carlisle CC, Rosenberg C, Kahn D, McRae R, Kramer NR: Simple predictors of uvulopalatopharyngoplasty in the treatment of obstructive sleep apnoea syndrome. Chest 2000;118:1025–1030.
30 Schwals RJ, Pasirstein M, Pierson R, Mackley A, Hachadoorian R, Arens R, Maislin G, Pack AI: Identification of upper airway anatomic risk factors for obstructive sleep apnoea with volumetric magnetic resonance imaging. Am J Respir Crit Care Med 2003;168:522–530.
31 Ciscar MA, Juan G, Martinez V, Ramón M, Lloret T, Mínguez J, Armengot M, Marín J, Basterra J: MRI of the pharynx and treatment efficacy of a mandibular advacement device in obstructive sleep apnoea syndrome. Eur Respir J 2001;17:79–86.
32 Mortimore IL, Marshall I, Wraith PK, Sellar RJ, Douglas NJ: Neck and total body fat deposition in non-obese and obese patients with sleep apnea compared with that in control subjects. Am J Respir Crit Care Med 1998;157: 280–283.
33 Rodenstein DO, Dooms G, Thomas Y, Liistro G, Stanescu DC, Culee C, Aubert-Tulkens G: Pharyngeal shape and size in snoring and sleep apnoea. Thorax 1990;45:722–727.
34 Ryan CF, Lowe A, Li D, Fleetham JA: Magnetic resonance imaging of the upper airway in obstructive sleep apneoa before and after chronic nasal continuous positive airway pressure therapy. Am Rev Respir Dis 1991;144:939–944.
35 Schwals RJ, Pack AI, Gupta KB: Upper airway and soft tissue changes induced by CPAP in normal subjects. Am J Respir Crit Care Med 1996;154:1106–1116.
36 Langin T, Pépin JL, Pendlebury S, Baranton-Cantin H, Ferreti G, Reyt E, Levy P: Upper airway changes in snorers and mild sleep apnoea sufferers after uvulopalatopharyngoplasty. Chest 1998;113:1595–1603.
37 Sanner BM, Heise M, Knoben B, Machnick M, Laufer U, Kikuth R, Zidek W, Hellmich B: MRI of the pharynx and treatment efficacy of a mandibular advacement device in obstructive sleep apnoea syndrome. Eur Respir J 2002;20:143–150.
38 Schwals RJ, Gefter WB, Hoffman EA, Gupta KB, Pack AI: Dynamic upper airway imaging during awake respiration in normal subjects and patients with sleep disordered breathing. Am Rev Respir Dis 1993;148:1385–1400.
39 Hudgel DW, Harasick T, Katz RL, Witt WJ, Abelson T: Uvulopalatopharyngoplasty in obstructive apnoea: value of preoperative localization of site of upper airway narrowing during sleep. Am Rev Respir Dis 1991;143:942–946.
40 Kwok W, Wiegand L, Channin DS, Wiegand DA: Development of the bi-directional ultrasound system for base of tongue imaging. Comput Biol Med 1994;24:295–304.

Prof. Daniel O. Rodenstein
Service de pneumologie, Cliniques universitaires Saint-Luc
Av. Hippocrate 10
BE–1200 Brussels (Belgium)
Tel. +32 2 764 28 86
Fax +32 2 764 28 31
E-Mail rodenstein@pneu.ucl.ac.be

Randerath WJ, Sanner BM, Somers VK (eds): Sleep Apnea.
Prog Respir Res. Basel, Karger, 2006, vol 35, pp 79–89

Upper Airway Obstruction in Snoring and Upper Airway Resistance Syndrome

Jason P. Kirkness[a,b] Vidya Krishnan[a] Susheel P. Patil[a] Hartmut Schneider[a]

[a]Johns Hopkins University, Department of Medicine, Division of Pulmonary and Critical Care Medicine, Johns Hopkins Sleep Disorders Center, Baltimore, Md., USA; [b]University of Western Australia, School of Anatomy and Human Biology, Faculty of Life and Physical Sciences, Perth, Australia

Abstract

Treatment options for snoring and upper airway resistance syndrome are hampered by either low compliance or low efficacy. Therefore, refinements in these therapeutic strategies are needed. The understanding of the pathogenic factors of upper airway obstruction and an individual's compensatory responses to defend ventilation in face of upper airway obstruction may help to develop more effective and less intrusive treatment alternatives. Undoubtedly, this may require more precise monitoring and pre- and post-treatment assessment of the factors that maintain upper airway patency and ventilation during sleep.

Snoring is a common phenomenon during sleep and associated with the obstructive sleep apnea/hypopnea syndrome (OSAHS), which has been identified as a risk factor for cardiovascular diseases [1]. Snoring is caused by upper airway obstruction, which is largely related to an increased propensity of the upper airway to collapse during sleep through a loss of neuromuscular tone in upper airway muscles. Frequently, compensatory neural responses to upper airway obstruction can adequately defend ventilation during sleep, and patients have a normal stable breathing pattern during sleep (primary snorer). Alternatively, compensatory responses to upper airway obstruction can intermittently fail, thereby reducing ventilation and inducing sleep fragmentation. These patients exhibit an unstable breathing pattern during sleep that is clinically referred to as either upper airway resistance syndrome (UARS) or obstructive hypopneas (fig. 1). Several intrinsic and extrinsic factors can either increase the risk for upper airway obstruction or blunt neuromuscular compensatory responses to upper airway obstruction. This chapter will focus on the pathophysiology of upper airway obstruction and its implications for the management of snoring and UARS.

Pathogenesis of Upper Airway Obstruction

In the last 20–30 years there has been an appreciable number of investigations of the mechanical properties of the upper airway, principally attempting to understand the pathophysiology of OSAHS. The main difficulty for the patient with OSAHS is collapse or partial obstruction of the pharyngeal airway that occurs during sleep in affected individuals [2]. To elucidate the mechanism of upper airway obstruction in obstructive sleep apnea (OSA), several approaches have been adopted to model the factors involved in the pathogenesis of pharyngeal collapse.

Upper Airway Function and Mechanics

The upper airway commences at the oral and nasal openings, while at the other end it divides into the tracheal and esophageal passageways. The upper airway has a complex geometry, and is enclosed by muscles and mobile nonmuscular structures that are able to alter airway configuration. The major respiratory function of the upper

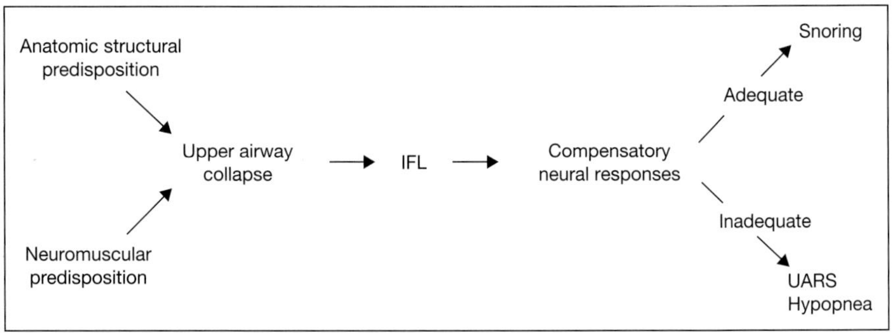

Fig. 1. Proposed pathogenesis of snoring and upper airway resistance syndrome (UARS). Anatomic and neuromuscular factors induce upper airway collapse and inspiratory airflow limitation (IFL). IFL induces compensatory neural responses, which may be adequate to stabilize breathing or inadequate or even absent with the subsequent development obstructed sleep disordered breathing.

airway is to permit air movement into and out of the lungs. In addition, the upper airway heats and humidifies inspired air, and is important in the regulation of both inspiratory and expiratory airflow. Under resting conditions including sleep, air flows through the nose, pharynx and larynx to the extrathoracic trachea. When airflow increases, as during heavy exercise or with nasal obstruction, breathing occurs through the mouth in addition to the nose, and hence the oral cavity is also part of the upper airway.

The upper airway is responsible for a major component of the total airway resistance in humans, providing 40–70% of the total pulmonary resistance during resting breathing. Nasal resistance is by far the largest component of the total upper airway resistance. Under quiet breathing during wakefulness in normal subjects, laryngeal and pharyngeal components are relatively small, but they are the most variable components of the total upper airway resistance. Upper airway size and resistance vary dynamically throughout the respiratory cycle and are also affected by the route of breathing (oral vs. nasal) [3], lung volume, level of ventilation, hypoxia and hypercapnia and behavioral state (conscious vs. unconscious and wakefulness vs. sleep). In addition, upper airway resistance can increase the work of the inspiratory muscles in producing airflow. Indeed, for patients with OSA and snorers, upper airway resistance may increase dramatically due to pharyngeal airway collapse and obstruction of inspiratory airflow [2].

Starling Resistor Model for Upper Airway Obstruction

Initial efforts for modeling upper airway obstruction focused on the interplay between extraluminal upper airway muscles that dilate and negative intraluminal pressures generated by the diaphragm that collapse the pharynx. It was originally postulated that upper airway patency was determined by the balance of pressures between the intraluminal and extraluminal space [2]. As intraluminal 'suction' pressures overcame the dilating forces around the pharyngeal lumen, the theory held that the pharynx would progressively collapse and ultimately occlude during sleep. Later studies, however, have minimized the role of intraluminal suction pressures in the pathogenesis of upper airway obstruction by demonstrating that upper airway occlusion could occur spontaneously, even when intraluminal pressures were positive [4]. These observations resolved a major question regarding the role of negative intraluminal pressures in the pathogenesis of OSA, and confirmed that negative pressures were not required for airway occlusion to occur. Rather, the markedly negative intraluminal pressures generated by the diaphragm during periods of upper airway obstruction were the consequence rather than the cause of upper airway occlusion.

To further elucidate the mechanism for upper airway obstruction, investigators have examined airflow dynamics during periods of obstruction, and found that pressure-flow relationships were identical to those previously described for other collapsible biologic conduits, i.e. the Starling resistor (fig. 1) [5]. This model provides a generalized approach for determining the critical pressure during inspiration, based on an analysis of pressure-flow relationships in the upper airway segment (fig. 2). A major feature of this model is that it describes the conditions leading to alterations in upper airway patency. Specifically, the model predicts that the airway would completely occlude whenever pressures both upstream (P_{us}) and downstream (P_{ds}) fall below a critical pressure (P_{crit}). Under these circumstances, no flow could pass through the airway as long as $P_{crit} > P_{us} > P_{ds}$. As the upstream pressure is raised above the critical pressure, however, the upper airway would no longer remain occluded. Rather, the Starling resistor model predicts that a flow-limited state would ensue as long as the downstream pressure remains below critical pressure ($P_{us} > P_{crit} > P_{ds}$) [6]. Inspiratory airflow limitation (IFL) is characterized by a plateauing of airflow and is associated

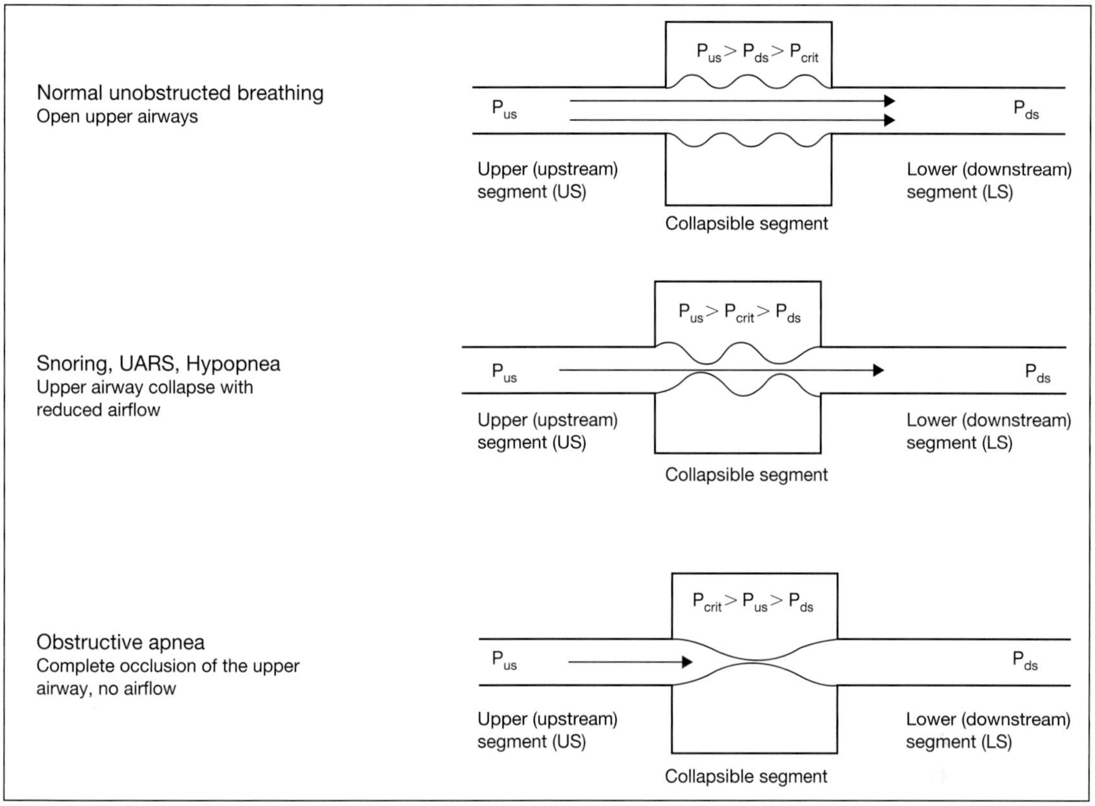

Fig. 2. The upper airway can be represented as a mechanical analogue of the Starling resistor model, consisting of a rigid tube with a collapsible segment. Upper (upstream, nasal) and lower (downstream, hypopharyngeal) segments have fixed diameters and defined resistances. Pressures in these segments are represented by P_{us} and P_{ds}, respectively. The collapsible segment has no resistance but is subject to the surrounding pressure, P_{crit}. Collapse occurs only when the surrounding pressure exceeds the downstream pressure (middle panel) and inspiratory airflow decreases compared to normal unobstructed breathing (upper panel). Complete occlusion occurs when P_{crit} exceeds both the upstream and downstream pressure (lower panel). Adapted from Gleadhill et al. [25].

with collapse of the pharynx and audible snoring. Under conditions of flow limitation, investigators have also demonstrated that flow through the upper airway rises linearly with elevations in upstream pressure, regardless of the downstream pressure level [7]. Thus, the Starling resistor model predicts that the airway will occlude when upstream and downstream pressures remain below a critical pressure, and that flow limitation will result in linear increases in airflow as the upstream pressure is raised above the critical pressure (the conditions leading to occlusion and flow limitation in the upper airway are identical to those corresponding to zones I and II for the pulmonary vasculature, respectively).

In further studies, the upstream nasal pressure has been manipulated systematically, and critical pressures were measured in groups of individuals manifesting varying degrees of upper airway obstruction during sleep (fig. 3) [7]. Critical pressures were markedly negative in normal individuals with evidence of airflow obstruction, whereas critical pressures were positive in apneic patients with complete upper airway occlusion. In patients with partial airflow obstruction during sleep (obstructive hypopnea, UARS, and asymptomatic snorers), critical pressures were between these two extremes (minimally to moderately negative) [7]. These observations suggested that varying degrees of upper airway obstruction during sleep were associated with quantitative differences in critical pressures, reflecting differences in upper airway collapsibility across the spectrum from health to disease.

Factors Influencing Ventilation in the Face of Upper Airway Obstruction

Inspired minute ventilation (V_I) during sleep is determined by anatomic factors and by the neural responses that

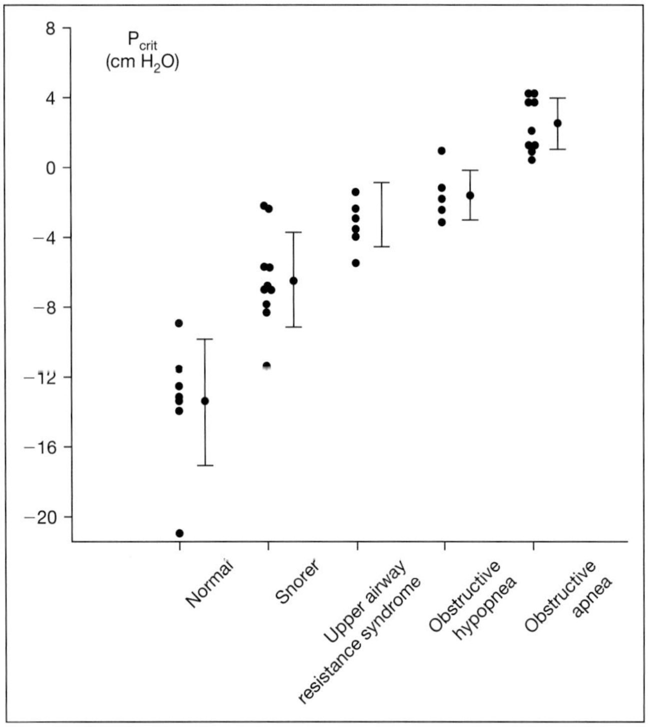

Fig. 3. Upper airway collapse (P_{crit}) and clinical expression. Critical closing pressures of the upper airway (P_{crit}) during sleep are plotted for groups of individuals that represent the clinical spectrum of obstructive sleep apnea – non-snoring, snoring, upper airway resistance syndrome (UARS), obstructive hypopnea, and obstructive apnea. P_{crit} increases with increasing disease severity over a relatively narrow range of pressures. Note overlap between UARS and obstructive hypopneas, suggesting that the two disorders are indistinguishable in the degree of upper airway function, or in the impact of upper airway obstruction on sleep continuity. Adapted from Schwartz et al. [7] and Gleadhill et al. [25].

stabilize breathing. The factors leading to hypoventilation have traditionally been described by the basic relationship:

$$V_I = \left[\frac{V_T}{T_I}\right] \cdot \left[\frac{T_I}{T_{TOT}}\right] \quad (1)$$

where V_I is the inspired minute ventilation, V_T is the tidal volume, T_I is the inspiratory time, T_{TOT} is the respiratory cycle length, and T_I/T_{TOT} is the inspiratory duty cycle [8]. The conceptual framework provided by equation 1 forms the basis for our approach of characterizing the respiratory phenotypes predisposing to hypoventilation during periods of upper airway obstruction. As shown in equation 1, reductions in ventilation (V_I) can be attributed to decreases in either the mean inspiratory flow (V_T/T_I) or inspiratory duty cycle (T_I/T_{TOT}). In early work, the mean inspiratory flow was found to be correlated with measurements of respiratory drive, whereas the inspiratory duty cycle was thought to be primarily determined by the timing characteristics of the respiratory pattern generators. Thus, reductions in ventilation could be attributed to decreases in ventilatory drive or inspiratory duty cycle.

Although the mechanisms involved in stabilizing ventilation during sleep in the presence of upper airway obstruction have not been well defined, upper airway obstruction is known to increase ventilatory drive, which should increase the mean inspiratory flow (eq. 1). If the upper airway collapses, however, such increases in drive could not lead to further increase in the mean inspiratory airflow because inspiratory flow would be limited to a maximal level that could not be exceeded as effort increases. Therefore, during periods of IFL, increases in ventilatory drive can no longer prevent the individual from hypoventilating during sleep. Instead of increasing ventilatory drive and/or mean inspiratory airflow, patients can only preserve ventilation in the face of upper airway obstruction by prolonging the inspiratory duty cycle [3]. In recent work, our group has suggested that both the maximum inspiratory flow during upper airway obstruction and inspiratory duty cycle constitute distinct respiratory phenotypic traits [9], as follows: Under conditions of IFL, equation 1 becomes:

$$V_I = [V_I \max]_{IFL} \cdot \left[\frac{T_I}{T_{TOT}}\right] \quad (2)$$

where $(V_I \max)_{IFL}$ represents the level of maximal inspiratory airflow, which approximates the mean inspiratory airflow in the flow limited condition. From equation 2 it is evident that minute ventilation could be stabilized during periods of upper airway obstruction in one of two ways (fig. 4).

First, the level of mean inspiratory airflow could be increased. As noted above, $(V_I \max)_{IFL}$ is determined solely by upper airway characteristics rather than the level of ventilatory drive. Any increase in the level of mean inspiratory airflow would be attributed to increases in upper airway neuromuscular responses or upper airway biochemical and physical properties.

Second, in the face of upper airway obstruction, an increase in ventilation could be accomplished by increasing the inspiratory duty cycle. As shown in figure 4, compensatory neural responses can help to maintain and stabilize ventilation during periods of upper airway obstruction by either restoring upper airway flow (inspiratory airflow) or prolonging the inspiratory duty cycle.

Taken together, the strengths of both compensatory neural responses will determine whether upper airway obstruction will be associated with stable breathing (snoring) or an unstable breathing pattern (UARS, hypopnea or apnea).

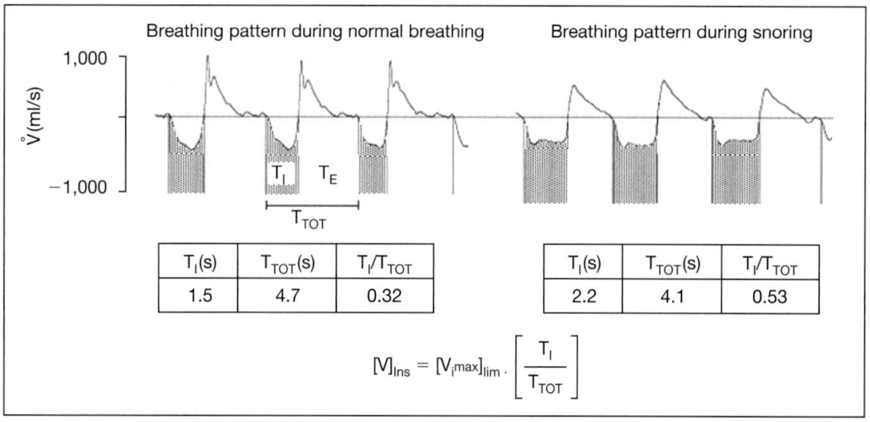

Fig. 4. Effect of upper airway obstruction on respiratory timing in a normal individual is illustrated in 1 subject. Upper airway obstruction was induced by lowering the nasal pressure from 5 cm H_2O (left panel) to –5 cm H_2O (right panel). Respiratory pattern indices (inspiratory time, T_I; total respiratory cycle length, T_{TOT}; inspiratory duty cycle, T_I/T_{TOT}) are shown for the baseline, unobstructed condition (left panel) and for the three breaths during the acute period of upper airway obstruction (right panel). The duty cycle increased substantially from the unobstructed period with the induction of upper airway obstruction. Adapted from Schneider et al. [3].

In the following section, we will discuss the factors that influence the neural compensatory drive.

Mechanisms that Predispose to Upper Airway Obstruction

Several factors have been associated with alterations in the properties of the upper airway. These factors include anatomic or structural, neurochemical factors, and those which modify the surface tension of the upper airway.

Anatomic Factors

Specific anatomic alterations including tonsillar hypertrophy [10], retrognathia and variations in craniofacial structure [11] have been linked to an increased risk of OSA. Similarly, computed tomographic and magnetic resonance imaging studies have provided evidence for increased fatty tissue deposition in the lateral walls of the pharynx and submucosal edema that result in narrowing of the pharyngeal lumen during wakefulness, and are thought to predispose to airway obstruction during sleep. Isono et al. [12] have provided evidence for this hypothesis in experiments utilizing general anesthesia and complete neuromuscular blockade to eliminate neuromuscular input to the upper airway during sleep. Based on analysis of the maximal pharyngeal area (MPA) and static pressure-area curves, they demonstrated that apneic patients had significant narrowing of the upper airway (MPA: 1.1 ± 0.8 vs. $2.1 \pm 0.9\,cm^2$) and a more collapsible upper airway as reflected by higher closing pressures (2.2 ± 3.0 vs. -4.4 ± 4.2 cm H_2O) in the velopharynx compared with control subjects [12].

Nevertheless, luminal narrowing alone may not be sufficient to produce collapse during sleep, since greater degrees of narrowing have been demonstrated in women who are resistant to upper airway collapse during sleep. Rather, such narrowing may elicit compensatory increases in upper airway neuromuscular activity that are required to maintain upper airway patency either during wakefulness or during sleep [13]. Taken together, these studies imply that snorers and apneic patients can be distinguished from normal patients on the basis of anatomic properties that predispose to upper airway obstruction when protective neuromuscular mechanisms wane at sleep onset.

Neural Factors

In addition to anatomic properties, it is well recognized that the upper airway is subject to neuromuscular factors that can also influence its patency. Upper airway obstruction is known to trigger various neuromuscular reflexes that activate upper airway dilator muscles and defend airway patency [14]. In animal studies of upper airway neuromuscular reflexes, these findings have led to the hypothesis that patients with OSA actually have increased levels of EMG activity that help maintain normal airway patency during wakefulness; however, when this compensating activity falls inappropriately at sleep onset airway occlusion may ensue. While these data attest to the importance of neural activation of upper airway muscles, the precise effect of EMG activity on upper airway function and ventilation during sleep has not been precisely defined.

To determine the impact of neuromuscular activity on upper airway patency, extensive studies in the isolated upper airway of animals have demonstrated that upper airway collapsibility is modulated by a complex interaction of neuromuscular and anatomic factors that influence pharyngeal collapsibility and airflow dynamics. Among these factors are pulmonary and upper airway mechanoreceptor pathways, as well as chemoreceptors, all of which have been shown to act individually or in combination to modify upper airway dilator muscle activity [15]. In addition, it is now thought that negative pressure reflexes of the upper airway may not respond appropriately to the markedly negative intraluminal pressure generated during periods of upper airway obstruction. Moreover, Mezzanotte et al. [14] have documented elevated genioglossal EMG activity in patients with OSA compared to normals during wakefulness, suggesting that the negative pressure reflex is selectively attenuated during sleep. Finally, it appears that upper airway sensory pathways may be impaired, since temperature, two-point discrimination and vibratory thresholds are disrupted in sleep apnea patients compared with normal individuals [16]. Sensory receptor dysfunction could also attenuate the response of upper airway dilator muscles to the markedly negative airway pressures generated during periods of upper airway obstruction. Further evidence for sensorimotor dysfunction is provided by graded histopathologic and immunochemical alterations in the palatopharyngeus and muscularis uvulae in sleep apnea patients, relative to asymptomatic snorers and normal individuals [17]. Findings of muscle fiber type redistribution and injury (fascicular atrophy and grouped atrophy in muscle fibers), have suggested that myopathic as well as sensory dysfunction may further compromise neuromuscular responses to upper airway obstruction.

Biomechanical Characteristics of the Upper Airway Mucosal Surface

The upper airway is lined by a liquid at the mucosal surface important to the patency of the upper airway. Many investigators have examined the role of surface tension in maintaining alveolar patency, whereas there are relatively few investigations of surface forces in upper airway patency. Wilson et al. [18] reported postmortem studies in infants which demonstrated that the intraluminal pressure required to re-open a closed upper airway was greater than the intraluminal pressure required to close the same airway. This difference between upper airway opening and closing pressure was ascribed to the force required to overcome surface tension effects between the walls of the closed airway. These findings suggest that surface forces operating in the liquid lining the upper airway exert an influence on upper airway patency. Since these first observations, there have been only a few studies that have addressed this concept. Olson and Strohl [19] demonstrated that stimulation of upper airway secretions in rabbits made the collapsed upper airway more difficult to re-open (i.e. because of increased upper airway opening pressure). This effect was ascribed to 'stickiness' of the induced upper airway secretions. In rabbits, instillation of surfactant into the upper airway has been shown to reduce the surface tension of the mucosal lining liquid and increase upper airway patency [20–22].

It has recently been shown in humans that the surface tension of upper airway lining liquid plays an important role in the control of upper airway patency [20–22]. For example, in both awake and anesthetized [21] humans lowering the surface tension of upper airway lining liquid with exogenous surfactant decreases the intraluminal pressure required to reopen a closed pharyngeal airway. In addition a number of studies have shown that the instillation of exogenous surfactant into the upper airway of patients with OSAHS reduces the severity of the associated sleep-disordered breathing [22–24]. Thus, alteration of the surface forces of the liquid lining the upper airway may provide a mechanism for influencing the collapsibility of the upper airway; however, the clinical value of this issue is yet to be resolved.

Taken together, anatomic structural properties, neuromuscular influences and biomechanical properties of the surface liquid could account for quantitative differences in critical pressure in humans manifesting various degrees of anatomic structural predisposition for upper airway obstruction during sleep. As outlined above, normal individuals are characterized by markedly negative critical pressures, reflecting diminished upper airway collapsibility during sleep, compared to progressive elevations in critical pressure in those with partial obstruction (snoring and obstructive hypopneas) and complete occlusion (obstructive apnea) [25]. Moreover, the critical pressures in normal sleeping individuals are markedly lower than those reported in normal anesthetized subjects after abolishing neuromuscular activity with a paralytic agent. The further reduction in critical pressure in the sleeping compared to the paralyzed state suggests that neuromuscular factors prevent collapse, and play an important role in maintaining upper airway patency during sleep.

Predisposing Factors for Hypoventilation in the Face of Upper Airway Obstruction

As outlined above, it is now evident that defects in both the upper airway and neuroventilatory control are pivotal for the development of obstructed sleep disordered breathing. Although neuromuscular control of upper airway function is crucial for the level of inspiratory airflow, the duty cycle has been identified as a distinct physiologic component for defending ventilation in response to upper airway obstruction. For example, the duty cycle contains a physiologic ceiling of approximately 0.6, at which no further increases of the duty cycle is possible [26]. If the duty cycle during unobstructed breathing is already above 0.5 as commonly seen in patients with underlying medical illnesses of the heart and lung, an individual would be able to increase the duty cycle and minute ventilation by only 20%, while a normal individual with a duty cycle of 0.3 at baseline may increase the duty cycle and ventilation by 200%.

Conversely, a hallmark of chronic obstructive pulmonary disease (COPD) and asthma is expiratory airflow limitation that leads to prolongations of the expiratory time, which in turn, shortens inspiratory time. As a consequence, these patients are also limited to increase their duty cycle, once they exhibit inspiratory upper airway obstruction, due to a ceiling effect imposed by their expiratory time requirement. However, it is currently unclear, whether this feature in patients with COPD may play a role for the increased prevalence of sleepiness and fatigue in these patients.

Gender might also affect ventilatory responses to upper airway obstruction, as testosterone, progesterone and estrogen are known to alter ventilatory control. Moreover, gender differences exist in lung function and metabolic demand, both of which may affect the ventilatory compensatory responses to upper airway obstruction.

Similarly, it has been shown that normal individuals exhibit substantial variation in the magnitude of duty cycle response, even when the baseline duty cycles are similar between subjects [3]. The response in inspiratory duty cycle in the setting of upper airway obstruction varied between 0.02 and 0.18, indicating that the duty cycle in response to upper airway obstruction may serve as an intermediate physiologic trait that may provide a link to specific genetic factors relevant to the expression of obstructive sleep disordered breathing [3].

Taken together, the duty cycle during unobstructed breathing may determine an individual's ability to respond adequately to upper airway obstruction. However, it is not clear whether such abnormalities exacerbate sleep related hypoventilation and UARS in normal patients with milder degrees of upper airway obstruction.

Upper Airway Resistance Syndrome

Definition

While primary snoring is by definition associated with a stable sleep and breathing pattern, UARS, similar to OSA, is defined by repetitive upper airway collapse resulting in IFL and subsequent arousals from sleep. Upper airway collapsibility, as reflected in the critical closing pressure (P_{crit}), of patients with UARS is intermediate between normal patients without sleep disordered breathing and patients with OSA [7, 25] establishing UARS on the spectrum of obstructive sleep disordered breathing. While OSA is associated with intermittent oxyhemoglobin desaturations and significant reductions in airflow, UARS does not share these features.

History of UARS

The term 'upper airway resistance syndrome' was first coined by Guilleminault and his colleagues in 1993. Over a decade earlier, they had published results of the first study of this clinical entity in children. In a retrospective study of 25 children with snoring, excessive daytime sleepiness, and behavioral disturbances, compared to 25 control children, they found that while subjects did not have overt OSA, the case subjects had more frequent episodes of IFL with significant intrathroacic pressure swings and subsequent arousals, compared to the control group. Treatment of case subjects with tonsillectomy and adenoidectomy resolved all daytime symptoms, implicating increased upper airway resistance in the pathophysiology of this clinical entity. Subsequent research in adults identified UARS as a significant cause of daytime hypersomnia.

UARS describes the constellation of daytime hypersomnolence due to respiratory arousals related to IFL, without overt apneas or hypopneas. Although controversy remains regarding the establishment of UARS as a distinct clinical entity. UARS is generally recognized as a subset of OSA syndrome, due to similarities in pathophysiology and treatment. Silent UARS, defined as UARS without clinically evident snoring, is present in 1% of patients evaluated for hypersomnolence in sleep laboratories [27]. Because of unique features in clinical presentation and diagnostic strategies, UARS continues to be an under-recognized and untreated form of sleep-disordered breathing.

IFL results in the generation of significant negative intrathoracic pressure with each breath. Gleeson and colleagues demonstrated a correlation between brief arousals and the magnitude of esophageal pressure swings, with a consistent arousal response when intrathoracic pressure reached a level of approximately –15 cm H_2O. Thus, frequent respiratory arousals associated with IFL can predictably result in sleep disruption and subsequent daytime hypersomnolence. While IFL is the hallmark of UARS and other obstructive sleep disorders, variation in clinical expression of IFL may also be determined by other patient

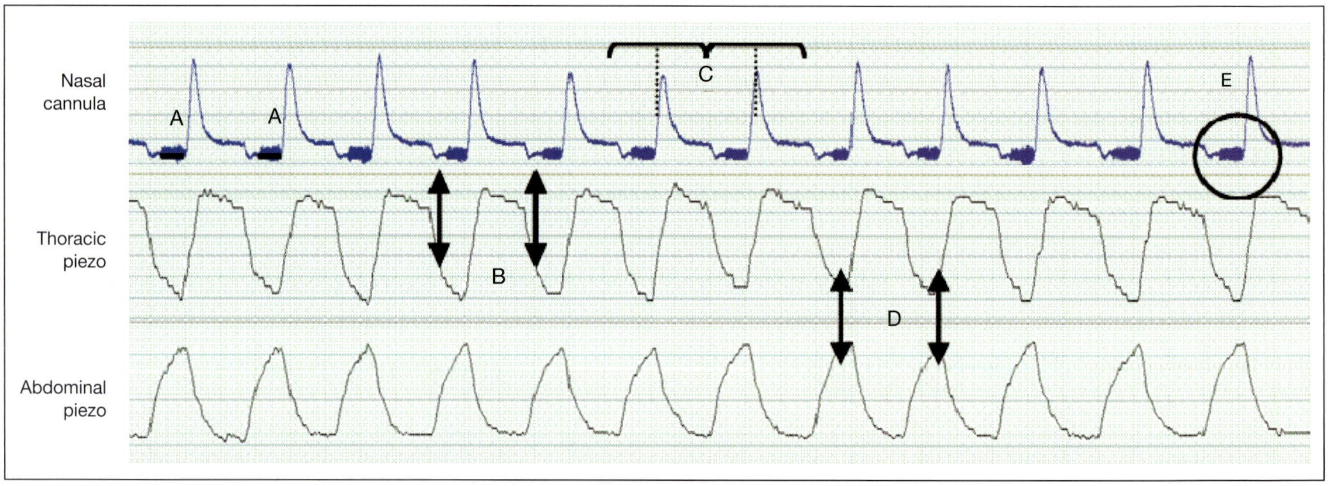

Fig. 5. Snapshot of polysomnography from a patient with inspiratory flow limitation. Signals of interest include airflow (via nasal cannula) and respiratory effort (via thoracic and abdominal piezo belts). Inspiratory flow limitation is characterized by constant or reduced inspiratory airflow (A) in the setting of continued or greater respiratory effort (B); prolongation of the inspiratory duty cycle (C); desynchrony of thoracic and abdominal movements with inspiratory (D), and snoring (E).

factors, such as comorbidity, gender and heritable alterations in ventilatory control as discussed above. This is also highlighted by the significant overlap of P_{crit} observed in patients with simple snoring, UARS, and obstructive sleep hypopneas [7, 25] suggesting that the clinical expression of IFL is determined by factors such as ventilatory protective mechanisms, degree of oxyhemoglobin desaturation with respiratory events, degree of hypercapnia, time since previous awakening or arousal, total sleep time, and temporal proximity to REM sleep [28].

Diagnosis

Diagnosis of UARS requires a heightened clinical suspicion of obstructive sleep disordered breathing along with sensitive diagnostic airflow measurements. Clinical history alone does not discriminate between types of obstructive sleep disordered breathing. Patients presenting with UARS often complain of excessive daytime sleepiness, snoring, fatigue, and morning headaches, similar to OSA. Physical examination may reveal an overcrowded pharynx, retrognathia, macroglossia, and other such features which would predispose to upper airway obstruction. Obesity can be a feature of patients with UARS, but is not necessary.

Nocturnal polysomnography is necessary to diagnose UARS. Esophageal balloon manometry, as a measure of intrathoracic pressure, and pneumotachography, a quantitative airflow measurement, have been the gold standard measurements for UARS. Although alternative measurements of respiratory effort (piezo belts, plethysmography) and airflow (nasal cannula, thermistors, thermocouples) are sufficient enough to detect IFL (fig. 5), they are often not sensitive or specific to detect UARS particularly due to the lack of either quantifying airflow or inspiratory effort. Reductions in airflow and progressively more negative intrathoracic pressure prior to an arousal was identified to be the hallmark of UARS (fig. 6). Frequent leg movements in the setting of IFL are often misclassified as periodic limb movements [29], when esophageal pressures and quantitative airflow measurements are not available.

Therapeutic Implications

Continuous positive airway pressure (CPAP) has been designed to overcome upper airway obstruction (positive critical pressure) by elevating upstream pressures at the nose or mouth [30]. CPAP has been a mainstay of therapy for OSA for nearly 20 years, and is effective in relieving obstruction in patients with OSAHS syndrome. However, snoring subjects and patients with UARS exhibit a very low compliance on CPAP due to (1) the inconvenience of wearing the cumbersome nasal masks, and (2) potentially subtherapeutic CPAP settings due to the difficulty in assessing an optimal therapeutic nasal pressure, and therefore often seek alternative less-intrusive treatment options.

There are several alternative approaches for relieving snoring, all of which can be subdivided into two basic principles. The first approach is to improve the structural

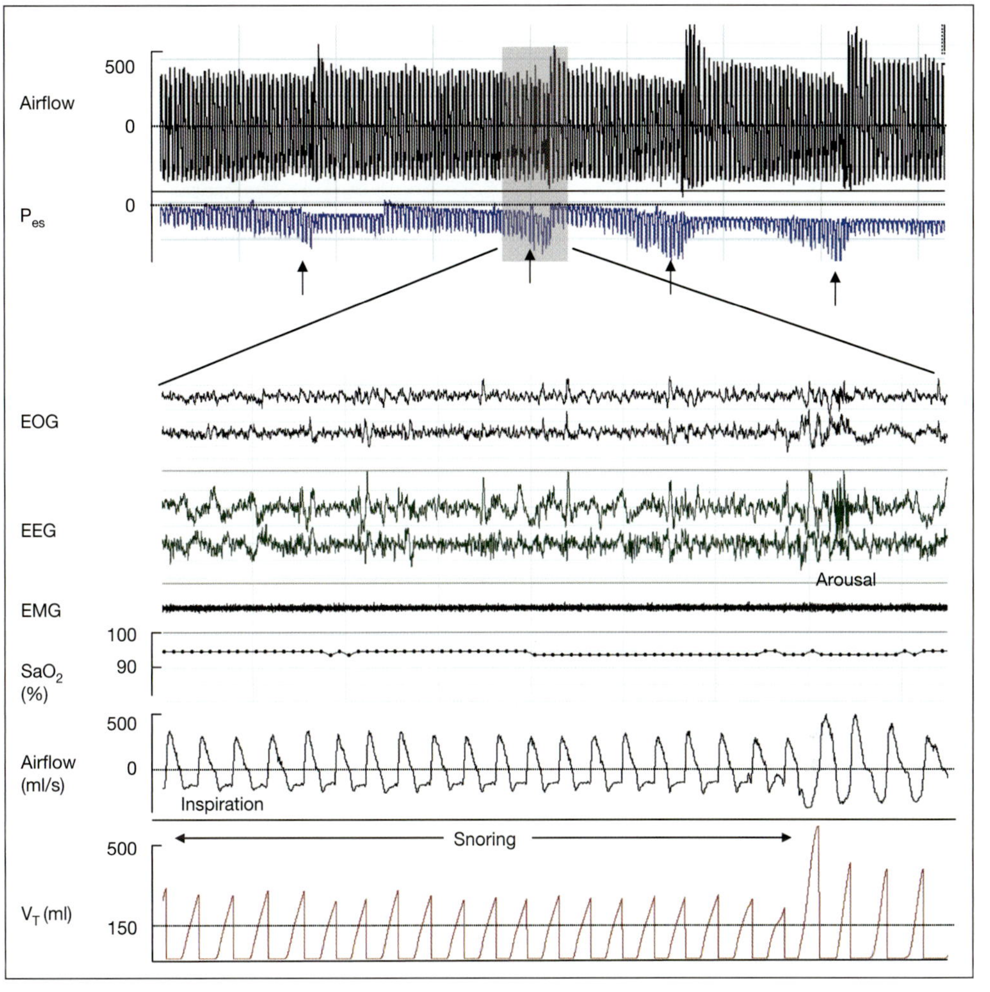

Fig. 6. Snapshot of polysomnography from a patient with upper airway resistance syndrome. In the upper panel a compressed (10 min) view of the airflow and esophageal pressure (P_{es}) signal. As can be seen, while minimal fluctuations occur in the airflow signals, there are intermittent progressive increases in P_{es} (upward arrows), indicating increases in upper airway resistance. As amplified in the panel below, periods of increased P_{es} were due to snoring with inspiratory flow limitation and reductions in tidal volume that led to an arousal from sleep. EOG = Electrooculogram; EEG = electroencephalogram; EMG = electromyogram; SaO_2 = oxygen saturation, V_T = tidal inspiratory volumes.

and neuromuscular properties of the upper airway, thereby lowering the critical closing pressure during sleep, the other is to protect neural compensatory responses to upper airway obstruction, thereby increasing ventilation and reducing the frequency of arousal from snoring.

The first alternative therapeutic approaches target to lower the critical pressure by either augmenting the structural or neuromuscular mechanisms required for the maintenance of airway patency. Current approaches to correcting alterations in upper airway mechanics include weight loss [31] and postural maneuvers [32]. Upper airway reconstructive surgery (uvulopalatopharyngoplasty, transpalatal resection, adenotonsillar resection), and a variety of procedures designed to move the hyoid, mandible and maxillary bones anteriorly [33] are also designed to lower critical closing pressure. These methods have been shown particularly effective in patients with milder degrees of upper airway obstruction but are limited by their intrusiveness and low efficacy in obese and older subjects. Surgical interventions are therefore not being recommended as first line treatment of snoring and UARS. Oral appliances, either mandibular advancement devices or tongue repositioning devices, function by

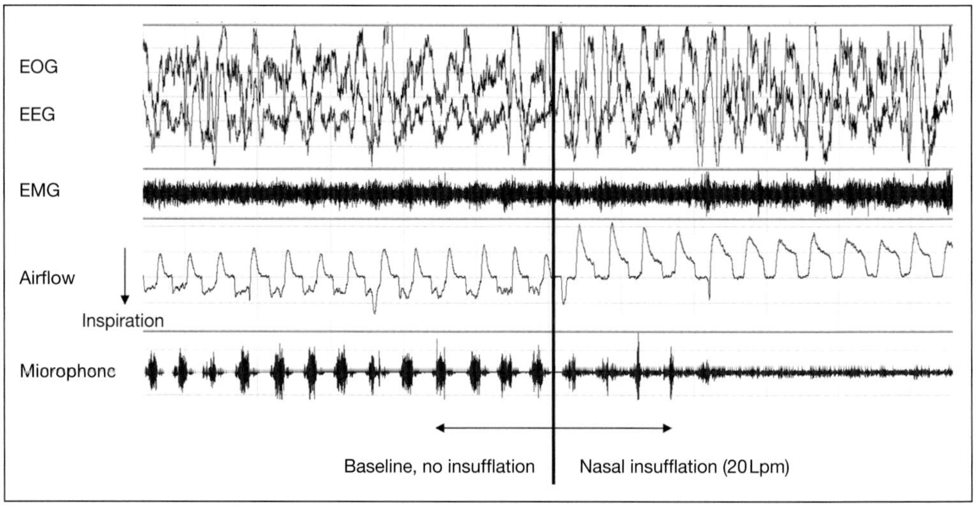

Fig. 7. Effect of nasal insufflation on inspiratory airflow limitation. The inspiratory flow contour indicates snoring (as highlighted in the recording of the sound signal by a microphone in the bottom tracing). With initiation of nasal insufflation, inspiratory flow contour normalizes and snoring abolishes (right panel). EOG = Electrooculogram; EEG = electroencephalogram; SaO_2 = oxygen saturation. From McGinley et al. [36].

mechanically increasing the posterior pharyngeal airspace, and can adequately treat partial upper airway collapse.

Pharmacologic strategies that either lower the surface tension or stimulate upper airway motor neuron pools with tricyclic antidepressants and serotonergic agents may offer partial relief of upper airway obstruction [34]. However, these methods also are limited by either a low efficacy or systemic side effects that inhibit its use in normal individuals who snore or patients with UARS.

The second alternative set of approaches are targeted at the improvement of ventilation during sleep. CNS depressants such as alcohol, benzodiazepines and opioids block compensatory neural responses in several ways, and should therefore be avoided in patients with snoring and UARS. First, although alcohol ingestion has been shown to decrease genioglossal muscle activity, thereby blunting reflex recruitment of the upper airway musculature and predisposing to worsening obstruction, these agents are also known to reduce arousal responses and ventilation during sleep. For example, the arousal responses to airway occlusion are known to be prolonged in normal sleeping subjects after alcohol ingestion, thereby increasing the risk of hypoventilation in face of upper airway obstruction. Finally, the combined effects of CNS depressants on the upper airway musculature and arousal responses could account for observed increases in the frequency and duration of sleep disordered breathing episodes, and worsening oxyhemoglobin desaturations after alcohol ingestion [35].

A new less-intrusive treatment for abolishing IFL by insufflating air through an open nasal cannula system was recently introduced [36]. Although this treatment seems to be effective in abolishing snoring (fig. 7), the precise mechanism and clinical efficacy remain to be resolved before recommending nasal insufflation for general use.

In summary, treatment options for snoring and UARS are hampered by either a low compliance or low efficacy. Therefore, refinements in these therapeutic strategies are needed. The understanding of the pathogenic factors of upper airway obstruction and an individual's compensatory responses to defend ventilation in face of upper airway obstruction may help to develop more effective and less intrusive treatment alternatives. Undoubtedly, this may require more precise monitoring and pre- and post-treatment assessment of the factors that maintain upper airway patency and ventilation during sleep.

References

1 Newman AB, Nieto FJ, Guidry U, Lind BK, Redline S, Pickering TG, Quan SF: Relation of sleep-disordered breathing to cardiovascular disease risk factors: the Sleep Heart Health Study. Am J Epidemiol 2001;154:50–59.

2 Remmers JE, deGroot WJ, Sauerland EK, Anch AM: Pathogenesis of upper airway occlusion during sleep. J Appl Physiol 1978;44:931–938.

3 Schneider H, Patil SP, Canisius S, Gladmon EA, Schwartz AR, O'Donnell CP, Smith PL, Tankersley CG: Hypercapnic duty cycle is an intermediate physiological phenotype linked to mouse chromosome 5. J Appl Physiol 2003;95:11–19.

4 Schneider H, Boudewyns A, Smith PL, O'Donnell CP, Canisius S, Stammnitz A, Allan L, Schwartz AR: Modulation of upper airway collapsibility during sleep: influence of respiratory phase and flow regimen. J Appl Physiol 2002;93:1365–1376.

5 Pride NB, Permutt S, Riley RL, Bromberger-Barnea B: Determinants of maximal expiratory flow from the lungs. J Appl Physiol 1967;23:646–662.

6 Smith PL, Wise RA, Gold AR, Schwartz AR, Permutt S: Upper airway pressure-flow relationships in obstructive sleep apnea. J Appl Physiol 1988;64:789–795.

7 Schwartz AR, Smith PL, Wise RA, Gold AR, Permutt S: Induction of upper airway occlusion in sleeping individuals with subatmospheric nasal pressure. J Appl Physiol 1988;64:535–542.

8 Milic-Emili J, Grunstein MM: Drive and timing components of ventilation. Chest 1976;70:131–133.

9 Tankersley C, Kleeberger S, Russ B, Schwartz A, Smith P: Modified control of breathing in genetically obese (ob/ob) mice. J Appl Physiol 1996;81:716–723.

10 Miyazaki S, Itasaka Y, Yamakawa K, Okawa M, Togawa K: Respiratory disturbance during sleep due to adenoid-tonsillar hypertrophy. Am J Otolaryngol 1989;10:143–149.

11 Hochban W, Kunkel M, Brandenburg U: Functional anatomy of the upper airway: Cephalometric and reflective acoustic studies. Pneumologie 1993;47(suppl 4):766–772.

12 Isono S, Remmers JE, Tanaka A, Sho Y, Sato J, Nishino T: Anatomy of pharynx in patients with obstructive sleep apnea and in normal subjects. J Appl Physiol 1997;82:1319–1326.

13 Aittokallio T, Saaresranta T, Polo-Kantola P, Nevalainen O, Polo O: Analysis of inspiratory flow shapes in patients with partial upper-airway obstruction during sleep. Chest 2001;119:37–44.

14 Mezzanotte WS, Tangel DJ, White DP: Waking genioglossal electromyogram in sleep apnea patients versus normal controls (a neuromuscular compensatory mechanism). J Clin Invest 1992;89:1571–1579.

15 Weiner D, Mitra J, Salamone J, Cherniack NS: Effect of chemical stimuli on nerves supplying upper airway muscles. J Appl Physiol 1982;52:530–536.

16 Kimoff RJ, Sforza E, Champagne V, Ofiara L, Gendron D: Upper airway sensation in snoring and obstructive sleep apnea. Am J Respir Crit Care Med 2001;164:250–255.

17 Friberg D, Ansved T, Borg K, Carlsson-Nordlander B, Larsson H, Svanborg E: Histological indications of a progressive snorers disease in an upper airway muscle. Am J Respir Crit Care Med 1998;157:586–593.

18 Wilson SL, Thach BT, Brouillette RT, Abu-Osba YK: Upper airway patency in the human infant: influence of airway pressure and posture. J Appl Physiol 1980;48:500–504.

19 Olson LG, Strohl KP: Airway secretions influence upper airway patency in the rabbit. Am Rev Respir Dis 1988;137:1379–1381.

20 Kirkness JP, Christenson HK, Garlick SR, Parikh R, Kairaitis K, Wheatley JR, Amis TC: Decreased surface tension of upper airway mucosal lining liquid increases upper airway patency in anaesthetised rabbits. J Physiol 2003;547:603–611.

21 Kirkness JP, Eastwood PR, Szollosi I, Platt PR, Wheatley JR, Amis TC, Hillman DR: Effect of surface tension of mucosal lining liquid on upper airway mechanics in anesthetized humans. J Appl Physiol 2003;95:357–363.

22 Kirkness JP, Madronio M, Stavrinou R, Wheatley JR, Amis TC: Relationship between surface tension of upper airway lining liquid and upper airway collapsibility during sleep in obstructive sleep apnea hypopnea syndrome. J Appl Physiol 2003;95:1761–1766.

23 Jokic R, Klimaszewski A, Mink J, Fitzpatrick MF: Surface tension forces in sleep apnea: the role of a soft tissue lubricant: a randomized double-blind, placebo-controlled trial. Am J Respir Crit Care Med 1998;157:1522–1525.

24 Morrell MJ, Arabi Y, Zahn BR, Meyer KC, Skatrud JB, Badr MS: Effect of surfactant on pharyngeal mechanics in sleeping humans: implications for sleep apnoea. Eur Respir J 2002;20:451–457.

25 Gleadhill IC, Schwartz AR, Schubert N, Wise RA, Permutt S, Smith PL: Upper airway collapsibility in snorers and in patients with obstructive hypopnea and apnea. Am Rev Respir Dis 1991;143:1300–1303.

26 Bates JH, Rossi A, Milic-Emili J: Analysis of the behavior of the respiratory system with constant inspiratory flow. J Appl Physiol 1985;58:1840–1848.

27 Kristo DA, Lettieri CJ, Andrada T, Taylor Y, Eliasson AH: Silent upper airway resistance syndrome: prevalence in a mixed military population. Chest 2005;127:1654–1657.

28 Berry RB, Gleeson K: Respiratory arousal from sleep: mechanisms and significance. Sleep 1997;20:654–675.

29 Exar EN, Collop NA: The association of upper airway resistance with periodic limb movements. Sleep 2001;24:188–192.

30 Smith PL, O'Donnell CP, Allan L, Schwartz AR: A physiologic comparison of nasal and oral positive airway pressure. Chest 2003;123:689–694.

31 Schwartz AR, Gold AR, Schubert N, Stryzak A, Wise RA, Permutt S, Smith PL: Effect of weight loss on upper airway collapsibility in obstructive sleep apnea. Am Rev Respir Dis 1991;144:494–498.

32 Penzel T, Moller M, Becker HF, Knaack L, Peter JH: Effect of sleep position and sleep stage on the collapsibility of the upper airways in patients with sleep apnea. Sleep 2001;24:90–95.

33 Riley RW, Powell NB, Guilleminault C: Maxillary, mandibular, and hyoid advancement for treatment of obstructive sleep apnea: a review of 40 patients. J Oral Maxillofac Surg 1990;48:20–26.

34 Veasey SC, Panckeri KA, Hoffman EA, Pack AI, Hendricks JC: The effects of serotonin antagonists in an animal model of sleep-disordered breathing. Am J Respir Crit Care Med 1996;153:776–786.

35 Issa FG, Sullivan CE: Alcohol, snoring and sleep apnea. J Neurol Neurosurg Psychiatry 1982;45:353–359.

36 McGinley BM, DeRosa P, Alan SR, Kirkness J, Patil S, Smith PL, Schneider H: A novel strategy for treating upper airway obstruction (UAO) with transnasal insufflation (TNI). Sleep 2005;28:A208.

Hartmut Schneider, MD, PhD
Johns Hopkins Sleep Disorders Center
5501 Hopkins Bayview Circle
Baltimore, MD 21224 (USA)
Tel. +1 410 550 4706
Fax +1 410 550 3374
E-Mail hschnei3@jhmi.edu

Randerath WJ, Sanner BM, Somers VK (eds): Sleep Apnea.
Prog Respir Res. Basel, Karger, 2006, vol 35, pp 90–96

Obstructive Sleep Apnea-Hypopnea Syndrome

Definitions and Pathophysiology

W. De Backer

Department of Pulmonary Medicine, University of Antwerp, Edegem, Belgium

Abstract

The narrowing or occlusion of the upper airway (UA) during sleep has been attributed to several factors. An abnormal anatomy of the UA, pathological and insufficient reflex activation of UA dilator muscles and increased collapsibility of the passive UA have all been demonstrated to occur and contribute to the UA collapse. More recently, it was also shown that UA collapse occurs during the terminal phase of the expiration preceding the apnea. When all data are taken into account, it is quite clear that OSAHS patients have a smaller and more collapsible airway. The airway is most at risk for complete collapse at the end of an expiration, where the tissue pressure may be larger than the intraluminal pressure. However, it is also clear that a larger airway is associated with less collapsibility or lower P_{crit}. Anatomical predisposition correlates with P_{crit} and artificial enlargement of the UA during inspiration also shifts the pressure-flow curve to the left. The UA collapse, partially determined by the cross sectional area during inspiration, finally occurs at the end of an expiration. We recently could confirm this latter finding and obtain some preliminary indications that modeling of the expiratory phase may be worthwhile in predicting the collapse and the outcome of some UA interventions.

Definitions

The obstructive sleep apnea-hypopnea syndrome (OSAHS) is characterized by recurrent episodes of partial or complete upper airway (UA) collapse during sleep. The collapse is highlighted by a reduction in or complete cessation of airflow despite ongoing inspiratory efforts. Due to the lack of adequate alveolar ventilation that results from the UA narrowing, oxygen saturation may drop and partial pressure of CO_2 may occasionally rise. The events are mostly terminated by arousals. Clinical consequences are excessive daytime sleepiness related to the sleep disruption. Minimal diagnostic criteria are defined for the OSAHS. Patients should have excessive daytime sleepiness that is not better explained by other factors or two or more of the following symptoms that also are not better explained by other factors: choking or gasping during sleep, recurrent awakenings from sleep, unrefreshing sleep, daytime fatigue, and impaired concentration. They should all have more than 5 obstructed breathing events per hour during sleep. An obstructive apnea or hypopnea can be defined as an event that lasts 10 s or longer and is characterized by a decrease from baseline in the amplitude of a valid measure of breathing during sleep that either reaches more than 50% or that is associated with an oxygen desaturation of 3% or an arousal. These definitions are recommended by the American Academy of Sleep Medicine (AASM) [1]. The Task Force of the AASM also states that there are common pathogenic mechanisms for obstructive apnea syndrome, central apnea syndrome, sleep hypoventilation syndrome and Cheyne-Stokes breathing. It was preferred to discuss them separately although they could be placed under the common denominator of 'sleep-disordered breathing syndrome'. The definition of OSAHS using 2 components, daytime symptoms and breathing pattern disturbances during sleep, may suggest that there is a tight correlation between both. However, unfortunately, this is not the case. The breathing pattern abnormalities, mostly described by an apnea-hypopnea index (AHI), only weakly correlate with quantified measures of sleepiness such as the Epworth Sleepiness Scale (ESS) [2]. This probably means that interindividual sensitivity, with some individuals coping better with sleep fragmentations than others, does compromise the relation between the AHI and scores of daytime sleepiness. Using a cut-off of 18 events/h including all apneas, hypopnea and flow limitation events (any series of two or more breaths, lasting >10 s, that had flattened or nonsinusoidal appearance on the inspiratory nasal cannula flow signal and ended abruptly with a return to breaths with sinusoidal shape), a sensitivity of 71% and a specificity of 60% for identifying subjects with excessive daytime sleepiness was obtained [3]. When using only the AI or the AHI (not counting flow limitations) the sensitivity/specificity was even far worse. Also, epidemiological studies show widespread sleepiness in the general population. Obviously epidemiological studies looking at the prevalence of OSAHS are all biased by the lack of a uniform definition. Using a very restrictive definition including only subjects with a fair amount of respiratory events who present with symptoms of sleepiness that warrant CPAP therapy, the prevalence is about 0.5% for middle-aged men with a normal BMI and 1.5% for the same group with an increased BMI [4]. The prevalence of an AHI of more than 5/h in a general population (without taking into account symptoms of sleepiness) was previously estimated to be 24% in a male population [5]. When symptoms of sleepiness were also taken into account, the prevalence decreased to 4% in men and 2% in women. In the more recently published Sleep Heart Health Study also a weak relation between the AHI and sleepiness was found: the ESS only rose from 7.2 to 9.3 when the AHI changed from less then 5/h to more then 30/h [6]. So, for clinical purposes it must be clear that the *total* RDI index (calculated from the sum of apneas, all flow hypopneas and all flow limitation events) should be taken into account, and that even then the correlation with daytime symptoms remains suboptimal.

Pathogenesis

The narrowing or occlusion of the UA during sleep has been attributed to several factors. An abnormal anatomy of the UA, pathological and insufficient reflex activation of UA dilator muscles and increased collapsibility of the passive UA have all been demonstrated to occur and contribute to the UA collapse. More recently it was also shown that UA collapse occurs during the terminal phase of the expiration preceding the apnea. We recently could confirm this latter finding and obtain some preliminary indications that modeling of the expiratory phase may be worthwhile in predicting the collapse and the outcome of some UA interventions.

Abnormal Anatomy of the UA

There are many studies indicating that the UA cross-sectional area is smaller in patients with obstructive sleep apnea (OSA). The narrowing of the UA, when studied during wakefulness, is often seen at the retropalatal and retroglossal area. Moreover, the configuration of the airway in OSA patients is different from normal controls with an anterior-posterior configuration [7]. In the airway of normal controls, a horizontal configuration is seen with the major axis in the lateral direction. During the inspiratory phase little narrowing is seen, suggesting that the activation of the UA dilator muscles accurately compensates for the negative intraluminal pressures. In apneic patients there was even some more enlargement during inspiration, possibly due to an increased UA muscle dilator activity. During expiration airway caliber initially increases due to the positive intraluminal pressure, again more pronounced in the apneic patients which present with the more distensible airways. However, at the end of the expiration, the airways narrow significantly and this narrowing is most pronounced in OSA patients. It becomes clear already from these studies, performed during wakefulness, that narrowing of the UA is most critical at the end of the expiration. Beyond narrowing of the airway by the lateral pharyngeal walls also tonsillar, uvula and tongue enlargement contribute to the occlusion of the UA during sleep. With more-detailed MRI techniques, it could be demonstrated that soft tissue enlargement predicts UA collapse. The volume of the tongue and the lateral walls were shown to be an independent risk factor for sleep apnea [8]. Also, ultrafast MRI imaging during sleep has confirmed these abnormalities. The variations in the velopharyngeal area during the respiratory cycle was greater in apneic patients than in controls and this was even more pronounced during sleep, suggesting an increased compliance of the velopharynx in these patients [9].

Insufficient Reflex Activation of UA Dilator Muscles

As already seen in the imaging studies, UA dilator muscle activation in OSA patients is quite adequate and even intensified during wakefulness. Several studies have confirmed this [10]. This activation is mainly due to reflex activation provoked by negative intrapharyngeal pressures that are more pronounced in OSA patients due to the smaller airway. This reflex is quite active during wakefulness but significantly declines during sleep. Especially during NREM sleep, this negative pressure reflex is substantially diminished or lost completely [11]. Studies of genioglossal muscle activity suggest that patients with OSA have a much greater reduction in the genioglossal EMG than normal subjects [12]. Due to the loss of this compensatory reflex activation of the UA dilator muscles, the UA of OSA patients may significantly narrow during inspiration when asleep.

Increased UA Collapsibility

Increased airway collapsibility significantly contributes to the UA collapse in OSA patients. Increasing levels of UA collapsibility lead to greater degree of airflow obstruction [13]. UA collapsibility can be determined from pressure-flow curves: the nasal mask pressure (P_n) below which the UA closes can be considered as the critical closing pressure or P_{crit}. The pressure flow relationship is dependent on the position of the patient and the sleep stage. Abbreviated methods have been developed to measure P_{crit} more conveniently during sleep [14]. Also negative pressure pulses (NPP) have been applied to measure UA collapsibility. It was demonstrated that collapsibility measured during wakefulness using NPP correlates significantly with collapsibility during sleep [15]. Very interesting data, however, were obtained by quantifying the static pressure-area relationship in the passive pharynx during general anesthesia with complete paralysis. Normal controls and 2 groups of mild and more severe OSA patients were compared. An endoscope inserted through the nose was positioned to visualize the velopharynx (retropalatal space) or the oropharynx (retroglossal space). The obtained images were then converted to obtain the pharyngeal cross-sectional area [16]. While the subject remained apneic for 2–3 min, the airway pressure was slowly reduced from 20 cm H_20 to the closing pressure, i.e. the pressure at which the (velo/oro)pharynx was seen to close completely. In patients, the site of primary closure is mostly the velopharynx. Closing pressure of the velopharynx was 0.90 (1.34) and 2.78 (2.78) cm H_2O for the mild and severe OSA patients compared to −3.77 (3.44) cm H_2O for the controls. Static pressure-area curves of the passive pharynx for the 3 groups studied are given in figure 1. Since these measurements are performed during apnea no indication could be obtained of the changes of collapsibility over the breathing cycle, although it is probably representative for the most relaxed periods of the expiration, presumably the end of the expiration in normally breathing sleepy patients.

Interestingly, pharyngeal collapsibility is influenced by abnormal craniofacial and soft tissue features. A significant correlation was found between P_{crit} and soft palate length, the distance from the hyoid bone to the posterior pharyngeal wall and the distance from the hyoid bone to the posterior nasal space [17]. In obese patients P_{crit} was related to the soft palate length, in nonobese patients the P_{crit} was determined by the distance of the hyoid bone to the mandibular plane. This may indicate that the anatomy of the UA determines P_{crit}. There are, however, also other indications that cross-sectional area of the UA, especially during inspiration, influences the P_{crit} and UA collapsibility. Indeed specific stimulation of the motor part of the hypoglossal nerve during inspiration not only lowers the AHI in OSA patients, but also significantly decreases the P_{crit} [18] as is given in figure 2. This is a very important observation since it implies that all local interventions that increase cross sectional area of the UA at the end of the inspiration have the potential to improve the sleep apnea syndrome by lowering the P_{crit}. It has also been shown that P_{crit} may be related to lung volume. UA size increases at higher lung volumes. The lung volume dependence of the UA size may also be greater in OSAHS patients.

Expiratory Collapse

Studies using endoscopic control of the UA size have demonstrated that the complete collapse of the UA in OSAHS patients occurs at the end of the expiration preceding the apneic event [19]. This was also seen in the UA imaging studies [7]. We recently used the forced oscillation technique (FOT) to study the airway impedance during sleep in OSAHS patients [20–22]. The basic principle of FOT is the application of pressure oscillations of small amplitude into the airways at a higher frequency than the natural breathing frequency. A loudspeaker generates the pressure oscillations whereas flow and pressure signals are recorded close to the airway opening by means of a pneumotachograph and a pressure transducer. The complex relationship between applied pressure and resulting flow, called impedance (Zrs), is determined by the mechanical properties of the airways, the lung tissue and the chest wall. Zrs, in general, is dependent on the frequency of oscillation. In a simplistic model, the in-phase relationship between

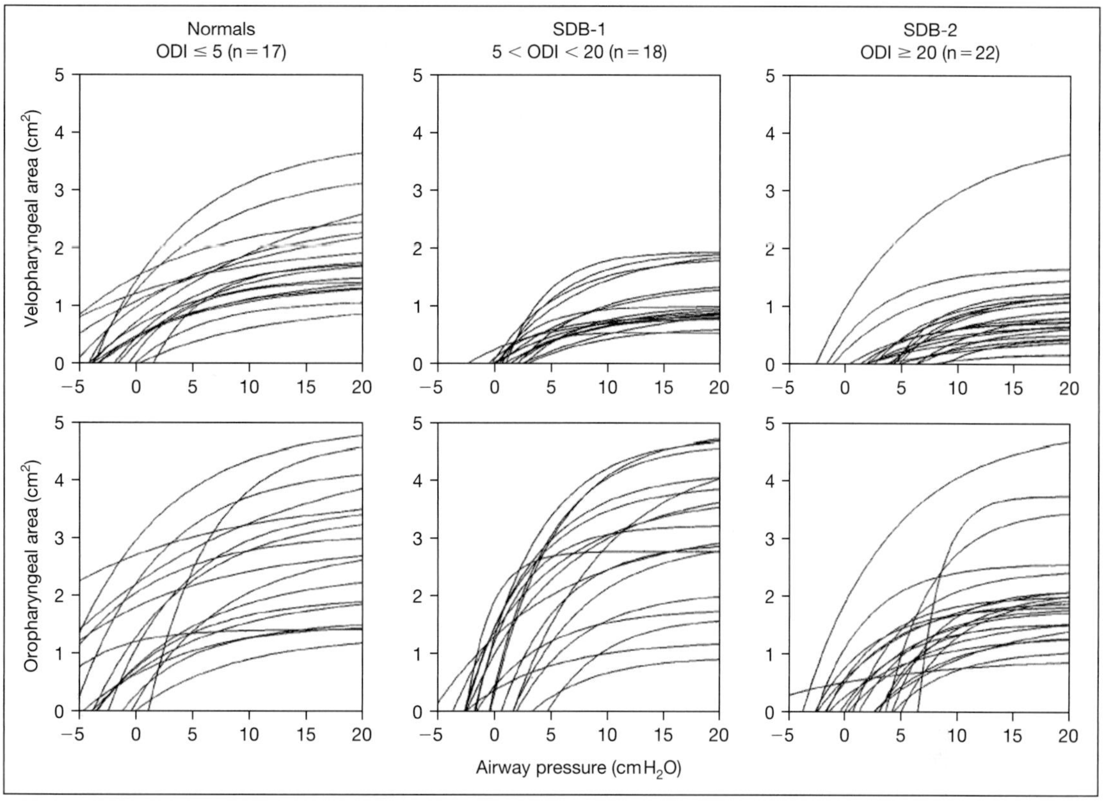

Fig. 1. Static pressure-area curves in normals and OSAHS patients measured over a pressure range of 20 cm H_2O during anesthesia [16].

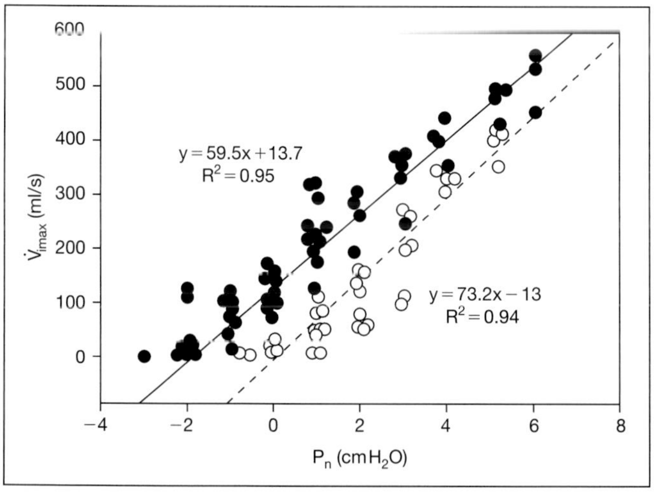

Fig. 2. Pressure flow curves with (full symbols) and without (open symbols) electrical stimulation (ES) of the hypoglossal nerve in a typical OSA patients. The intercept (and P_{crit}) decreases with ES [18].

pressure and flow, the resistance or real part of impedance (Rrs), is determined by the resistive properties of the respiratory system. The 90° out-of-phase relationship, reactance or imaginary part of impedance (Xrs) is determined by the elastic properties of the respiratory system at low frequency and by the inertive elements at high frequency. In 8 patients, we measured the respiratory impedance during and before the apnea. A typical pattern of Zrs over several breathing cycles is seen in figure 3 and the progressive increase of the Zrs during the second part of the expiration preceding the apnea is seen in more detail in figure 4. The impedance often rises during inspiration but always drops during the following expiration until collapse occurs during the end of an expiration (with Zrs amounting to the level observed during the apnea). This clearly confirms the observations from the imaging studies where cross sectional area of the UA is seen lowest at the end of the expiration.

Modeling of the Expiratory Collapse

Since the expiratory phase preceding the apnea is crucial in the pathogenesis and the understanding of the UA collapse, we tried to model the UA during this phase using finite elements techniques [23]. The 3-D model was constructed by converting a CT scan to a CAD (computer-aided design) model (fig. 5). The boundary conditions for

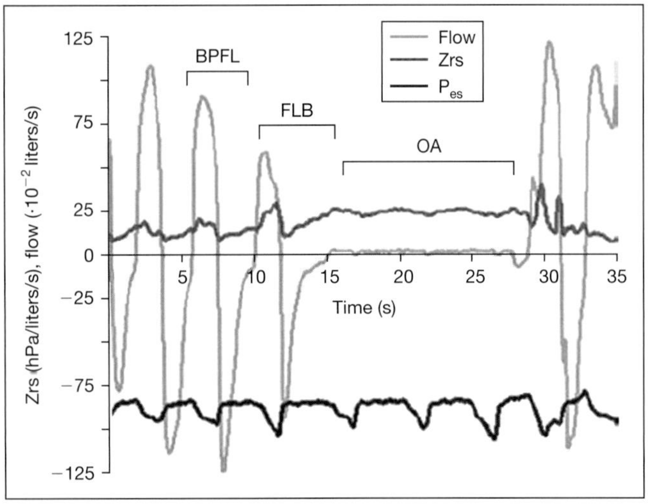

Fig. 3. Respiratory impedance (Zrs) before and during an obstructive apnea (OA) measured with the forced oscillation technique [22].

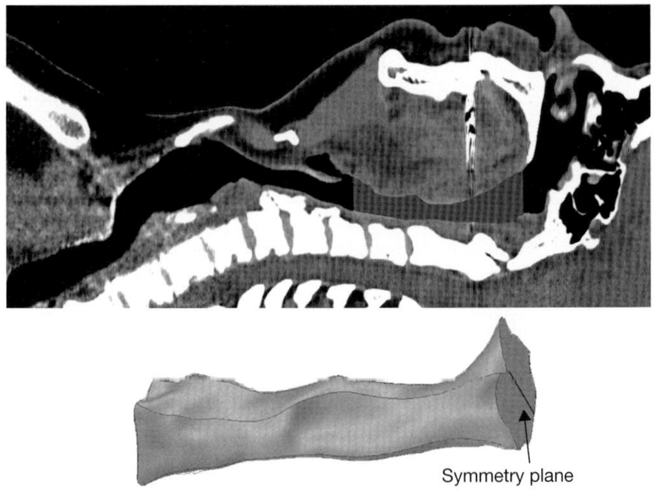

Fig. 5. Conversion of a CT scan of the upper airway into a CAD model.

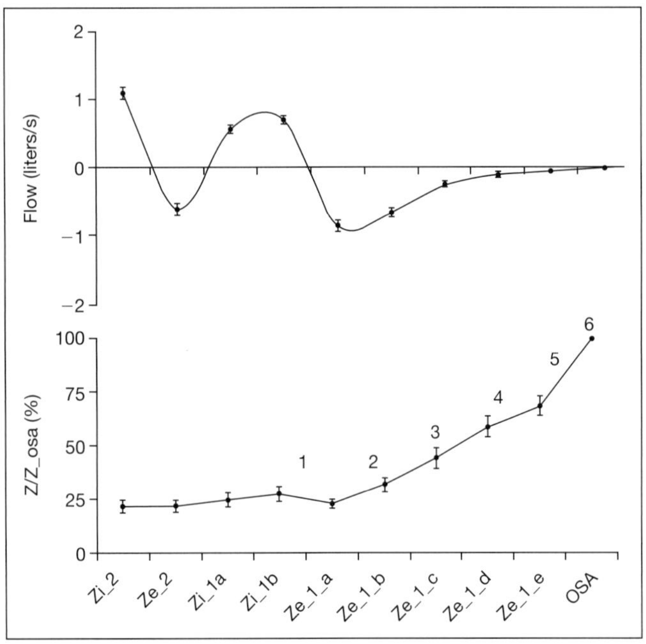

Fig. 4. Pattern of increase in respiratory impedance (Zrs) during the expiration preceding the apnea (OSA) [23].

this analysis approximate a normal expiration, where the displacement of the UA wall is limited. At the inlet, a transient velocity is defined, while at the outlet a transient pressure is defined. All data are based on in patient measurements obtained during sleep studies. By applying realistic boundary conditions and material properties, it was possible to generate a model that is in agreement with data obtained with the FOT (fig. 4). The pressure contours during the expiration are given in figure 6. Clearly, they correlate with the FOT data and confirm that after an initial rise in pressure during expiration, pressure drops and wall collapse occurs which is almost complete at the end of the expiration.

Interactions and Overall Pathogenic Model

When all data are taken into account, it is quite clear that OSAHS patients have a smaller and more collapsible airway. The airway is most at risk for complete collapse at the end of an expiration, where the tissue pressure may be larger than the intraluminal pressure. However, it is also clear that a larger airway is associated with less collapsibility or lower P_{crit}. Anatomical predisposition correlates with P_{crit} [17] and artificial enlargement of the UA during inspiration also shifts the pressure-flow curve to the left [18]. The UA collapse, partially determined by the cross-sectional area during inspiration, finally occurs at the end of an expiration. This process can be modeled for individual patients based on their anatomic properties obtained by UA CT and UA flow pressure profiles obtained during sleep [23]. With the same model, it can also be predicted that prolongation of expiratory time promotes collapse. Therefore, with more loop gain and PCO_2 dropping for a longer time period below the apneic threshold, expiratory time may prolong and collapse may be elicited. It was shown that OSAHS patients may have a higher loop gain [24]. We previously could also show that OSAHS patients may have a higher chemical drive (hypercapnic

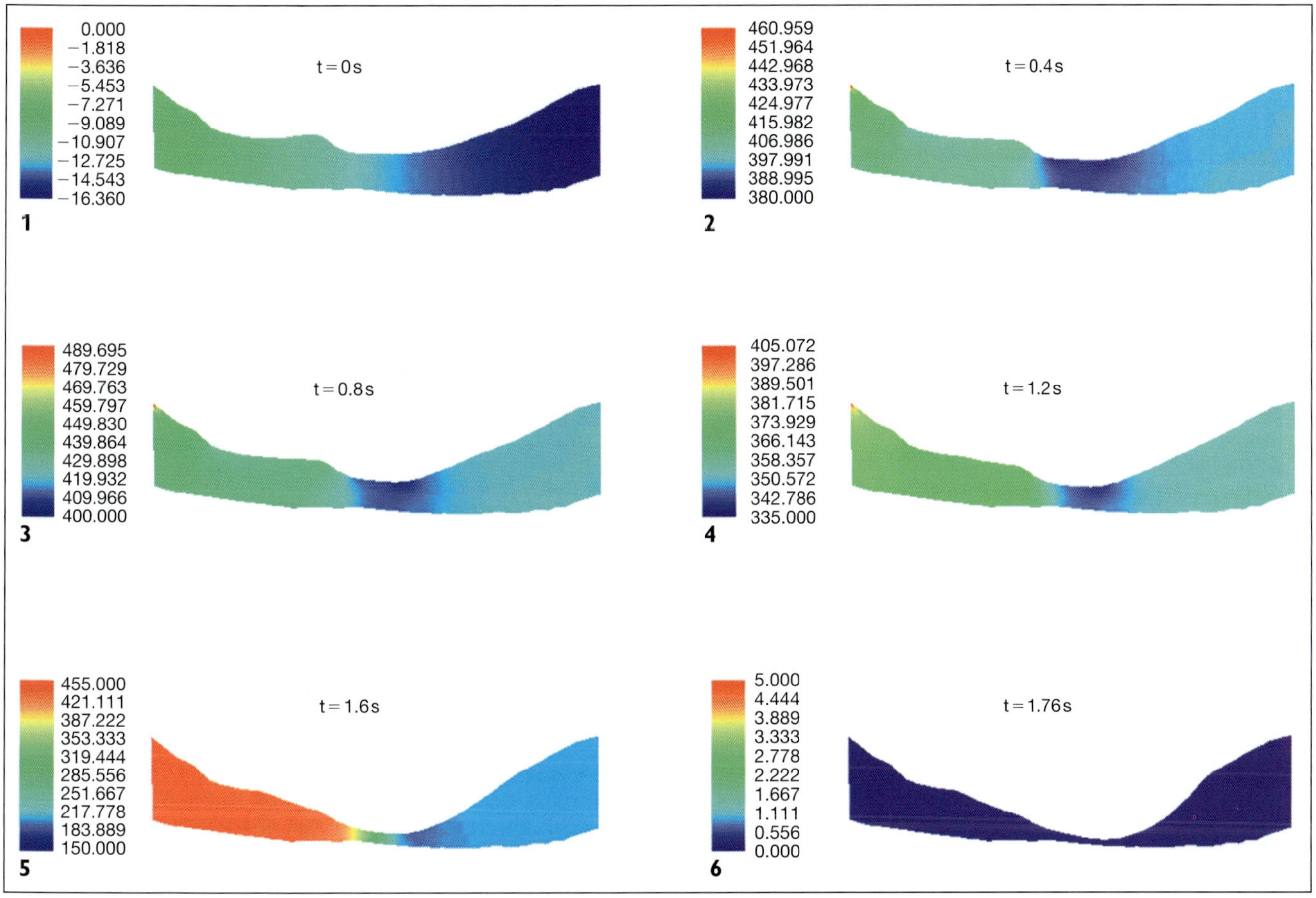

Fig. 6. Pressure contours during expiration (start = 0 s, end is 1.76 s) in the upper airway (left: hypopharynx; right: nasopharynx; top: tongue; bottom: dorsal pharyngeal wall) resulting in an apnea. Blue colors represent the lowest pressure.

ventilatory response) that can contribute to the increased loop gain [25]. Treatment with CPAP lowers this CO_2 drive over time. Of course any intervention that stabilizes the breathing pattern will ultimately also lower the tendency to collapse. This is the case for acetazolamide that lowers the CO_2 threshold and therefore stabilizes the breathing pattern. Acetazolamide is clearly effective for central sleep apnea [26] but can also have some effect in OSAHS patients.

Conclusion

There is still no final agreement on the definitions to be used to describe patients with the OSAHS syndrome. From a practical point of view, we have to focus on patients that need therapy. The choice of the therapy and also the introduction of new therapies depend on the insight into the pathogenetic mechanisms in general and more importantly for the patient under consideration. For patients with milder forms of the OSAHS, where alternative treatment options for nCPAP can be considered, it might be worthwhile to obtain insight into the critical closing pressure, the site of collapse and the UA anatomy. Then, a more substantiated choice of local therapy can be made. In the near future we will also be able to model the UA from individuals so that we can predict the outcome of local interventions [27]. Such models, however, still need update and larger scale evaluation, but may represent a very intriguing new approach that can improve therapeutic outcomes.

References

1 The Report of an American Academy of Sleep Medicine Task Force: Sleep-Related Breathing Disorders in Adults: recommendations for syndrome definition and measurement techniques in clinical research. Sleep 1999;22:667–689.

2 Stradling JR, Davies RJ: Sleep. 1. Obstructive sleep apnoea/hypopnoea syndrome: definitions, epidemiology, and natural history. Thorax 2004;59:73–78.

3 Hosselet J, Ayappa I, Norman RG, Krieger AC, Rapoport DM: Classification of sleep-disordered breathing. Am J Respir Crit Care Med 2001;163:398–405.

4 Stradling JR, Crosby JH: Predictors and prevalence of obstructive sleep apnoea and snoring in 1001 middle aged men. Thorax 1991;46:85–90.

5 Young T, Palta M, Dempsey J, Skatrud J, Weber S, Badr S: The occurrence of sleep-disordered breathing among middle-aged adults. N Engl J Med 1993;328:1230–1235.

6 Gottlieb DJ, Whitney CW, Bonekat WH, et al: Relation of sleepiness to respiratory disturbance index: the Sleep Heart Health Study. Am J Respir Crit Care Med 1999;159:502–507.

7 Schwab RJ, Gefter WB, Hoffman EA, Gupta KB, Pack AI: Dynamic upper airway imaging during awake respiration in normal subjects and patients with sleep disordered breathing. Am Rev Respir Dis 1993;148:1385–1400.

8 Schwab RJ, Pasirstein M, Pierson R, et al: Identification of upper airway anatomic risk factors for obstructive sleep apnea with volumetric magnetic resonance imaging. Am J Respir Crit Care Med 2003;168:522–530.

9 Ciscar MA, Juan G, Martinez V, et al: Magnetic resonance imaging of the pharynx in OSA patients and healthy subjects. Eur Respir J 2001;17:79–86.

10 Fogel RB, Malhotra A, Pillar G, et al: Genioglossal activation in patients with obstructive sleep apnea versus control subjects: mechanisms of muscle control. Am J Respir Crit Care Med 2001;164:2025–2030.

11 De Backer W: Upper airway reflexes and obstructive sleep apnoea. Eur Respir J 1993;6:9–10.

12 Mezzanotte WS, Tangel DJ, White DP: Influence of sleep onset on upper-airway muscle activity in apnea patients versus normal controls. Am J Respir Crit Care Med 1996;153:1880–1887.

13 Gleadhill IC, Schwartz AR, Schubert N, Wise RA, Permutt S, Smith PL: Upper airway collapsibility in snorers and in patients with obstructive hypopnea and apnea. Am Rev Respir Dis 1991;143:1300–1303.

14 Boudewyns A, Punjabi N, Van de Heyning PH, et al: Abbreviated method for assessing upper airway function in obstructive sleep apnea. Chest 2000;118:1031–1041.

15 Malhotra A, Pillar G, Fogel R, Beauregard J, Edwards J, White DP: Upper-airway collapsibility: measurements and sleep effects. Chest 2001;120:156–161.

16 Isono S, Remmers JE, Tanaka A, Sho Y, Sato J, Nishino T: Anatomy of pharynx in patients with obstructive sleep apnea and in normal subjects. J Appl Physiol 1997;82:1319–1326.

17 Sforza E, Bacon W, Weiss T, Thibault A, Petiau C, Krieger J: Upper airway collapsibility and cephalometric variables in patients with obstructive sleep apnea. Am J Respir Crit Care Med 2000;161:347–352.

18 Oliven A, O'Hearn DJ, Boudewyns A, et al: Upper airway response to electrical stimulation of the genioglossus in obstructive sleep apnea. J Appl Physiol 2003;95:2023–2029.

19 Morrell MJ, Arabi Y, Zahn B, Badr MS: Progressive retropalatal narrowing preceding obstructive apnea. Am J Respir Crit Care Med 1998;158:1974–1981.

20 Oostveen E, MacLeod D, Lorino H, et al: The forced oscillation technique in clinical practice: methodology, recommendations and future developments. Eur Respir J 2003;22:1026–1041.

21 Vanderveken OM, Oostveen E, Boudewyns AN, Verbraecken JA, Van de Heyning PH, De Backer WA: Quantification of pharyngeal patency in patients with sleep-disordered breathing. ORL J Otorhinolaryngol Relat Spec 2005;67:168–179.

22 Oostveen E, Vanderveken O, Verbraecken J, De Backer W: Progressive upper airway narrowing occurs during expiration prior to obstructive, central and mixed apneas. Am J Respir Crit Care Med 2005;2:A610.

23 De Backer J, Gorle C, Vanderveken O, Wittesaele W, Verbraecken J, Oostveen E, Wuyts F, Van de Heyning P, De Backer W: Modeling of upper airway collapse in OSA patients based on computational fluid dynamics. Am J Respit Crit Care Med 2005;2:A491.

24 Younes M, Ostrowski M, Thompson W, Leslie C, Shewchuk W: Chemical control stability in patients with obstructive sleep apnea. Am J Respir Crit Care Med 2001;163:1181–1190.

25 Verbraecken J, De Backer W, Willemen M, De Cock W, Wittesaele W, Van de Heyning P: Chronic CO_2 drive in patients with obstructive sleep apnea and effect of CPAP. Respir Physiol 1995;101:279–287.

26 DeBacker WA, Verbraecken J, Willemen M, Wittesaele W, DeCock W, Van de Heyning P: Central apnea index decreases after prolonged treatment with acetazolamide. Am J Respir Crit Care Med 1995;151:87–91.

27 De Backer J, Gorle C, Vanderveken O, Wittesaele W, Wuyts F, Parizel P, Van de Heyning P, De Backer W: Assessment of a mandibular advancement device (MAD) in a sleep apnea patient using computational fluid dynamics (CFD). Am J Respir Crit Care Med 2005;2:A491.

Prof. Dr. W. De Backer
Department of Pulmonary Medicine
University Hospital Antwerp
Wilrijkstraat 10
BE–2650 Edegem (Belgium)
Tel. +32 3 8213447, Fax +32 3 8214447
E-Mail wilfried.de.backer@uza.be

Randerath WJ, Sanner BM, Somers VK (eds): Sleep Apnea.
Prog Respir Res. Basel, Karger, 2006, vol 35, pp 97–104

Oxidative Stress – The Culprit of Obstructive Sleep Apnea Syndrome

Lena Lavie Peretz Lavie

Lloyd Rigler Sleep Apnea Research Laboratory, Ruth and Bruce Rappaport Faculty of Medicine, Technion Institute of Technology, Haifa, Israel

Abstract

Obstructive sleep apnea, characterized by intermittent and recurrent pauses in respiration during sleep resulting in a decreased oxygen saturation and sleep fragmentation, is closely associated with cardiovascular morbidity. There is accumulated evidence that hypoxia/reoxygenation, such that is characteristic of sleep apnea, promotes the formation of reactive oxygen species that activate critical redox-sensitive signaling pathways and transcription factors. This facilitates the expression of sets of genes that encode proteins essential to adaptation to hypoxia, as well those that elicit inflammatory pathways such as adhesion molecules and inflammatory cytokines. Consequently, inflammatory and immune responses are aggravated, thus resulting in the activation of endothelial cells/leukocytes/platelets. These activated cells express adhesion molecules and pro-inflammatory cytokines that in turn may further exacerbate inflammatory responses and cause endothelial cell injury and dysfunction. These may lead to the development of cardio- and cerebrovascular morbidities in sleep apnea. Evidence supporting the existence of endothelial dysfunction and early clinical signs of atherosclerosis in patients with sleep apnea provides firm support to the above chain of events. This newly acquired insight into the pathophysiology of cardiovascular morbidity in OSA has important implications regarding the diagnosis and treatment of the syndrome.

Obstructive sleep apnea (OSA) syndrome, a breathing disorder which is characterized by intermittent and recurrent pauses in respiration during sleep resulting in a decreased oxygen saturation and sleep fragmentation, is a prevalent syndrome [1]. One in 4 men and 1 in 10 women have at least 5 apneas or hypopneas in each hour of sleep and 4% of adult men and 2% of adult women have sleep apnea syndrome defined as at least 5 respiratory events per hour of sleep combined with characteristic symptoms such as excessive daytime sleepiness, chronic fatigue or neurocognitive decline [2]. Breathing disorders in sleep have emerged in recent years as an independent risk factor for cardiovascular morbidity and mortality. This association has been demonstrated in cross-sectional, population-based, and prospective studies, as well as in intervention studies [3, 4]. Although the underlying mechanisms of the association between breathing disorders in sleep and cardiovascular morbidity are not fully elucidated, accumulated evidence indicates that atherosclerosis and its underlying mechanisms – oxidative stress and inflammation – play a major role [5]. Thus, recent research pointed at apneas-related oxidative stress, inflammatory cell activation and metabolic consequences of the nocturnal events as important mediators of the underlying cardiovascular morbidities. We here review the evidence linking OSA with oxidative stress and inflammation, and outline the chain of events that start with nocturnal intermittent hypoxia (IH) and through oxidative stress and activation of inflammatory pathways culminating in cardiovascular morbidity. We will also discuss the clinical implications of this chain of events with respect to the diagnosis and treatment of breathing disorders in sleep.

Oxidative Stress in Sleep Apnea

What Is Oxidative Stress?

Oxidative stress represents a common threat and a hazard to all aerobic organisms, and may drastically affect the development of various pathological conditions. Basically it is characterized by an imbalance between oxidant producing systems and anti-oxidant defense mechanisms, resulting in excessive formation of reactive oxygen species (ROS). ROS molecules can oxidize various macromolecules as lipids, proteins, carbohydrates and DNA and thus can alter their functions leading to various seemingly unrelated pathologies. Excessive ROS formation was documented in conditions such as hypoxia/reoxygenation or hypoxia/reperfusion, inflammatory diseases, diabetes, hypercholesterolemia, hyperhomocysteinemia, smoking, obesity and in cases of exposure to heavy metals, ionizing irradiation and strenuous exercise [6, 7]. Therefore, enzymatic and nonenzymatic anti-oxidant systems have evolved to eliminate excess ROS and to maintain and regulate the balance between pro-oxidant and anti-oxidant mechanisms (redox state).

At the same time, under physiological conditions, ROS are generated during normal cellular respiration at low levels, as by-products of oxygen metabolism. A wealth of data implicates their formation within the cells as signaling molecules. Thus, increased ROS molecules such as superoxide, hydrogen peroxide and hydroxyl radical induce a plethora of signaling pathways that activate transcriptional factors responsible for the regulation of proper responses to the oxidative insults, by inducing redox adaptive gene expression [7, 8].

Hypoxia/Reoxygenation and Oxidative Stress in Sleep Apnea

The primary source of altered redox balance in patients with OSA stems from their unique pathophysiology – the IH these patients undergo through sleep – which results in repetitive episodes of hypoxia/reoxygenation [5]. Oxidative stress is a prominent feature of ischemia/reperfusion or hypoxia/reoxygenation and is manifested by increased ROS production and altered metabolic and molecular processes, resulting in cellular and tissue injury [6]. Yet, due to their pivotal role, ROS and oxidative stress in OSA may activate redox-sensitive signaling pathways which initiate adaptive responses to hypoxia and/or inflammatory pathways [7, 8]. Consequently, endothelial cells, leukocytes, and platelets are activated [9]. These activated cells can further contribute to oxidative stress through a further release of ROS and increased expression of adhesion molecules on leukocytes, platelets, and endothelial cells, thereby facilitating endothelial cell-leukocyte interactions that in turn further amplify inflammatory responses [10]. Moreover, circulating activated leukocytes which express adhesion molecules can also block microvascular capillaries by attaching to endothelial cells, a phenomenon referred to as 'no-flow' [6], thus resulting in cerebro- and cardiovascular morbidities [9].

Experimental Evidence: Intermittent Hypoxia-Dependent Oxidative Stress

There is currently substantial evidence demonstrating that the IH characteristic of patients with OSA indeed affects several enzymatic pathways in a similar manner to the experimentally induced hypoxia/reperfusion in tissue culture and animal models. It primarily includes mitochondrial dysfunction, and xanthine oxidase and NADPH oxidase activation.

(1) Mitochondrial dysfunction is a well-established source of excess ROS formation due to hypoxia/reperfusion. In patients with OSA, mitochondrial dysfunction was demonstrated through measurement of changes in cytochrome oxidase redox state during the obstructive sleep apneas [11]. Specifically, McGown et al. [11] have shown that the oxidation state of the mitochondrial cytochrome oxidase which is responsible for the final metabolism of molecular oxygen to produce adenosine triphosphate (ATP) in the respiratory chain was altered, as were cerebral oxygenation levels, arterial saturation and cerebral blood flow velocity. Additionally, in vitro studies give further support and delineate the mechanisms by which mitochondria become dysfunctional under intermittent hypoxic conditions. For instance, by subjecting PC12 cells to IH in vitro, Yuan et al. [12] have shown that superoxide anion levels were increased in mitochondria. This was evidenced by the decreased aconitase enzyme activity and the increased levels of hydrogen peroxide, a stable dismutated product of superoxide anions. Also, complex I of the mitochondrial electron transport chain was markedly inhibited in IH exposed cells. These findings clearly implicate the mitochondrial electron transport chain in the generation of superoxide anions as a result of IH.

(2) Xanthine oxidase is a well-established source of ROS during hypoxia/reperfusion. In patients with OSA its involvement is indirectly implicated by elevated levels of

metabolic by-products in this pathway, including uric acid and adenosine (reviewed in [5]).

(3) NADPH oxidase is the primary enzyme utilized by inflammatory phagocytic cells for generating ROS as a protective mechanism against microbial invasion [6]. Isoforms of this enzyme, however, are ubiquitously present among a variety of cells including endothelial cells that produce low levels of ROS for signaling purposes. Several stimuli can activate the NADPH oxidase of leukocytes and endothelial cells including hypoxia/reoxygenation. In patients with OSA, both neutrophils and monocytes were shown to be activated and to release 2- to 3-fold higher amounts of ROS, suggesting the involvement of NADPH oxidase [13, 14]. Of note, the NADPH oxidase isoform which is expressed by activated endothelial cells was implicated in the pathogenesis of hypertension that also confers a risk factor for cardiovascular disease and stroke [15].

A recent study by Zhan et al. [16] confirmed increased neuronal NADPH oxidase mRNA and protein levels in wake-active brain regions of mice subjected to long-term IH. However, in transgenic $Gp91^{phox}$ (a critical subunit of NADPH oxidase) deficient mice, or under pharmacologic inhibition of NADPH oxidase, long-term IH did not induce oxidative stress or a proinflammatory response. Collectively, these data demonstrate the importance of this enzyme as a critical source of superoxide affecting oxidative and proinflammatory responses after exposure to IH. Thus, inhibiting NADPH oxidase can be considered as one possible modality to prevent oxidation-mediated morbidities in obstructive sleep apnea.

Additional sources including enzymes such as cyclooxygenase, lipooxyganase, nitric oxide synthase and heme oxygenases, should be considered as well.

Outcomes of Oxidative Stress in Sleep Apnea

Oxidation of Lipids, Proteins and DNA in OSA

Oxidation of macromolecules as lipids, proteins, DNA and carbohydrates clearly attests to increased oxidative stress in patients with OSA. Of these, lipids are the most prone to oxidation. In OSA, increased lipid peroxidation that was attenuated by the use of nasal continuous positive airway pressure (nCPAP) was demonstrated [17]. Moreover, the reported increased lipid peroxidation was specifically found to be apnea/hypopnea index (AHI – the number of apneas plus hypopneas divided by hours of sleep) severity dependent. Also, it was less affected by co-morbidities as hypertension and cardiovascular diseases, or by age and Body Mass Index (BMI) [17]. The fact that lipid peroxidation, which is a surrogate marker of atherosclerosis and cardiovascular morbidity, was found to be AHI severity dependent emphasizes the possible involvement of ROS in amplifying atherosclerotic processes in patients with OSA.

Additionally, increase in DNA oxidation was demonstrated in patients with OSA by documenting increased urinary excretion of 8-hydroxy-2′-deoxyguanosine [18]. Interestingly, in several studies utilizing animal models of chronic intermittent hypoxia (CIH) protein and nucleic acid oxidation as well as lipid peroxidation were demonstrated [16, 19]. Importantly, in a recent report Chen et al. [20], utilizing rats, emphasized the contribution of IH and oxidative stress to myocardial function. In this animal model, increased myocardial lipid peroxidation and decreased activity of the anti-oxidant enzyme Cu/Zn superoxide dismutase were correlated with blood pressure and left ventricular myocardial dysfunction.

Decreased Antioxidant Activity in OSA

Disruption of the tightly regulated cellular oxidation-reduction (redox) state, maintained between oxidant producing systems and anti-oxidant defense mechanisms, can also be affected by decreased antioxidant capacities. As noted earlier, in patients with OSA this balance was shown to be perturbed by excess ROS formation; however, decreased anti-oxidant capacity has also been documented (reviewed in [21]). Additionally, a lower activity of paraoxonse-1 (PON-1) (an anti-oxidant enzyme that is located exclusively on high-density lipoprotein and protects both low- and high-density lipoprotein from oxidative modification) was found in patients with OSA. This decreased PON-1 activity was more pronounced in patients who also had cardiovascular co-morbidities [17]. Also, PON-1 activity was significantly negatively correlated with AHI but not with BMI or age [unpubl. observations], thus further emphasizing the specific effects of OSA morbidity on oxidative stress. In the clinical setting, PON-1 activity was shown to decrease in patients with acute MI, hypercholesterolemia, and diabetes mellitus [22]. More recently, HDL was shown to be dysfunctional in preventing the formation and inactivation of oxidized lipids in OSA [23].

Collectively, the accumulated data emphasize the existence of an altered balance between oxidant and anti-oxidant capacities, by demonstrating on the one hand increased ROS production and on the other, decreased antioxidant activity. Thus, oxidative stress is implicated as being as one of the fundamental mechanisms that underlie the increased prevalence of cardiovascular morbidities in OSA.

Redox-Sensitive Signaling Pathways and Transcription Factors

Once oxidative stress ensues, it activates a plethora of signaling pathways that may initiate inflammatory responses ultimately leading to atherosclerosis [6, 8, 9, 24]. As noted earlier, oxidative stress was shown to be exaggerated in a severity dependent manner in patients with OSA. This implies that in the setting of OSA, ROS molecules can also act as signaling molecules and promote activation of an array of signaling pathways and activate a host of redox-sensitive transcription factors which regulate gene expression [8]. As a consequence, this may promote inflammation and endothelial dysfunction – a subclinical condition of atherosclerosis – the outcomes of which are cardio- and cerebrovascular morbidities. It is not clear, however, in OSA, how ROS are perceived by the cells and how they regulate the activation of intracellular pathways which initiate and regulate redox-sensitive transcription factor activation. Moreover, thus far, there is no direct evidence demonstrating increased redox-sensitive transcription factor activation in OSA.

However, the experimental evidence documenting redox regulated transcription factors and their gene products in response to sustained hypoxia are overwhelming. The addition of exogenous oxidant molecules such as superoxide and hydrogen peroxide induces a large number of gene products functioning to restore homeostasis [8]. Thus, the main redox-regulated transcription factors that are most likely to be involved in OSA are hypoxia-inducible factor-1α (HIF-1α), activator protein-1 (AP-1, which results from heterodimerization of c-Fos and c-Jun proteins) and nuclear factor kappa-B (NFκB). Importantly, most of the evidence gathered at the level of animal or in vitro studies is mainly a result of short or prolonged sustained hypoxia, or a single challenge of an ischemic insult followed by a various time periods of reoxygenation, whereas the number of studies employing IH in patterns mimicking OSA is limited. Thus, the question how IH, such that is inflicted by OSA, affects transcriptional activation, largely remains to be elucidated. Yet, the fact that gene products of redox-sensitive transcription factors such as erythropoietin, vascular endothelial growth factor (VEGF), inflammatory cytokines and adhesion molecules, are enhanced in OSA, indirectly suggests that AP-1, NFκB and HIF-1α are upregulated [5].

However, the most convincing data regarding the effects of IH on transcription factor activation are derived from in vitro studies, which have shown up regulation of HIF-1α, AP-1 and NFκB. In two elegant studies by Yuan et al. [12, 25], subjecting cultured cells to IH in vitro, in intervals mimicking sleep apnea, resulted in AP-1 and HIF-1α activation. In the first study, by exposure of PC12 cells to IH (cycles of 15 s hypoxia/4 min normoxia), a significant elevation of c-Fos (functionally coupled to AP-1) mRNA as well as transcriptional activation was evident. Moreover, IH was more potent and induced a longer lasting activation of c-Fos than comparable cumulative duration of continuous hypoxia. IH also increased AP-1 activity and tyrosine hydroxylase mRNA – an AP-1-regulated downstream gene. Using superoxide dismutase mimetic, a potent scavenger of superoxide anions, prevented IH-induced c-Fos, AP-1 and tyrosine hydroxylase activations. These data clearly suggest that IH-induced c-Fos-mediated transcriptional activation involves oxidative stress.

In the second study Yuan et al. [25] investigated the effects of IH on HIF-1α activation, and which signaling pathways were involved. By subjecting PC12 cells to IH (60 cycles consisting of 30 s hypoxia, followed by 4 min normoxia), a significant increase in HIF-1α protein of nuclear extracts was found. Yet, unlike in sustained hypoxia, signaling via protein kinases (PCK-α, PCK-γ) was not required, whereas the Ca^{2+}/calmodulin-dependent kinase activity was increased 5-fold in the cells subjected to IH. These observations suggest that IH induces HIF-1α transcriptional activity via a novel signaling pathway involving Ca^{2+}/calmodulin-dependent kinase [25]. More recently, Ryan et al. [26] demonstrated increased NFκB activation after subjecting HeLa cells to acute IH as compared to normoxia or to sustained hypoxia, by subjecting the cells to cycles of 5 min hypoxia/10 min normoxia.

Collectively, these in vitro studies clearly support the notion that the redox-sensitive transcription factors HIF-1α, NFκB and AP-1, could be elevated in OSA as well. More importantly, however, the specific signaling pathways affected by IH, need to be elucidated in order to better understand the pathology of OSA.

Inflammatory Responses in OSA

Activation of redox-sensitive transcription factors – as described above – can initiate and propagate inflammatory responses by subjecting a cell, a tissue, or the whole organism, to IH. Some of the gene products upregulated by NFκB and AP-1 include adhesion molecules and pro-inflammatory cytokines. These have been shown to participate and aggravate inflammatory responses at the vasculature [8, 24]. Thus, the ROS produced in response to IH presumably from endothelial cells and leukocytes can promote accumulation of leukocytes and platelets in the vasculature, which is facilitated by overexpression of adhesion molecules in both blood cells and endothelial cells.

Adhesion Molecules and Leukocytes/Endothelial Cells Interactions

The understanding of leukocytes/endothelial cells interactions and consequently adhesion molecule expression in response to hypoxia/reoxygenation has been largely increased in recent years, based on experimental evidence primarily derived from animal models utilizing intravital microscopy. In these studies, microscopic visualization of events that occur within microvessels allowed to determine the sequence of the interactions between blood cells and endothelial cells and the contribution of each of the adhesion molecules in promoting these interactions in response to hypoxia/reoxygenation [10, 27]. Furthermore, investigating mice that are genetically deficient in a specific adhesion molecule has further shown that the adhesion molecules involved elicited a prothrombotic and a pro-inflammatory phenotype in the microvascular circulation that was also oxidative stress dependent [27]. For instance, within minutes of reperfusion, P-selectin, which is normally stored in the Weibel-Palade bodies in endothelial cells, was expressed on the surface of the endothelium, thus supporting an early oxidant-dependent leukocyte recruitment. In the second stage, which is mediated by transcription dependent upregulation of adhesion molecules, leukocytes were recruited hours after reperfusion, involving E-selectin over-expression on the endothelium [27]. Unlike in OSA, that has multiple short cycles of hypoxia/reperfusion lasting a whole night sleep, such an experimental paradigm investigated one hypoxia/reperfusion cycle. Yet, from such elaborated studies we can gain insights into adhesion molecule expression and blood cells/endothelial cells interactions.

Indeed, the interactions between leukocytes – monocytes and various subpopulations of cytotoxic T lymphocytes – in OSA were thoroughly investigated [13, 21, 28–30]. Albeit, in these studies, the authors utilized leukocytes of patients with OSA undergoing repetitive hypoxia/reperfusion episodes in vivo in patients' circulation during sleep.

One of the striking differences noted between monocytes of patients with OSA and controls was the expression of adhesion molecules. Notably, the CD15 complex on selectins (of the family of adhesion molecules which mediates rolling) and CD11c, a β-subunit of the integrins (and a counter-receptor for ICAM-1 on endothelial cells) were elevated, and treatment with nCPAP that ameliorated the hypoxia, downregulated their expression [13]. Increased CD15 expression on monocytes was also found to be associated with the severity of the syndrome [31], and was corroborated by increased adhesion to endothelial cells of venous and artery origin, which supports an activated phenotype.

Evidently, investigating several cytotoxic T lymphocyte subpopulations revealed an activated and a cytotoxic phenotype as well. Increased adhesion to endothelial cells and increased cytotoxicity were shown by the CD8+, CD4+ and γδ cytotoxic T lymphocytes as compared to controls [28–30]. Interestingly, unlike in CD4+, the killing abilities of CD8+ T lymphocytes were found to be AHI severity dependent, and each of the T cell subpopulations investigated utilized different killing mechanisms to injure the endothelial cells [21].

Markers of Endothelial Cell Activation in OSA

The presence of soluble isoforms of the various adhesion molecules that are shed from activated endothelial cells, were also detected in the circulation of OSA patients. These included P- and E-selectin, intracellular adhesion molecule-1 (ICAM-1), and vascular cell adhesion molecule-1 (VCAM-1), which are regarded as markers of active atherosclerotic diseases, and as predictors of future cardiovascular disease. In fact, in OSA, the increased expression of ICAM-1, VCAM-1 and E-selectin was attenuated by nCPAP treatment (reviewed in [21]).

Collectively, the increased expression of adhesion molecules, the increased avidity to endothelial cells, and the stronger cytotoxicity against endothelial cells, are all markers of activation of the various leukocyte subpopulations. These can be considered indicators of the possible ongoing processes that may damage the endothelium, predisposing it to cardiovascular morbidity in OSA.

Pro-Inflammatory Cytokines

Pro-inflammatory cytokines are also gene products of redox-sensitive transcription factor activation which participate and amplify inflammatory responses. These pleiotropic molecules function to regulate macrophage activation, scavenger receptor expression and metalloproteinase secretion, modulate smooth muscle cell proliferation, nitric oxide production and apoptosis, and induce endothelial cell activation. The most investigated pro-inflammatory cytokines tumor necrosis factor-α (TNF-α), interleukin-6 (IL-6) and interleukin-8 (IL-8), are regulated by oxygen tension and free radicals via activation of NFκB and AP-1 and possibly via HIF-1α as well [32]. Apparently, once the inflammatory response is initiated, these cytokines can in turn activate NFκB further exacerbating the inflammatory response. In OSA, elevated levels of inflammatory cytokines were found in the circulation [21, 33] and in various cytotoxic T lymphocytes [29, 30]. Importantly, the balance between pro-inflammatory and anti-inflammatory cytokines is disrupted in patients with OSA. In lymphocytes for instance, while the levels of the pro-inflammatory cytokine TNF-α were increased, the levels of the anti-inflammatory cytokine interleukin-10 (IL-10) were also increased; yet, this IL-10 elevation was not proportional to the elevation seen in TNF-α [30]. Such an IL-10 increase could perhaps act as a compensatory mechanism to alleviate the deleterious effects of TNF-α. A cytokine imbalance between the levels of TNF-α and IL-10 was suggested to be involved in the pathogenesis of several vascular morbidities as stroke and after cardiac surgery with cardiopulmonary bypass [34], which further supports increased inflammatory-atherogenic processes in patients with OSA.

Endothelial Dysfunction in Sleep Apnea

Recent years have seen a growing awareness that impairment of endothelial-dependent vasomotion is a reliable marker of atherosclerosis [35]. Thus, a large number of conditions known to be risk factors for atherosclerosis such as hyperlipidemia, hyperhomocysteinemia, smoking, diabetes and hypertension, are associated with endothelial dysfunction, which is mediated by decreased nitric oxide bioavailability [35]. As outlined before, increased endothelial-leukocyte adhesion mediated by increased production of adhesion molecules and upregulation of pro-inflammatory cytokines that predispose to endothelial dysfunction have been demonstrated in OSA. It is therefore not surprising that patients with OSA, free of any overt cardiovascular diseases, have displayed endothelial dysfunction [36]. This has been shown using a variety of techniques such as flow-mediated ultrasonographic measurements of brachial artery dilation, forearm blood flow responses to intra-arterial infusions of acetylcholine, venodilatory responsiveness to bradykinin, and by measuring the response of the peripheral arterial tone to hyperemia. Endothelial dysfunction in OSA patients was also found to be severity dependent, and it could be reversed by nCPAP treatment [37]. Of note, in a group of OSA patients having also cardiovascular morbidity, this association between the severity of OSA and endothelial dysfunction was stronger than in patients with OSA alone [38]. In agreement with the impairment in the endothelium-dependent arterial vasodilatation, there is evidence on decreased availability of circulating nitric oxide in sleep apnea patients that could also be restored by nCPAP treatment [39].

Thus, sleep apnea is associated with a maladaptive endothelium that plays a major role in the early stages of atherosclerosis and is prognostic of future cardiovascular events.

Early Signs of Atherosclerosis

In addition to detecting impaired arterial vasomotion, earlier phases of atherosclerosis are also characterized by other indicators that can be measured noninvasively. These include measuring carotid intima-media thickness (IMT) by ultrasonography, measuring coronary calcium by means of computed tomography and studying the elastic properties of arteries and arterial remodeling [40]. Carotid IMT that is widely used as a noninvasive surrogate end-point to measure progression of atherosclerosis has been studied in OSA by several researchers. All reported on increased IMT in patients with severe OSA compared with healthy controls [41]. The severity of OSA as indexed by hypoxemia was reported to be the most important predictor of carotid IMT. Also, severe OSA was found to be associated with arterial plaque formation [42], calcified artery atheromas [43], atherosclerotic lesions [44] and higher pulse wave velocity [41].

Implications for Diagnosis and Treatment of Sleep Apnea

Based on the above evidence it can be safely assumed that sleep apnea accelerates atherogenic processes. This acceleration most probably starts to accrue during the very first nights that hypoxemic events appear, regardless of the patient's symptoms. Patients, however, are generally referred for diagnosis only when the characteristic symptoms of snoring or excessive daytime sleepiness start to affect them or their bed partners, generally around the age of 50. Although there are no well-controlled studies on the natural evolution of sleep apnea, there is evidence that apneas are already prevalent in the third decade of life. Based on the Wisconsin Study, 17% of men aged 30–39 have a form of sleep apnea classified as mild or beyond and 6.2% have sleep apneas classified as moderate or beyond [1]. Specific high risk populations such as the obese and habitual snorers have no doubt much higher rates. Prospective studies [45] have shown that people displaying disordered breathing during sleep were more likely to develop incident hypertension within a span of 4 years. Likewise, we reported [46] that although untreated OSA patients, investigated 5 years apart, did not show any change in BMI nor the severity of OSA, but nevertheless showed an increase in the rate of cardiovascular morbidity which was most evident in patients who had more severe sleep apnea at the initial diagnosis. These observations suggest that the damage to the cardiovascular system in patients with OSA is progressive and accumulates over time. Furthermore, results of mortality studies of patients with breathing disorders in sleep demonstrated an age decline trend in mortality with the highest risk of mortality in patients younger than the age of 50 [47].

In summary, a diagnosis and treatment of OSA at the age of 50 that is delayed by 10–20 years from the time patients had first displayed breathing disorders in sleep, is too late to reverse the accumulated damage to the cardiovascular system, and is too late for many of the patients who are at maximal risk of dying. To prevent this damage, diagnosis and treatment of breathing disorders in sleep should be done at the earliest age possible. Thus, there is an urgent need to lower the age of diagnosis from age 50 to between 25 and 30.

Conclusion

This review summarized the data that demonstrate the existence of increased oxidative stress which promotes systemic inflammation in sleep apnea and have paved the way for establishing sleep apnea as an independent risk factor for cardiovascular morbidities. It is suggested that hypoxia/reoxygenation, such that is characteristic of sleep apnea, promotes the formation of ROS, and can be deleterious to cells and tissues. However, ROS activate critical redox-sensitive signaling pathways and transcription factors, thus resulting in increased expression of sets of genes that encode proteins essential to adaptation to hypoxia. Yet, redox-sensitive transcription factors as NFκB and AP-1 that elicit inflammatory pathways are activated as well, thereby affecting inflammatory and immune responses that facilitate the activation of endothelial cells, leukocytes and platelets. These activated cells express adhesion molecules and pro-inflammatory cytokines that in turn may cause endothelial cell injury and dysfunction leading to the development of cardio- and cerebrovascular morbidities in OSA. Evidence supporting the existence of endothelial dysfunction and early clinical signs of atherosclerosis in OSA provides firm support to the above chain of events. This newly acquired insight into the pathophysiology of cardiovascular morbidity in OSA emphasizes the urgent need for an early diagnosis and treatment of the syndrome.

References

1 Young T, Palta M, Dempsey J, Skatrud J, Weber S, Badr S: The occurrence of sleep-disordered breathing among middle-aged adults. N Engl J Med 1993;328:1230–1235.

2 Malhotra A, White DP: Obstructive sleep apnoea. Lancet 2002;360:237–245.

3 Wolk R, Somers VK: Cardiovascular consequences of obstructive sleep apnea. Clin Chest Med 2003;24:195–205.

4 Phillips B: Sleep-disordered breathing and cardiovascular disease. Sleep Med Rev 2005;9:131–140.

5 Lavie L: Obstructive sleep apnoea syndrome: an oxidative stress disorder. Sleep Med Rev 2003;7:35–51.

6 Babior BM: Phagocytes and oxidative stress. Am J Med 2000;109:33–44.

7 McCord JM: The evolution of free radicals and oxidative stress. Am J Med 2000;108:652–659.

8 Liu H, Colavitti R, Rovira II, Finkel T: Redox-dependent transcriptional regulation. Circ Res 2005;97:967–974.

9 Lefer DJ, Granger DN: Oxidative stress and cardiac disease. Am J Med 2000;109:315–323.

10 Panes J, Granger DN: Leukocyte-endothelial cell interactions: molecular mechanisms and implications in gastrointestinal disease. Gastroenterology 1998;114:1066–1090.

11 McGown AD, Makker H, Elwell C, Al Rawi PG, Valipour A, Spiro SG: Measurement of changes in cytochrome oxidase redox state during obstructive sleep apnea using near-infrared spectroscopy. Sleep 2003;26:710–716.

12 Yuan G, Adhikary G, McCormick AA, Holcroft JJ, Kumar GK, Prabhakar NR: Role of oxidative stress in intermittent hypoxia-induced immediate early gene activation in rat PC12 cells. J Physiol 2004;557:773–783.

13 Dyugovskaya L, Lavie P, Lavie L: Increased adhesion molecules expression and production of reactive oxygen species in leukocytes of sleep apnea patients. Am J Respir Crit Care Med 2002;165:934–939.

14 Schulz R, Mahmoudi S, Hattar K, Sibelius U, Olschewski H, Mayer K, et al: Enhanced release of superoxide from polymorpho nu clear neutrophils in obstructive sleep apnea: impact of continuous positive airway pressure therapy. Am J Respir Crit Care Med 2000;162: 566–570.

15 Lassegue B, Griendling KK: Reactive oxygen species in hypertension: an update. Am J Hypertens 2004;17:852–860.

16 Zhan G, Serrano F, Fenik P, Hsu R, Kong L, Pratico D, Klann E, Veasey SC: NADPH oxidase mediates hypersomnolence and brain oxidative injury in a murine model of sleep apnea. Am J Respir Crit Care Med 2005;172: 921–929.

17 Lavie L, Vishnevsky A, Lavie P: Evidence for lipid peroxidation in obstructive sleep apnea. Sleep 2004;27:123–128.

18 Yamauchi M, Nakano H, Maekawa J, et al: Oxidative stress in obstructive sleep apnea. Chest 2005;127:1674–1679.

19 Xu W, Chi L, Row BW, Xu R, Ke Y, Xu B, Luo C, Kheirandish L, Gozal D, Liu R: Increased oxidative stress is associated with chronic intermittent hypoxia-mediated brain cortical neuronal cell apoptosis in a mouse model of sleep apnea. Neuroscience 2004;126: 313–323.

20 Chen L, Einbinder E, Zhang Q, Hasday J, Balke CW, Scharf SM: Oxidative stress and left ventricular function with chronic intermittent hypoxia in rats. Am J Respir Crit Care Med 2005;172:915–920.

21 Lavie L: Sleep-disordered breathing and cerebrovascular disease: a mechanistic approach. Neurol Clin 2005;23:1059–1075.

22 Durrington PN, Mackness B, Mackness MI: Paraoxonase and atherosclerosis. Arterioscler Thromb Vasc Biol 2001;21:473–480.

23 Tan KC, Chow WS, Lam JC, Lam B, Wong WK, Tam S, Ip MS: HDL dysfunction in obstructive sleep apnea. Atherosclerosis 2005 Jun 20 [Epub ahead of print].

24 Libby P: Inflammation in atherosclerosis. Nature 2002;420:868–874.

25 Yuan G, Nanduri J, Bhasker CR, Semenza GL, Prabhakar NR: Ca^{2+}/calmodulin kinase-dependent activation of hypoxia inducible factor 1 transcriptional activity in cells subjected to

intermittent hypoxia. J Biol Chem 2005; 280: 4321–4328.
26 Ryan S, Taylor CT, McNicholas WT: Selective activation of inflammatory pathways by intermittent hypoxia in obstructive sleep apnea syndrome. Circulation 2005;112: 2660–2667.
27 Stokes KY, Granger DN: Hypercholesterolemia: its impact on ischemia-reperfusion injury. Expert Rev Cardiovasc Ther 2005;3:1061–1070.
28 Dyugovskaya L, Lavie P, Hirsh M, Lavie L: Activated CD8+ T-lymphocytes in obstructive sleep apnoea. Eur Respir J 2005;25:820–828.
29 Dyugovskaya L, Lavie P, Lavie L: Phenotypic and functional characterization of blood gammadelta T cells in sleep apnea. Am J Respir Crit Care Med 2003;168:242–249.
30 Dyugovskaya L, Lavie P, Lavie L: Lymphocyte activation as a possible measure of atherosclerotic risk in patients with sleep apnea. Ann N Y Acad Sci 2005;1051:340–350.
31 Lavie L, Dyugovskaya L, Lavie P: Sleep apnea related intermittent hypoxia and atherogenesis: adhesion molecules and monocytes/endothelial cells interactions. Atherosclerosis 2005;183: 183–184.
32 Haddad JJ, Harb HL: *L*-Gamma-glutamyl-*L*-cysteinyl-glycine (glutathione; GSH) and GSH-related enzymes in the regulation of pro- and anti-inflammatory cytokines: a signaling transcriptional scenario for redox(y) immunologic sensor(s)? Mol Immunol 2005; 42:987–1014.
33 Vgontzas AN, Papanicolaou DA, Bixler EO, et al: Sleep apnea and daytime sleepiness and fatigue: relation to visceral obesity, insulin resistance, and hypercytokinemia. J Clin Endocrinol Metab 2000;85:1151–1158.
34 Nakamura K, Ueno T, Yamamoto H, Iguro Y, Yamada K, Sakata R: Relationship between cerebral injury and inflammatory responses in patients undergoing cardiac surgery with cardiopulmonary bypass. Cytokine 2005;29:95–104.
35 Davignon J, Ganz P: Role of endothelial dysfunction in atherosclerosis. Circulation 2004; 109(23 suppl 1):III27–32.
36 Lavie L: Sleep apnea syndrome, endothelial dysfunction, and cardiovascular morbidity. Sleep 2004;27:1053–1055.
37 Ip MS, Tse HF, Lam B, Tsang KW, Lam WK: Endothelial function in obstructive sleep apnea and response to treatment. Am J Respir Crit Care Med 2004;169:348–353.
38 Itzhaki S, Lavie L, Pillar G, Tal G, Lavie P: Endothelial dysfunction in obstructive sleep apnea measured by peripheral arterial tone response in the finger to reactive hyperemia. Sleep 2005;28:594–600.
39 Lavie L, Hefetz A, Luboshitzky R, Lavie P: Plasma levels of nitric oxide and *L*-arginine in sleep apnea patients: effects of nCPAP treatment. J Mol Neurosci 2003;21:57–63.
40 Pearson TA: New tools for coronary risk assessment: what are their advantages and limitations? Circulation 2002;105:886–892.
41 Drager LF, Bortolotto LA, Lorenzi MC, Figueiredo AC, Krieger EM, Lorenzi-Filho G: Early signs of atherosclerosis in obstructive sleep apnea. Am J Respir Crit Care Med 2005;172:613–618.
42 Kaynak D, Goksan B, Kaynak H, Degirmenci N, Daglioglu S: Is there a link between the severity of sleep-disordered breathing and atherosclerotic disease of the carotid arteries? Eur J Neurol 2003;10:487–493.
43 Friedlander AH, Friedlander IK, Yueh R, Littner MR: The prevalence of carotid atheromas seen on panoramic radiographs of patients with obstructive sleep apnea and their relation to risk factors for atherosclerosis. J Oral Maxillofac Surg 1999;57:516–521.
44 Aboyans V, Lacroix P, Virot P, Tapie P, Cassat C, Rambaud G, Laskar M, Bensaid J: Sleep apnoea syndrome and the extent of atherosclerotic lesions in middle-aged men with myocardial infarction. Int Angiol 1999;18:70–73.
45 Peppard PE, Young T, Palta M, Skatrud J: Prospective study of the association between sleep-disordered breathing and hypertension. N Engl J Med 2000;342:1378–1384.
46 Fisher D, Pillar G, Malhotra A, Peled N, Lavie P: Long-term follow-up of untreated patients with sleep apnoea syndrome. Respir Med 2002;96:337–343.
47 Lavie P, Lavie L, Herer P: All-cause mortality in males with sleep apnoea syndrome: declining mortality rates with age. Eur Respir J 2005;25:514–520.

Lena Lavie, PhD
Unit of Anatomy and Cell Biology
Ruth and Bruce Rappaport Faculty of Medicine
Technion, POB 9649, 31096 Haifa (Israel)
Tel. +972 4 829 5234
Fax +972 4 834 3934
E-Mail lenal@tx.technion.ac.il

Randerath WJ, Sanner BM, Somers VK (eds): Sleep Apnea.
Prog Respir Res. Basel, Karger, 2006, vol 35, pp 105–112

Genetics Aspects of the Obstructive Sleep Apnea/Hypopnea Syndrome

Renata L. Riha

Department of Sleep Medicine, University of Edinburgh, Royal Infirmary Edinburgh, Edinburgh, UK

Abstract

Obstructive sleep apnea/hypopnea syndrome is a common condition affecting approximately 0.3–4% of the middle-aged population. A hereditary component to the condition has long been identified but the genetic basis has been difficult to elucidate. Not least of the difficulties resides in a single definition of the phenotype. In an attempt to unravel some of the components, which might contribute to the expression of the syndrome, 'intermediate phenotypes' such as craniofacial structure, obesity and upper airway control have been utilized. A number of gene polymorphisms have been explored in association with these and two genome-wide scans have identified potential regions, which may be of interest in further defining the 'intermediate phenotypes'. This chapter focuses largely on human studies with an update on the most recent work in the area.

Obstructive sleep apnea/hypopnea syndrome (OSAHS) affects approximately 0.3–4% of the middle-aged population and is defined on the basis of symptoms of daytime sleepiness and objective measures of disordered breathing during sleep [1]. OSAHS occurs throughout the entire lifespan, from neonates to the elderly. In adults, the frequency of disordered breathing during sleep increases with age and is poorly associated with an increased incidence of daytime sleepiness or other symptoms of OSAHS [2, 3].

A number of studies have shown that OSAHS runs in families. Mechanisms contributing to the etiology of OSAHS include genetically and environmentally induced changes in craniofacial dimensions, differential deposition of adipose tissue, abnormalities in upper airway control and differential susceptibility to sleepiness. All of these potential co etiologies have come under increasing scrutiny on a genetic level. With the completion of the Human Genome Project and the establishment of a single nucleotide polymorphism (SNP) gene map, enormous progress has been made in clarifying the genetic causes of phenotypic differences in the human population.

Here, we will deal with current knowledge regarding OSAHS and genetic factors with a focus on human studies.

OSAHS Phenotype

A precise characterization of the OSAHS phenotype is difficult. Therein lies the primary problem in conducting genetic studies on this disorder.

There is no one specific human morphology that is typical such as is the case in mendelian (single gene) disorders, e.g. Duchenne's muscular dystrophy. OSAHS remains a condition that must be classified on a physiological basis and on objective or subjective evaluation of sleepiness manifest as a daytime symptom. Currently, the most widely accepted definition of OSAHS is provided by The American Academy of Sleep Medicine Task Force [4]. Although this constitutes a good general working definition of the disorder and can be applied satisfactorily in a research setting, it is pragmatic rather than soundly evidence based and does not take into account age-related or gender-related changes in sleepiness and sleep-disordered breathing. There are very few normative data for either in the population and the results obtained are highly dependent on the technology used to measure breathing during sleep or sleepiness [2, 3, 5].

Variations in definitions hinder comparison between studies and may make replication studies examining genetic factors difficult to evaluate.

Owing to the inherent nosological problems with the definition of OSAHS, genetic studies have largely focused on its component parts, the 'intermediate phenotypes', which contribute to its clinical expression such as craniofacial changes, obesity, fat distribution, metabolic derangements and control of ventilation.

Is Obstructive Sleep Apnea/Hypopnea Syndrome Hereditary?

It has been suggested that hereditary factors invoke 40% of the variance in the occurrence of OSAHS in the population [6].

Initially, case reports were suggestive of a familial link for OSAHS, but they were not representative of the population at large (e.g. [7]).

Douglas [8] performed a prospective study of first-degree relatives of 20 consecutive nonobese patients with OSAHS. In studying a total of 40 relatives, they found that 10 of them had more than 15 apneas/hypopneas per hour of sleep and 8 had more than five 4% desaturations per hour. A further study using cephalometry suggested that relatives of probands with OSAHS had more backset maxillae and mandibles compared to age and sex-matched controls [9]. Twin studies have found greater concordance for snoring among monozygotic compared to dizygotic twins [10]. Familial aggregation and segregation analysis of snoring and symptoms of OSAHS applied to 584 pedigrees with 2,019 cased enrolled in the Tucson Epidemiologic Study of Obstructive Airways disease demonstrated mendelian dominant or co-dominant transmission [11]. However, this analysis also found that a non-genetic model would fit the data equally well, suggesting that environmental factors probably contribute to the development of OSAHS. More recently, Buxbaum et al. [12] performed a segregation analysis on a sample of 177 Caucasian families and 125 African-American families. This demonstrated transmission of a putative candidate gene for OSAHS (defined solely by apnea/hypopnea index, AHI) that was variable depending on whether the mathematical/statistical model was age- or BMI-adjusted for the Caucasians and independent of BMI for African-Americans.

AHI is variable within subjects on a nightly basis and subject to recording and scoring error. Therefore, it is not an immutable characteristic that substitutes for phenotype. Furthermore, a previous study showed that BMI is just as important in the etiology of OSAHS in African Americans as it is in American Caucasians [13].

Although there may be racial differences in the presentation of OSAHS [14], it is often taken for granted that the human species is divided into homogeneous groups or races among which biological differences are large [15]. Studies of allele frequencies *do not* support this view, as differences between members of the same population account for 85% of the total diversity. Differences among continents represent roughly 1/10 of human molecular diversity, which does not suggest that racial subdivision of our species reflects any major discontinuity in our genome [15].

Craniofacial Morphology

The craniofacial complex is probably one of the most important heritable determinants of OSAHS. A number of morphological features have been described including changes in cranial base dimensions, displacement of the hyoid bone inferiorly, macroglossia, adenotonsillar hypertrophy, bulkier soft tissue in the upper airway resulting in narrowing and increases in lower facial height [16–18].

Retroposed maxillae and specifically short mandibles have been consistently shown to predispose to OSAHS [17, 18]. Such differences in jaw size can be inherited or acquired – e.g., following nasal occlusion in childhood [19]. There are also a number of syndromes such as the Carpenter syndrome and Apert's syndrome, which are associated with craniofacial anomalies leading to OSAHS. Here the genetic locus has been identified but the confounder remains the multitude of associated anomalies, which characterize these syndromes.

The craniofacial complex is comprised of a number of components which are interdependent in their growth patterns and which are so closely linked, that the growth and shape of one component will influence the rest.

A hierarchy of control genes is activated in sequence, which specifies how the cells in a domain should develop. These controls are influenced by local feedback and intercommunication mechanisms between cells and tissues. The effect of other genes on contiguous tissue will also influence expression of the gene of interest with resultant effects on each other. Genes have been identified through animal studies (mouse mutants), human craniofacial syndromes and expression studies of signaling molecules during facial development [20]. It is now well recognized that growth of the craniofacial complex continues throughout adulthood; that significant sexual dimorphism exists with men being larger at all ages with more growth; that women have periods of increased growth often associated with pregnancy, and that mandibular orientation and occlusal relations change throughout the life cycle [21].

Environmental mechanisms affecting growth include deleterious orofacial muscle habits such as thumb-sucking and abnormal tongue posturing; nasopharyngeal disease and disturbed respiratory function which may produce mouth-breathing; oral/gingival tumors; dental caries with loss of teeth and loss of permanent teeth. Polymorphisms in genes controlling final adult height and stature may affect craniofacial growth. These include the vitamin D receptor, beta-2-adrenergic receptor, growth hormone, insulin-like growth factor (IGF-1), insulin-like growth factor receptor and growth hormone receptor (GHR). Specifically, IGF-1 has been shown to be an important and independent regulator of maxillofacial and mandibular growth postnatally [22].

GHR gene SNPs have been associated with postnatal bone and soft tissue growth as well as with obesity [23]. A recent study aimed to quantitatively evaluate the relationship between craniofacial morphology and the Pro561Thr (P561T) variant in the GHR gene in a normal Japanese population [24]. Subjects without P561T had a significantly longer mandibular ramus as measured cephalometrically suggesting that the GHR gene P561T variant may be associated with mandibular height growth as well as being a genetic marker for it. Riha et al. [unpubl.] examined the GHR P561T polymorphism (within 10 kb of the +561 T/G SNP) in 400 subjects and found no association with cephalometric variables in those with OSAHS compared to those without it.

Studies using genome-wide linkage to look at mandibular structure and size have so far not been undertaken in humans.

Obesity

Obesity is the most commonly identified risk factor for OSAHS [25]. Obesity is thought to contribute to the development/expression of OSAHS due to reduction in nasopharyngeal caliber secondary to fat deposition or as a result of hypoventilation due to a decrease in chest wall compliance. Heritability for Body Mass Index (BMI) in large sample sizes has been estimated to lie between 25 and 40% [26].

The susceptibility to becoming obese therefore seems to be determined significantly by genetic factors, but a favorable 'obesogenic' environment is necessary for phenotypic expression [27].

The regulation of appetite and energy expenditure comprises an extremely complex system with a large number of redundant pathways biased towards weight gain. Obesity develops when energy intake exceeds energy expenditure over time. Accumulated information regarding obesity susceptibility genes is so extensive, that it is currently published in updated form on an annual basis as *The Human Obesity Gene Map* and is now available as a website (http://obesitygene.pbrc.edu). The most current update [27] incorporates published results on single-gene mutation obesity cases, Mendelian disorders exhibiting obesity as a feature, quantitative trait loci (QTLs) from human genome-wide scans and animal crossbreeding experiments as well as association and linkage studies with candidate genes and other markers. In total, more than 300 genes, markers and chromosomal regions have been associated or linked with human obesity phenotypes.

So far, only a few single gene mutations causally related to obesity have been convincingly detected in a small number of people. These include the leptin receptor gene, the leptin gene, the pro-opiomelanocortin gene, the prohomone convertase 1 gene and the melanocortin MC_4 receptor gene. A recent meta-analytic review of the linkage association of the 3 currently known leptin receptor gene polymorphisms in a total of 3,263 individuals (>74% Caucasian) showed no statistically significant association with waist circumference or body mass index at the $p = 0.05$ level [28]. The role of leptin in OSAHS has been emphasized in recent sleep research. However, its role in normal and obese physiology has not been elucidated. Because of its pleiotropic effects on metabolic and appetite regulation, control of ventilation and sleep homeostasis, it cannot be fully integrated in a single pathway that results in OSAHS alone. Other genes that have been sequenced and screened in the search for what predisposes to obesity include the agouti gene, the uncoupling proteins (UCP1–3), all the melanocortin receptor genes, the neuropeptide Y receptor 1 and 5 genes, TNF-α, peroxisome proliferation-activated receptor-gamma (PPAR-γ) and the β_3-adrenoceptor genes among many others. None of the genetic associations reported so far has been proven to be the consequence of a mutation affecting the function or amount of a gene product. Many of the studies reporting single gene polymorphisms associations also need to be supported by cellular work identifying the functional consequences of the reported polymorphisms and it would be of greater clinical relevance if the environmental circumstances necessary for the full phenotypic consequence of these genes and their expression were identified.

Sleepiness

Epidemiological studies have shown that sleepiness does not necessarily correlate with the severity of sleep-disordered breathing and that there is a differential susceptibility to somnolence between individuals [29]. Mechanisms involved in sleep promotion need to be considered as part of the process aimed at elucidating the reasons for the observed differences and as a predisposition to the syndrome of OSAHS.

Sleep is regulated by neuronal and humoral mechanisms that are interdependent [30]. The mediation of a large number of neurohumoral factors by IL-1 and TNF-α appears to be central to the sleep activation pathway and their roles in OSAHS have been the subject of much work [31]. Other cytokines thought to induce sleep include IL-10, IL-6, interferon; IL-2, IL-4, GM-CSF and FGF [32].

TNF-α is elevated in OSAHS independently of obesity and may play a role in daytime sleepiness experienced by the obese even in the absence of OSAHS [33]. There is some evidence to suggest that TNF-α gene polymorphisms may be associated with hypertension [34] as well as with obesity [35]. TNF-α is implicated in bone growth and remodeling, which may affect craniofacial growth [36].

Differences among patients with OSAHS in terms of excessive daytime somnolence may in part be accounted for by differences in cytokine production, which in turn may be mediated by genetic polymorphisms. One study to date has shown increased prevalence of the higher-secreting SNP (−308A) in the TNF-α gene in subjects with OSAHS compared to controls and in siblings with OSAHS compared to those without it [37].

Hypocretin (Orexin)

Animal studies and most recently human studies have identified that the neuropeptide hypocretin is integral to sleep pathways [38]. Most patients with narcolepsy have undetectable levels of hypocretin in the cerebrospinal fluid and a marked decrease in hypocretin immunoreactivity and transcript levels in the perifornical hypothalamus [39]. It has been postulated that the same pathways that cause sleepiness in narcolepsy may potentially be implicated in the induction of sleepiness in the normal population as well as in OSAHS. However, the pathogenesis and clinical expression of the two disorders is so different that it is unlikely that a gene polymorphism in the hypocretin system is involved. Furthermore, hypocretin is involved also in the pathogenesis of cataplexy, which does not occur in OSAHS.

Upper Airway in OSAHS

Sleep-related reductions in pharyngeal muscle activity lead to snoring and upper airway obstruction, which in turn lead to arousal from asleep. These arousals in turn activate the pharyngeal muscles thereby restoring airway patency and more effective breathing.

The genioglossus muscle, innervated by the hypoglossal nerve, is considered to be the major upper airway dilator. NREM sleep and especially REM sleep are associated with the withdrawal of tonic excitation of the hypoglossal motor neurons via reduced firing of predominantly serotonergic medullar raphe neurons and less so by noradrenergic locus coeruleus neurons [40].

Molecular dissection techniques have most recently shown the 5HT2A receptor to be the predominant receptor subtype in hypoglossal motor neurons [41] and pharmacologic trials support this receptor subtype as well as 5-HT2c (found in much smaller quantities) as the predominant post-synaptic facilitator of hypoglossal motor neurons, thereby being instrumental to the regulation of upper airway tone [42].

Clinically, attempts have been made to alleviate obstructive apneas by using selective serotonin reuptake inhibitors (SSRI) [43]. The results have been mixed, with incomplete responses to the SSRIs despite demonstration of increased genioglossal activity as measured by EMG in the awake state.

In light of current knowledge in this area, it would be of potential value to explore whether gene polymorphisms in the 5-HT2A receptor may play a role in the modulation of serotonin metabolism affecting upper airway responsiveness. A preliminary study by Riha [unpubl.] showed no difference in a population of over 400 subjects in the distribution of the T102C SNP in the 5HTR2A gene between those with and without OSAHS. The issue is complicated by imprinting, which plays a large role in the expression of this gene, and the fact that the study was underpowered to detect a difference (over 3,000 subjects would have been required). More promising results may be obtained by examining the serotonin transporter (5-HTT) molecule, which is the initial site of action of SSRIs. A recent study on a small Turkish population showed no association of the serotonin transporter gene polymorphism with OSAHS [44].

Control of Ventilation

Genetic influences may play a role in determining the wide variability in the magnitude of response to hypoxia and hypercapnia in the adult human. Studies in adult monozygotic twins have shown concordance in responses to hypoxia, but not consistently to hypercapnia [45, 46]. A high degree of heritability of peripheral chemoreceptor response to hypoxia and hyperoxia in monozygotic twins during infancy compared with dizygotic twins exposed to similar environmental conditions has also been shown [47].

An examination of the ventilatory drive in OSAHS patients and their healthy relatives as well as healthy unrelated controls has been undertaken by a number of investigators with no convincing differences demonstrated [48, 49]. Based on this information, it is difficult to conclude that there is one single abnormality in ventilation in sleep disordered breathing, making search for a candidate gene currently untenable. Knowledge with regard to neural control of breathing in vertebrates is still in its infancy. Gene deletion models and their effects on ventilatory responses in transgenic mice have been investigated at length but the genes examined potentially play their most important role during early embryonic development and for a brief and transient period only, e.g. Hox and Krox-20 [50].

The outstanding issue remains whether respiratory control is implicated in the pathogenesis of OSAHS. Although there are abnormalities of respiratory control in OSAHS, these reverse with CPAP [51, 52]. Thus, the changes may be secondary rather than causative. This makes search for a genetic abnormality in respiratory control likely to be low yield.

Apolipoprotein E – A Role in OSAHS?

Apolipoprotein E (APOE = gene; ApoE = protein) occurs in all lipoproteins and its major role is thought to be the conversion of LDL proteins to IDLs [53]. The 3 major isoforms of human apo E (apoE2; apoE3 and apoE4) are coded for by 3 alleles (epsilon 2, 3, 4). The APOE3 allele is the most frequent, especially in populations with a long-established agricultural economy such as those in the Mediterranean basin where the frequency of the allele is 0.849–0.898. The APOE4 allele frequency remains higher in populations such as the Pygmies (0.407), Aborigines of Malaysia (0.240) and Australia (0.260) [54].

Allelic variants in APOE were first examined on the basis of its role as an 'injury-response' macromolecule in peripheral nerves and neuromuscular junctions in the context of pharyngeal dilator muscle patency in OSAHS [55]. In this Finnish population, there was no significant difference in distribution of either APOE alleles or genotypes between cases and controls. A second study in an American population looked exclusively at the presence or absence of apolipoprotein E4 alleles in a group of patients who had all undergone polysomnography and were classified as all having sleep apnea (AHI >5) [56]. A normal control group was not used and subjects were grouped as either APOE4-positive (n = 222) or APOE4-negative (n = 569). There was a significantly higher mean AHI in the E4-positive group (6.5SE0.6 vs. 4.8SE0.3) and there was a higher percentage of patients with AHI >15 in the E4-positive group (12 vs. 7%). However, the median values between groups were not significantly different: 1.3 (0–121) in the E4-negative group vs. 2 (0–81) in the E4-positive group. A third study in 718 Japanese-American men in Hawaii aged between 79 and 97 years demonstrated a prevalence of 18% of the E4 allele [57]. Moderate to severe sleep disordered breathing (AHI >15) was present in 42% of this sample of men and adjustment for age, BMI, smoking and use of antihypertensive medication did not reveal an association between E4 and an AHI >15. The most recent study in 1,775 American subjects aged between 40 and 100 years, showed one APOE e4 allele present in 25% of subjects with only 1.3% being E4/E4 homozygotes [58]. Only 19% of the population had an AHI >15 events/h. The strongest association of APOE e4 was found in subjects aged less than 65 years (OR 3.08, CI 1.43–6.64) and was stronger with hypertension or cardiovascular disease.

Apo E is inconsistently associated with the presence of atherosclerosis, Alzheimer's disease and potentially neuropathy and the association with sleep apnea is even more problematic. No controls without OSAHS have been examined in the positive studies. Furthermore, OSAHS is associated with a number of comorbidities that have independently been shown to associate with increased frequency of the E4 allele, such as atherosclerosis, and coronary artery disease. There also appears to be no biologically plausible mechanism currently under consideration that would link ApoE with the development of OSAHS.

OSAHS as a Complex Trait

OSAHS appears to be a polygenic disorder with a complex phenotype, so it is not surprising that there have been relatively few studies investigating genetic markers in association with global phenotype per se.

Early studies looked at HLA markers. A Japanese study [59] showed an association of the HLA-A2 antigen with OSAHS. Another study in an American population showed no association of HLA-DR2, commonly found in the narcoleptic population, with OSAHS [60]. Numbers in both studies were very small. A more recent study examining

HLA antigens in 41 children with OSAHS found HLA-B65 to be significantly more frequently expressed in this group compared to controls [61]. Overall, however, the data did not suggest that HLA played a key role in the pathogenesis of OSAHS.

More recently, attempts have been made to associate various gene polymorphisms with OSAHS. Data from a Han Chinese population was examined for an association of the angiotensin system genes (modulation of hypoxic responses at altitude; effects on hypertension) with OSAHS [62]. Findings suggested that the angiotensin G/T polymorphism was potentially involved in the development of central obesity and thereby may have contributed to the expression of OSAHS and hypertension. Application of this result to over a thousand American subjects in the Wisconsin Sleep Cohort revealed that the ACE gene insertion/deletion polymorphism was dose-dependently associated only with the degree of blood pressure recorded and not with sleep-disordered breathing [63].

Another factor potentially accelerating the development of cardiovascular disease is haptoglobin, an antioxidant and immunomodulatory protein encoded by 2 alleles. A study examining 465 subjects with OSAHS compared to 757 controls showed the risk of cardiovascular disease in sleep apnea patients <55 years with haptoglobin 2–2 was greater than 2.32-fold compared to haptoglobin 2–1 [64].

The first study to look at cytokine gene polymorphisms in OSAHS has shown that the (−308A) TNF-α polymorphism occurs significantly more frequently in subjects with OSAHS compared to population controls and in siblings with OSAHS compared to siblings without OSAHS [37].

To date, 2 genome-wide scans in a population with OSAHS have been published. Palmer et al. [65] performed a 9-cM genome scan for OSAHS and obesity in 66 European-American pedigrees comprising 349 subjects. OSAHS was phenotyped on the basis of AHI alone. The pedigrees were chosen on the basis of either an affected individual with overnight, in-home measurement of breathing using a portable monitor (Edentec®) or a proband who was a neighborhood control individual. Multipoint variance-component linkage analysis was performed for the OSAHS-associated quantitative phenotypes of AHI and BMI. The analysis identified candidate regions on chromosomes 1p (LOD score 1.39), 2p (LOD score 1.64), 12p (LOD score 1.43) and 19p (LOD score 1.40) for linkage with AHI. BMI was linked to the following regions: chromosome 2p (LOD 3.08), 7p (LOD score 2.53) and 12p (LOD score 3.41). Further statistical modeling indicated that evidence for linkage to AHI was removed after adjustment for BMI, excepting regions on chromosomes 2p (adjusted LOD score 1.33) and 19p (adjusted LOD score 1.45). When BMI linkages were adjusted for AHI the LOD scores were roughly halved.

A further 9-cM whole genome scan was conducted in 59 African-American pedigrees [66]. Once again, OSAHS was defined on AHI alone and analysis identified linkage on chromosome 8q (LOD score 1.29) [64]. Body mass index was linked to chromosomes 4q (LOD = 2.63) and 8q (LOD = 2.56). Adjustment for AHI greatly reduced linkages to BMI and vice versa.

Why findings between the two studies differ is difficult to explain. It should also be noted that LOD scores of less than 2 are not considered to demonstrate significant linkage under most circumstances so the results must be interpreted with caution.

Conclusions

OSAHS is a complex, polygenic disease with a number of etiologies interacting to produce a single phenotype. OSAHS is not just a sporadic, but also a familial condition. The degree of environmental influence on its development is currently unknown but is almost certainly considerable including effects on obesity and craniofacial structure.

The major factor affecting progress in genetic studies remains a solid definition of the OSAHS phenotype. Further investigation should be undertaken into whether the OSAHS phenotype remains static throughout life, or whether it changes with time and under different environmental conditions. At present, we are limited to studying the phenotype at a single point in time – when it calls itself to clinical attention, generally in middle age.

Longitudinal studies, firstly identifying those who have OSAHS in childhood and following them through and secondly, continuing to follow those with sleep disordered breathing identified in adult life could be useful in clarifying this issue. There may be large differences in underlying genotype, for instance, between those progressing into old age with asymptomatic sleep disordered breathing, compared to those who develop symptoms and require treatment. We may discover that we are dealing with a range of diseases that manifest as a single phenotype at a particular point in time in the individual's life rather than a single disorder (genotype). Further study is needed to determine the best variables to be used to define phenotype, including age and gender related cut-offs to be used.

Perhaps it is premature at present to utilize genome-wide scans in OSAHS owing to phenotype complexity. Choosing candidate genes for OSAHS in case-control studies is also difficult because a large number of disparate co-etiologies need to be considered. These include obesity, craniofacial structure, upper airway control and sleepiness. Each of these etiologies in turn is regulated by a wide variety of genes and mechanisms that may be pleiotropic and may interact and influence each other. The role of epigenetic phenomena is underestimated and highlights influences that are difficult to measure with accuracy.

OSAHS is a complex disorder and future work attempting to unravel its genetic basis may be better served by utilizing a combination of investigative methods. At present, much remains to be done in elucidating the precise role of genes involved in the regulation of craniofacial growth as well as upper airway control. Once the basic biochemical and physiological processes have been completely understood, then the underlying genetic factors will be rapidly identified.

References

1 Douglas NJ: Clinician's Guide to Sleep Medicine. London, Arnold, 2002.
2 Duran J, Esnaola S, Rubio R, Iztueta A: Obstructive sleep apnea-hypopnea and related clinical features in a population-based sample of subjects aged 30 to 70 yr. Am J Respir Crit Care Med 2001;163:685–689.
3 Bixler EO, Vgontzas AN, Ten Have T, Tyson K, Kales A: Effects of age on sleep apnea in men. I. Prevalence and severity. Am J Respir Crit Care Med 1998;157:144–148.
4 Sleep-Related Breathing Disorders in Adults: Recommendations for syndrome definition and measurement techniques in clinical research. The Report of an American Academy of Sleep Medicine Task Force. Sleep 1999;22: 667–689.
5 Young T, Palta M, Dempsey J, Skatrud J, Weber S, Badr S: The occurrence of sleep-disordered breathing among middle-aged adults. N Engl J Med 1993;328:1230–1235.
6 Redline S, Tishler PV: The genetics of sleep apnea. Sleep Med Rev 2000;4:583–602.
7 Strohl KP, Saunders NA, Feldman NT, Hallett M: Obstructive sleep apnea in family members. N Engl J Med 1978;299:969–973.
8 Douglas NJ, Luke M, Mathur R: Is the sleep apnoea/hypopnoea syndrome inherited? Thorax 1993;48:719–721.
9 Mathur R, Douglas NJ: Family studies in patients with the sleep apnea-hypopnea syndrome. Ann Intern Med 1995;122:174–178.
10 Ferini-Strambi L, Calori G, Oldani A, Della MG, Zucconi M, Castronovo V, Gallus G, Smirne S: Snoring in twins. Respir Med 1995;89:337–340.
11 Holberg CJ, Natrajan S, Cline MG, Quan SF: Familial aggregation and segregation analysis of snoring and symptoms of obstructive sleep apnea. Sleep Breath 2000;4:21–30.
12 Buxbaum SG, Elston RC, Tishler PV, Redline S: Genetics of the apnea hypopnea index in Caucasians and African Americans. I. Segregation analysis. Genet Epidemiol 2002;22:243–253.
13 Redline S, Tishler PV, Hans MG, Tosteson TD, Strohl KP, Spry K: Racial differences in sleep-disordered breathing in African-Americans and Caucasians. Am J Respir Crit Care Med 1997;155:186–192.
14 Wong ML, Sandham A, Ang PK, Wong DC, Tan WC, Huggare J: Craniofacial morphology, head posture, and nasal respiratory resistance in obstructive sleep apnoea: an inter-ethnic comparison. Eur J Orthod 2005;27:91–97.
15 Barbujani G, Magagni A, Minch E, Cavalli-Sforza LL: An apportionment of human DNA diversity. Proc Natl Acad Sci USA 1997;94: 4516–4519.
16 Schwab RJ, Gupta KB, Gefter WB, Metzger LJ, Hoffman EA, Pack AI: Upper airway and soft tissue anatomy in normal subjects and patients with sleep-disordered breathing: significance of the lateral pharyngeal walls. Am J Respir Crit Care Med 1995;152: 1673–1689.
17 Tangugsorn V, Skatvedt O, Krogstad O, Lyberg T: Obstructive sleep apnoea: a cephalometric study. I. Cervico-craniofacial skeletal morphology. Eur J Orthod 1995;17:45–56.
18 Riha RL, Brander P, Vennelle M, Douglas NJ: A cephalometric comparison of patients with the sleep apnea/hypopnea syndrome and their siblings. Sleep 2005;28:315–320.
19 Trask GM, Shapiro GG, Shapiro PA: The effects of perennial allergic rhinitis on dental and skeletal development: a comparison of sibling pairs. Am J Orthod Dentofacial Orthop 1987;92:286–293.
20 Mina M: Regulation of mandibular growth and morphogenesis. Crit Rev Oral Biol Med 2001;12:276–300.
21 Behrents RG: The biological basis for understanding craniofacial growth during adulthood. Prog Clin Biol Res 1985;187:307–319.
22 McCarthy TL, Centrella M: Local IGF-I expression and bone formation. Growth Horm IGF Res 2001;11:213–219.
23 Ohlsson C, Bengtsson BA, Isaksson OG, Andreassen TT, Slootweg MC: Growth hormone and bone. Endocr Rev 1998;19:55–79.
24 Yamaguchi T, Maki K, Shibasaki Y: Growth hormone receptor gene variant and mandibular height in the normal Japanese population. Am J Orthod Dentofacial Orthop 2001;119:650–653.
25 Hoffstein V, Szalai JP: Predictive value of clinical features in diagnosing obstructive sleep apnea. Sleep 1993;16:118–122.
26 Bouchard C: Obesity in adulthood: the importance of childhood and parental obesity. N Engl J Med 1997;337:926–927.
27 Perusse L, Rankinen T, Zuberi A, Chagnon YC, Weisnagel SJ, Argyropoulos G, Walts B, Snyder EE, Bouchard C: The human obesity gene map: the 2004 update. Obes Res 2005; 13: 381–490.
28 Heo M, Leibel RL, Fontaine KR, Boyer BB, Chung WK, Koulu M, Karvonen MK, Pesonen U, Rissanen A, Laakso M, Uusitupa MI, Chagnon Y, Bouchard C, Donohoue PA, Burns TL, Shuldiner AR, Silver K, Andersen RE, Pedersen O, Echwald S, Sorensen TI, Behn P, Permutt MA, Jacobs KB, Elston RC, Hoffman DJ, Gropp E, Allison DB: A meta-analytic investigation of linkage and association of common leptin receptor (LEPR) polymorphisms with body mass index and waist circumference. Int J Obes Relat Metab Disord 2002;26:640–646.
29 Cluydts R, De Valck E, Verstraeten E, Theys P: Daytime sleepiness and its evaluation. Sleep Med Rev 2002;6:83–96.
30 Krueger JM, Obal F Jr, Fang J: Humoral regulation of physiological sleep: cytokines and GHRH. J Sleep Res 1999;1(suppl 8):53–59.
31 Vgontzas AN, Papanicolaou DA, Bixler EO, Kales A, Tyson K, Chrousos GP: Elevation of plasma cytokines in disorders of excessive daytime sleepiness: role of sleep disturbance and obesity. J Clin Endocrinol Metab 1997; 82:1313–1316.
32 Redwine L, Hauger RL, Gillin JC, Irwin M: Effects of sleep and sleep deprivation on interleukin-6, growth hormone, cortisol, and melatonin levels in humans. J Clin Endocrinol Metab 2000;85:3597–3603.
33 Vgontzas AN, Papanicolaou DA, Bixler EO, Hopper K, Lotsikas A, Lin HM, Kales A, Chrousos GP: Sleep apnea and daytime sleepiness and fatigue: relation to visceral obesity, insulin resistance, and hypercytokinemia. J Clin Endocrinol Metab 2000;85: 1151–1158.
34 Demirbas B, Guler S, Cakir B, Culha C, Aral Y: Plasma tumor necrosis factor-alpha levels and insulin resistance in nondiabetic hypertensive subjects. Horm Res 2002;58: 283–286.
35 Pausova Z, Deslauriers B, Gaudet D, Tremblay J, Kotchen TA, Larochelle P, Cowley AW, Hamet P: Role of tumor necrosis factor-alpha gene locus in obesity and obesity-associated hypertension in French Canadians. Hypertension 2000;36:14–19.

36 Cheng X, Kinosaki M, Murali R, Greene MI: The TNF receptor superfamily: role in immune inflammation and bone formation. Immunol Res 2003;27:287–294.
37 Riha RL, Brander P, Vennelle M, McArdle N, Kerr SM, Anderson N, Douglas NJ: Tumour necrosis factor-α (-308) gene polymorphism in the obstructive sleep apnoea/hypopnoea syndrome. ERJ 2005;26:673–678.
38 Mignot E: A commentary on the neurobiology of the hypocretin/orexin system. Neuropsychopharmacology 2001;25:S5–S13.
39 Nishino S: The hypocretin/orexin system in health and disease. Biol Psychiatry 2003; 54:87–95.
40 Parkis MA, Bayliss DA, Berger AJ: Actions of norepinephrine on rat hypoglossal motoneurons. J Neurophysiol 1995;74:1911–1919.
41 Zhan G, Shaheen F, Mackiewicz M, Fenik P, Veasey SC: Single cell laser dissection with molecular beacon polymerase chain reaction identifies 2A as the predominant serotonin receptor subtype in hypoglossal motoneurons. Neuroscience 2002;113:145–154.
42 Fenik P, Veasey SC: Pharmacological characterization of serotonergic receptor activity in the hypoglossal nucleus. Am J Respir Crit Care Med 2003;167:563–569.
43 Kraiczi H, Hedner J, Dahlof P, Ejnell H, Carlson J: Effect of serotonin uptake inhibition on breathing during sleep and daytime symptoms in obstructive sleep apnea. Sleep 1999;22:61–67.
44 Ylmaz M, Bayazit YA, Ciftci TU, Erdal ME, Urhan M, Kokturk O, Kemaloglu YK, Inal E: Association of serotonin transporter gene polymorphism with obstructive sleep apnea syndrome. Laryngoscope 2005;115:832–836.
45 Kobayashi S, Nishimura M, Yamamoto M, Akiyama Y, Kishi F, Kawakami Y: Dyspnea sensation and chemical control of breathing in adult twins. Am Rev Respir Dis 1993;147: 1192–1198.
46 Arkinstall WW, Nirmel K, Klissouras V, Milic-Emili J: Genetic differences in the ventilatory response to inhaled CO_2. J Appl Physiol 1974;36:6–11.
47 Thomas DA, Swaminathan S, Beardsmore CS, McArdle EK, MacFadyen UM, Goodenough PC, Carpenter R, Simpson H: Comparison of peripheral chemoreceptor responses in monozygotic and dizygotic twin infants. Am Rev Respir Dis. 1993;148:1605–1609.
48 Fortin G, del Toro ED, Abadie V, Guimaraes L, Foutz AS, Denavit-Saubie M, Rouyer F, Champagnat J: Genetic and developmental models for the neural control of breathing in vertebrates. Respir Physiol 2000;122:247–257.
49 Radwan L, Maszczyk Z, Koziej M, Franczuk M, Koziorowski A, Kowalski J, Zielinski J: Respiratory responses to chemical stimulation in patients with obstructive sleep apnoea. Monaldi Arch Chest Dis 2000;55: 96–100.
50 Marcus CL, Gozal D, Arens R, Basinski DJ, Omlin KJ, Keens TG, Ward S: Ventilatory responses during wakefulness in children with obstructive sleep apnea. Am J Respir Crit Care Med 1994;149:715–721.
51 Moura SM, Bittencourt LR, Bagnato MC, Lucas SR, Tufik S, Nery LE: Acute effect of nasal continuous positive air pressure on the ventilatory control of patients with obstructive sleep apnea. Respiration 2001;68:243–249.
52 Verbraecken J, Willemen M, De Cock W, Wittesaele W, Govaert K, Van de HP, De Backer W: Influence of longterm CPAP therapy on CO(2) drive in patients with obstructive sleep apnea. Respir Physiol 2000;123: 121–130.
53 Davignon J, Gregg RE, Sing CF: Apolipoprotein E polymorphism and atherosclerosis. Arteriosclerosis 1988;8:1–21.
54 Corbo RM, Scacchi R: Apolipoprotein E (APOE) allele distribution in the world: Is APOE*4 a 'thrifty' allele? Ann Hum Genet 1999;63:301–310.
55 Saarelainen S, Lehtimaki T, Kallonen E, Laasonen K, Poussa T, Nieminen MM: No relation between apolipoprotein E alleles and obstructive sleep apnea. Clin Genet 1998; 53:147–148.
56 Kadotani H, Kadotani T, Young T, Peppard PE, Finn L, Colrain IM, Murphy GM Jr, Mignot E: Association between apolipoprotein E epsilon4 and sleep-disordered breathing in adults. JAMA 2001;285:2888–2890.
57 Foley DJ, Masaki K, White L, Redline S: Relationship between apolipoprotein E epsilon4 and sleep-disordered breathing at different ages. JAMA 2001;286:1447–1448.
58 Gottlieb DJ, DeStefano AL, Foley DJ, Mignot E, Redline S, Givelber RJ, Young T: APOE epsilon4 is associated with obstructive sleep apnea/hypopnea: the Sleep Heart Health Study. Neurology 2004;63:664–668.
59 Yoshizawa T, Akashiba T, Kurashina K, Otsuka K, Horie T: Genetics and obstructive sleep apnea syndrome: a study of human leukocyte antigen (HLA) typing. Intern Med 1993; 32:94–97.
60 Rubin RL, Hajdukovich RM, Mitler MM: HLA-DR2 association with excessive somnolence in narcolepsy does not generalize to sleep apnea and is not accompanied by systemic autoimmune abnormalities. Clin Immunol Immunopathol 1988;49:149–158.
61 Brunetti L, Francavilla R, Leonardo Miniello V, Leone M, Rana M, Colazzo D, Logrillo P, Favoino B, Armenio L: Influence of HLA antigens and OSAS in childhood: a preliminary report. J Sleep Res 2005;14:157–162.
62 Zhang J, Zhao B, Gesongluobu, Sun Y, Wu Y, Pei W, Ye J, Hui R, Liu L: Angiotensin-converting enzyme gene insertion/deletion (I/D) polymorphism in hypertensive patients with different degrees of obstructive sleep apnea. Hypertens Res 2000;23:407–411.
63 Lin L, Finn L, Zhang J, Young T, Mignot E: Angiotensin-converting enzyme, sleep-disordered breathing, and hypertension. Am J Respir Crit Care Med 2004;170:1349–1353.
64 Lavie L, Lotan R, Hochberg I, Herer P, Lavie P, Levy AP. Haptoglobin polymorphism is a risk factor for cardiovascular disease in patients with obstructive sleep apnea syndrome. Sleep 2003;26:592–595.
65 Palmer LJ, Buxbaum SG, Larkin E, Patel SR, Elston RC, Tishler PV, Redline S: A whole-genome scan for obstructive sleep apnea and obesity. Am J Hum Genet 2003;72:340–350.
66 Palmer LJ, Buxbaum SG, Larkin EK, Patel SR, Elston RC, Tishler PV, Redline S: Whole genome scan for obstructive sleep apnea and obesity in African-American families. Am J Respir Crit Care Med 2004;169:1314–1321.

Renata L. Riha, MD
Department of Sleep Medicine
Royal Infirmary Edinburgh
51 Little France Crescent
Little France EH16 4SA
Edinburgh (UK)
Tel. +44 131 242 1837
Fax +44 131 2421776
E-Mail rlriha@hotmail.com,
rriha1@staffmail.ed.ac.uk

Randerath WJ, Sanner BM, Somers VK (eds): Sleep Apnea.
Prog Respir Res. Basel, Karger, 2006, vol 35, pp 113–117

Upper Airway Muscles in Obstructive Respiratory Sleep Disorders

Eva Svanborg

Department of Clinical Neurophysiology, University Hospital, Linköping, Sweden

Abstract

This chapter concerns studies of pharyngeal muscles, especially concerning histopathological changes observed in patients with obstructive sleep apnea syndrome (OSAS) and habitual snoring. The concept of OSAS as a progressive disease is presented as well as the possible causes for this. These include signs of local nervous lesions in the upper airway, both motor and sensory. The focus in this review is put on evidence for motor neuron lesions in the upper airway muscles such as the phenomena of type grouping and grouped atrophy in histological sections, and how this may be related to muscle strength. There are signs of lesions to the motor neurons supplying the upper airway muscles in patients with OSAS and to a lesser degree also in patients with habitual snoring that are consistent with neurogenic lesions. This supports the hypothesis that the progression from habitual snoring to the clinical disease of OSAS could be attributed to neurogenic changes.

The pharynx is essentially a muscular tube which serves three purposes: respiration, swallowing and speech. It lacks substantial bony or rigid support and is therefore highly collapsible. The patency of the pharynx during respiration is almost completely dependent on the activity of the pharyngeal dilator muscles. The most important striated upper airway muscles involved in respiration are:

In the palate
- Palatoglossus (anterior tonsillar pillar), moves the palate downwards-forwards, thus promoting nasal airflow.
- Palatopharyngeus (posterior tonsillar pillar), which moves the palate downwards.
- Levator and tensor veli palatini. These muscles elevate and tighten the soft palate, promoting oral respiration. They are tonically active during the whole respiratory cycle, and are therefore important for airway patency during both inspiration and expiration. Their activity is diminished during sleep.

In the floor of the oral cavity
- Genioglossus protrudes the tongue. It contracts with each inspiration, i.e. it exhibits phasic activity, remaining essentially the same during wakefulness and the different sleep stages. This muscle is considered the most powerful of all pharyngeal dilators.
- Geniohyoideus elevates and protrudes the hyoid bone, and is active at inspiration in the same manner as the genioglossus muscle.

Muscle Activation Patterns

At inspiration, the negative pharyngeal pressure caused by the inflation of the lungs tends to suck the airway closed. This is normally counteracted by activation of the dilating muscles, which thus stiffen the upper airway [1].

These muscles are referred to as inspiratory phasic upper airway muscles. Several studies on the activation patterns of these muscles, the genioglossus in particular, have been conducted. An increased inspiratory activity is also present in mm. palatoglossus, palatopharyngeus and levator palatini. Their activity is much reduced during expiration when the pressure inside the airway becomes positive. Other muscles, such as the tensor veli palatini, do not consistently show increased activity at inspiration but instead maintain a relatively constant level of activity throughout the respiratory cycle [2]. These tonically active muscles are referred to as postural and are of course also important for the patency of the airway. In the supine position, when gravity is negatively influencing the width of the upper airway, an increased activity has been demonstrated in the palatoglossus and palatopharyngeus muscles [3, 4].

The activity of these muscles is increased by several stimuli. Negative pressure is considered the strongest stimulant, but also rises in pCO_2, falling of pO_2 and the sensation of cold (e.g. inhaled air) are important [5, 6]. The responses to negative pressure and temperature have the character of reflexes. These are probably mediated via sensory neurones in the pharyngeal mucosa, since the muscles in question appear to lack muscle spindles [7], and since the responses may be abolished by a combination of local anesthesia of the upper airway and superior laryngeal nerve block [8].

During sleep, there is always a diminished activity of the tonically active muscles. This causes an increased pharyngeal resistance even in normal subjects. This is the most likely explanation why apneas only take place during sleep in obstructive sleep apnea syndrome (OSAS). In OSAS, there are repeated episodes of narrowing of the pharynx during sleep. During an obstructive sleep apnea, the upper airway dilating muscle activity is not sufficient to overcome the negative inspiratory pressure created by the thoracic pump. Consequently, the upper airway collapses. During an apnea, the timing of events is such that initially the genioglossal activity goes down, and towards the end the activity increases again [9, 10]. The activity in the genioglossus muscle has also been shown to be significantly more reduced in OSAS patients than in normal subjects during sleep [11]. Pharyngeal reopening always coincides with increased activity in the genioglossus muscle, and often with arousal, when the activity of the postural muscles increases. Apnea resolution does not occur until inspiratory EMG activity reaches its peak in all dilating muscles, irrespective of whether an arousal occurs or not [12]. An intriguing observation in this context is that during wakefulness, the peak genioglossal activity is higher in OSAS patients than in normal subjects [13]. However, genioglossal activity in OSAS patients is substantially reduced at sleep onset compared to normal subjects [14]. This has been interpreted as loss of a neuromuscular compensation mechanism, present during wakefulness.

Muscle Fiber-Type Characteristics in OSAS

Skeletal muscles are composed of fibers of different types, each type being characterized by the isoform of the myosin heavy chain. Slow fibers are referred to as type I, and they are resistant to fatigue due to their highly oxidative metabolism. Type IIX and IIB fibers are easily fatigable. Fast IIA fibers exhibit intermediate fatigue resistance. Fatigue-resistant fibers are characterized by small fiber diameter, an abundance of capillaries, and a high aerobic oxidative enzyme activity. Upper airway muscles have less type IIB fibers and more type I and IIA than limb muscles, and also a smaller fiber size, which is typical for muscles which often have to remain active for long periods. Patients with OSAS and/or severe snoring have an increased amount of type IIA and less type IIB and type I [15, 16].

Heavy-resistance training, as in body-building, may produce preferential type II hypertrophy. However, some motor units with predominantly hypertrophic fibers also occur in several peripheral neurogenic disorders, probably as a result of overuse of the remaining healthy motor units. The changes described above in OSAS could result from increased use of the upper airway dilators to maintain airway patency. To counteract the increased intraluminal pressure caused by a narrow upper airway, these muscles simply have to work harder than those in a nonapneic person. This might also account for an increased fatigability during sleep.

Degeneration of motor neurons leads to decreased electromechanical activity in the muscle fibers they supply, and also to a lack of trophic factors from the nerves to the muscle fibers. The principal morphological change in a denervated muscle fiber is shrinking of its diameter. All muscle fibers belonging to the same motor unit are of the same histochemical type. In a normal muscle, they are evenly distributed over a rather large area, creating a mosaic pattern of fibers from different units. When reinnervation takes place, as it always tends to do to some extent even in a slowly progressive neurogenic disorder, the regenerating axon attempts to innervate all muscle fibers it comes close to. Fibers adjacent to each other are then activated by the same axon and will therefore be of the same histochemical type [17]. This creates a histological pattern known as 'type grouping'. The new motor units also tend to be much larger that the original ones, i.e. containing a higher number of

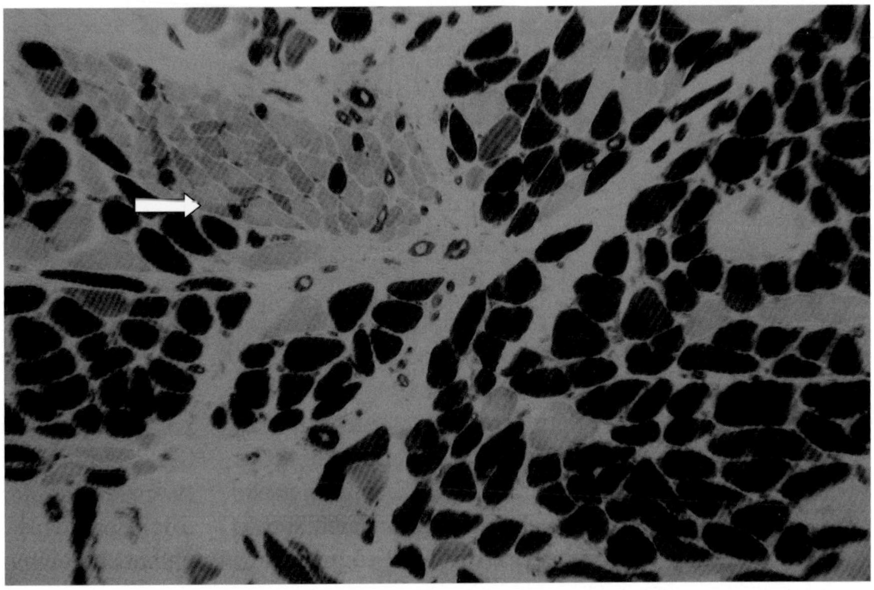

Fig. 1. Cross-section from m. palatopharyngeus of a patient with OSAS, stained with myofibrillar ATPase, after acid preincubation with pH 4.6. Type I fibers stain black, type IIA light, and type IIB grey. There is a complate dominance of type II fibers. The thick white arrow points to a fascicle with atrophic fibers of the same type. This is an example of the phenomenon of fascicular atrophy. This unit and the adjacent with grey fibers of even size are also examples of type grouping.

muscle fibers. If the axon dies, the whole motor-unit will degenerate; creating a histological picture termed 'fascicular atrophy'. Figure 1 illustrates these processes in an upper airway muscle from a patient with sleep apnea. When a nervous lesion occurs over an extended period of time, the rule is that there will be parallel processes of reinnervation and denervation, creating patterns of both type grouping and grouped atrophy in histological sections from the same muscle. Since those muscle motor units which are still functioning have to carry the load of the atrophied ones, the rule is also that a number of units with hypertrophic fibers will be seen. This is simply the effect of hard exercise and not a pathological phenomenon. It also is important to remember that occasional large motor-units with hypertrophic fibers must not be mistaken for increased strength in the studied muscle. The hypothesis behind some of the studies mentioned below was therefore that the inability of the dilating upper airway muscles to maintain airway patency during sleep is the effect of peripheral nerve lesions, causing a partial paresis, worsening over time.

Studies Concerning Possible Motor Neuron Lesions in the Upper Airway Muscles:

- Woodson et al. [18] used light and electron microscopy, and found atrophied and hypertrophied muscle fibers in the soft palate of 8 patients with sleep apnea and severe snoring, but not in 4 nonsnoring controls. There were also frequent focal degeneration of myelinated nerve fibers in their severely apneic patients.
- Edström et al. [19], in 1992, performed the first study which showed typical histological signs of peripheral nerve lesions in pharyngeal muscle tissue from OSAS patients. The above-described phenomena of type grouping, grouped atrophy and great variability of muscle fiber size (simultaneous atrophy and hypertrophy) were found.
- Friberg et al. [20] employed the same techniques as in the above mentioned work by Edström et al. [19], but in this study heavy snorers were also included. Histological findings indicating a progressive 'snorer's disease' was found in the palatopharyngeus muscle. Some degree of pathology was present in the majority of snorers, but with marked worsening in the OSAS patients. The individual score of abnormality was significantly correlated to the percentage periodic obstructive breathing of total sleep time, but not to the oxygen desaturation index. The most important cause for the histological muscle changes could therefore be the amount of time during which the upper airway is subjected to the trauma of snoring and apneas, whereas the qualitative factor of hypoxia is less important.
- Lindman and Stål [7] investigated the histopathology in biopsies from the palatopharyngeus muscle and the

uvula in patients with sleep-disordered breathing and reference samples from autopsy material. The muscle samples from the patients, especially those from the palatopharyngeus, showed several morphological abnormalities; increased amount of connective tissue, an abnormal variability in fiber size, an increased proportion of small-sized fibers, and an increased frequency of fibers containing developmental MyHC isoforms. These findings all point towards a process of simultaneous denervation and degeneration, i.e. a neuromuscular disorder.

- Boyd et al. [21] performed morphometric analysis of upper airway tissue of OSAS patients, and showed that there were clear signs of simultaneous reinnervation (increase in intramuscular nerve fibers) and denervation (positive immunostaining). Immunoreactivity tests showed that there was a dramatic increase in intramuscular nerve fibers in OSA patients compared with control subjects, which is a clear sign of reinnervation. There was also direct evidence of denervation based on positive immunostaining.
- Svanborg [22] has reviewed the possibility to diagnose muscular aberrations using various EMG techniques, including concentric needle EMG, with comparison to the structural changes revealed by histological methods.

Etiology of Obstructive Sleep Apnea Syndrome

Lugaresi et al. [23] in Bologna conducted the first studies of patients with hypersomnia and sleep apneas at the end of the sixties. Already then, they observed that many patients reported similar histories. Heavy snoring had been present for years, often since the patient's youth. In middle age, the spouse noted that the snoring became intermittent with breathing pauses. At the same time, diurnal somnolence became apparent. In the late stages of the disease, respiratory insufficiency, cardiomegaly and polycythemia could also occur. Lugaresi et al. [23] coined the term 'heavy snorer's disease' to describe this course of events. It was hypothesized that the abnormal respiratory efforts during snoring every night for years could cause anatomical changes in the upper airway that would eventually lead to occlusion. This could cause a vicious circle; the more occluded the upper airway would be, the heavier the inspiratory efforts would be, with even further narrowing as a result. The typical evolution of events in 'heavy snorer's disease' is corroborated by the fact that OSAS is an unusual diagnosis before middle age. It has also been shown in several later studies, with objective recordings of indices of respiratory distress, that a progress takes place in many cases, in particular those with a mild-to-moderate disease [24, 25].

Obstructive sleep apnea can develop as the result of a variety of physiologic characteristics. Most OSAS patients have an anatomically small upper airway due to overweight with fat deposits in the pharynx, an aberrant facial skeleton or soft tissue enlargement. In these cases, their upper airway dilator muscles are obviously unable to adequately respond to rising intrapharyngeal negative pressure and increasing CO_2 during sleep. The patient's arousal threshold in response to respiratory stimulation is also important, as is instability in ventilatory control. Primary muscular hypotonia could also be a cause (OSA is overrepresented in neuromuscular diseases). However, OSAS/snorers disease is in many cases a progressive disorder, and the above mentioned mechanisms do not offer a substantial explanation for this development. Weight increase does not always provoke impairment of obstructive respiration. In one study, there was no certain correlation between increases in the apnea/hypopnea index and body weight [24], and in another, marked worsening of obstructive breathing was found in some patients despite weight loss [25]. After adolescence, the tonsils gradually decrease in relative size, and skeletal aberrations as a rule do not worsen in adulthood. Concomitant clinical neuromuscular disorders are rare in OSAS cases. Some other factor could therefore also be responsible for progression, as will be discussed below.

The majority of patients report that they have been habitual snorers for years before apneas become apparent. Snoring implies vibrations of the tissues that produce the sound. In occupational medicine, it has been shown that long-standing tissue vibration may cause local nerve lesions [26, 27]. Vibrations could, however, also cause primary structural changes in tissue. Sinclair and Roach [28] tested the effect of vibratory stress on dog bronchi. Turbulent airflow was created by a cannula acting as a stenosis, producing vibrations in the wall, similar to what happens in the upper airway during obstructive breathing. There was a significant alteration in the structural properties. A 'yielding' in the direction of maximum vibration was observed with a corresponding structural rearrangement (radius decreased, length increased). The bronchi also became less resistant to collapse under negative pressures.

One hypothesis is therefore that snoring vibrations, repeated every night for several years, cause neuronal lesions in the upper airway. This, in turn, could result in a gradual collapse of the pharyngeal tube due to partial paresis of the dilating muscles. Another additive cause of airway collapse could be an impaired reflex. The sensation of cold air triggers the dilating muscles to contract at inspiration.

It is reasonable that both motor and sensory neurons should be damaged, if vibration of the upper airway is the cause. Evidence for sensory nervous lesions has indeed been given in several previous studies. Larsson et al. [29] found pathologically decreased temperature sensitivity on the tonsillar pillars in patients with OSAS in comparison to non-snoring subjects. Kimoff et al. [30] showed decreased sensitivity to vibration in the upper airway of both snorers and OSAS patients, with significant improvement after CPAP-treatment. Nguyen et al. [31] found a virtually inverse dose-response relationship between AHI and laryngeal sensitivity to air puffs.

In conclusion, the dilating muscles of the pharynx are vitally important for maintenance of airway patency during sleep. Many studies have shown malfunction and structural abnormalities in the upper airway muscles in patients with obstructive respiratory sleep disorders. These changes could, at least in part, be due to neurogenic lesions.

References

1 Van Lunteren E: Muscles of the pharynx: structural and contractile properties. Ear Nose Throat J 1993;72:2733–2739.
2 Tangel DJ, Mezzanotte WS, White DP: The influence of sleep on tensor palatini EMG and upper airway resistance in normal subjects. J Appl Physiol 1991;70:2574–2581.
3 Mortimore IL, Mathur R, Douglas NJ: Effect of posture, route of respiration, and negative pressure on palatal muscle activity in humans. J Appl Physiol 1995;79:448–454.
4 Mortimore IL, Douglas N: Palatal muscle EMG response to negative pressure in awake sleep apneic and control subjects. Am J Respir Crit Care Med 1997;156:867–873.
5 Mathew OP: Upper airway negative pressure effects on respiratory activity of upper airway muscles. J Appl Physiol 1984;56:500.
6 Horner R, Innes J, Murphy K, Guz A: Evidence for reflex upper airway dilator muscle activation by sudden negative airway pressure in man. J Physiol 1991;436:15–29.
7 Lindman R, Stal PS: Abnormal palatopharyngeal muscle morphology in sleep-disordered breathing. J Neurol Sci 2002;195:11–23.
8 Horner RL, Innes JA, Holden HB, Guz A: Afferent pathway(s) for pharyngeal dilator reflex to negative pressure in man: a study using upper airway anaesthesia. J Physiol 1991;436:31–44.
9 Guilleminault C, Hill MW, Simmons FB, Dement WC: Obstructive sleep apnea: electromyographic and fiberoptic studies. Exp Neurol 1978;62:48–67.
10 Suratt P, McTier RF, Wilhoit SC: Upper airway muscle activation is augmented in patients with obstructive sleep apnea compared with that in normal subjects. Am Rev Respir Dis 1988;137:889–894.
11 Fogel RB, White DP: Obstructive sleep apnea. Adv Intern Med 2000;45:351–389.
12 Carlson DM, Onal E, Carley DW, Lopata M, Basner RC: Palatal muscle electromyogram activity in obstructive sleep apnea. Am J Respir Crit Care Med 1995;152:1022–1027.
13 Mezzanotte WS, Tangel DJ, White DP: Waking genioglossal electromyogram in sleep apnea patients versus normal controls (a neuromuscular compensatory mechanism). J Clin Invest 1992;89:1571–1579.
14 Onal E, Lopata M: Periodic breathing and the pathogenesis of occlusive sleep apneas. Am Rev Respir Dis 1982;126:676–680.
15 Smirne S, Iannaccone S, Ferini-Strambi L, Comola M, Colombo E, Nemni R: Muscle fibre type and habitual snoring. Lancet 1991;337:597–599.
16 Sériès FJ, Simoneau SA, St Pierre S, Marc I: Characteristics of the genioglossus and musculus uvulae in sleep apnea hypopnea syndrome and in snorers. Am J Respir Crit Care Med 1996;153:1870–1874.
17 Carpenter S, Carpati G: Pathology of Skeletal Muscle. New York, Churchill-Livingstone, 1984, pp 460–470.
18 Woodson BT, et al: Histopathologic changes in snoring and obstructive sleep apnea syndrome. Laryngoscope 1991;101:1318–1322.
19 Edström L, Larsson H, Larsson L: Neurogenic effects on the palatopharyngeal muscle in patients with obstructive sleep apnea. J Neurol Neurosurg Psychiatry 1992;55:916–920.
20 Friberg D, Ansved T, Borg K, Carlsson-Nordlander B, Larsson H, Svanborg E: Histological indications of a progressive snorers disease in an upper airway muscle. Am J Respir Crit Care Med 1998;157:586–593.
21 Boyd JH, Petrof BJ, Hamid Q, Fraser R, Kimoff RJ: Upper airway muscle inflammation and denervation changes in obstructive sleep apnea. Am J Respir Crit Care Med 2004;170: 541–546.
22 Svanborg E: Impact of obstructive sleep apnea syndrome on upper airway respiratory muscles. Respir Physiol Neurobiol 2005;147: 263–272.
23 Lugaresi E, Mondini S, Zucconi M, Montagna P, Cirignotta F: Staging of heavy snorers' disease: a proposal. Bull Eur Physiopathol Respir 1983;19:590–594.
24 Lindberg E, Elmasry A, Gislason T, Janson C, Bengtsson H, Hetta J, Nettelbladt M, Boman G: Evolution of sleep apnea syndrome in sleepy snorers: a population-based prospective study. Am J Respir Crit Care Med 1999;159: 2024–2027.
25 Svanborg E, Larsson H: Development of nocturnal respiratory disturbance in untreated patients with obstructive sleep apnea syndrome. Chest 1993;104:340–343.
26 Takeuchi T, Futatsuka M, Imanishi H, Yamada S: Pathological changes observed in the finger biopsy of patients with vibration-induced white finger. Scand J Work Environ Health 1986;12:280–283.
27 Brismar T, Ekenvall L: Nerve conduction in the hands of vibration exposed workers. Electroencephalogr Clin Neurophysiol 1992; 85:173–176.
28 Sinclair S, Roach MR: Effect of vibration on isolated dog bronchi. J Appl Physiol 1975;38: 780–785.
29 Larsson H, Carlsson-Nordlander B, Lindblad LE, Norbeck O, Svanborg E: Temperature thresholds in the oropharynx of patients with obstructive sleep apnea syndrome. Am Rev Respir Dis 1992;146:1246–1249.
30 Kimoff RJ, Sforza E, Champagne V, Ofiara L, Gendron D: Upper airway sensation in snoring and obstructive sleep apnea. Am J Respir Crit Care Med 2001;164:250–255.
31 Nguyen D, Jobin V, Payne R, Beauregard J, Naor N: Laryngeal and velopharyngeal sensory impairment in obstructive sleep apnea. Sleep 2005;28:585–593.

Eva Svanborg, MD, PhD
Department of Clinical Neurophysiology
University Hospital
SE–581 85 Linköping (Sweden)
Tel. +46 13 22 20 30
Fax +46 13 22 45 41
E-Mail evasv@inr.liu.se

Randerath WJ, Sanner BM, Somers VK (eds): Sleep Apnea.
Prog Respir Res. Basel, Karger, 2006, vol 35, pp 118–136

Obstructive Sleep Apnea: Clinical Presentation, Diagnosis and Treatment

Susie Yim Amy Jordan Atul Malhotra

Sleep Disorders Program at BIDMC, Sleep Medicine and Pulmonary and Critical Care Divisions, Brigham and Women's Hospital, and Harvard Medical School, Boston, Mass., USA

Abstract

Obstructive sleep apnea is a common disorder. Most patients are referred to sleep clinics because of snoring, excessive daytime sleepiness and witnessed apneas. Obesity, male sex, older age, and family history are recognized risk factors for sleep apnea. The cardiovascular and neurocognitive sequelae of OSA makes early diagnosis and treatment of this disease important. CPAP remains the treatment of choice. Even though treatment improves quality of life and can improve cardiovascular endpoints, adherence and acceptance of CPAP remains problematic but on par with treatment of other chronic medical conditions. The natural history of untreated sleep apnea and a description of its clinical course has not been fully elucidated. However, more research is needed to help clarify if sleep apnea has different phenotypes and clinical courses in different patient populations.

Clinical Presentation

Definitions

In obstructive sleep apnea/hypopnea syndrome (OSAHS), the upper airway collapses during sleep causing episodic airflow obstruction. In an attempt to re-establish airflow, the afflicted individual makes progressively larger respiratory efforts until there is arousal from sleep and resumption of breathing. In order to characterize and diagnose obstructive sleep apnea (OSA), the terms apnea and hypopnea have been used to define these events. An apnea is the cessation of airflow of at least 10 s in duration. Hypopneas, however, have been harder to characterize and much debate still persists as to what constitutes a hypopnea. The American Academy of Sleep Medicine Task Force defines hypopnea as one of the following three: >50% reduction in airflow, <50% reduction in airflow associated with a desaturation of >3%, or a moderate reduction in airflow with associated arousal by electroencephalogram [1]. Detecting changes in airflow has become more sensitive with the use of nasal pressure measurements instead of oronasal thermistors. The clinical relevance of hypopneas, therefore, has become even more confusing. Although the range of normal is still being defined, it has been generally accepted that during sleep, normal individuals may have up to at least five to ten airflow reductions or cessation events an hour.

The apnea-hypopnea index (AHI) is the number of apneas and hypopneas per hour. This index has been used to define and characterize the severity of the sleep apnea syndrome (table 1), although its ability to predict OSA-related complications has been modest at best. An AHI of >5–10 events per hour is used to characterize patients with OSA. As the AHI increases, two main consequences occur.

The first is that patients have an increased number of arousals. These arousals disturb sleep architecture resulting in nonrestorative sleep and daytime somnolence. Recurrent arousals combined with intermittent hypoxia lead to worsening neurocognitive functioning and compromise in daytime attention. In fact, patients with sleep apnea syndrome

Table 1. Severity indices of OSA

	AHI, events/h	O_2 saturation, %
Normal	<5	>95
Mild	5–19	>85
Moderate	20–39	>65
Severe	>40	<65

are at markedly increased risk of motor vehicle accidents when compared to matched controls [2]. Patients with sleep apnea have also been found to have difficulty with memory, intellectual capacity and motor coordination. Performing tasks that require psychomotor vigilance such as visual reaction and auditory learning are impaired in patients with sleep apnea.

The second consequence of OSA is that to the cardiovascular system. While the hemodynamic effects of arousals are still being elucidated, each arousal occurs in the setting of episodic hypoxemia and a surge of sympathetic tone. Repetitive hypoxemia may cause injury to tissues and is thought to play a role in the development of cardiovascular disease (see below). In addition, fluctuations in sympathetic tone during the night may also contribute to increasing daytime systemic hypertension, as will be discussed. This link between hypertension and sleep apnea is increasingly apparent in both large human prospective epidemiological studies and human interventional trials [3–6]. With each apneic event per hour of sleep, the odds of having daytime hypertension increases by approximately 1% and if the events are associated with a 10% oxygen desaturation, the odds increase by 13% [4]. Although the effect of sleep apnea on systemic hypertension is becoming clearer, its role in pulmonary hypertension is more confusing. Older observations that patients with sleep apnea had increasing pulmonary hypertension with associated right heart dysfunction and cor pulmonale are misleading. Recent studies have shown that OSA alone is not sufficient to cause severe pulmonary hypertension but that daytime derangements in arterial blood gases must be present as well. Therefore, to attribute severe pulmonary hypertension to OSA, there must be another abnormality to cause daytime hypoxemia and hypercapnia such as obesity hypoventilation syndrome or emphysema [7]. However, more recent data suggest that OSA can lead to mild to moderate pulmonary hypertension in the absence of parenchymal lung disease. Of note, this form of pulmonary hypertension is reversible with OSA therapy. In addition, these patients exhibit marked hypoxic vasoreactivity such that pulmonary artery pressures can elevate considerably in the face of hypoxic stimuli. Thus, substantial elevations in pulmonary arterial pressures can be observed in patients with underlying OSA who then develop hypoxemia, e.g. from mild pneumonia. The role of sleep apnea in coronary artery disease (CAD), stroke, and other cardiovascular diseases is currently being investigated, and will be discussed subsequently.

Clinical Importance of OSAHS

Wake up America: A National Sleep Alert, 1993 Report of the National Commission on Sleep Disorders Research [8]: 'By any measuring stick, the deaths, illness, and damage due to sleep deprivation and sleep disorders represent a substantial problem for American society.'

Sleep disorders are emerging as a substantial public health problem. In 1987, the US Congress passed legislation requiring the National Institutes of Health to establish a plan for researching sleep disorders. In response, the National Commission on Sleep Disorders Research was founded in 1988 to conduct a comprehensive study of the status on current knowledge, research, and resources available for addressing sleep disorders. The Commission published its findings in the 1993 report 'Wake up America.' This study estimated that OSAHS affects approximately 20 million Americans, making it more prevalent than asthma in adults. The cost of sleep apnea is substantial with estimates of USD 42 million a year in hospital bills. Yet despite these statistics, OSAHS remains a largely unrecognized and undiagnosed disorder. It is not because these patients do not seek medical treatment. A telephone survey of 5,000 individuals in the United Kingdom found that 31% of those with breathing pauses during sleep sought medical attention more than 6 times in the previous year [9]. This is true in the United States as well. When patients seeing their primary care physician were asked to complete a survey regarding symptoms associated with OSAHS, 32% had a high pretest probability for OSAHS [10]. The failure of medical professionals to recognize OSAHS is likely due to the limited training in sleep medicine. In the United Kingdom for instance, medical students receive only 5 min of sleep medicine teaching throughout their training [11]. The United States does not fare much better, where, on average, less than 2 h of the curriculum are devoted to sleep medicine [12]. Even among highly trained pulmonologists, formal sleep medicine training is limited with many learning 'on their own' [13]. A study of 60 chest physicians at the American College of Chest Physicians annual meeting in 1998 revealed that even though 65% of the respondents directed or were on staff

Table 2. Classic symptoms of sleep apnea

Snoring
Excessive daytime sleepiness
Witnessed apneas

in a sleep laboratory, only 3% had completed any type of formal sleep medicine training and 18% had American Board of Sleep Medicine certification [14].

However, times are changing as sleep disorders become more prominent in both the public eye and the medical profession. OSAHS and its effects on productivity, cognition, coordination, quality of life, and cardiovascular health are important to be able to recognize since this is a treatable disease. Because OSAHS is so common, its clinical presentation and diagnosis is crucial for any physician to know. Almost every medical specialty will come across patients with symptoms associated with or exacerbated by OSAHS [15]. Sleep physicians, specifically, will most likely see patients who are referred because of snoring, excessive daytime sleepiness (EDS), or witnessed apneas (table 2).

Snoring

Snoring is very common. In the United Kingdom, a telephone survey revealed that 40% of the total population snored regularly with an increased prevalence in men [9]. Snoring can be intrusive and can cause strain on the relationships between bed partners, even threatening marriages. Often times, it is the bed partner who will raise concern over the snoring bringing the patient to medical attention. The bed partner is sometimes even more invested in obtaining a diagnosis and treatment for snoring. Studies of bed partners have shown that if snoring is due to OSAHS, then treatment will improve both the bed partner's and the patient's quality of life [16]. Yet the patient's own perception of his or her snoring can be very inaccurate with the majority of snorers denying it when asked. One pulmonologist recalls a patient and his wife who came into his office seeking treatment for excessive snoring. The patient did not believe his wife and when she produced a tape recording of his loud snoring, he yelled 'You're lying. That is not me!' as he stormed out of the office. This story illustrates the importance of bed partner reports since these may be the only clues to diagnosing OSAHS. Snoring is one of the most common symptoms of OSAHS, occurring in up to 70–95% of patients with the syndrome [17]. However, because it is so common, snoring is not specific for OSAHS. However, the severity of snoring can be helpful as patients with very loud snoring are more likely to have sleep apnea than those with soft snoring. On the other hand, lack of snoring makes OSAHS much less likely with reports of only 3–6% of nonhabitual snorers having OSAHS [18].

Excessive Daytime Sleepiness

Like snoring, daytime sleepiness is relatively common, in part because there are a myriad of causes for sleep deprivation. It is estimated that approximately 20–30% of people with or without OSAHS suffer from daytime sleepiness [19]. To complicate matters, self-reported sleepiness is often inaccurate and likely underestimates the degree of sleepiness [20]. This may be due to lack of awareness or environmental pressures to ignore sleepiness. Caffeine, a modestly traded commodity, is a frequent 'masking' agent and can substantially complicate assessments of sleepiness. For example, doctors in training, truck drivers, and shift workers often work despite substantial sleep deprivation caused by long job hours. Patients with OSAHS, however, do not suffer from lack of sleep time. They experience daytime sleepiness because of the sleep fragmentation caused by intermittent apneas and hypoxia. Yet despite the widespread prevalence of EDS, 80–90% of those who present to sleep clinics with this symptom will be diagnosed with a sleep disorder [21]. This may be because patients with the most severe symptoms present to sleep clinics. On the other hand, patients who are sleepy due to lifestyle-inflicted sleep deprivation may not come to clinical fruition very often.

Because daytime sleepiness can often be confused with lethargy or fatigue, the distinction must be made in order to pursue the correct diagnosis. 'Sleepiness' is the urge to fall asleep during normal activities, usually those that may not require complete concentration, such as driving, watching television, conversing, or listening to lectures. Fatigue or lethargy, on the other hand, is not always associated with an increased propensity to sleep. Patients who feel fatigue, lethargy, or exhaustion may feel tired but not necessarily have hypersomnolence. Conditions such as anemia, congestive heart failure (CHF), depression, or hypothyroidism may present with fatigue. Making the distinction between sleepiness and tiredness may ultimately lead to a different diagnosis. True sleepiness is usually caused by inadequate sleep duration, sleep fragmentation, or increased sleep drive. However, patients with OSAHS use words such as fatigue, tiredness, or lack of energy to describe their own symptoms of sleepiness. In a study of patients with sleep apnea, complaints of fatigue, tiredness or lack of energy

Table 3. The Epworth Sleepiness Scale

Rate the likelihood of falling asleep or dozing off in the following situations, in contrast to feeling just tired
Refer to your usual way of life in recent times
0 = Would never doze
1 = Slight chance of dozing
2 = Moderate chance of dozing
3 = High chance of dozing
Situation Score
1. Sitting and reading
2. Watching television
3. Sitting inactive in a public place (e.g. church)
4. As a passenger in a car for an hour without a break
5. Lying down to rest in the afternoon when circumstances permit
6. Witting and talking to someone
7. Sitting quietly after lunch without alcohol
8. In a car, while stopped for a few minutes in traffic

were commonly used by sleep apneics to describe sleepiness especially among women [22]. Therefore, to exclude the diagnosis of OSAHS because a patient may describe his/her symptoms as fatigue more than sleepiness may lead to missed diagnoses.

There are several tools available to measure the degree of sleepiness. These include the Epworth Sleepiness Scale (ESS; table 3), the Multiple Sleep Latency Test (MSLT), the Maintenance of Wakefulness Test (MWT), and the Osler test. There is no gold standard as they all likely measure somewhat different phenomena. The easiest tool to use is the ESS because it is simple to administer, quick, inexpensive, and has a high test-retest reliability [23]. It consists of a self-administered questionnaire where patients rate on a scale of 0–3 their likelihood of falling asleep during everyday activities. A score of 6–7 indicates normal somnolence, a score of 8–12 indicates mild sleepiness, a score of 13–17 indicates moderate sleepiness, and a score of 18 or higher indicates severe sleepiness. The drawbacks to the ESS are that it does not always correlate with the severity of sleep apnea and because it relies on self-reporting, can often be inaccurate or vulnerable to misreporting.

Objective tests eliminate self-reporting but are often time consuming to administer and may not necessarily reflect the activities of daily living. During the MSLT, the subject is instructed to try to sleep at multiple times during the day, during which length of time to sleep onset and presence of REM sleep is assessed. The MWT test differs in that the subject is asked to stay awake. The Osler test asks the subject to press a switch each time a light turns on and a computer scores the number of correct answers. The advantage of the Osler test over the other two is that is does not require an electroencephalogram. This test has been found to correlate with the others when tested in comparison [24].

Witnessed Apneas

A bed partner may witness breathing pauses or apneas during the patient's sleep, or the patient may report waking up choking or feeling acutely panicked during the night. This is one of the more common reasons for referral to a sleep clinic. However, the accounts of witnessed apneas may often be incorrect as even trained medical staff are not very good at recognizing respiratory events in patients with OSAHS [25]. Apneas can also occur in the non-OSAHS population. Finally, it is important to distinguish between nocturnal shortness of breath from witnessed apneas. Other conditions such as CHF, asthma, and laryngospasm may present with nighttime symptoms of dyspnea. Paroxysmal noctural dyspnea can have some of the same characteristics as apneas with a similar sensation of 'choking'. Often patients with OSAHS may only be breathless for a brief moment whereas the other conditions have prolonged dyspnea. Also, there are usually other more obvious signs and symptoms associated with the conditions listed above.

Although patients may present with EDS, snoring, or witnessed apneas, none of these symptoms alone allow for an accurate diagnosis. Sleep doctors have often been wrong when asked to make the diagnosis on history and physical exam. However, a combination of these symptoms, such as snoring and witnessed apneas, are more predictive of OSAHS. To improve the likelihood even more, recognition of certain risk factors may help to establish a diagnosis.

Risk Factors

Anatomy

Narrowing of the upper airway is the most recognized risk factor for OSAHS. Unlike most mammals, humans do not have a rigid bony support for the pharyngeal airway, hence the patency of the upper airway relies on muscle activation and soft tissue structures. The smaller upper airway causes a reflexive increase in muscle activity to maintain patency during wakefulness. When these protective reflexes are lost during sleep, the upper airway is prone to collapse. Multiple imaging studies using computed tomography, magnetic resonance imaging, fluoroscopy, and acoustic reflection have demonstrated that patients with OSAHS indeed have a small pharyngeal airway with the smallest area occurring at the velopharynx. Patients with

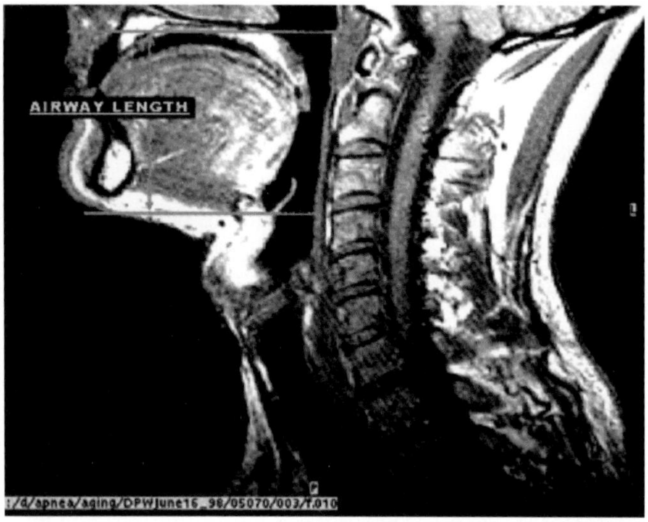

Fig. 1. The pharyngeal airway length from the top of the hard palate to the epiglottis.

Table 4. Risk factors for sleep apnea

Anatomy
Small upper airway
Craniofacial abnormalities
Macroglossia
Hypertrophied tonsil and adenoids
Increased nasal resistance
Obesity
Male sex
Increased age
Genetics
Alcohol, opioid, or benzodiazepine use
Smoking

OSAHS have larger tongues, soft palates, parapharyngeal fat pads, and lateral walls around the pharynx [26]. There are also speculated differences in the direction of the long axis. It is thought that the orientation is anterior-posterior instead of inferior-superior, which may place the pharyngeal dilator muscles at a mechanical disadvantage making them less effective in keeping the airway patent [27]. Finally, in normal subjects, increased distance between the hyoid bone and the mandibular plane (and other surrogates for pharyngeal airway length) have been shown to increase the propensity for airway collapse [28] (fig. 1).

Conditions such as obesity (see below), craniofacial abnormalities (retrognathia, micrognathia, midface or mandibular hypoplasia), macroglossia, hypertrophied tonsils and adenoids (especially in children), and increased uvula size can lead to smaller upper airways. Therefore, it is not the obese patient alone who suffers from OSAHS. Other diseases such as Down's syndrome, which can lead to both midface hypoplasia and macrogloassia, or acromegaly, which can lead to macroglossia, can present with OSAHS.

Although obesity is a major risk factor for OSAHS, location of fat deposition, not BMI alone is a more likely predictor of OSAHS. There is an increase in excess fat in areas anterolateral to the upper airway in both obese and nonobese patients with OSAHS [29]. This is perhaps why neck circumference has been shown to be a strong predictor of OSAHS [30]. Neck circumferences greater than 48 cm are associated with a high risk of OSAHS while circumferences less than 37 cm are lower risk for OSAHS. Despite these data, physicians should be aware that OSA is being increasingly recognized in lean individuals who have small neck circumferences.

Although the velopharynx is the most common site of airway narrowing, nasal anatomy also plays a role in OSAHS. When there is increased nasal resistance, the diaphragm will produce more negative pressure potentially causing the pharyngeal airway to collapse. Therefore, nasal polyps, deviated septa, and congestion can exacerbate or lead to OSAHS. In fact, patients with rhinitis and OSAHS have a decrease in their AHI when treated with an intranasal corticosteroid [31] (table 4).

Obesity

Obesity is a well known risk factor for OSAHS. Many studies over the years have shown a clear correlation between OSAHS and excess body weight. Even modest gains in weight have led to increased severity of OSAHS. The Wisconsin Sleep Cohort has shown that patients with mild OSAHS have a 6-fold increase in risk for developing moderate or severe OSAHS if they gain only 10% of their body weight [32]. And among those who are most overweight (BMI of >40), 70% suffer from OSAHS. Therefore, it seems that weight gain increases the chance of developing OSAHS and can worsen the severity of OSAHS in those who already have it. Why obesity can lead to OSAHS is not completely understood, but probably relates to a smaller pharyngeal airway, dysfunctional upper airway muscles, and decreased lung volumes. While weight loss among patients who have had bariatric surgery or who have participated in weight reduction studies can lead to substantial decreases in OSA severity [33], it often does not eliminate OSAHS altogether. Current studies have been limited by small numbers, short observation periods, and lack of correlation with symptoms. Also, whether there is a difference in weight loss achieved through reduced caloric intake vs. increased caloric output remains unclear. Nevertheless, weight loss, if maintained long term, will likely be the best means for reducing prevalence and severity of OSAHS and remains a large public health challenge.

Yet obesity and BMI alone do not always correlate with severity of OSAHS. There are many nonobese people who suffer from OSAHS, who likely remain undiagnosed, and many obese patients without OSAHS. The 'Pickwickian' stereotype does not always hold true. Neck circumference, waist-hip ratio, and degree of central obesity may be better predictors of OSAHS in men than obesity in general [33]. There is, however, no real consensus on the most predictive body habitus for OSAHS because of large variations in body morphology and difficulties in objective accurate measurements of phenotype. Most weight loss interventions, therefore, have focused on weight or BMI reductions rather than changes in fat distribution.

Sex

The general stereotype of the obese male as having OSAHS emphasizes male gender as being an important risk factor. Among patients studied in a sleep center, the male to female ratio is often 8–10:1. However epidemiologic studies have shown that in the general population, this ratio is often lower (2:1). Nevertheless, the increased prevalence in males remains undeniable. The reason for the male predominance remains uncertain. In the Wisconsin Sleep Cohort study, postmenopausal women were three times more likely to have moderate to severe OSAHS when compared to premenopausal women matched for age and BMI [34]. Other population-based studies have shown similar results. Although hormonal changes are important to women and the subsequent development of OSAHS, they still do not account for the differences in sex. In general, hormonal therapy for men has failed to reduce the AHI. Differences in upper airway shape and fat deposition may account for some of the differences between men and women but there have been no conclusive studies. There may be many other factors such as differences in chronic diseases, occupational exposures, or health behaviors that may be playing a role.

Age

The relationship between OSAHS and age is complex. Children ages 3–5 years old have relatively high prevalence of sleep apnea because of their narrow airways and enlarged tonsils and adenoids. The prevalence then decreases during adolescents and young adulthood. Among middle-aged and elderly adults, the prevalence increases again. Several large cohort studies have shown that among men and women >60 years of age, the prevalence of sleep apnea increases anywhere from two- to threefold higher than middle-aged populations [35–40]. However, this relationship between age and the increased prevalence of OSAHS is not clearly understood.

One explanation is that with any disease that is nonfatal, increased prevalence over time may be due to accumulation of cases and not necessarily due to an increased incidence. If increased age actually contributes to the etiology of OSAHS, one would expect the prevalence of OSAHS to continue to rise with age. This however, has not been shown in several studies. In the Sleep Heart Health Study, much of the increase in prevalence of OSAHS occurred before age 65 and then plateaued [39]. Either the incidence declines or mortality increases to explain this phenomenon. The natural history of OSAHS, however, is still not defined. We do not know the incidence rate of this disease with any age group and so far OSAHS has not been clearly shown to cause death. Of note, OSAHS is often linked with potentially serious comorbidities that may also contribute to the 'survivor effect' in these epidemiological data. Increased mortality from other diseases associated with OSA may mask true prevalence of OSA in the elderly. The relationship between age and OSAHS therefore, remains speculative at this point.

Is OSAHS in elderly adults a different condition than OSAHS in middle-aged adults? BMI in elderly adults is not clearly correlated with increased prevalence of OSAHS as it is in middle-aged adults. In an 18-year, longitudinal study of elderly adults, only a weak association between BMI and AHI was found [41]. Other common characteristics of OSAHS, such as snoring, are also not as prevalent in elderly adults. This may be due to loss of bed partners who, as discussed, are the main reporters of the patient's snoring. Another explanation is that central sleep apnea, which is less associated with snoring, may be more prevalent in older populations, although data supporting this theory are minimal. Again, more data are needed to try and define this disease in elderly populations and to clarify if there are confounding factors, such as survivor effects, differences in diagnosis in elderly adults, or co-morbid conditions to name a few.

Race and Genetics

OSAHS has largely been studied in Western Caucasian populations. The prevalence of this disease in other countries is just beginning to be explored; therefore, the importance of racial or genetic differences is not yet understood.

As with most epidemiologically based studies, determining genetic etiologies of disease is difficult to differentiate from differences in lifestyle and diet. However, some of the data now available are intriguing. For instance, several population studies in the United States suggest that OSAHS is more prevalent among African-Americans. In a population study of adults over 65 years old, Ancoli-Israel et al. [42] observed 2.5-fold increased odds of having an AHI greater than 30 events per hour in African-Americans. In subjects less than 25 years old, the Cleveland Family Study found that the prevalence of OSAHS in African-Americans was higher after controlling for BMI and other factors [126]. However, other studies, such as the Sleep Heart Health Study, did not find the same association between African-Americans and OSAHS [39]. Clearly, more research is needed to further clarify whether race impacts the prevalence of OSAHS.

There have been several studies of OSAHS in Hong Kong among Chinese males and females. From these studies, it is estimated that the prevalence of OSAHS (when the definition of AHI >5 events per hour with daytime sleepiness is used) is 4% in males and 2% in females [43, 44]. Unlike Caucasian populations, obesity is not strongly correlated with OSAHS in Asians. The relationship between obesity and OSAHS is also not evident in other races, including African-Americans, in the Cleveland Family Study. Similarly, in New Zealand, increasing BMI correlated with increased severity of OSAHS in white but not Polynesian men [45]. Whether race contributes to differences in the phenotype of OSAHS patients is currently being investigated.

There are likely specific genetic factors that influence the etiology and presentation of OSAHS as well. OSAHS can cluster in families. The syndrome is substantially more prevalent in offspring of patients with OSAHS. The relative risk for OSAHS may be two- to fourfold greater in first-degree relatives. Even in the unaffected offspring of OSAHS patients, there is increased vulnerability to upper airway collapse. In provocative tests with inspiratory resistive loading, the unaffected offspring had increased upper airway collapse when compared with controls [46]. Although no specific pattern of inheritance has emerged, genetics likely plays a role in the etiology of OSAHS and may have differing penetrance in certain subjects. One study showed an increased risk for OSAHS in nonobese relatives of sleep apneics [47], suggesting that factors other than obesity contribute to the genetics of the syndrome.

Other Risk Factors

There are many other risk factors that have been associated with OSAHS. Alcohol and drugs that cause CNS depression (such as opioids and benzodiazepines) are likely to exacerbate OSAHS. Endocrine disorders such as hypothyroidism can lead to OSAHS due to myxedema and decreased upper airway muscle function. Acromegaly can cause macroglossia. Cerebrovascular accidents and neuromuscular diseases (including muscular dystrophies, myopathies, and neuropathies) can cause both central and obstructive sleep disordered breathing. Smoking is also a possible risk factor for OSAHS in epidemiological studies. Smokers are three times more likely to have OSAHS when compared to lifelong nonsmokers or former smokers [48]. This is probably due to the increased upper airway inflammation from smoking. Former smokers do not have increased risk for sleep apnea, implying that this risk is reversible.

Presentation to Other Subspecialties

As discussed earlier, patients with OSAHS seek more medical attention when compared to controls. Prior to the diagnosis of OSAHS, these patients see more doctors and are hospitalized more than controls [15]. What are they being treated for? A chart review of over 700 Canadian residents with OSAHS showed that in the 5 years prior to diagnosis, many of these patients were being treated for ischemic heart disease, CHF, hypertension, cardiac arrhythmias, chronic obstructive lung disease, and depression [15]. The association between cardiovascular disease and OSAHS is becoming clearer. Hypertension, to date, is the most well-documented and studied consequence of OSAHS. The risk of systemic hypertension rises with increased severity of OSAHS as measured by the respiratory disturbance index (RDI) [49]. A 4-year follow-up of the Wisconsin cohort showed a dose-response association between AHI and hypertension. An odds ratio of 4.54 for hypertension was associated with an AHI ≥15 events per hour [50]. A causal link between OSA and hypertension is now generally accepted based on mechanistic animal studies, large well-controlled cross-sectional and longitudinal epidemiological studies, and most recently based on human interventional studies. Patients with refractory hypertension (requiring at least 3 antihypertensive medications) may be particularly at risk of OSA, and may benefit substantially from therapy.

The correlation between ischemic heart disease and OSAHS is less defined. In the Sleep Heart Health Study, OSAHS was found to be an independent risk factor for CAD although the increase was modest [51]. ST-segment changes in sleep apneics with concomitant CAD are common and have been related to both hypoxemia and sympathetic surges after apneic episodes [52]. Sleep apnea may also be a poor prognostic indicator in patients with CAD with a mortality rate of 38% reported in one study [53]. The direct cause-effect relationship between OSAHS and CAD, however, is still debatable. It is apparent that OSAHS can exacerbate underlying CAD, but whether repetitive hypoxemia, hypercapnia, and surges in sympathetic tone observed during apneic episodes contribute to atherosclerosis is currently being investigated. OSAHS is now being associated with inflammation, endothelial injury, coagulation abnormalities, and metabolic abnormalities. The mechanisms of how OSAHS relates to these abnormalities and the genesis of CAD is under rigorous examination and will have a large impact on the treatment and diagnosis of OSAHS in patients with CAD in the future.

As with CAD, both diastolic and systolic CHF has been associated with OSAHS. The Sleep Heart Health Study found a stronger correlation between CHF and OSAHS than CAD and OSAHS. The relative odds ratios for CHF in subjects with sleep apnea was 2.38 [51]. However, whether OSAHS causes CHF or whether CHF causes OSAHS or whether they simply correlate with one another is unclear. Hypertension, increased catecholamines, and hypoxemia caused by OSAHS could all contribute to CHF. On the other hand, worsening upper airway edema from CHF could decrease upper airway size leading to increased collapsibility and result in OSA. Periodic breathing associated with CHF because of increased chemosensitivity, prolonged circulation times, and hyperventilation has been proposed to destabilize the upper airway [52]. Whether treatment of OSAHS with continuous positive airway pressure (CPAP) improves CHF among patients with sleep disordered breathing is currently being studied, although early reports appear promising.

Arrhythmias have also been associated with OSAHS, the most common being sinus bradycardia. Ventricular premature beats, premature ventricular contractions, and in some cases ventricular tachycardia have also been described. Some data have suggested that theses arrhythmias resolve with treatment of OSAHS [54].

Although cardiologists commonly see sleep apnea patients, there are many other subspecialties that come across these patients. Neurocognitive effects of OSAHS have been well documented with decreases in cognition and attention. Patients with OSAHS have higher incidences of traffic accidents and work-related accidents and are therefore likely to be seen by emergency room physicians, orthopedists, etc. Symptoms of sleep deprivation can often appear similar to those of depression, although a direct correlation is unclear. In a Canadian study, patients with OSAHS who were treated for depression were often prescribed antidepressants but not psychotherapy [15]. Although speculative, it is possible that these patients may have been misdiagnosed since symptoms such as decreased concentration, and daytime sleepiness can be mistaken for depression. More recent studies have shown that patients report amelioration of their depressive symptoms after treatment with CPAP even if they were already on an antidepressant [55]. Again, although sleep apnea is unlikely to cause depression, it can worsen underlying symptoms and is therefore important for clinicians to recognize.

As many neurologists know, sleep apnea has also been associated with stroke. The Sleep Heart Health Study showed that in OSAHS patients, there was a modest increase in stroke prevalence [51]. Among people who have suffered from stroke, sleep apnea has been reported in 43–91% of patients [52]. However, observations that prevalence and severity of sleep apnea did not differ among patients with stroke vs. transient ischemic attacks [56], and that frequency of obstructive apneas did not decline 3 months after a stroke [57] have led some investigators to believe that OSAHS is likely present prior to stroke in most patients. Most recently, a prospective observational cohort study has been published in *NEJM* that has shown OSA to be a risk factor in the development of stroke or death, independent of known confounding variables [127]. Of note, more severe OSA was more likely to lead to stroke than milder OSA. Despite these compelling data, the generalizability of this study has been questioned since all patients were referred to a sleep laboratory. In addition, there was no evidence of a beneficial effect of CPAP treatment, although this was not the primary focus of the report. As with CHF, the direct cause-effect relationship between sleep apnea and stroke and sleep apnea remains blurred. Moreover, randomized trials are needed to establish the role of sleep apnea therapy in preventing stroke.

Anesthesiologists are also becoming more familiar with the perioperative management of patients with OSAHS. Due to smaller airways, these patients are more likely to be difficult intubations. In severe cases, drugs administered during conscious sedation (opioids and benzodiazepines) have led to respiratory arrests in nonintubated patients. Unlike sleep, anesthesia produces an unarousable state. The normal protective reflexes against asphyxia are blunted or even lost. Anesthesia has been shown to decrease arousal to inspiratory load, hypercapnic and hypoxic stimuli, which are normally at least somewhat preserved during sleep [58]. After induction of anesthesia, the postoperative management of OSAHS patients can be challenging. For instance, they may not tolerate extubation if they are somnolent and not fully awake. Many anesthesiologists have witnessed apneas in these

Table 5. Presentation to other subspecialties with associated diagnoses and symptoms

Cardiology – ischemic heart disease, CHF, hypertension, arrythmias
Pulmonology – chronic obstructive lung disease, aspiration pneumonia, respiratory failure, pulmonary hypertension
Neurology – stroke, poor cognition
Anesthesiology – difficult intubation, respiratory failure
Otolaryngologists – snoring, nasal obstruction, hoarse voice
Gastroenterology – gastroesophageal reflux disease
Psychiatry – depression
Urology – nocturia, impotence, erectile dysfunction

patients during recovery. Extra precautions should be taken in OSAHS patients, such as early initiation of CPAP, if required, or placing the patient in the lateral decubitus position to help minimize airway collapse. These patients will need vigilant nursing care, especially if they remain somnolent postoperatively, to avoid an airway emergency. Unfortunately, the area of perioperative management of OSA is currently lacking in solid data.

Otolaryngologists are also very familiar with OSAHS patients not only because of the surgical overlap in treatment of this population, but because they may initially present to them with complaints of snoring, nasal obstruction, sore throat or hoarse voice. Interestingly urologists also see many OSAHS patients with complaints of nocturia, impotence, and erectile dysfunction.

There is an increased prevalence of gastroesophageal reflux disease (GERD) in these patients not only because of obesity but because the increased negative intrathoracic pressure created during periods of apneas worsens GERD. Pulmonologists see these patients for a myriad of reasons including aspiration pneumonias, shortness of breath, respiratory failure, and pulmonary artery hypertension (table 5).

Summary

In summary, because sleep apnea is a common disorder all physicians will come across patients who have the syndrome and will have to be cognizant of the symptoms to make an accurate diagnosis. Most patients are referred to sleep clinics because of snoring, EDS and witnessed apneas. Recognition of risk factors such as obesity, male sex, older age, and family history may help to differentiate sleep apneics. However, because of the cardiovascular and neurocognitive sequelae of OSAHS, many of these patients will initially report to other providers with symptoms of CAD, CHF, hypertension, depression, decreased cognition, and sexual dysfunction. Sleep apnea can also cause complications during anesthesia. Because OSAHS is a treatable disease, early recognition of these patients is important. Treatment may help prevent further complications and increase quality of life.

CPAP Treatment

CPAP has been the mainstay of treatment for OSAHS since its initial description in 1981. Sullivan et al. [59] tested 5 subjects with nasal CPAP at varying levels of pressure (from 4.5 to 10 cm H_2O) and found that it acted as a 'pneumatic splint' for the upper airway, preventing collapse. These subjects had a night of consolidated sleep when the nasal CPAP was applied. Since Sullivan's initial description, CPAP has been used on countless patients for treatment of OSAHS. There has been strong evidence to support that treatment with CPAP has improved breathing during sleep, concentration, alertness, neurocognitive functions, mood, breathing during sleep and even some cardiovascular outcomes. Despite this, adherence and patient acceptance of CPAP has been limited. By some estimates, one third of patients who are eligible for CPAP refuse to use it [62]. Nevertheless, it is currently the treatment of choice. Understanding of its mechanism(s) of action, outcomes, and adverse effects is necessary for any sleep physician. Likewise, understanding reasons for acceptance and adherence is also essential since no treatment can be effective if the patient does not use it.

Mechanism of Action

As proposed by Sullivan et al. [59], the idea that CPAP provides a 'pneumatic stent' for the pharyngeal airway has been widely accepted. Subsequent studies have supported this theory. In early work by Alex et al. [61], esophageal pressure and inspiratory airflow measurements were made on awake normal subjects on CPAP. It was found that there was an increase in mean inspiratory airflow for a given esophageal pressure when CPAP was applied, despite a decrease in upper airway muscle activity. This decrease in upper airway muscle activity with CPAP has been further elucidated. In awake subjects with OSAHS, genioglossus muscle activity is augmented in response to negative pressure [62]. When CPAP is applied, the negative pressure stimulus is eradicated, resulting in decreased genioglossus muscle activity. A more open pharyngeal airway puts less demand on the upper airway dilator muscles. This explains the decrease in genioglossus muscle activity with positive pressure. To summarize, if the flow increases but esophageal pressure (which approximates pleural pressure) remains the same, then resistance must be decreased, despite a decrease in upper airway muscle activity. It has been proposed that by acting as a mechanical splint, CPAP reduces upper airway resistance.

However, the mechanism by which CPAP prevents upper airway collapse is slightly more complicated. Lung volumes play a role in upper airway stability. A study of awake obese subjects with sleep apnea showed that the pharyngeal cross-sectional area significantly decreased as lung volumes diminished from total lung capacity (TLC) to functional residual volume (FRC) [63]. The decrease in airway size was more pronounced in sleep apnea patients when compared to controls. This study, however, was done on awake subjects and, therefore, may not be truly reflective of what happens during sleep. In addition, the coordination between respiratory and airway muscle groups is complex. For example, the genioglossus becomes active prior to diaphragmatic contraction or inspiratory airflow thus preventing the upper airway from collapse by the negative pressure that is subsequently generated [128, 129]. During expiration, however, the genioglossus relaxes when positive pressure makes the airway less prone to collapse. The observation that upper airway size diminishes as lung volume decreases from TLC to FRC may be a result of behavioral changes in upper airway muscle activation during the respiratory cycle rather than changes in lung volume per se.

To elucidate the effect of lung volume on the upper airways, Sériès et al. [64] looked at upper airway resistance with passive changes in lung volume using an iron lung. This method tried to eliminate confounders that may be present during active breathing. Measurements of both nasal and pharyngeal airway resistance showed that when positive extrathoracic pressure was applied, resulting in lower lung volumes, upper airway resistance increased. It was noted however, that when negative extrathoracic pressure was applied, resulting in larger lung volumes, pharyngeal resistance decreased more appreciably than nasal resistance. This observation supported previous theories that mechanical forces, such as caudal traction on the trachea, may lead to increased upper airway patency with larger lung volumes [65]. Unlike the pharyngeal airway, the nasal airway is not influenced by caudal traction of the trachea.

With both passive and active changes in lung volumes, pharyngeal airway size decreases with lower lung volumes. Most of these previous studies, however, were done on awake subjects. The influence of lung volume on the upper airway during NREM sleep required more investigation. Stanchina et al. [66] studied normal subjects during NREM sleep and altered their lung volume passively with positive and negative extrathoracic pressure. With lower lung volumes, subjects had increased upper airway resistance and collapsibility. Of note, the genioglossus muscle had increased activity with low lung volumes, but this was not adequate to maintain airway patency.

To summarize, CPAP prevents upper airway collapse in subjects with sleep apnea by stenting open the airway. However, because lung volumes influence upper airway resistance, size, and collapsibility, the increase in lung volumes seen with CPAP likely has an additional effect on upper airway patency. To what extent changes in upper airway resistance are influenced by lung volume or by the 'pneumatic stenting' effect of CPAP has been studied by Sériès et al. [67]. Using positive extrathoracic pressure to maintain the same lung volume, increases in CPAP resulted in a progressive decline in upper airway resistance in normal subjects. Although decreases in resistance were seen with multiple modalities that increased lung volumes (such as applying end expiratory pressure, or negative extrathoracic pressure), these changes were not as impressive as when CPAP was applied. Although this study suggests that splinting of the airway is the main mechanism of action of CPAP, most investigators agree that lung volume plays a substantial role and is likely important.

Acceptance and Adherence to CPAP

Although the natural history of OSAHS is still being elucidated, to our best knowledge it is an ongoing, unremitting disease process. Nonsurgical treatment is not curative, therefore, whatever treatment that is offered will likely be lifelong. Although CPAP is a very effective treatment of this disease, acceptance and adherence to it has been challenging to say the least. Acceptance of CPAP has been a substantial problem since its inception. It is admittedly an awkward device and can cause significant discomfort during sleep. Multiple investigators have tried to determine what factors are associated with improved adherence and acceptance. Over the years, it has been shown that sleep apnea patients with EDS and severe hypoxemia during sleep were more likely to accept CPAP [130]. Patients with other symptoms such as snoring, poor memory, and cognition were less likely to accept CPAP. Also, who initiates the sleep consultation is an important predictor of acceptance. For instance, if the patient initiated the referral, rather than the spouse, CPAP acceptance increases. Presumably this is because it is harder for a patient to accept treatment if he or she does not recognize that they have a problem. However, once a patient accepts treatment, having a partner or spouse initiate the referral predicted better adherence [68]. This is probably because the partner or spouse encourages daily CPAP use and provides positive reinforcement. Even if patients initially used CPAP, long-term acceptance of this treatment has been problematic as well. Within several months of follow-up, one third of patients who initially accepted CPAP discontinued it [69].

Once a patient accepts CPAP as a treatment, adherence is another issue. Reports of adherence vary, depending on which definition one uses. However, all studies are in agreement that adherence is suboptimal. Initial studies of CPAP adherence were encouraging with reports of up to 85% of patients claiming daily use [70]. These initial papers relied on self-questionnaires that were vulnerable to misreporting. This was found to be true when CPAP machines were fitted with monitoring devices that recorded the number of hours used. The objective information obtained proved that adherence was poor and since then adherence has been a major issue in the treatment for OSAHS. One study found that only 46% of subjects studied used CPAP for at least 4 hours on 70% of the days monitored [71]. Subsequent studies have shown that CPAP is used, on average, for only 4.7 h a night [72]. Larger, long-term studies have shown that 20% of patients stop CPAP all together [73]. It has been a challenge to figure out why patients do not adhere to CPAP treatment and how best to improve this. However, all is not lost. If patients adhere to treatment for the first 3 months, they are likely to continue CPAP use in a 5-year follow-up [73]. Other studies have shown that patient use during the first 2 weeks of CPAP initiation predicted long-term use [74]. It has become increasingly clear that practitioners have a small window of opportunity to influence long-term adherence to CPAP.

Why is CPAP not being used? It is natural to assume that the severity of OSAHS may play some role in the adherence to CPAP with the more severe patients being more apt to use the treatment. Yet reports on the correlation between adherence and disease severity have been conflicting. Some studies have shown that with higher AHIs, use of CPAP is more reliable [75]. On the other hand, several studies have shown that there is no correlation [73, 76]. Other predictors such as symptomatic relief have also been variable with some reports of EDS being a major predictor of adherence, while others cite quality of life measurements. Still other studies have shown that perhaps it is not the severity of disease or improvement in quality of life that predicts future CPAP use, but a patient's initial experience with the device that matters. Lewis et al. [77] studied 80 patients with CPAP for approximately 1 month and found that those patients who reported initial problems with the machine were most likely to discontinue or not adhere to it. They also found that patients with recent life events and those who lived alone were also less likely to adhere to CPAP treatment. All of these studies point to the complexity of issues associated with CPAP usage and how many non-OSAHS-related factors can play a large part in adherence. However, to place CPAP adherence in perspective, adherence to other treatment modalities for chronic medical conditions is comparable to CPAP. For example, metered-dose inhaler use in patients with obstructive lung disease is similar to CPAP usage (estimated use 37–52%) [78, 79]. Even with less obtrusive therapies, adherence to medical therapy is a substantial problem (table 6).

Table 6. Factors affecting adherence to CPAP

Symptomatic relief
Initial experience with CPAP
Side effects – nasal congestion, airleaks
Recent life events
Social support system

How can CPAP adherence be improved? This has been an area of great interest to many investigators. The realization that initial CPAP use determined long-term use has led to several educational/psychological interventions to try and improve the CPAP initiation experience. With CPAP education at home, partner involvement, and a 3-night trial of CPAP at a sleep center, Hoy et al. [80] showed improvement in long-term usage compared to patients who received standard therapy. This type of intervention, however, is difficult for any sleep center to maintain since it requires considerable resources. With increasing numbers of patients being diagnosed with OSAHS, the system would be quickly overwhelmed if every patient were to have this type of intensive support. However, if the practicing physician is aware of this intensive initial support, selected patients may benefit from this type of early therapy. There is a growing number of options to improve adherence. One should be aware, however, that effectiveness of these interventions may also be influenced by the patient's level of education, cultural background, and ethnicity. A study of OSAHS patients in Hong Kong showed that intensive supportive therapy provided by videotapes, respiratory nurse visits, and physician visits did not increase CPAP adherence [81].

Many complaints regarding CPAP have to do with airleaks, mask discomfort, upper airway dryness, and feelings of claustrophia. Higher pressures may have some impact on these discomforts. For instance, higher pressures may cause greater air leaks. However, many of the patients who complain of noisy machines and nocturnal awakenings have less severe disease and likely use lower CPAP levels [82]. CPAP levels per se are a predictor of CPAP use in only some studies, but not in others, potentially related to the confounding influences of disease severity.

Nevertheless, many of the interventions to improve adherence and acceptance have focused on how to deliver lower pressures. Autotitrating PAP, which is discussed elsewhere, was developed to deliver optimal pressures throughout the night recognizing that the amount of pressure needed can vary depending on sleep stage and body position. By doing so, less pressure can be delivered throughout the night, which in turn may be more tolerable for the patient. However, although some reports show that there was a preference for auto-CPAP devices over fixed CPAP or no treatment, there is no conclusive evidence that auto-PAP improves adherence. Even with less conservative estimates, subjects may use auto-PAP for about 15–20 min longer when compared to the fixed CPAP users [83]. A meta-analysis of auto-PAP vs. CPAP showed there was no significant reduction in sleepiness or AHI with auto-PAP and adherence did not increase (average use increased by 0.20 h per night) [84]. Even though auto-PAP does not improve adherence, there are selected groups of people who may benefit from it, such as those who have very variable pressure requirements throughout the night. Subjects who require high pressure levels or who have not been able to use fixed CPAP may tolerate and hence, use auto-PAP more [85, 86].

Bi-level PAP has also been studied in improving adherence. The thought is that by decreasing expiratory positive airway pressure, subjects may feel more comfortable with positive airway pressure in general and therefore use it more often. Like the studies with auto-PAP, studies of bi-level PAP have not shown a significant improvement in adherence or acceptance, although in one study more patients withdrew from the fixed CPAP group [87]. The cost of bi-level PAP devices is also a concern and can be substantially higher than CPAP, making it difficult to justify its routine use. As with auto-PAP, there are likely select groups of people who are more comfortable on bi-level PAP. For instance, patients who feel excessive pressure or discomfort during expiration may feel more comfortable with lower expiratory pressures. Universal use, however, to improve adherence in general is not indicated at this time.

A new technique (Cflex) has been recently released for clinical use. By using a proprietary algorithm, the manufacturers (Respironics, Inc.) provide reduced pressure in early exhalation while maintaining the prescribed level by end exhalation. The resulting 'pressure relief' is tolerated well by some patients. Because pharyngeal collapse tends to occur at end-exhalation, the reductions in applied pressure in early exhalation do not appear to impact efficacy. Although randomized trials are clearly needed, some observational data do suggest some benefits over standard CPAP. This algorithm has also been adapted into bi-level devices (Bi-flex) and to auto-tiration devices (Auto-flex); however, improvements in outcome with these techniques remain unproven.

Table 7. Methods to improve CPAP adherence

Intensive educational/psychological support
Humidification
Auto-titrating CPAP
Bi-level PAP
Cflex

Improving upper airway dryness has also been shown to improve adherence and acceptance. Many patients complain of dryness and daytime rebound nasal congestion. With nasal CPAP, mouth leaks may lead to one-way airflow and progressive drying of the nasal mucosa. Humidification helps to alleviate these symptoms. Small studies using humidification have shown slight increases in adherence when humidified nasal CPAP was used vs. placebo [88]. However, these results do not warrant routine initial use of humidification since it can be costly and requires maintenance. On the other hand, because the window to establish therapy is narrow, we generally recommend initial humidification if costs are not prohibitive. Other strategies such as a chin strap or full face mask may be as efficacious and as easy to implement (table 7).

Indications for CPAP Treatment

What are the indications for treatment with CPAP? A consensus statement published in *Chest* in 1999 recommended that CPAP be given to all OSAHS patients who are symptomatic (EDS, impaired cognition, mood disorders, insomnia, cardiovascular disease, or stroke) with an RDI of >5 events per hour [89]. It was also recommended that all patients with an RDI $\geq$ 30 events per hour be treated regardless of whether they are symptomatic or not, given the increased risk of hypertension described by the Wisconsin Sleep Cohort Study [90]. The American Academy of Sleep Medicine, however, set forth a slightly different set of guidelines [91]. They have recommended that patients with an apnea index (AI) of >20 events per hour or an AHI of >30 events per hour should receive CPAP regardless of symptoms. For patients with EDS, an AHI of >10 events per hour or a respiratory arousal index of >10 per hour warrants treatment. The difference between the *Chest* consensus statement and the American Academy of Sleep Medicine practice parameters is subtle but brings up a few interesting questions. What should we use to measure the severity of sleep apnea? Should it be the AI (mean number of apneas per hour), AHI (mean number of apneas and hypopneas per hour), the respiratory arousal index or the RDI (mean number of arousals per hour)? Although AHI and RDI are often used interchangeably, they are not exactly the same. An RDI can include respiratory effort-related arousals (RERA) which is neither an apnea nor hypopnea. However, with the use of nasal pressure diagnostic technology, the majority of these 'RERAs' are actually mild hypopneas making this distinction somewhat semantic. When should we start treatment with CPAP? An AI > 20 events per hour, AHI > 30 events per hour, RDI > 30 events per hour, AHI > 10 events per hour with symptoms, RDI > 5 events per hour with symptoms? A study of community-dwelling adults showed that 21% had EDS with an RDI of <5 events per hour [92]; should these people be treated as well? And what should we include as symptoms: EDS only, or should we include cognitive deficits, mood disorders, and cardiovascular symptoms? Currently, Medicare in the United States will pay for CPAP treatment in those patients who have an AHI ≥ 15 events per hour or AHI of 5–14 events per hour with symptoms of EDS, impaired cognition, hypertension, ischemic heart disease, history of stroke, mood disorders, and insomnia [93].

However, treatment with CPAP remains controversial. Even though CPAP is widely accepted as the treatment of choice for OSAHS, its efficacy has been questioned. Until recently, comparison studies evaluated CPAP against conservative management, pill placebo, or suboptimal CPAP with varying results. With the invention of 'sham' CPAP, more clinical trials are emerging with somewhat surprising results. As mentioned, there are two sets of guidelines advocating treatment of severe sleep apnea, with an AHI ≥ 30 events per hour, regardless of whether the patient has symptoms or not. Yet a multi-centered, randomized, placebo-controlled trial of asymptomatic patients (i.e. no daytime sleepiness) with AHI ≥ 30 events per hour showed no benefit with CPAP treatment after 6 weeks when compared to placebo (sham CPAP) [94]. Critics of the study point out that measuring sleepiness as an outcome in nonsleepy subjects may not be meaningful and that 6 weeks of therapy may be an inadequate amount of time to see changes with therapy. In addition, there were some important trends towards improvement in blood pressure in this study (i.e. of similar magnitude to studies with sleepy patients) that may have been significant with increased sample size.

The realization that AHI and symptoms do not always correlate, however, exemplifies the complexity of sleep disorders. There are people who are not apparently affected by sleep fragmentation for unclear reasons. It has been suggested that response to sleep deprivation and sleep fragmentation may be individually or genetically determined [95]. Future research is needed to understand whether these 'asymptomatic' patients are misperceiving their degree of impairment or whether they are somehow biologically protected.

Symptomatic patients with moderate to severe sleep apnea, however, do benefit from treatment. A randomized controlled trial using sham CPAP vs. optimal CPAP in patients with moderate to severe sleep apnea (average AHI was about 50 events per hour) showed considerable improvement in daytime sleepiness, vigilance, and general productivity [96]. Using a sham CPAP that mimicked CPAP in noise, humidity and perceived airflow, ensured that these results could be interpreted fairly and did indeed show that CPAP was effective.

At the other end of the spectrum are studies of mild symptomatic OSAHS showing significant improvement after treatment with CPAP. Patients with an AHI of 5–15 events per hour who complained of EDS, had improved subjective sleepiness, cognition, feelings of depression, and quality of life when treated with CPAP [97]. Unlike the previous study, however, an oral pill was used for comparison rather than a sham CPAP. Not unexpectedly, even though the subjects had improvements in their symptoms with CPAP, the majority of them preferred the oral placebo. Again, we are reminded of the challenge of getting patients to accept CPAP as a treatment modality.

Outcomes of CPAP Treatment

Daytime Sleepiness

As stated, several studies comparing CPAP to sham CPAP and other placebos have shown that CPAP does improve symptoms of EDS. Many of these studies have shown both subjective improvements in sleepiness (using questionnaires such as the ESS), and objective improvement in alertness (using multiple sleep latency testing, or psychomotor vigilance task testing). Although the Epworth Scale has been criticized by some, it does represent the most robust technique available for measuring improvement with CPAP in OSA. There is evidence to suggest that in patients with symptomatic OSAHS, missing one night of CPAP reverses almost all of the previous improvements in alertness and sleepiness [98].

Performance

Sleep fragmentation caused by OSAHS affects memory, learning, and performance. Measurements using questionnaires or task testing after CPAP use have shown improvements in performance with CPAP. Where the effect on poor performance becomes dangerous is when sleepy subjects operate machinery. It has been well known that subjects with OSAHS have a higher risk of motor vehicle accidents [99], most likely from poor daytime performance and alertness. Studies have shown that men with an AHI > 5 events per hour have significant increased risk of having at least one accident in 5 years. Worse yet, men and women with and AHI > 15 events per hour have higher odds of multiple accidents within 5 years [99].

Trying to delineate the contribution of OSAHS on motor vehicle accidents remains a challenge. Targeting specific populations, such as commercial vehicle drivers, has revealed that OSAHS is prevalent and correlates with increased risk of accidents. Studies have shown a 15.8% prevalence of OSAHS amongst commercial vehicle drivers, although these figures vary widely among patients [100]. The sleepiest 5% of these drivers have two to three times increased odds of having an accident or even multiple accidents [100]. There is evidence that treatment does decrease the risk. When treated with CPAP, subjects were involved in less motor vehicle accidents when compared to controls. Treated subjects decreased their risk of accidents to normal [101]. A meta-analysis calculated that in the United States more than 800,000 drivers were involved in OSAHS-related accidents, costing approximately USD 15.9 billion and 1,400 deaths. If all drivers with OSAHS were treated, USD 11.1 billion could be saved and 980 lives per year [102].

Cardiovascular Effects

The correlation between sleep apnea and cardiovascular disease is well known and is being better clarified with ongoing research. Hypertension is the most well-documented cardiovascular consequence of sleep apnea. Two large studies, the Sleep Heart Health Study, and the Wisconsin Sleep Cohort Study have shown a relationship between AHI and hypertension [103, 90]. That is, as AHI increases, the odds of hypertension increase as well. These findings have been validated in a prospective 4-year follow up of the Wisconsin Sleep Cohort which also shows a dose-response association between AHI and hypertension [3]. There is also evidence that patients with refractory hypertension have an extraordinarily high prevalence of OSAHS (up to 87%) [106]. The effect of treatment with nasal CPAP has been studied in several small randomized controlled trials. Some showed no change in blood pressure [94, 108], while others showed up to a 10-mm-Hg fall in mean blood pressure with CPAP [109]. It appears that subjects who are sleepy, on antihypertensives, and who have more severe disease are likely to see the greatest improvements in blood pressure with CPAP treatment (table 8).

Table 8. Adjusted odds ratio for hypertension at a follow-up sleep study [50] according to the AHI at baseline

Baseline AHI, events/h	Odds ratio adjusted for baseline hypertension
0	1.0
0.1–4.9	1.66 (1.35–2.03)
5.0–14.9	2.74 (1.82–4.12)
≥15.0	4.54 (2.46–8.36)

As noted, sleep apnea has also been correlated with ischemic heart disease, arrhythmias, congestive hear failure, and death due to cardiovascular disease. Because CPAP has been shown to improve symptoms of daytime sleepiness, cognitive functioning, and hypertension, large, long-term randomized controlled trials with a no treatment control arm seem unethical. However, because of difficulty with adherence in sleep apneics, a natural cohort of untreated individuals can be observed. Marin et al. [110] observed treated and untreated male sleep apneics for 10 years and found that those with severe untreated OSAHS had an increased risk of fatal and nonfatal cardiovascular events. CPAP reduced this risk and in fact, those who were adherent to CPAP had the same risk as the general population for cardiovascular events. Although these data are tantalizing, the question remains whether these findings represent a benefit to CPAP or whether the use of CPAP selects for a more adherent population with improved outcome based on motivation, adherence with medications, education, etc. There are also some data from small trials that suggest that CPAP treatment also reduces cardiac arrhythmias [111] and improves CHF [112], although larger trials to confirm these findings are needed. Overall, there is increasing evidence that sleep apnea patients who also suffer from concomitant cardiovascular disease should be treated with nasal CPAP.

Side Effects

As mentioned earlier, adherence to CPAP depends upon the patient's initial experience with the device. If the practitioner can minimize side effects as early as possible, then the patient is more likely to use CPAP. Congestion and rhinorrhea are some of the most common symptoms of CPAP. Often, these symptoms are caused by nasal dryness which may cause an increase in inflammatory mediators. Humidification may help to alleviate these symptoms and if possible, should be started early if costs are not prohibitive. Patients who are on medications that cause mucosal dryness, or who suffer from nasal congestion, or who have had previous surgery may find humidification helpful in preventing worsening rhinorrhea.

Symptomatic treatment with nasal steroids or ipratropium spray may also help alleviate nasal congestion. Making the distinction between vasomotor rhinitis and allergic rhinitis may help in choosing the most effective nasal spray. Other strategies like using a chin strap or a full face mask may also help alleviate reactive congestion and rhinorrhea by preventing mucosal drying.

Other complaints center around poorly fitting masks or skin breakdown around the masks. Using different types of masks or nasal pillows has helped to improve patient comfort. Poorly fitting masks can also lead to air leaks which can cause dry eyes, loud noises, and suboptimal pressure delivery. Patients who report airleaks often state they have poor sleep quality and do not feel symptomatic benefit from treatment. Trying different masks can help improve these symptoms but can take some patience and time. Additional care should also be taken in patients who have concomitant lung disease, such as bullous emphysema, who may be vulnerable to barotrauma from excessive positive airway pressures. This is quite rare, but should be recognized as a possible complication of CPAP.

In summary, CPAP remains the treatment of choice for patients with OSAHS, especially in patients with symptoms of daytime sleepiness. Acceptance and adherence of CPAP remains problematic but is on par with treatment with other chronic medical conditions. By improving the initial experience of CPAP, patients are more likely to adhere to treatment. CPAP can improve neurocognitive functioning, performance, daytime sleepiness, and cardiovascular outcomes. The benefits of CPAP are still being elucidated, but current evidence suggests that this mode of treatment can improve not only quality of life but mortality from cardiovascular disease.

Sleep Apnea: Prognosis

The clinical course of OSAHS is still the subject of ongoing investigation. Currently, OSAHS is not thought to be a fatal disease; however, several studies have shown an increase in mortality amongst untreated sleep apneics, recognizing that such studies are frequently confounded by comorbidities. So far, the most common cause of death is due to cardiac disease. Repeated apneas cause hypoxemia, hypercapnia, surges in sympathetic tone, episodic hypertension, cardiac arrhythmias, and increases in ventricular wall stress. Over time these insults likely contribute to cardiovascular disease. OSAHS has also been associated with hypercoagulability, systemic inflammation, endothelial dysfunction, impaired glucose metabolism and the metabolic syndrome. It appears that even though OSAHS in and of itself is not fatal, the effect it has on cardiovascular disease contributes to increased mortality. Current research is clarifying the effect of OSAHS on the cardiovascular system to better understand if OSAHS is simply a marker for cardiovascular risk, exacerbates underlying cardiac disease, or actually causes cardiovascular injury.

Clinical Course

Although there is an association between increased age and OSAHS, the natural history of the disease is not clearly defined. We know that with middle age, there is an increased prevalence of OSAHS when compared to young adults. Then as age increases, the prevalence of OSAHS increases. However, the prevalence plateaus at around 65 years old [39]. What we do not know is if the plateau in prevalence is due to a decline in incidence or an increase in mortality in the elderly population. The clinical course is also not known. Do people get worsening sleep apnea as they get older or do they maintain the same level of severity throughout their course? Is sleep apnea in elderly patients a different disease? Because aging is frequently complicated by weight gain, the isolated effect of aging on the natural history of sleep apnea is somewhat difficult to study.

Mortality

The mortality data on OSAHS are still emerging. Because OSAHS is associated with obesity, cardiovascular disease, and hypertension, drawing a clear relationship between OSAHS and mortality is difficult. Studies have been hampered by small numbers making them potentially vulnerable to confounders. Earlier reports did not find a significant correlation between OSAHS and death [114]. However, later several small studies demonstrated an association between OSAHS and death. Seppala et al. [115] found an increase in mortality among male snorers. Habitual snorers were more likely to die in their sleep and were at higher risk for morning death. Among sleep apnea patients, Partinen et al. [116] found that those treated conservatively with weight loss were more likely to die when compared to those who had received tracheostomies. Likewise, He et al. [117] found that sleep apneics with an AI > 20 had a higher mortality than those with an AI < 20. They found this mortality difference was especially true for patients <50 years old. Since then, more studies have shown an increase in mortality especially in middle-aged sleep apneics. Lavie et al. [118] looked at 1,620 adults with OSAHS and found that there was an increase in mortality during the fourth and fifth decades when compared to the general population. They found that the most common cause of death was due to myocardial infarction. Interestingly, however, AI was not a significant predictor for cardiopulmonary or cardiovascular deaths even though it was a predictor for all cause mortality. Reasons for this observation are speculative. Lavie et al. [118] pointed out that perhaps it is the combination of conditions such as lung disease and OSAHS or heart disease and OSAHS that increases the risk of dying rather than OSAHS alone. Alternatively, noncardiopulmonary causes of death, such as motor vehicle accidents, may be associated with higher AIs skewing the relationship between AI and cardiopulmonary deaths.

Surprisingly, Lavie et al. [118] also noted that in sleep apneics older than 70 years old, the risk of death was actually lower than that of the general population. It is hard to believe that OSAHS could be protective. Perhaps elderly sleep apneics referred to the sleep clinics in the study by Lavie et al. may have been a healthier population or a survivor population. Nevertheless, the relationship between age, OSAHS, and mortality has been unexpected in other studies as well. The hypothesis that OSAHS contributes to mortality in the elderly population has not clearly panned out. Early studies by Ancoli-Israel et al. [119] found that the RDI was an independent risk factor for mortality in institutionalized elderly women. However, they did not find a relationship between RDI and mortality for men in the same institution. Later studies by Ancoli-Israel et al. [120] found that in a community-dwelling elderly population, RDI was also not an independent predictor of death. However, those with an RDI ≥ 30 events per hour had shorter survival, dying up to 2 years earlier. Ancoli-Israel et al. drew similar conclusions as Lavie et al. that OSAHS may hasten death in those patients with other underlying conditions such as cardiopulmonary disease, but is not necessarily a predictor of mortality itself in the elderly population.

As the evidence linking OSAHS to cardiovascular disease grows stronger, the question of how patients with OSAHS die is being investigated. Gami et al. [121] looked at whether OSAHS increases the risk of sudden death from cardiac causes during sleep. From midnight to 6 am the relative risk of sudden death from cardiac disease in patients with OSAHS was 2.57. This is in stark contrast to what occurs in the general population and in people without OSAHS. In these populations, sudden death occurs in the early morning hours from 6 am to noon and, in fact, there is a decrease in risk from sudden death at night. However, this study points out that the mean age at sudden death was the same in both the sleep apneics and the control groups (around 70 years old). Therefore, whether sleep apnea increases overall risk of sudden death is still not answered. This study was also not able to address what happens to younger populations. What we do know is that sleep apnea patients are at increased risk of sudden death at night as compared with the daytime. Observations that OSAHS is associated with autonomic and electrocardiographic abnormalities such as increases in Q-T intervals during periods of apnea [122], decreased heart rate variability [123], cardiac arrhythmias, increased sympathetic activity, and coagulation abnormalities may explain why sleep apnea patients are at a higher risk of sudden death during their sleep.

Because epidemiological studies have been troubled by small numbers, study limitations, and confounding factors, the clear link between mortality and OSAHS has not been established even though much evidence points to an increase in mortality from cardiovascular disease among sleep apneics. Observational studies have tried to answer the question of whether OSAHS increases mortality in general and whether it causes increased risk of cardiovascular events (both fatal and nonfatal) in particular. Because many patients with OSAHS are nonadherent to treatment with CPAP, long-term observational studies of treated vs. nontreated sleep apneics have been possible. Marti et al. [124] found that patients in a historical cohort of sleep apneics who received no treatment had a higher mortality than those who received some form of treatment which included CPAP, surgery, or diet. The risk of death was higher in patients <50 years old and highest in those who had a history of severe chronic obstructive lung disease. A few more observational studies specifically addressing whether untreated OSAHS influences cardiovascular outcomes and whether CPAP in particular changes these outcomes have been published. Marin et al. [110] observed treated and untreated male sleep apneics for 10 years and found that those with severe untreated OSAHS had an increased risk of fatal and nonfatal cardiovascular events. CPAP reduced this risk and, in fact, those who were adherent to CPAP had the same risk as the general population for cardiovascular events.

In summary, the natural history of sleep apnea and the description of its clinical course have not been fully described. It appears that OSAHS may increase mortality from cardiovascular disease, but whether it is a cause of cardiovascular injury still remains to be seen. CPAP reverses the increased risk of cardiovascular events or death. The modest increase in mortality seems most evident in middle-aged populations, while elderly populations do not appear to suffer from an increase in mortality because of OSAHS. More research is needed to help clarify if sleep apnea has different phenotypes and clinical courses in different populations.

References

1 American Academy of Sleep Medicine Task Force: Sleep-related breathing disorders in adults: recommendations for syndrome definition and measurement techniques in clinical research. Sleep 1999;22:667–689.
2 Teran-Santos J, Jimenez-Gomez A, Cordero-Guevara J: The association between sleep apnea and the risk of traffic accidents. Cooperative Group Burgos-Santander. N Engl J Med 1999;340:847–851.
3 Peppard P, Young T, Palta M, Skatrud J: Prospective study of the association between sleep disordered breathing and hypertension. N Engl J Med 2000;342:1378–1384.
4 Lavie P, Here P, Hoffstein V: Obstructive sleep apnea syndrome as a risk factor for hypertension. Brit Med J 200;320:479–482.
5 Pepperell JC, Ramdassigh-Dow S, Crosthwaite N, Mullins R, Jenkinson D, Stradling JR, Davies RJ: Ambulatory blood pressure after therapeutic and subtherapeutic nasal continuous positive airway pressure for obstructive sleep apnoea: a randomized parallel trial. Lancet 2002;359:204–210.
6 Weiss JW, Remsburg S, Garpestad E, Ringler J, Sparrow D, Parker JA: Hemodynamic consequences of obstructive sleep apnea. Sleep 1996;19:388–397.
7 Lavie P, Pillar G, Malhotra A: Sleep Disorders: diagnosis, management and treatment. A handbook for clinicians. Martin Dunitz Ltd, London, 2002.
8 National Commisson on Sleep Disorders Research. Wake Up America: A National Sleep Alert. Vol 1: Executive summary and executive report. Bethesda, MD: National Institutes of Health, 1993.
9 Ohayon MM, Guillemiault C, Priest RG, et al: Snoring and breathing pauses during sleep: telephone interview survey of a United Kingdom population sample. BMJ 1997;314: 860–863.
10 Netzer NC, Hoegel JJ, Loube D, et al: Prevalence of symtoms and risk of sleep apnea in primary care. Chest 2003;124: 1406–1414.
11 Stores G, Crawford C: Medical student education in sleep and its disorders. J R Coll Physicians Lond 1998;32:149–153.
12 Rosen RC, Rosekind M, Rosevear C, et al: Physician education in sleep and sleep disorders: a national survey of U.S. medical schools. Sleep 1993;16:249–254.
13 American Thoracic Society/American Sleep Disorders Association/American College of Chest Physicians/APCCMPD. Statement about training of pulmonary physicians in sleep disorders. New York, NY: American Thoracic Society, 1994.
14 Phillips B, Collop N, Goldberg R: Sleep medicne practices, training and attitudes: a wake-up call for pulmonologists. Chest 2000;117:1603–1607.
15 Smith R, Ronald J, Delaive K, et al: What are obstructive sleep apnea patients being treated for prior to this diagnosis? Chest 2002;121: 164–172.
16 Parish JM, Lyng PJ: Quality of life of bed partners of patients with obstructive sleep apnea or hypopnea after treatment with continuous positive airway pressure. Chest 2003;124: 942–947.
17 Whyte KF, Allen MB, Jeffrey AA, et al: Clinical features of the sleep apnea/hypopnea syndrome. Q J Med 1989;72:659–666.
18 Young T, Palta M, Dempsey J, et al: The occurrence of sleep-disordered breathing among middle-aged adults. NEJM 1993;328:1230–1235.
19 Duran J, Esnoala S, Rubio R, Iztueta A: Obstructive sleep apnea-hypopnea and related clinical features in a population-based sample of subjects ages 30–70 yr. Am J Respir Crit Care Med 2001 Mar;163(3 Pt 1): 685–689.
20 Gottlieb DJ, Whitney CW, Bonekat WH, et al: Relation of sleepiness to respiratory disturbance index: the Sleep Heart Health Study. Am J Respir Crit Care Med 1999;159:502–509.
21 App WE: Boatwrigth GW, Ostrander SE, et al: Disorder of excessive daytime somnolence: a case series of 1000 patients. J Ky Med Assoc 1990;88:393–396.
22 Chervin RD: Sleepiness, fatigue, tiredness, and lack of energy in obstructive sleep apnea. Chest 2000;118:372–379.
23 Johns MW: Reliability and factor analysis of the Epworth Sleepiness Scale. Sleep 1992; 15:376–381.
24 Bennett LS, Stradling JR, Davies RJ: A behavioural test to assess daytime sleepiness in obstructive sleep apnoea. J Sleep Res 1997;6: 142–145.
25 Haponik EF, Smith PL, Meyers DA, et al: Evaluation of sleep disordered breathing. Is polysomnography necessary? Am J Med 1984;77:671–677.
26 Schwab RJ, Gupta KB, Gefter WB, et al: Upper airway and soft tissue anatomy in no mal subjects and patients with sleep-disordered breathing. Significance of the lateral pharyngeal walls. Am J Respir Crit Care Med 1995;152:1673–1689.
27 Leiter JC: Upper airway shape: Is it important in the pathogenesis of obstructive sleep apnea? Am J Respir Crit Care Med 1996;153: 894–898.
28 Malhotra A, Juwang Y, Fogel RB, et al: The male predisposition to pharyngeal collapse: importance of airway length. Am J Respir Crit Care Med 2002;166:1388–1395.
29 Mortimore IL, Marshall I, Wraith PK, et al: Neck and total body fat deposition in nonobese and obese patients with sleep apnea compared with that in control subjects. Am J Respir Crit Care Med 1998; 157: 280–283.
30 Stradling JR, Crosby JH: Predictors and prevalence of obstructive sleep apnea and snoring in 1001 middle aged men. Thorax 1991Feb;46(2):85–90.
31 Kiely JL, Nolan P, McNicholas WT: Intranasal corticosteroid therapy for obstructive sleep apnoea in patients with co-existing rhinitis. Thorax 2004;59(1):50–55.
32 Peppard PE, Young T, Palta M, Dempsey J, Skatrud J: Longitudinal study of moderate weight change and sleep-disordered breathing. JAMA 2000;284:3015–3021.
33 Young T, Peppard PE, Gottlieb DJ: Epidemiology of obstructive sleep apnea: a population health perspective. Am J Respir Crit Care Med 2002;165:1217–1239.
34 Young T, Finn L, Austin D, Peterson A: Menopausal status and sleep-disordered breathing in the Wisconsin Sleep Cohort study. Am J Respir Crit Care Med 2002;167: 1181–1185.
35 Bixler E, Vgontazas A, Ten Have T, Tyson K, Kales A: Effects of age on sleep apnea in men. Am J Respir Crit Care Med 1998;157:144–148.
36 Bixler E, Vgontzas A, Lin H, Ten Have T, Rein J, Vela-Bueno A, Kales A: Prevalence of sleep-disordered breathing in women. Am J Respir Crit Care Med 2001;163:608–613.
37 Durán J, Esnaola S, Rubio R, Iztueta A: Obstructive sleep apnea-hypopnea and related clinical features in a population-based sample of subjects aged 30 to 70 yr. Am J Respir Crit Care Med 2001;163:685–689.
38 Redline S: Epidemiology of sleep-disordered breathing. Semin Respir Crit Care Med 1998;19:113–122.
39 Young T, Shahar E, Nieto FJ, Redline S, Newman AB, Gottlieb DJ: Walsleben JA, Enright PL, Samet JM: Predictors of sleep-disordered breathing in community dwelling adults: the Sleep Heart Health Study. Arch Intern med 2002;162:893–900.

40 Ancoli-Israel S, Kripke D, Klauber M, Mason W, Fell R, Kaplan O: Sleep-disordered breathing in community-dwelling elderly. Sleep 1991;14:486–495.
41 Ancoli-Israel S, Gehrman P, Kripke DF, Stepnowsky C, Mason W, Cohen-Zion M, Marler M: Long-term follow-up of sleep disordered breathing in older adults. Sleep Med 2001;2:511–516.
42 Ancoli-Israel S, Klauber M, Stepnowsky C, Estline E, Chinn A, Fell R: Sleep-disordered breathing in African-American elderly. Am J Respir Crit Care Med 1995;152:1946–1949.
43 Ip M, Lam B, Lauder I, Tsang K, Chung K, Mok Y, Lam W: A community study of sleep-disordered breathing in middle-aged Chinese men in Hong Kong. Chest 2001;199:62–69.
44 Ip MSM, Lam B, Mok YW, Ip TY, Lam WK: Prevalence of sleep disordered breathing in middle-aged Chinese women in Hong Kong. Am J Respir Crit Care Med 2001;163:A636.
45 Coltman R, Taylor D, Whyte K, Harkness M: Craniofacial form and obstructive sleep apnea in Polynesian and Caucasian men. Sleep 2000;23:943–950.
46 Pillar G, Schnall RP, Peled N, Oliven A, Lavie P: Impaired respiratory response to resistive loading during sleep in healthy offspring of patients with obstructive sleep apnea. Am J Respir Crit Care Med 1997;155(5): 1602–1608.
47 Redline S, Tosteson T, Tishler PV, Carskadon MA, Millman RP: Studies in the genetics of obstructive sleep apnea. Familial aggregation of symptoms associated with sleep-related breathing disturbances. Am Rev Respir Dis 1992;145:440–444.
48 Wetter DW, Young TB, Bidwell TR, et al: Smoking as a risk factor for sleep-disordered breathing. Arch Intern Med 1994;154: 2219–2224.
49 Lavie P, Herer P, Hoffstein V: Obstructive sleep apnoea syndrome as a risk factor for hypertension: population study. BMJ 2000;320:479–482.
50 Peppard PE, Young T, Palta M, Skatrud J: Prospective study of the association between sleep-disordered breathing and hypertension. N Engl J Med 2000;342(19):1378–1384.
51 Shahar E, Whitney CW, Redline S, Lee ET, Newman AB, Javier Nieto F, O'Connor GT, Boland LL, Schwartz JE, Samet JM: Sleep-disordered breathing and cardiovascular disease: cross-sectional results of the Sleep Heart Health Study. Am J Respir Crit Care Med 2001;163:19–25.
52 Leung RS, Bradly TD: Sleep apnea and cardiovascular disease. Am J Respir Crit Care Med 2001;164:2147–2165.
53 Peker Y, Hedner J, Kraiczi H, Loth S: Respiratory disturbance index: an independent predictor of mortality in coronary artery disease. Am J Respir Crit Care Med 2000;162:81–86.
54 Harbison J, O'Reilly P, McNicholas WT: Cardiac rhythm disturbances in the obstructive sleep apnea syndrome: effects of nasal continuous positive airway pressure therapy. Chest 2000;118,591–595.
55 Schwartz DJ, Kohler WC, Karatinos G: Symptoms of depression in individuals with obstructive sleep apnea may be amenable to treatment with continuous positive airway pressure. Chest 2005;128:1304–1309.
56 Bassetti C, Aldrich MS: Sleep apnea in acute cerebrovascular diseases: final report on 128 patients. Sleep 1999;22:217–223.
57 Parra O, Arboix A, Bechich S, Garcia-Eroles L, Montserrat JM, Lopez JA, Ballester E, Guerra JM, Sopena JJ: Time course of sleep-related breathing disorders in first-ever stroke or transient ischemic attack. Am J Respir Crit Care Med 2000;161:375–380.
58 Loadsman JA, Hillman DR: Anaesthesia and sleep apnoea. Br J Anaesth 2001;86:254–266.
59 Sullivan CE, Issa FG, Berthon-Jones M, et al: Reversal of obstructive sleep apnoea by continuous positive airway pressure applied through the nares. Lancet 1981;1:862–865.
60 Rauscher H, Popp W, Wanke T, Zwick H: Acceptance of CPAP therapy for sleep apnea. Chest 1991;100:1019–1023.
61 Alex CG, Aronson RM, Onal E, Lopata M: Effects of continuous positive airway pressure on upper airway and respiratory muscle activity. J Appl Physiol 1987;62:2026–2030.
62 Berry RB, White DP, Roper J, Pillar G, Fogel RB, Stanchina M, Malhotra A: Awake negative pressure reflex response of the genioglossus in OSA patients and normal subjects. J Appl Physiol 2003;94:1875–1882.
63 Hoffstein V, Zamel N, Phillipson EA: Lung volume dependence of pharyngeal cross-sectional area in patients with obstructive sleep apnea. Am Rev Respir Dis 1984;130:175–178.
64 Sériès F, Cormier Y, Desmueules M: Influence of passive changes of lung volume on the upper airways. J Appl Physiol 1990;68: 2159–2164.
65 Van der Graaf WB: Thoracic influence on upper airway patency. J Appl Physiol 1988; 65:2124–2131.
66 Stanchina ML, Malhotra A, Fogel R, Trinder J, Edwards JK, Schory K, White DP: The influence of lung volume on pharyngeal mechanics, collapsibility, and genioglossus muscle activation during sleep. Sleep 2003;26(7): 851–856.
67 Sériès F, Cormier Y, Couture J, et al: Changes in upper airway resistance with lung inflation and positive airway pressure. J Appl Physiol 1990;68:1075–1079.
68 Lewis KE, Seale L, Bartle IE, Watkins AJ, Ebden P: Early predictors of CPAP use for the treatment of obstructive sleep apnea. Sleep 2004 1:27(1):134:8.
69 Rolfe I, Olson LG, Saunders NA: Long-term acceptance of continuous positive airway pressure in obstructive sleep apnea. Am Rev Respir Dis 1991;144(5):1130–1133.
70 Sanders MH, Gruendl CA, Rogers RM: Patient compliance with nasal CPAP therapy for sleep apnea. Chest 1986;90:330–333.
71 Kribbs NB, Pack AI, Kline LR, Smith PL, Schwartz AR, Schubert NM, Redline S, Henry JN, Getsy JE, Dinges DF: Objective measurement of patterns of nasal CPAP use by patients with obstructive sleep apnea. Am Rev Respir Dis 1993;147(4):887–895.
72 Engleman HM, Martin SE, Douglas NJ: Compliance with CPAP therapy in patients with the sleep apnoea/hypopnoea syndrome. Thorax 1994;49:263–266.
73 McArdle N, Devereux G, Heidarnejad H, Engleman HM, Mackay TW, Douglas NJ: Long-term use of CPAP therapy for sleep apnea/hypopnea syndrome. Am J Respir Crit Care Med 1999;159:1108–1114.
74 Popescu G, Latham M, Allgar V, Elliott MW: Continuous positive airway pressure for sleep apnoea/hypopnoea syndrome; usefulness of a 2 week trial to identify factors associated with long term use. Thorax 2001;56:727–733.
75 Lloberes P, Marti S, Sampol G, Roca A, Sagales T, Munoz X, Ferre M: Predictive factors of quality-of-life improvement and continuous positive airway pressure use in patients with sleep apnea-hypopnea syndrome: study at 1 year. Chest 2004;126(4):1241–1247.
76 Reeves-Hoche MK, Meck R, Zwillich CW: Nasal CPAP: an objective evaluation of patient compliance. Am J Respir Crit Care Med 1994;149(1):149–154.
77 Lewis KE, Seale L, Bartle IE, Watkins AJ, Ebden P: Early predictors of CPAP use for the treatment of obstructive sleep apnea. Sleep 2004;1:27:134–138.
78 Tashkin DP, Rand C, Nides M, et al: A nebulizer chronology to monitor compliance with inhaler use. Am J Med 1991;91:33S–36S.
79 Mawhinney H, Spector SL, Kinsman RA, et al: Compliance in clinical trials of two non-bronchodilator, antiasthma medications. Ann Allergy 1991;66:294–299.
80 Hoy CJ, Vennelle M, Kingshott RN, Engleman HM, Douglas NJ: Can intensive support improve continuous positive airway pressure use in patients with the sleep apnea/hypopnea syndrome? Am J Respir Crit Care Med 1999;159:1096–1100.
81 Hui DS, Chan JK, Choy DK, Ko FW, Li TS, Leung RC, Lai CK: Effects of augmented continous positive airway pressure education and support on compliance and outcome in a Chinese population. Chest 2000;117:1410–1416.
82 Douglas NK, Engleman HM: CPAP therapy: outcomes and patient use. Thorax 1998;53: 47–48.
83 Haniffa M, Lasserson TJ, Smith I: Interventions to improve compliance with continous positive airway pressure for obstructive sleep apnoea. The Cochrane Library, (3) 2005.
84 Ayas NT, Patel SR, Malhotra A, et al: Auto-titrating versus standard continuous positive airway pressure for the treatment of obstructive sleep apnea: results of a meta-analysis. Sleep 2004;27:249–253.
85 Rostig S, Synofik C, Peter JH, Vogelmeier C, Becker HF. [Bo26] [Poster:707] Auto-adjusting versus conventional nCPAP therapy in obstructive sleep apnea patients with low treatment compliance. www.abstracts2view.com 2003.
86 Massie CA, McArdle N, Hart RW, Schmidt-Nowara WW, Lankford A, Hudgel DW, Gordon N, Douglas NJ: Comparison between automatic and fixed positive airways pressure therapy in the home. Am J Respir Crit Care Med 2003;167(1):20–23.
87 Reeves-Hoche MK, Hudgel DW, Meck R, Witteman R, Ross A, Zwillich CW: Continuous

versus bilevel positive airway pressure for obstructive sleep apnea. Am J Respir Crit Care Med 1995;151(2 Pt 1):443–449.
88 Neill AM, Wai HS, Bannan SPT, Beasley CR, Weatherall M, Campbell AJ: Humidified nasal continuous positive airway pressure in obstructive sleep apnoea. Eur Respir J 2003;22:258–262.
89 Loube DI, Gay PC, Strohl KP, Pack AI, White DP, Collop NA: Indications for positive airway pressure treatment of adult obstructive sleep apnea patients: a consensus statement. Chest 1999;115:863–866.
90 Young T, Peppard P, Palta M, et al: Population-based study of sleep-disordered breathing as a risk factor for hypertension. Arch Intern med 1997;157:1746–1752.
91 Indication For Polysomnography Task Force, American Sleep Disorders Association Standards Of Practice Committee. An American sleep disorders association report: Practice parameters for the indications for polysomnography and related procedures. Sleep 1997;20(6):406–422.
92 Gottlieb DJ, Whitney CW, Bonekat WH, et al: Relation of sleepiness to respiratory disturbance index: the sleep heart health study. Am J Respir Crit Care Med 1999;159: 502–507.
93 Meicare. Medicare guidelines. http://www.cms.hhs.gov/medlearn/matters/mmarticles/2005/MM3843.pdf\
94 Barbe F, Mayoralas LR, Duran J, et al: Treatment with continuous positive airway pressure is not effective in patients with sleep apnea but no daytime sleepiness. Ann Intern med 2001;134:1015–1023.
95 Pack AI: Who should get treated for sleep apnea? Ann Intern Med 2001;134(11): 1065–1067.
96 Montserrat JM, Montserrat F, Hernandez L, et al: Effectiveness of CPAP treatment in daytime function in sleep apnea syndrome: a randomized controlled study with an optimized placebo. Am J Respir Crit Care Med 2001; 164:608–613.
97 Engleman HM, Kingshott RN, Wraith PK, Mackay TW, Deary IJ, Douglas NK: Randomized placebo-controlled crossover trial of continuous positive airway pressure for mild sleep apnea/hypopnea syndrome. Am J Respir Crit Care Med 1999;159:461–467.
98 Kribbs NB, Pack AI, Kline LR, Getsy JE, Schuett JS, Henry JN, Maislin G, Dinges DF: Effects of one night without nasal CPAP treatment on sleep and sleepiness in patients with obstructive sleep apnea. Am Rev Respir Dis 1993;147(5):1162–1168.
99 Young T, Blustein J, Finn L, Palta M: Sleepiness, driving, and accidents: sleep-disordered breathing and motor vehicle accidents in a population-based sample of employed adults. Sleep 1997;20(8):608–613.
100 Howard ME, Desai AV, Grunstein RR, et al: Sleepiness, sleep-disordered breathing, and accident risk factors in commercial vehicle drivers. Am J Resp Crit Care Med 2004;170: 1014–1021.
101 George CF: Reduction in motor vehicle collisions following treatment of sleep apnoea with nasal CPAP. Thorax 2001;56:508–512.
102 Sassani A, Findley LJ, Kryger M, Goldlust E, George C, Davidson TM: Reducing motor-vehicle collisions, costs, and fatalities by treating obstructive sleep apnea syndrome. Sleep 2004;27(3):453–458.
103 Nieto FJ, Young TB, Lind BK, Shahar E, Samet JM, Redline S, D'Agostino RB, Newman AB, Lebowitz MD, Pickering TG: Association of sleep-disordered breathing, sleep apnea, and hypertension in a large community-based study. Sleep Heart Health Study JAMA 2000;283:1829–1836.
104 Young T, Peppard P, Palta M, Hla KM, Finn L, Morgan B, Skatrud J: Population-based study of sleep disordered breathing as a risk factor for hypertension. Arch Intern Med 1997;157:1746–1752.
105 Peppard PE, Young T, Palta M, Skatrud J: Prospective study of the association between sleep-disordered breathing and hypertension. N Engl J Med 2000;342:1378–1384.
106 Logan AG, Perlikowski SM, Mente A, Tisler A, Tkacova R, Nirouman M, Leung RS, Bradley TD: High prevalence of unrecognized sleep apnoea in drug-resistant hypertension. J Hypertension 2001;19(12):2271–2277.
107 Barbe F, Mayoralas LR, Duran J, et al: Treatment with continuous positive airway pressure is not effective in patients with sleep apnea but no daytime sleepiness. A randomized, controlled trial. Ann Intern Med 2001; 134: 1015–1023.
108 Monasterio C, Vidal S, Duran J, et al: Effectiveness of continuous positive airway pressure in mild sleep apnea-hypopnea syndrome. Am J Respir Crit Care Med 2001;164:939–943.
109 Becker C, Jerrentrup A, Ploch T, et al: Effect of nasal continuous positive airway pressure treatment on blood pressure in patients with obstructive sleep apnea. Circulation 2003; 107:68–73.
110 Marin JM, Carrizo SJ, Vicente E, Agusti AG: Long-term cardiovascular outcomes in men with obstructive sleep apnoea-hypopnoea with or without treatment with continuous positive airway pressure: an observational study. Lancet 2005;365:1046–1053.
111 Harbison J, O'Reilly P, McNicholas WT: Cardiac rhythm disturbances in the obstructive sleep apnea syndrome: effects of nasal continuous positive airway pressure therapy. Chest 2000;118(3):591–595.
112 Malone S, Liu PP, Holloway R, Rutherford R, Xie A, Bradley TD: Obstructive sleep apnoea in patients with dilated cardiomyopathy: effects of continuous positive airway pressure. Lancet 1991;338:1480–1484.
113 Young T, Shahar E, Nieto FJ, Redline S, Newman AB, Gottlieb DJ, Walsleben JA, Enright PL, Samet JM: Predictors of sleep-disordered breathing in community dwelling adults: the Sleep Heart Health Study. Arch Intern Med 2002;162:893–900.
114 Gonzalez-Rothi RJ, Foresman GA, Block AJ: Do patients with sleep apnea die in their sleep? Chest 1988;94:531–538.
115 Seppala T, Partinen M, Penttila A, Aspholm R, Tiainen E, Kaukianen A: Sudden death and sleeping history among Finnish men. J Intern Med 1981;141:985–992.
116 Partinen M, Jamieson A, Guilleminault C: Long-term outcome for obstructive sleep apnea syndrome patients. Mortality. Chest 1988;94:1200–1204.
117 He J, Kryger MH, Zorick FJ, Conway W, Roth T: Mortality and apnea index in obstructive sleep apnea. Experience in 385 male patients. Chest 1988;94:9–14.
118 Lavie P, Herer P, Peled R, Berger I, Yoffe N, Zomer J, Rubin AE: Mortality in sleep apnea patients: a multivariate analysis of risk factors. Sleep 1995;18(3):149–157.
119 Ancoli-Israel S, Klauber MR, Kripke DF, Parker L, Cobarrubias M: Sleep apnea in female patients in a nursing home: increased risk of mortality. Chest 1989;96:1054–1058.
120 Ancoli-Israel S, Kripke DF, Klauber MR, Fell R, Stepnowsky C, Estline E, Khazeni N, Chinn A: Morbidity, mortality and sleep-disordered breathing in community dwelling elderly. Sleep 1996;19(4):277–282.
121 Gami AS, Howard DE, Olson EJ, Somers VK: Day-night pattern of sudden death in obstructive sleep apnea. N Engl J Med 2005; 352:1206–1214.
122 Gillis AM, Stoohs R, Guilleminault C: Changes in the QT interval during obstructive sleep apnea. Sleep 1991;14:346–350.
123 Narkiewicz K, Montano N, Coliati C, vande Borne PJ, Dyken ME, Somers VK: Altered cardiovascular variability in obstructive sleep apnea. Circulation 1998;98:1071–1077.
124 Marti S, Sampol G, Munoz X, Torres F, Roca A, Lloberes P, Sagales T, Quesada P, Morell F: Mortality in severe sleep apnoea/hypopnoea syndrome patients: impact of treatment. Eur Respir J 2002;20:1511–1518.
125 Marin JM, Carrizo SJ, Vicente E, Agusti AG: Long-term cardiovascular outcomes in men with obstructive sleep apnoea-hypopnoea with or without treatment with continuous positive airway pressure: an observational study. Lancet 2005;365:1046–1053.
126 Redline S: Epidemiology of sleep-disordered breathing. Semin Respir Crit Care Med 1998; 19:113–122.
127 Parra O, Arboix A, Bechich S, et al: Time course of sleep-related breathing disorders in first-ever stroke of transient ischemic attack. Am J Respir Crit Care Med 2000;161:375–380.
128 Horner RL: Impact of brainstem sleep mechanisms on pharyngeal motor control. Respir Physiol 2000;119:113–121.
129 van Lunteren E: Muscles of the pharynx: structural and contractile properties. Ear Nose Throat J 1993;72:27–29, 33.
130 Meurice JC, Dore P, Paquereau J, et al: Predictive factors of long-term compliance with nasal continuous positive airway pressure treatment in sleep apnea syndrome. Chest 1994;105:429–433.

Atul Malhotra, MD
Sleep Disorders Program at BIDMC
Sleep Medicine and Pulmonary and
Critical Care Divisions
Brigham and Women's Hospital
75 Francis Street, Boston, MA 02115 (USA)
Tel. +1 617 732 6488
Fax +1 617 732 7337
E-Mail amalhotral@partners.org

Randerath WJ, Sanner BM, Somers VK (eds): Sleep Apnea.
Prog Respir Res. Basel, Karger, 2006, vol 35, pp 137–144

Automatic Positive Airway Pressure Titration and Treatment

Winfried J. Randerath

Institute for Pneumology at the University Witten/Herdecke, Clinic for Pneumology and Allergology, Center of Sleep Medicine and Respiratory Care, Bethanien Hospital, Solingen, Germany

Abstract

Continuous positive airway pressure therapy (CPAP) represents the standard treatment for obstructive sleep apnea syndrome (OSAS). With the aim of achieving optimal adaptation of the treatment pressure to the actual requirement of the patients and improving compliance, auto-adjusting CPAP (APAP) devices were developed. They react to respiratory flow, flattening of the inspiratory flow contour, snoring, generator speed or the upper airway impedance. In recent years, the devices have proven to effectively treat respiratory disturbances, improve sleep profile and the self-assessment of the patients equally as good as the gold standard constant CPAP. APAP reduces the treatment pressure substantially. Although an improvement of the patient's compliance has not been shown consistently, most patients prefer APAP vs. constant CPAP. APAP devices use different algorithms depending on the primary purpose of the application. Therefore, a clear distinction between automatic titration and treatment is of major relevance. While titration devices aim at the finding of one single pressure which is fixed to a constant CPAP device, automatic treatment means the chronic use of APAP at home for optimal adaptation of the treatment pressure to the actual requirements of the patient. A high constant CPAP level, huge pressure variability, insufficient compliance with constant CPAP may be indications for APAP treatment. The main reason for automatic titration is standardization of the initiation process.

Treatment of obstructive sleep apnea syndrome (OSAS) with continuous positive airway pressure (CPAP) was introduced in clinical practice at almost the same time as the syndrome was recognized as a major clinical issue [1]. CPAP still represents the standard of treatment for OSAS. Nevertheless, adaptation of the therapy requires large efforts in education and personal resources. Great experience is needed to find the best equipment (CPAP device, mask, humidifier) for the individual patient, to optimize the treatment according to the patient's needs or to side effects. Moreover, an experienced technician or nurse is required to perform the polysomnography and manual titration during the night. Although CPAP has proven to be effective in most patients with OSAS, several problems raised during the application of CPAP in large patient groups:

(1) Adaptation of therapy by manual titration needs additional time and attention of the technician besides the supervision of the patient and the polysomnographic parameters. The technicians have to focus on several polysomnographies in most sleep labs simultaneously, therefore it cannot be excluded that a number of respiratory disturbances might be overseen.

(2) Differences in the level of experience and education of the technician and difficulties with standardization of the titration procedure might lead to different therapeutic results.

(3) Up to 30% of the patients reject constant CPAP therapy, e.g. for local side effects.

(4) The level of the upper airways obstruction varies within one night in different sleep stages or body positions, from night to night due to spontaneous variability or lifestyle, such as alcohol consumption, or in the longer term due to nasal obstructions (rhinitis) or changes of the body weight. Therefore, it seems difficult to define one single pressure level for optimal treatment in any situation throughout the treatment course [2].

In the light of these problems, self-adjusting CPAP devices (automatic devices, APAP) were developed since the mid-1990s [3–9]. The aim was to optimally adapt the treatment pressure to the actual requirements of the patient according to the varying level of upper airway obstruction. APAP can be applied for two aspects [10], both crucially important for the conception of the algorithm:

(1) On the one hand, APAP devices can be used for *automatic titration*. They are intended to find the one single optimal pressure level for continuous treatment with a constant CPAP device at home. As under manual titration, the pressure level should be as low as possible but has to completely suppress the respiratory disturbances in any situation throughout the course of therapy.

(2) On the other hand, algorithms for *automatic treatment* are not intended to find a constant pressure level but have to continuously adapt a treatment pressure every night, in every situation to the actual level of obstruction. The aim is to reduce the mean treatment pressure and to improve the patient's acceptance.

These two aspects focus in different directions. At the end of this chapter, it will be discussed if they can be reached sufficiently with one algorithm. First of all, the technical aspect of automatic CPAP devices, their efficacy and the indications for APAP therapy will be discussed.

Technical Aspects of Automatic CPAP Devices

APAP devices react to variations of respiratory flow, flattening of the inspiratory flow contour ($APAP_{FLAT}$), snoring, or generator speed, thus indirectly determining the degree of obstruction [2–7]. Furthermore, a system was developed to directly measure the complex resistance, the impedance, of the upper airways with the aid of the forced oscillation technique ($APAP_{FOT}$), thus making it independent of respiratory effort and flow characteristics [8, 9, 11]. Based on these parameters, APAP devices detect respiratory disturbances which induce elevations of the treatment pressure. When the obstruction is overcome, the devices reduce the treatment pressure at different speeds and different frequencies.

Lofaso et al. [12] described an automatic device which measured snoring based on pressure variations in the mask. A high-frequency pressure sensor analyzed frequencies between 30 and 280 Hz. It classified variations of the amplitude as snoring and changed the treatment pressure exclusively based on the detection of the snoring signals. Scharf et al. [13] used a device which analyzed the breathing pattern by flow and pressure sensor and classified apneas, hypopneas or mixed apneas according to the reduction of the amplitude. The analysis of the flow limitation, the flattening of the respiratory flow curve, is widely spread in APAP devices ($APAP_{FLAT}$). Condos et al. [14] described variations of the flow contour on the different levels of the upper airways obstruction. Ayappa et al. [15] found that flow limitation indicated the recurrence of obstruction earlier than snoring when CPAP was decreased. Teschler et al. [7] studied an APAP device based mainly but not exclusively on the analysis of the flow contour.

While the parameters snoring, flow, flattening and esophageal pressure depend directly on the patient's effort, the measurement of the impedance by the forced oscillation technique is independent of the activity of the patient. An oscillatory flow with low amplitude is superimposed to the breathing flow of the patient. A pressure signal is measured at the mask which is composed of the actual CPAP pressure and the pressure variations induced by the oscillatory flow. The latter is used for the measurement of impedance. The APAP device increases or decreases the treatment pressure according to the relative changes of the oscillatory flow. In contrast to the effort-dependent parameters, the impedance can be measured even if the patient does not breath at all. Farré et al. [16] demonstrated that the forced oscillation can simultaneously be applied to CPAP in clinical routine.

Hoster et al. [17] experimentally compared the sensitivity of different parameters for the measurement of the upper airway obstruction in young healthy persons (fig. 1). The volunteers breathed through a tube which was narrowed step by step down to a diameter of 1 mm. Flow, flattening and esophageal pressure reacted in similar ways. There was no significant change of the figures up to a stenosis of 20–28 mm^2. When the stenosis was narrowed further, a sharp decrease of the flow and flattening and a increase of the esophageal pressure were measured. In contrast, the impedance reacted substantially differently. There was a continuous increase of the impedance beginning at a stenosis of 130 mm^2. Thus, the forced oscillation technique presented as most sensitive in this study.

It has been difficult to compare the behavior of APAP devices in response to different breathing disturbances. Therefore, Farré et al. [18] implemented a bench test to

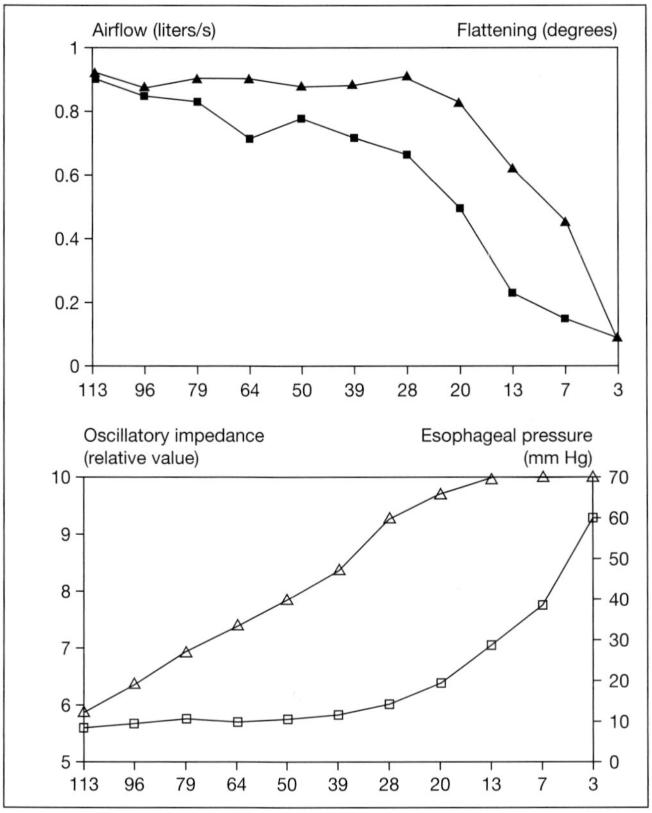

Fig. 1. Variations of flow (▲), flattening (■), esophageal pressure (□) and impedance (△) during experimental breathing. A tube was narrowed gradually to a diameter of 1 mm. Flow, flattening, and esophagical pressure did not change relevantly up to a square of 20–28 mm^2. The impedance signal increased much earlier and was therefore more sensitive in detecting early obstructions [17, modified].

simulate normal breathing, apneas, hypopneas, flow limitation and snoring and to describe the different responses of APAP devices. They used a computer-controlled breathing waveform generator, which consisted of a servo-controlled pump to generate flow, a loudspeaker to generate snoring, and orifices to simulate leakages. The APAP devices reacted considerably differently. Two of five devices did not detect apneas sufficiently. All devices showed pressure increases to hypopnea or flow limitations and reacted correctly to the simulated snoring. However, in the presence of leakages some devices reacted to apneas but reduced the rate of pressure increase in response to hypopneas, while others did not respond to apneas but to hypopneas. Problems were found with devices based on snoring alone, especially in case of leakages.

However, this first bench test was not able to simulate upper airway obstruction and was therefore unable to test the forced oscillation technique. Therefore, Rigau [unpubl. data, 2003] and Schwaiboldt [unpubl. data, 2005] used a modified simulator to reproduce flow and airway obstruction. They tested eight devices based on flow, flow shapes, snoring or upper airway resistance. Once again, remarkable differences were found. Only two devices, one based on flattening, the other on forced oscillation technique, were able to stabilize the virtual patient's respiration to an AHI ≤5/h over the long-term.

These studies point out that there are relevant differences between the APAP devices according to their technique and algorithms (fig. 2). Thus, the devices are not generally interchangeable [19]. The reactions in the individual patients have to be tested under supervision in the sleep lab.

The clinical use of APAP devices may be limited by several problems:

(1) Flow- or flattening-derived devices ($APAP_{FLAT}$) do not discriminate between central or obstructive disturbances in case of complete interception of the airflow.

(2) The device based on impedance alone ($APAP_{FOT}$) could not detect leakages or other artificial increases of the upper airway resistance, which led to unintentional pressure increases.

Therefore, a new APAP device was developed which unified the advantages of the forced oscillation technique, the flattening and snoring. Therefore, it allows the detection of leakages, central breathing disturbances, and initial obstructions (such as flattening or snoring). Moreover, discrimination of inspiration and expiration is possible. The algorithm excludes pressure reactions to pure expiratory obstructions which often result from mouth leakage due to the position of the soft palate. Based on this technique, not only a treatment but also a titration algorithm has been developed. The first results prove the good efficacy of this APAP device based on the combination of flow and impedance in both algorithms [Galetke, unpubl. data, 2005].

Efficacy of the APAP Therapy in Chronic Treatment

Numerous studies were performed to evaluate the clinical efficacy of APAP devices in the treatment of OSAS. Most data are available for the APAP devices based on flow, flattening or impedance. In a large group of unselected consecutive patients with OSAS, $APAP_{FOT}$ was similar to constant CPAP in all polysomnographic aspects. The patients were treated in a randomized, double-blind study for 6 weeks with both constant CPAP and $APAP_{FOT}$. The

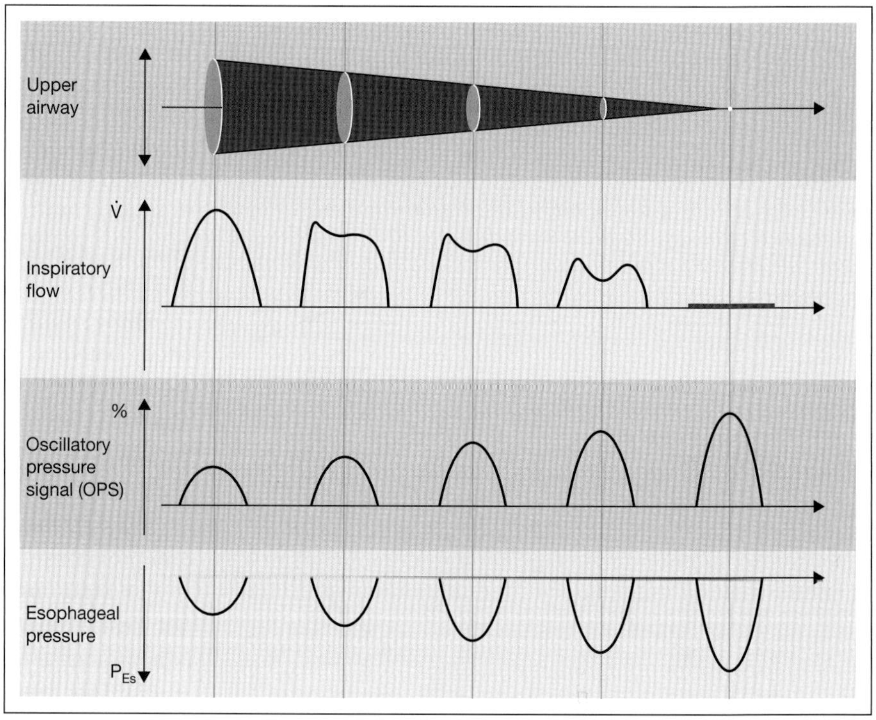

Fig. 2. Schematic presentation of the differences between impedance and flow during an increasing obstruction of the upper airways in OSAS, which is represented in the upper line. During the course, the esophageal pressure becomes increasingly negative. The impedance of the forced oscillation technique increases similarly and reaches its highest level at closure of the airway. The amplitude of the flow signal reduces and the peak is flattened. When the obstruction is complete no flow can be measured, so that a differentiation between central and obstructive apneas is impossible.

CPAP pressure and the mean APAP pressure increased in correlation with the Body Mass Index. However, there was a substantial reduction of the treatment pressure with $APAP_{FOT}$ by 1.5–2.5 mbar reaching 6 mbar in individual cases. The pressure range of the APAP device should be as wide as possible to reach the best pressure reduction [20]. Berry et al. [10] evaluated the available literature in a review of the *American Academy of Sleep Medicine* in 2002. They found evidence that APAP devices effectively suppress respiratory disturbances in a huge majority of the patients. While they are equally as effective as constant CPAP, in general the mean treatment pressure can be reduced significantly [10].

When APAP was introduced in clinical practice, it was anticipated that the pressure variation might impair the sleep quality. However, those fears were not confirmed using modern automatic devices in recent years. On the contrary, most studies showed an improvement of sleep parameters as compared with the baseline. Moreover, APAP reduced arousals and improved REM and slow-wave sleep as well as constant CPAP [10].

Although APAP has proven to be as effective as constant CPAP, an improvement in patients' compliance could not be demonstrated consistently [6, 20–25]. However, it is remarkable that constant CPAP reaches very high levels of compliance under the conditions of controlled studies which might not be representative of the real life situation [20]. However, in several studies the majority of patients (up to 75%) preferred APAP against constant CPAP. $APAP_{FOT}$ was preferred by a huge majority of unselected difficult-to-treat patients as compared with bilevel therapy [20, 21]. Similar data were presented by Marrone et al. [22] who verified the patients' self-assessment using objective parameters. The patients used the preferred devices (CPAP or APAP) for longer time periods. 14 of 22 patients who preferred the flow-derived device as compared to CPAP showed a daily compliance of 4.8 $\pm$ 1.8 h/day under CPAP while it reaches 5.5 $\pm$ 1.5 h/day under APAP. Interestingly, the baseline AHI was significantly lower in those patients who preferred constant CPAP.

Several studies evaluated the clinical symptoms of OSAS, the quality of life and the sleepiness based on - self-assessment questionnaires and electrophysiological tests. Senn et al. [26] compared constant CPAP with two different APAP devices based on the detection of apneas and hypopneas or snoring and variations of the flow contour, respectively. They found an improvement of the symptoms and quality-of-life scores and the performance in maintenance of the wakefulness test without any difference between the treatment modes. Massie et al. [25] described an improvement in the vitality score and mental health score of the SF-36 test but not in the Epworth sleepiness scale under APAP. The authors focused on patients with a constant CPAP level ≥10 mbar. The patients reported more recreation sleep, better sleep quality and less discomfort with APAP vs. CPAP.

In conclusion, chronic treatment with APAP offers additional treatment options which are equally effective in terms of respiratory and polysomnographic parameters as compared to constant CPAP. While an improvement in patients' compliance has not been shown consistently, APAP reduces the treatment pressure substantially and is preferred by most patients [27].

Indications for Chronic APAP Treatment

Despite the advantages of APAP treatment, it cannot be recommended routinely for economic reasons. However, while there are no generally accepted criteria for APAP treatment at the moment, evidence increases for which patients APAP treatment might be beneficial. APAP is often used in patients with high variability of pressure requirements depending on body position, sleep stages or night-to-night variability. Moreover, in patients who are insufficiently treated with constant CPAP, bilevel treatment is often applied [28]. These patients may be candidates for APAP treatment, too.

Therefore, the efficacy of $APAP_{FOT}$ was compared to bilevel therapy in patients with difficult-to-treat OSAS. Patients with primary CPAP intolerance, a high CPAP pressure (≥12 mbar), or with mixed sleep apnea syndrome with a proportion of central respiratory disturbances of ≥10% were randomly treated with both APAP or bilevel therapy in a cross-over design. Substantial improvement in the respiratory disturbances and arousals were observed in the overall group and the individual indication groups. The mean AHI was lowered to values of around 10/h, with no significant differences between the modalities. As compared to earlier investigations comparing $APAP_{FOT}$ with constant CPAP, this study differed by the higher baseline AHI and difficult-to-treat disease status in which CPAP was ineffective or not tolerated by the patients. In a large majority of patients (20 of 27), the AHI could be reduced to <10/h with at least one of the two modalities [21].

Additionally, in patients with high pressure requirements (≥10 mbar), Massie et al. [25] found a significantly greater compliance under APAP as compared to constant CPAP. Moreover, in this population APAP improved the perception of sleep quality and treatment comfort.

Ficker et al. [11] studied 8 OSAS patients with constant CPAP and APAP in randomized order. There were no differences in the results of the Epworth sleepiness scale or the polysomnographic data. However, the mean CPAP pressure was significantly lower with APAP as compared to constant CPAP. Especially the pressure applied in the lateral body position was significantly lower with APAP than that employed in conventional CPAP.

Although the night-to-night variability of OSAS is a well-known phenomenon, the clinical relevance of the problem was unclear. Therefore, the pressure profile of a 6-week treatment period with APAP was analyzed in 20 patients with the aim of quantifying the pressure variability. The deviations of the treatment pressure from the mean value defined a variability index (VI). Breathing was assumed to be stable if neither the mean of the VI nor >10% of the treatment nights exceeded a defined threshold (pressure variation of ±1.5 mbar). Only 3 of 20 patients fulfilled both criteria of pressure stability. The VI exceeded the threshold in mean in 50% of the patients and in more than 10% of the nights in 7 of the remaining 10 patients. Based on these findings one can conclude that *stability* of the pressure requirement is the exception and that *variability* is the rule [29].

Automatic Treatment versus Automatic Titration

Besides important differences clear discrimination between automatic titration and treatment is often lacking in the literature. The aim of *chronic automatic therapy* is to apply the optimal treatment pressure each and every night, in every situation, in every sleep state, and in the case of additional interfering factors such as nasal obstructions or muscle relaxants (drugs, alcohol). The treatment pressure should be as low as possible in each situation and should be increased only in the actual case of obstruction.

Automatic titration does not principally differ from manual titration. Both have to define one single pressure level which is sufficient for every situation. Therefore, the pressure value has to be adapted to the worst obstruction, e.g. in the supine position or during REM sleep. The constant CPAP level titrated manually or automatically, regularly exceeds the mean pressure under automatic treatment. It could be shown that the automatically titrated constant CPAP allows for a sufficient improvement of sleep quality and suppression of respiratory disturbances [30, 31]. However, it is obvious that a level, titrated in a single night, will not optimally fulfill the varying requirements dictated by changes of body weight or nasal obstruction during the course of disease.

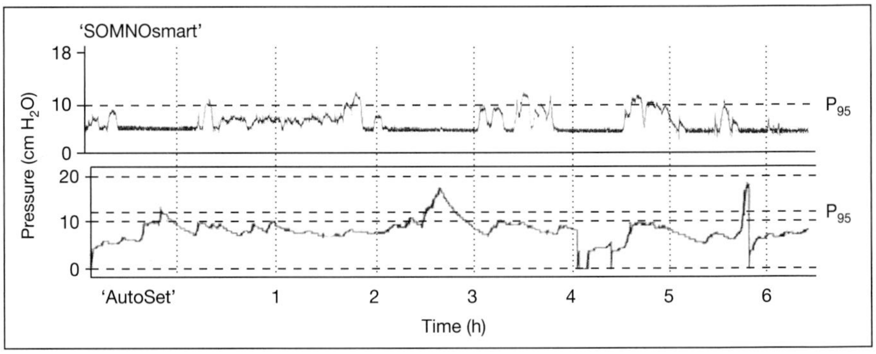

Fig. 3. Differences between the pressure profile under automatic treatment and automatic titration. The SOMNOsmart® ($APAP_{FOT}$) curve shows longer periods of minimal pressure resulting in lower P_{mean}. On the other hand, the P_{95} from the AutoSet can be recommended for constant CPAP therapy [32, with permission].

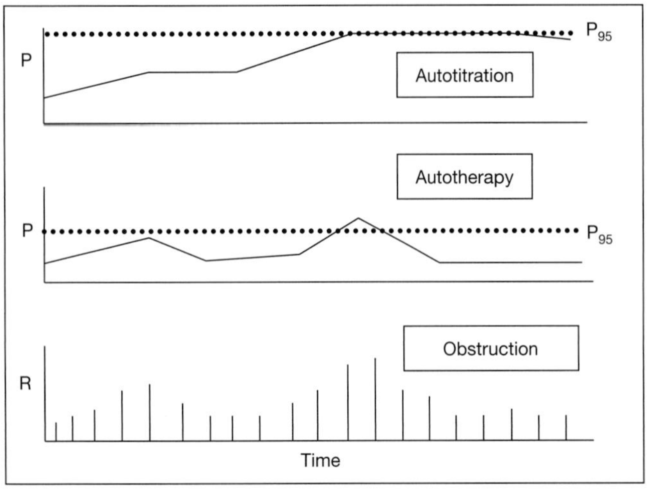

Fig. 4. Schematic presentation of the difference between automatic titration and treatment. Automatic titration aims at finding a single pressure level for constant CPAP. Thus, the algorithm increases pressure whenever an obstruction can be found but rarely reduces it. On the other hand, automatic therapy is intended to treat patients with the lowest treatment pressure throughout any night of his course. Hence, it will increase pressure if necessary but will reduce pressure whenever possible.

The reports read out of the APAP devices describe the pressure profile of a single night or longer time periods. They mostly include maximum pressure (P_{max}), mean pressure (P_{mean}) and 95th percentile (P_{95}). The latter describes the pressure figure which is exceeded ≤5% of the time. Teschler et al. [7] demonstrated that the P_{95} read out from a titration device could be recommended for constant CPAP. Based on these findings, different APAP devices were compared. Kessler et al. [32] randomly studied 16 patients on 2 consecutive nights. They performed titration studies in the sleep lab without supervision using two automatic devices. As the P_{95} under $APAP_{FLAT}$ exceeded $APAP_{FOT}$, different figures for constant CPAP had to be recommended (fig. 3).

Pevernagie et al. [33] compared the same devices in a randomized cross-over split-night study in 30 patients with OSAS. They found relevant increases of the P_{95} under $APAP_{FLAT}$ during wake-to-sleep transition while it fell under $APAP_{FOT}$. Moreover, the pressure variability was higher under $APAP_{FOT}$ as compared to $APAP_{FLAT}$. While the authors found a lower snoring index with $APAP_{FLAT}$ there was no difference in the respiration or sleep profile between the two devices. These data indicate the difference between the algorithms of automatic titration and treatment. The $APAP_{FOT}$ device was designed for chronic automatic treatment. For this reason, treatment pressure is set to the lowest possible level throughout long periods of the night, resulting in significantly lower P_{95} and P_{mean}, as compared to titration algorithms. Automatic titration increases the treatment pressure step by step but rarely lowers it. Therefore, a higher variability of the treatment pressure results from treatment devices (fig. 4).

Indications for Automatic Titration

Automatic titration is discussed for several reasons: On the one hand, there is a long time delay between the suspicion of OSAS and the start of the treatment due to long waiting lists in some countries. On the other hand, the diagnostic procedure and treatment initiation in the sleep lab is thought to be too expensive.

Studying the use of APAP, some critical issues have to be taken into concern:

APAP devices which cannot discriminate between central and obstructive disturbances may increase the treatment pressure inappropriately in case of central apneas, hypopneas or periodic breathing and, therefore, aggravate the situation.

Any positive airway pressure treatment, APAP, CPAP, bilevel, may not sufficiently treat hypoventilation disorders.

A supplementation of oxygen or noninvasive ventilation might be necessary in these cases.

Juhasz et al. [34] described central apneas and arrhythmias in patients with pre-existing heart failure or lung diseases.

Marrone et al. [35] found that CPAP titration by automatic devices alone results in imperfect titration in >10% of the patients. Only polysomnographic recording ensures titration reliability in all patients.

For these reasons, unattended treatment initiation cannot be recommended. The diagnostic evaluation and the first treatment night have to prove that the patients do not suffer relevant central disturbances or develop them under treatment. Up to now, the studies on automatic titration excluded patients with relevant cardiovascular or pulmonary disorders, such as heart failure or chronic pulmonary diseases. Therefore, there is no evidence of the efficacy and safety of automatic titration in this group of patients. Those APAP devices which detect central disturbances and avoid pressure increases might be used safely in these patients. Patients with cardiovascular or pulmonary diseases should be adapted to any positive airway pressure treatment under attention in the sleep lab.

Moreover, there is a lack of evidence that automatic titration might be efficient for economic reasons. The rapid prescription of a treatment device does not fulfill the quality standards of the treatment of OSAS. Optimal diagnostic work-up, follow-up, mask adaptation and patient education are essential. Several disadvantages have to be taken into account for the correct calculation of costs and effectiveness: insufficient treatment, additional titration nights, direct and indirect costs due to insufficient compliance, time-consuming advice to the patient about the titration device and sensors [see paper by Hein 'Portable Monitoring Systems', this vol, pp 47–50]. Unattended CPAP titration at home cannot be recommended by now as it does not allow for polysomnographic and visual control of optimal pressure adaption or for solving problems with the devices or mask. The constant CPAP pressure should be recommended not only based on the reading of the software, but also on the correlation of the polysomnography with the raw data of the respiratory disturbances and the pressure profile.

Nevertheless, automatic titration may allow one to standardize the treatment initiation. The technicians have to supervise several polysomnographies in most sleep labs. Moreover, besides monitoring they have to attend the patients in case of problems and to correct the sensors if necessary. The level of education and experience differs within the team. The interpretation of minor respiratory disturbances such as flattening during the running study is a major issue even for experienced sleep specialists. Automatic titration might overcome all these problems. The devices allow for reliable reactions to respiratory disturbances. Thus, the titration becomes independent of the technician's attention and experience and may be cost-effective as repetitions of titration studies might be reduced.

In conclusion, the clinician has to define why the use of an automatic device is intended. If the purpose is to find a constant CPAP pressure, an automatic titration algorithm could be used and the P_{95} can be recommended for fixed CPAP. If chronic automatic treatment is indicated, a treatment device should be chosen to optimally reduce the treatment pressure and adapt it to the actual need of the patient.

Regarding autoadjusting CPAP, the American Academy of Sleep Medicine gives the following recommendations [36]:

APAP titration and APAP treatment are not currently recommended for patients with congestive heart failure, significant lung disease, daytime hypoxemia and respiratory failure of any cause, or prominent nocturnal desaturation other than from OSAS.

A diagnosis of OSAS must be established by an acceptable method which, in most cases, is polysomnography. Split-night studies and the use of unattended APAP – neither for titration nor for treatment in CPAP-naïve patients – are not recommended.

Certain APAP devices may be used during attended titration to identify by polysomnography a single pressure for use with standard CPAP for the treatment of OSA.

Once an initial successful attended CPAP or APAP titration has been determined by polysomnography, certain APAP devices may be used in the self-adjusting mode for unattended treatment of patients with OSA.

All patients being treated with fixed CPAP on the basis of APAP titration or being treated with APAP must be followed to determine treatment effectiveness and safety, and must be re-evaluated if symptoms do not resolve or the CPAP or APAP treatment otherwise appears to lack efficacy.

References

1 Sullivan CE, Issa FG, Berthon-Jones M, Eves L: Reversal of obstructive sleep apnea by continuous positive airway pressure applied through the nares. Lancet 1981;i:862–865.

2 Sharma S, Wali S, Pouliot Z, Peters M, Neufeld H, Kryger M: Treatment of obstructive sleep apnea with a self-titrating continuous positive airway pressure (CPAP) system. Sleep 1996;19:497–501.

3 Behbehani K, Yen FC, Lucas EA, Burk JR: A sleep laboratory evaluation of an automatic positive airway pressure system for treatment of obstructive sleep apnea. Sleep 1998;21: 485–491.

4 Stradling JR, Barbour C, Pitson DJ, Davies RJ: Automatic nasal continuous positive airway pressure titration in the laboratory: patient outcomes. Thorax 1997;52:72–75.

5 Lloberes P, Ballester E, Montserrat JM, Botifoll E, Ramirez A, Reolid A, Gistau C, Rodriguez-Roisin R: Comparison of manual and automatic CPAP titration in patients with sleep apnea/hypopnea syndrome. Am J Respir Crit Care Med 1996;154:1755–1758.

6 d'Ortho MP, Grillier-Lanoir V, Levy P, Goldenberg F, Corriger E, Harf A, Lofaso F: Constant vs. automatic continuous positive airway pressure therapy: home evaluation. Chest 2000;118:1010–1017.

7 Teschler H, Berthon-Jones M, Thompson AB, Henkel A, Henry J, Konietzko N: Automated continuous positive airway pressure titration for obstructive sleep apnea syndrome. Am J Respir Crit Care Med 1996; 154:734–740.

8 Randerath WJ, Parys K, Feldmeyer F, Sanner B, Rühle KH: Self-adjusting nasal continuous positive airway pressure therapy based on measurement of impedance: a comparison of two different maximum pressure levels. Chest 1999;116:991–999.

9 Randerath W, Galetke W, David M, Siebrecht H, Sanner B, Ruhle KH: Prospective randomized comparison of impedance-controlled auto-CPAP ($APAP_{FOT}$) with constant CPAP. Sleep Med 2001;2:115–124.

10 Berry RB, Parish JM, Hartse KM: The use of auto-titrating continuous positive airway pressure for treatment of adult obstructive sleep apnea. An American Academy of Sleep Medicine review. Sleep 2002;25:148–173.

11 Ficker JH, Fuchs FS, Wiest GH, Asshoff G, Schmelzer AH, Hahn EG: An auto-continuous positive airway pressure device controlled exclusively by the forced oscillation technique. Eur Respir J 2000;16:914–920.

12 Lofaso F, Lorino AM, Duizabo D, Najafi Zadeh H, Theret D, Goldenberg F, Harf A: Evaluation of an auto-nCPAP device based on snoring detection. Eur Respir J 1996;9:1795–1800.

13 Scharf MB, Brannen DE, McDannold MD, Berkowitz DV: Computerized adjustable versus fixed NCPAP treatment of obstructive sleep apnea. Sleep 1996;19:491–496.

14 Condos R, Norman RG, Krishnasamy I, Peduzzi N, Goldring RM, Rapoport DM: Flow limitation as a noninvasive assessment of residual upper-airway resistance during continuous positive airway pressure therapy of obstructive sleep apnea. Am J Respir Crit Care Med 1994;150:475–480.

15 Ayappa I, Norman RG, Hosselet JJ, Gruenke RA, Walsleben JA, Rapoport DM: Relative occurrence of flow limitation and snoring during continuous positive airway pressure titration. Chest 1998;114:685–690.

16 Farré R, Rotger M, Montserrat JM, Navajas D: A system to generate simultaneous forced oscillation and continuous positive airway pressure. Eur Respir J 1997;10:1349–1353.

17 Hoster M, Schlenker E, Raddatz M, Ruhle KH: Oszillatorische Impedanz, Ösophagusdruck und Atemfluss bei Stenoseatmung. Modell für die extrathorakale Obstruktion; in Ruhle KH (ed): Oszillatorische Impedanz beischlafbezogenen Atemregulationsstörungen. Stuttgart, Thieme, 1996, pp 13–18.

18 Farré R, Montserrat JM, Rigau J, Trepat X, Pinto P, Navajas D: Response of automatic continuous positive airway pressure devices to different sleep breathing patterns: a bench study. Am J Respir Crit Care Med 2002;166:469–473.

19 Stammnitz A, Jerrentrup A, Penzel T, Peter JH, Vogelmeier C, Becker H: Automatic CPAP titration with different self-setting devices in patients with obstructive sleep apnoea. Eur Respir J 2004;24:273–278.

20 Randerath WJ, Schraeder O, Galetke W, Feldmeyer F, Ruhle KH: Autoadjusting CPAP therapy based on impedance efficacy, compliance and acceptance. Am J Respir Crit Care Med 2001;163:652–657.

21 Randerath W, Galetke W, Rühle KH: Autoadjusting CPAP based on impedance versus bilevel pressure in difficult-to-treat sleep apnea syndrome: a prospective randomized crossover study. Med Sci Monit 2003;9: 353–358.

22 Marrone O, Resta O, Salvaggio A, Giliberti T, Stefano A, Insalaco G: Preference for fixed or automatic CPAP in patients with obstructive sleep apnea syndrome. Sleep Med 2004;5: 247–251.

23 Meurice JC, Marc I, Series F: Efficacy of auto-CPAP in the treatment of obstructive sleep apnea/hypopnea syndrome. Am J Respir Crit Care Med 1996;153:794–798.

24 Hudgel DW, Fung C: A long-term randomized crossover comparison of auto-titrating and standard nasal continuous positive airway pressure. Sleep 2000;23:1–4.

25 Massie CA, McArdle N, Hart RW, Schmidt-Nowara WW, Lankford A, Hudgel DW, Gordon N, Douglas NJ: Comparison between automatic and fixed positive airway pressure therapy in the home. Am J Respir Crit Care Med 2003;167:20–23.

26 Senn O, Brack T, Matthews F, Russi EW, Bloch KE: Randomized short-term trial of two autoCPAP devices versus fixed continuous positive airway pressure for the treatment of sleep apnea. Am J Respir Crit Care Med 2003;168:1506–1511.

27 Ayas NT, Patel SR, Malhotra A, Schulzer M, Malhotra M, Jung D, Fleetham J, White DP: Auto-titrating versus standard continuous positive airway pressure for the treatment of obstructive sleep apnea: results of a meta-analysis. Sleep 2004;27:249–253.

28 Reeves-Hoché MK, Hudgel DW, Meck R, Witteman R, Ross A, Zwillich CW: Continuous versus bilevel positive airway pressure for obstructive sleep apnea. Am J Respir Crit Care Med 1995;151:443–449.

29 Randerath W, Rocholl C, Feldmeyer F, Galetke W: Variability of the treatment pressure under continuous positive airway pressure treatment in obstructive sleep apnea syndrome. Pneumologie 2002;56:425–431.

30 Berkani M, Lofaso F, Chouaid C, d'Ortho MP, Theret D, Grillier-Lanoir V, Harf A, Housset B: CPAP titration by an auto-CPAP device based on snoring detection: a clinical trial and economic considerations. Eur Respir J 1998;12: 759–763.

31 Gagnadoux F, Pelletier-Fleury N, Philippe C, Rakotonanahary D, Fleury B: Home unattended vs. hospital telemonitored polysomnography in suspected obstructive sleep apnea syndrome: a randomized crossover trial. Chest 2002;121:753–758.

32 Kessler R, Weitzenblum E, Chaouat A, Iamandi C, Alliotte T: Evaluation of unattended automated titration to determine therapeutic continuous positive airway pressure in patients with obstructive sleep apnea. Chest 2003;123:704–710.

33 Pevernagie DA, Proot PM, Hertegonne KB, Neyens MC, Hoornaert KP, Pauwels RA: Efficacy of flow- vs impedance-guided autoadjustable continuous positive airway pressure: a randomized cross-over trial. Chest 2004;126:25–30.

34 Juhasz J, Schillen J, Urbigkeit A, Ploch T, Penzel T, Peter JH: Unattended continuous positive airway pressure titration: clinical relevance and cardiorespiratory hazards of the method. Am J Respir Crit Care Med 1996;154:359–365.

35 Marrone O, Insalaco G, Salvaggio A, Bonsignore G: Role of different nocturnal monitorings in the evaluation of CPAP titration by autoCPAP devices. Respir Med 2005;99:313–320.

36 Littner M, Hirshkowitz M, Davila D, Anderson WM, Kushida CA, Woodson BT, Johnson SF, Merrill SW: Standards of Practice Committee of the American Academy of Sleep Medicine: practice parameters for the use of auto-titrating continuous positive airway pressure devices for titrating pressures and treating adult patients with obstructive sleep apnea syndrome. An American Academy of Sleep Medicine report. Sleep 2002;25:143–147.

Prof. Dr. Winfried J. Randerath
Institute for Pneumology at the University Witten/Herdecke
Clinic for Pneumology and Allergology
Center of Sleep Medicine and Respiratory Care, Bethanien Hospital
Aufderhöherstrasse 169–175
DE–42699 Solingen (Germany)
Tel. +49 212 63 6000
Fax +49 212 63 6005
E-Mail randerath@klinik-bethanien.de

Randerath WJ, Sanner BM, Somers VK (eds): Sleep Apnea.
Prog Respir Res. Basel, Karger, 2006, vol 35, pp 145–150

Humidification in Sleep-Related Breathing Disorders

Adam V. Benjafield Glenn N. Richards

Clinical and Research Services, ResMed Ltd, North Ryde, Australia

Abstract

Humidification of inspired air is critical for the protection of the airways and alveoli of the lung. The nose is a highly efficient conditioner of inspired air with a large mucosal surface area and an airpath designed to create turbulent flow. Normal upper airway function can be interfered with by the use of positive airway pressure (PAP) therapy, leading to symptoms such as nasal congestion, dry nose or throat, sore throat and epistaxis. These symptoms are caused by mouth leaks, which during PAP treatment lead to high unidirectional nasal airflow. This has a cooling and drying effect on the nasal mucosa which leads to mucosal inflammation, rebound nasal congestion and an increase in nasal resistance creating a potential vicious circle. The symptoms are a common side effect of PAP therapy and may decrease both compliance and the effective pressure delivered to the oropharynx. Adequate humidification of inspired air attenuates these increases in nasal resistance, symptoms, and may increase compliance with therapy. The types of humidifiers available, their limitations, alternatives to humidification and the current prescription practice for humidification will also be discussed.

Normal Nasal Physiology and Function

The nasal airway performs two main functions in respiration, filtration of particulate matter and conditioning of inspired air. Normal mucociliary function in proximal lung airways depends on adequately conditioned air, and in the presence of dry air there is increased mucus viscosity, slowing of mucociliary transport, cilial dysfunction and epithelial cell death. This in turn inevitably leads to atelectasis and pneumonia, a sequence of events that was quickly appreciated by pioneering physicians attempting long-term ventilation through bypassed upper airways.

The anatomy of the nasal airway ensures very efficient conditioning of inspired air by causing turbulent airflow and maximizing the contact between air and mucosa (fig. 1). Room air entering the nasal airway at 20°C and 50% relative humidity will be approximately 32°C and 100% humidified by the time it reaches the nasopharynx. Conditioning is normally completed in the trachea at a point known as the isothermic saturation boundary. This point may shift distally with high minute ventilation such as with exercise, and if it reaches proximal airways may trigger the phenomena of exercise-induced asthma.

The energy and water required for air conditioning is supplied through a rich submucosal vascular network. There is rapid movement of water across the mucosa with the approximately 150 μl of fluid that covers the nasal mucosa being replaced every 90 s. A counter current system is used to maximize efficiency. During inspiration the mucosa is cooled as it gives up heat and moisture, but during expiration the air is warmer than the mucosa and approximately a third of the water and heat lost in inspiration are recovered. The total loss of water per day is approximately 300–400 ml and is known as the respiratory insensible water loss.

The nasal mucosa is highly specialized with the system of glands, goblet cells and blood vessels under the influence

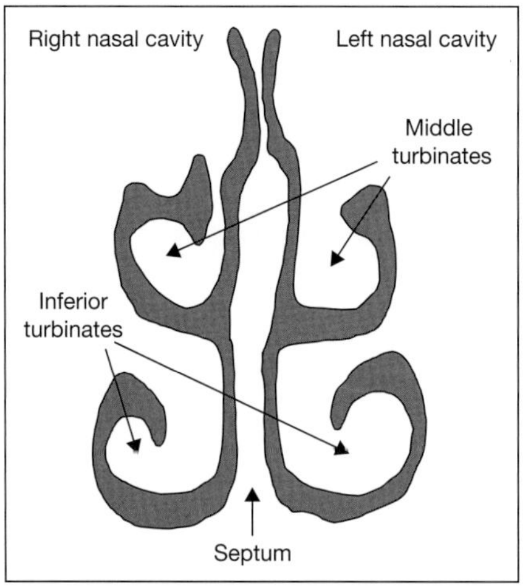

Fig. 1. Schematic representation of a coronal CT of the nasal passage.

of an autonomic neural network that delicately adjusts the secretory control system to changes in demand due to changing breathing patterns and environment. Blood vessels run in the long axis of the turbinates with the venous system lying superficial to the arterial system with interconnections through numerous anastomoses. Within the turbinates and parts of the septum there exist erectile tissue rich in capacitance vessels. Filling of capacitance vessels and blood flow is regulated by sympathetic postganglionic vasomotor fibers, and nasal glands by postganglionic parasympathetic fibers from the pterygopalatine ganglion. Rich local neural networks exist and while the afferent receptors are not well understood, it appears that they respond to osmolarity of the mucosal surface. Normal nasal secretions consist of 2–3% mucin, 1–2% salts, with the remainder being water [1]. If the requirement for conditioning increases, evaporation of water increases salt concentration at the mucosal surface. This stimulates afferent nerves with resulting increases in submucosal blood flow, enlargement of capacitance vessels and increasing secretion from nasal glands.

An efficient air conditioning system necessarily has high resistance to airflow, and the nasal airway is no exception. Nasal resistance is approximately half of total airway resistance with the narrowest part of the respiratory tract being at the nasal valve, a physiologic site at the proximal end of the turbinates. Changes in the caliber of the capacitance vessels at this site in response to changes in demand for humidification may cause large changes in nasal resistance. Other factors that may normally influence nasal resistance include the nasal cycle, which is a phenomenon in which nasal resistance alternates from one nostril to the other at an interval of approximately 90 min, supine posture which increases resistance, and stimulation of ventilation by exercise, hypoxia or hypercapnia, which decrease resistance. Rhinitis of any cause increases resistance and it can be reduced by treatment with atropine, sympathomimetic decongestants and steroids.

Considerable understanding of normal and abnormal nasal physiology has been derived from experimenting with a phenomena well known to alpine enthusiasts – skiers nose. Nasal hypersecretion in lift queues is a frequent problem due to the normal nasal physiologic systems being overwhelmed and then unable to adapt to a sudden decrease in demand due to reduced ventilation. Experimental models of cold dry air exposure have demonstrated the importance of unidirectional airflow, the appearance of inflammatory mediators on nasal mucosa if it becomes hyperosmolar, and the reversal of the process by humidification [2–4]. This research, originally undertaken to enhance understanding of exercise induced asthma, has serendipitously provided important insights into some of the adverse effects of PAP therapy.

Nasal Symptoms and PAP Therapy

The nasal breathing route is preferred by most, but it has higher resistance than the alternative, mouth breathing, and thus causes higher work of breathing. If nasal resistance becomes abnormally high the normal response is to switch to mouth breathing to reduce work of breathing. Measurement of partitioning between mouth and nasal breathing is difficult as the instrumentation required may influence breathing route, but it has been shown that increases in nasal resistance, or airflow (which indirectly increases resistance) as with graded exercise, normally causes an increased proportion of breathing through the mouth. Long term increases in nasal resistance as seen in chronic rhinitis may cause mouth breathing to be learnt, so that if rhinitis resolves, mouth breathing may continue.

The preferred route of breathing for many patients with OSA is through the mouth. We conducted a survey of 600 new patients attending a sleep service in Australia and found that two thirds had a history of chronic nasal symptoms before starting therapy. There is evidence that nasal disease may sometimes play a causative role in OSA, with patients suffering from allergic rhinitis having a higher AHI during episodes of rhinitis. The mouth is nearly as efficient as the nose as a humidifier, and mouth breathing has no known long-term adverse effects apart from OSA. However, if PAP therapy is required, mouth breathing may have unwanted consequences.

Mouth leaks during PAP therapy are common and offer a rational mechanism for the development of adverse upper airway symptoms as they cause high unidirectional nasal airflow, progressive drying of the upper airway mucosa, release of inflammatory mediators, increased nasal mucosal blood flow, increased nasal resistance and daytime upper airway symptoms [3, 5, 6].

The degree of mouth leak with PAP therapy depends on the pressure in the nasal mask, the nasal resistance and the extent of jaw opening. With a well-fitting mask, the mean flow through the mask (i.e. difference between inspiration and expiration volumes) is small, in the order of 0–12 liters/min. At CPAP pressures over 10 cm H_2O, pinhole leaks between the lips give measured leaks of 24–60 liters/min [6]. Sealing the lips abolishes this increase. Leaks via the mouth in excess of 40 liters/min are commonly encountered in clinical practice since PAP devices are designed to deliver large flows.

We conducted a series of experiments during which normal subjects deliberately simulated a mouth leak of 50 liters/min for 10 min while using CPAP [6]. Nasal resistance was measured, using posterior rhinomanometry, to assess activation of compensatory nasal physiologic mechanisms to mucosal drying. This stimulus induced a fourfold increase in nasal resistance that reduced rapidly for 10 min then more slowly over 30 min but had not returned to baseline at the conclusion of the test (fig. 2). All subjects also experienced discomfort during the stimulus followed by rhinorrhea and a persistent sensation of nasal congestion that lasted longer than the 40 min of the test. Repetitive challenges of mouth leak, to simulate the occurrence of multiple mouth leaks during the course of a night, demonstrated that there was no tachyphylaxis (fig. 3) [6]. Mouth leaks of 3 min in duration repeated every 10 min caused increases in nasal resistance of similar magnitude each time. Nasal resistance did not reach baseline between challenges, causing a gradual increase in baseline resistance over time. An unpublished series of experiments on a group with chronic nasal disease demonstrated a higher baseline resistance and a much greater response to the stimulus such that it became difficult to measure nasal resistance. Subjects with established nasal disease appear to be significantly more susceptible to the effects of nasal mucosal drying than those without symptoms.

The same subjects were tested using protocols that used air at differing temperatures and humidities. Fully humidified air at temperatures ranging from 23°C (similar to the output of commercially available heated humidifiers) to 37°C were found to prevent the response to the stimulus. Cold passover humidifiers, which provide little added humidity at high flows, were ineffective at preventing increases in nasal resistance. These findings were extended by another group [5], employing an identical protocol but measuring nasal mucosal blood flow using a Doppler method, who found increases in nasal blood flow were attenuated with the use of fully humidified air.

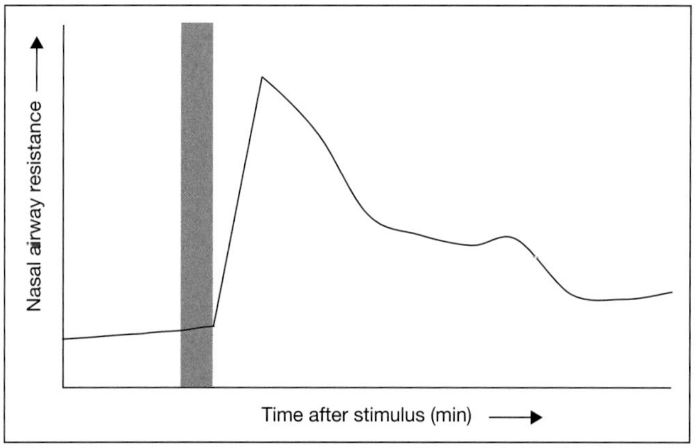

Fig. 2. Increase of nasal resistance after stimulus and gradual decrease of nasal resistance over 20 min. Shaded area represents stimulus of 10 min.

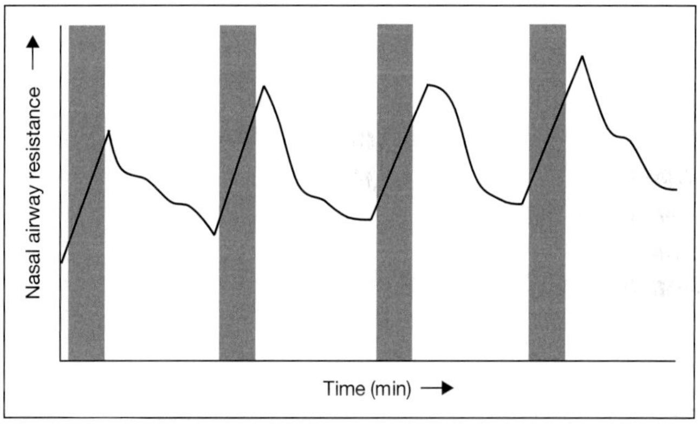

Fig. 3. Mean nasal resistance after repeated challenges of mouth leak with room air at 50 liters/min. Shaded areas represent the four periods of mouth leak for 3 min each.

The results of the above observations and experiments suggest that nasal symptoms during PAP therapy are likely to be due to mouth leaks. They suggest that a mechanism similar to that described in cold dry air challenges is involved in the development of upper airway symptoms but also raise some possibilities, which are unique to PAP therapy, that deserve consideration. As increased nasal resistance predisposes to mouth breathing, and during PAP therapy mouth breathing leads to increased nasal resistance,

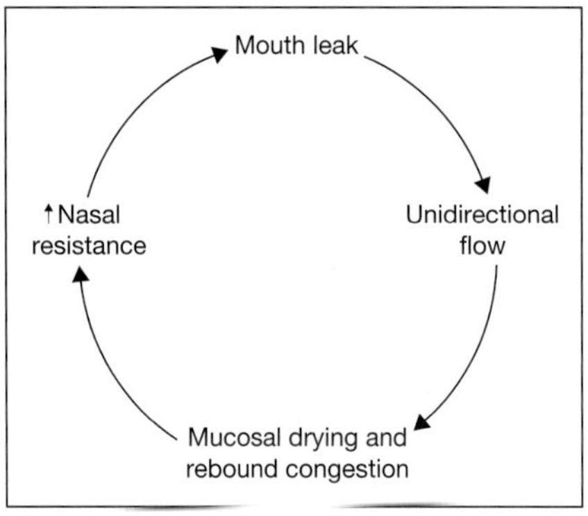

Fig. 4. The vicious circle for the development of nasal symptoms when using PAP therapy.

a vicious circle may occur (fig. 4) which is self sustaining. For patients starting therapy with PAP the only way to prevent this circular escalation is to seek added treatment such as humidification that disrupts the sequence of events, to persist hoping that it will spontaneously resolve, or to stop PAP therapy. It is likely that some choose the last option. Additionally, the degree of increase in nasal resistance may reduce efficacy of PAP therapy. A change in nasal resistance of 10–15 cm H_2O/liter/s at flow rates observed during normal tidal breathing, would equate to a pressure drop of 5–7.5 cm H_2O across the nose [6]. This degree of change in resistance was observed frequently during the experiments described above. CPAP titration for OSA is performed to determine a mask pressure that is assumed is transmitted to the anatomic site on which the positive pressure acts – the oropharynx. These results demonstrate that the nasal airway is dynamic, and suggest that patients experiencing nasal symptoms may experience a critical reduction in CPAP delivered to their oropharynx, which can result in suboptimal treatment of their disease.

Clinical Evidence

Patients commencing CPAP for OSA frequently find it inconvenient and may experience a range of difficulties that interfere with their ability to use the therapy. Several studies have documented a high frequency of complaints including discomfort from the mask, upper airway symptoms, sleep disruption due to noise and the presence of equipment, and difficulty exhaling. Upper airway symptoms including nasal congestion, dry nose or throat, sore throat and epistaxis affect 30–70% of patients and may limit long-term acceptance [7–10]. Approximately 20–30% of patients prescribed CPAP do not use it long term. The reasons that cause patients to decline PAP therapy are often complex, and it is unusual for one single factor to be identified, but side effects are generally important.

Four studies have addressed the effects of humidification on acceptance rates of CPAP therapy for OSA. Massie et al. [11] studied 38 new CPAP users comparing heated humidification, cold passover humidification and no humidification using a randomized crossover design. They found significantly increased use of CPAP (35 min per night) in those using heated humidification compared to no humidification, a reduction in reported upper airway side effects, and increased satisfaction with treatment. Use of cold passover humidification was ineffective. There was a strong seasonal influence demonstrated, with significantly larger increases in CPAP use noted in winter months compared to spring months. Neill et al. [12], using a very similar crossover design, compared heated humidification with placebo humidification in 37 new CPAP users. They found a modest improvement (24 min per night) in CPAP use over a three week period in those using heated humidification, and a reduction in symptoms compared to placebo.

Rakotonanahary et al. [13] studied a cohort of 82 new CPAP users for a medium duration of 347 days. 46 subjects (56%) developed upper airway symptoms and were started on cold passover humidification, with 23 experiencing persistent symptoms and subsequently starting heated humidification. The group using heated humidification had significantly greater mean CPAP use (5.4 h) than those using cold passover humidification (4.6 h). Mador et al. [14] performed a randomized parallel study of one year duration comparing a group who received heated humidification at the onset of CPAP therapy, with a control group who received heated humidification only if they developed upper airway symptoms refractory to other measures. Despite chronic upper airway symptoms being very common in both groups before initiation of CPAP only a quarter of control subjects complained of more than mild symptoms when on treatment. Half of the subgroup of controls who developed troublesome symptoms were successfully treated with simple measures and half were crossed over to heated humidification. There was no difference between the groups in use of CPAP, quality of life, or sleepiness although there were fewer upper airway symptoms in the group using heated humidification. These results suggest that routine use of heated humidification at CPAP initiation does not lead to better outcomes than treatment of symptoms as they arise.

The current literature generally supports the use of heated humidification in the large minority of patients who develop new or worsened upper airway symptoms during PAP therapy for OSA. Heated humidification is effective at preventing and treating upper airway symptoms associated with therapy, although improvements in use of PAP therapy may be modest. Patients generally make a decision about long-term acceptance early in the course of therapy with use at 1 month predicting use at 3 months [9], and suboptimal usage able to be identified after 4 nights [15]. Early intervention for side effects is prudent, but in clinical practice nasal symptoms may be present for an extended time before any treatment is initiated. The studies demonstrating a positive effect of humidification on CPAP acceptance have introduced humidification early, and it cannot be assumed that these effects will be recognized if the addition of humidification is significantly delayed.

There is no convincing evidence supporting the use of humidification in patients using noninvasive ventilation. However, upper airway side effects are common in patients using this therapy and in some there is the additional concern of worsening sputum retention if the nasal humidification system is overwhelmed resulting in the isothermic saturation boundary moving distally. In addition, if nasal resistance increases in these patients and causes increasing mouth leak, treatment efficacy may be compromised. It is therefore common clinical practice for patients using noninvasive ventilation to be routinely prescribed heated humidification.

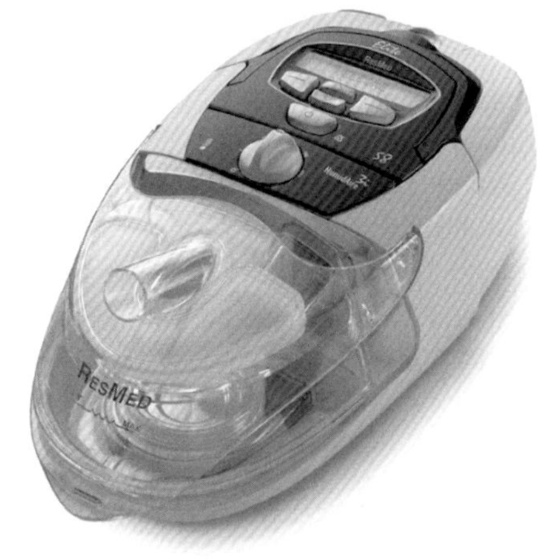

Fig. 5. An example of a heated humidification unit integrated with a CPAP unit. Copyright ResMed Limited 2005.

Treatment of Upper Airway Symptoms

Treatment of pre-existing nasal disease should always be considered in patients starting CPAP therapy, but is frequently neglected. Effective therapy may reduce a tendency to mouth breathe, and reduce the sensitivity of the nasal mucosa to drying, thereby significantly reducing nasal symptoms.

Full face masks offer a potential treatment as they prevent the high unidirectional nasal airflow caused by mouth leaks [16, 17]. Many patients find them difficult to use and less comfortable than a nasal mask, which has restricted their use for this indication. However, with improvements in design they are becoming an attractive alternative to heated humidification for some patients with upper airway symptoms. Some clinicians have advocated the use of oily nose drops, with the aim being to reduce nasal drying by providing a barrier to evaporation. The use of oily drops has not been subject to a clinical study, except where they were used as a control, and were found to be less effective than heated humidification [18]. Chin straps have been widely used to reduce mouth leaks, but the effect on nasal symptoms has not been studied. They may reduce but not eliminate mouth leaks, and are not always well tolerated, but are an inexpensive option for some patients.

The principle treatment of upper airway symptoms caused or exacerbated by PAP therapy is humidification. There are three types of devices available, heat and moisture exchangers (HMEs), cold passover humidifiers, and heated humidifiers. HMEs are membranes placed in the distal part of the CPAP tubing or the mask inlet that retain expired heat and moisture to humidify subsequent inspired air. These are ineffective for symptoms caused by mouth breathing because expired air does not pass through the membrane. Cold passover humidifiers use a reservoir of water at room temperature in the airpath with a large surface area to maximize evaporation. Humidity output is modest and reduces significantly during periods of high airflow associated with mouth leak. They have not been found to be effective in reducing increases in nasal resistance or nasal blood flow in normal subjects, or improving symptoms or CPAP use in clinical studies.

Heated humidification uses the same setup as cold passover humidification, except that the reservoir of water is heated to above 40°C. The water bath may be separate, or more commonly integrated with the CPAP device (fig. 5). Heated humidifiers are capable of producing fully saturated air at the mask at just above room temperature even with high airflow and effectively prevent nasal responses to high unidirectional airflow. The amount of water lost on respiring non-humidified air has been reported to be decreased by 44% with heated humidification compared with 16%

with cold passover humidification [19]. Heated humidifiers are the only humidification method that has been shown to reduce nasal symptoms or increase CPAP use in clinical studies.

Tube condensation is a problem frequently encountered with heated humidifiers and occurs because air rapidly cools between the humidifier and mask, reducing its ability to transport water. Condensation increases in conditions that promote heat loss from the tube such as cold ambient conditions or drafts, and can be reduced by decreasing the humidifier temperature, insulating the tube or increasing ambient temperature. Problems with condensation can generally be overcome with advice and some minor adjustment of the humidifier output. The possibility of iatrogenic respiratory infection from pathogens growing in the water bath is frequently raised as an issue, but there are no reported cases of this having occurred. There are a number of reasons that make this possibility unlikely. Patients using CPAP or non-invasive ventilation have intact upper airway defenses against infection in contrast to those who are intubated, the temperature of the water bath in most heated humidifiers is bacteriocidal to the majority of pathogens, and heated humidifiers produce molecules of water which are too small to transport pathogens. So unless water is accidentally spilled into the tube, there is no means of transport from the humidifier bath to the upper airway. Some clinicians advocate the use of sterile water for heated humidifiers to avoid the possibility of iatrogenic infection, but this is an unnecessary and expensive option.

The use of heated humidification in CPAP therapy for OSA has increased rapidly over the last decade. In the USA, it is estimated that two thirds of patients prescribed CPAP are also prescribed humidification. Some of this has been driven by reimbursement issues and the availability of integrated humidification with many CPAP devices, rather than clinical need. The use of cold passover humidifiers, which were once widely used, has declined considerably over this time. In Europe, the proportion prescribed heated humidification is somewhat lower at approximately a third of patients. To some extent the use of humidification is determined by the ambient conditions, with prescriptions being higher in locations with climatic extremes and the frequent use of central heating than in equatorial climates with less variation in temperature and higher ambient humidity.

References

1 Ingelstedt S: Studies on the conditioning of air in the respiratory tract. Acta Otolaryngol 1956;56:1–80.

2 Cruz AA, Togias AG, Lichtenstein LM, Kagey-Sobotka A, Proud D, Naclerio RM: Local application of atropine attenuates the upper airway reaction to cold, dry air. Am Rev Respir Dis 1992;146:340–346.

3 Strohl KP, Arnold JL, Decker MJ, Hoekje PL, McFadden ER: Nasal flow-resistive responses to challenge with cold dry air. J Appl Physiol 1992;72:1243–1246.

4 Togias AG, Naclerio RM, Proud D, Fish JE, Adkinson NF, Jr., Kagey-Sobotka A, Norman PS, Lichtenstein LM: Nasal challenge with cold, dry air results in release of inflammatory mediators. Possible mast cell involvement. J Clin Invest 1985;76:1375–1381.

5 Hayes MJ, McGregor FB, Roberts DN, Schroter RC, Pride NB: Continuous nasal positive airway pressure with a mouth leak: effect on nasal mucosal blood flux and nasal geometry. Thorax 1995;50:1179–1182.

6 Richards GN, Cistulli PA, Ungar RG, Berthon-Jones M, Sullivan CE: Mouth leak with nasal continuous positive airway pressure increases nasal airway resistance. Am J Respir Crit Care Med 1996;154: 182–186.

7 Engleman HM, Asgari-Jirhandeh N, McLeod AL, Ramsay CF, Deary IJ, Douglas NJ: Self-reported use of CPAP and benefits of CPAP therapy: a patient survey. Chest 1996;109: 1470–1476.

8 Hoffstein V, Viner S, Mateika S, Conway J: Treatment of obstructive sleep apnea with nasal continuous positive airway pressure: patient compliance, perception of benefits, and side effects. Am Rev Respir Dis 1992; 145:841–845.

9 Kribbs NB, Pack AI, Kline LR, Smith PL, Schwartz AR, Schubert NM, Redline S, Henry JN, Getsy JE, Dinges DF: Objective measurement of patterns of nasal CPAP use by patients with obstructive sleep apnea. Am Rev Respir Dis 1993;147:887–895.

10 Pepin JL, Leger P, Veale D, Langevin B, Robert D, Levy P: Side effects of nasal continuous positive airway pressure in sleep apnea syndrome: study of 193 patients in two French sleep centers. Chest 1995;107:375–381.

11 Massie CA, Hart RW, Peralez K, Richards GN: Effects of humidification on nasal symptoms and compliance in sleep apnea patients using continuous positive airway pressure. Chest 1999;116:403–408.

12 Neill AM, Wai HS, Bannan SP, Beasley CR, Weatherall M, Campbell AJ: Humidified nasal continuous positive airway pressure in obstructive sleep apnoea. Eur Respir J 2003;22: 258–262.

13 Rakotonanahary D, Pelletier-Fleury N, Gagnadoux F, Fleury B: Predictive factors for the need for additional humidification during nasal continuous positive airway pressure therapy. Chest 2001;119:460–465.

14 Mador MJ, Krauza M, Pervez A, Pierce D, Braun M: Effect of heated humidification on compliance and quality of life in patients with sleep apnea using nasal continuous positive airway pressure. Chest 2005;128: 2151–2158.

15 Weaver TE, Kribbs NB, Pack AI, Kline LR, Chugh DK, Maislin G, Smith PL, Schwartz AR, Schubert NM, Gillen KA, Dinges DF: Night-to-night variability in CPAP use over the first three months of treatment. Sleep 1997;20:278–283.

16 Martins de Araujo MT, Vieira SB, Vasquez EC, Fleury B: Heated humidification or face mask to prevent upper airway dryness during continuous positive airway pressure therapy. Chest 2000;117:142–147.

17 Mortimore IL, Whittle AT, Douglas NJ: Comparison of nose and face mask CPAP therapy for sleep apnoea. Thorax 1998;53:290–292.

18 Wiest GH, Lehnert G, Bruck WM, Meyer M, Hahn EG, Ficker JH: A heated humidifier reduces upper airway dryness during continuous positive airway pressure therapy. Respir Med 1999;93:21–26.

19 Randerath WJ, Meier J, Genger H, Domanski U, Ruhle KH: Efficiency of cold passover and heated humidification under continuous positive airway pressure. Eur Respir J 2002;20: 183–186.

Dr. G.N. Richards
ResMed Ltd, 97, Waterloo Road
North Ryde, NSW 2113 (Australia)
Tel. +61 2 9886 5000
Fax +61 2 9889 1483
E-Mail glennr@resmed.com.au

Randerath WJ, Sanner BM, Somers VK (eds): Sleep Apnea.
Prog Respir Res. Basel, Karger, 2006, vol 35, pp 151–159

Oral Appliances in the Treatment of Obstructive Sleep Apnea and Snoring

Marie Marklund

Department of Orthodontics, Umeå University, Umeå, Sweden

Abstract

This overview summarizes current knowledge of effects, side effects and indications for oral appliances in the treatment of patients with obstructive sleep apnea (OSA) and snoring. Mandibular repositioning appliances (MRAs) in various designs represent the most evaluated type of oral appliance. MRAs relocate the lower jaw forward and downward in order to prevent sleep-induced pharyngeal collapse. Short-term success rates with MRAs of over 80% of selected OSA patients have been reported, but figures vary. MRAs are indicated for patients with mild to moderate OSA, men with supine-dependent OSA and women. Patients with initial treatment success may benefit from MRAs over a long time, provided that they do not gain weight and wear high quality devices. There are few randomized controlled trials of treatment effects from MRAs on OSA, particularly regarding symptoms. MRA design, methodology and the teamwork between dentists and physicians has an influence on the treatment outcome. Continuous positive airway pressure is the primary treatment for patients with more severe OSA because of its superior effects compared with MRAs. Another drawback of MRAs is their dependence on healthy teeth and the risk of dental side effects. It is concluded that MRAs are indicated for selected patients with OSA, but more research is needed.

Highly effective treatments are required for patients with obstructive sleep apnea (OSA) who suffer from a varying severity of nightly breathing stops with poor oxygenation, irresistible daytime sleepiness and cognitive deficits in combination with longer-term increased risks for other disorders such as cardiovascular disease and accidents. The multicausal character of OSA, including factors such as gender, obesity, age, endocrine disorders and morphologic abnormalities indicates that a battery of treatments is desirable.

Oral appliances represent an attractive, simple and non-invasive treatment option for patients with OSA and snoring. Mandibular repositioning appliances (MRAs) in various designs are the most widespread and evaluated types of oral appliances [1, 2], and the effects and side effects of MRAs are therefore the main topic of this overview. Tongue-retaining devices, which intend to hold the tongue forward into an anterior bulb by suction, exemplify another, less effective type of oral appliance [1, 2]. MRAs widen the upper airway by holding the mandible forwards and downwards in order to avoid OSAs and snoring [1, 2]. Already at the beginning of the 20th century, Pierre Robin introduced a predecessor to the present MRA, the 'monoblock', to facilitate breathing in children with extremely retropositioned lower jaws and problems to keep their airways unobstructed during sleep. Similar types of devices have been extensively used in orthodontics in children and adolescents for the treatment of distal occlusion, i.e. the lower dentition retropositioned in relation to the upper dentition, since the repositioning of the lower jaw by the device will produce corrective forces on the teeth when the mandible makes efforts to relocate backwards and upwards again. Only during the last two decades, MRAs

Table 1. Results from crossover studies comparing MRA with placebo treatments or CPAP [3–12]

	Recruited patients	Both arms	Inclusion criteria	AHI, RDI or ODI mean value (SD) [SEM]						Objective snoring
				Baseline	Placebo device	Placebo tablet	MRA	% success	CPAP	largest reduction
MRA vs. *placebo device*										
Gotsopoulos et al. [2002]	85	73	RDI ≥ 10[a]	27 [2]	25 [2]		12 (2)	36%[b]		MRA
Johnston et al. [2002]	21	20	ODI ≥ 10	32 (21)	38 (25)		23 (23)	33%[c]		
Mehta et al. [2001]	28	24	AHI ≥ 10[a]	27 (17)	30 [2]		14 [2]	38%[b]		MRA
MRA vs. *CPAP*										
Barnes et al. [2004]	114	80	AHI 5–30	21 [1.3]		20 [1.1]	14 [1.1]		4.8 [0.5]	
Engleman et al. [2002]	51	48	AHI ≥ 5[a]	31 (26)			15 (16)	19%[b]	8 (6)	
Randerath et al. [2002]	20	20	AHI 5–30[a]	18 (7.7)			14 (11)	30%[c]	3.2 (2.9)	CPAP
Tan et al. [2002]	24	21	AHI 10–49	22 (10)			8.0 (11)	70%[c]	3.1 (2.8)	
Ferguson et al. [1997]	24	20	AHI 15–55[a]	24–25			14 (15)	55%[d]	4.0 (2.2)	
Ferguson et al. [1996]	27	21	AHI 15–50	18–20			9.7 (7.3)	48%[d]	3.6 (1.7)	

Values for AHI, RDI and ODI represent mean values (SD) [SEM]. [a] + symptoms; [b] AHI < 5; [c] AHI < 10; [d] AHI < 10 + relief of symptoms.

have become a widespread treatment modality for adult patients with OSA and snoring.

High percentages of treatment success in OSA, of over 80% of selected patients have been reported, but the figures are highly variable in the few randomized controlled studies (table 1) and many case series that have been conducted so far [1–12]. The randomized controlled trials have shown clear reductions of OSAs from MRAs, whilst the effects on symptoms and snoring as well as the longer-term health effects and side effects have been less tested [3–11]. A recent Cochrane review has stated that the evidence for MRA treatment is limited and that continuous positive airway pressure (CPAP) should be regarded as the first treatment of choice [12]. At present, MRAs are therefore primarily indicated for patients with snoring or mild to moderate OSA, men with supine-dependent OSA and women, and as a secondary treatment in patients who do not tolerate CPAP and have no other OSA treatment [1, 2, 13, 14].

Side effects from MRAs are common in the shorter term, e.g. increased salivation and tender teeth, but these are considered negligible among patients who continue using the device [1, 2, 13]. Longer-term dental side effects are mainly manifested as bite changes, which may occur in one fifth of the patients after 2 years and thereafter progress with time [1, 2, 13, 15]. Once in a while these adverse events result in recommendations to discontinue MRA treatment and the need for another therapy for sleep apnea, although many patients consider that the advantages of the device outweigh the negative effects on the teeth. Methods to avoid these adverse events will be of importance for the long-term usage of MRAs in clinical practice. New data show that the initial bite characteristics and the design of MRA predict the bite changes during longer-term treatment [15].

Teamwork between dentists who are specialized in sleep apnea treatments and physicians and the continuous education in the discipline are essential for optimal results with this method [1]. A great number of patients are treated with oral appliances today, despite the fact that there is a need for more evidence for this method. Some patients have continued to use their devices for a long time, since the treatment was introduced in the middle of the 1980s. It is therefore likely that the benefits from the treatment are more obvious for many patients and their therapists than the scientific evidence shows so far, a fact which encourages more research in the field.

Mechanism of Action

Oral appliances target the sleep-induced decrease in upper airway dimensions, which is suggested to cause OSAs in patients with undersized upper airways [1, 2, 13, 16]. A retropositioned or small lower jaw or increased soft tissue volume may cause the reduced upper airway size. Pharynx is longer and laterally constricted and the soft palate and tongue may be enlarged in OSA patients [16]. The lateral narrowing in the upper airway consists of a combination of increased amount of fat tissue and muscle volume [16]. During sleep in the supine position, the upper airway is particularly small when the lower jaw and soft palate move backwards from gravitational forces. The velopharyngeal area is the most changeable and vulnerable site of the upper airway in OSA patients [16]. A collapse in this region leads to subsequently increased risks of airway narrowing at more caudally located sites.

MRAs stabilize the lower jaw forward and downward with the intention to indirectly reposition the tongue and soft palate in the same direction in order to increase upper airway dimensions and reduce the effects of the sleep-induced decrease in pharyngeal dilator muscle activity [1, 2, 16]. It has been shown, that MRAs enlarge the upper airway, in oro-, velo- and hypopharynx and reduce the pharyngeal collapsibility [1, 2]. There is predominantly a lateral enlargement of the upper airway, but also an anterior-posterior expansion has been observed [1, 2, 16, 17]. In this way, the tongue gets more space and becomes flatter and more stretched out, equivalent to the mandibular advancement [17]. The hyoid bone and the mandible approach [1]. The mechanical fixation of the lower jaw forward by the device is probably of importance for the mechanism of the device. The pharyngeal resistance has been found to diminish during the passive repositioning of the mandible, but not during an active protrusion of the lower jaw [18]. Possibly, muscles which stiffen the upper airway relax by the device and this may also cause the increased lateral dimensions in the pharynx. There are also indications that MRAs increase the activity in some other upper airway dilator muscles such as the genioglossus muscle [1]. A reduced nasal resistance during mandibular advancement may further contribute to the mechanism of the device.

Successfully treated patients receive a larger increase of upper airway dimensions than patients who experience treatment failure with MRAs, independent of the degree of mandibular advancement and disease severity [17]. The soft palate moves more forward and pharynx becomes less flexed in good responders compared with nonresponders [17]. Women increase their airway dimensions more than men do when they move their lower jaws forwards [19]. On the contrary, OSA patients who have a long soft palate, an inferiorly positioned hyoid bone, an enlarged lower face height or a small mandible have a reduced chance to widen their airways by MRAs.

In summary, MRAs increase the upper airway dimensions and reduce the pharyngeal collapsibility. OSA patients will therefore be able to withstand more negative pressure during breathing at night and reduce their risk of suffering from sleep-induced OSAs compared with untreated conditions.

The Mandibular Repositioning

The degree of mandibular repositioning by MRA is a crucial question, since this procedure is closely linked to the treatment effect of the device. Larger forward displacements of the mandible have given larger reductions in OSAs [20], oxygen desaturations and pharyngeal collapsibility compared with smaller advancements, often in a dose-dependent way [14, 20]. Nonadvanced devices are inefficient or may aggravate OSA. Clinical recommendations of more than 5 mm mandibular advancement, percentage values of above 50 or 75% of maximum protrusion or maximal comfortable protrusion are common for MRAs. The vertical displacement by MRA is usually advised to be kept to a minimum, since large openings cause a backward rotation of the lower jaw and this relocation may impinge on upper airway dimensions. Still, advancements within a wide range, from 0 to 12 mm have been related to treatment success [14, 20]. Openings of 4–14 mm have produced similar apnea reductions, although the patients preferred the smaller opening [1, 2]. Probably, the structural response in the pharynx from the mandibular repositioning is modulated by factors such as the pretreatment pharyngeal or craniomandibular morphology, gender and disease severity.

A forward and downward relocation of the mandible is certainly necessary for optimal effects from an MRA. The amount of mandibular displacement that is required for the individual patient can, so far, not be predicted and has to be titrated during the initial treatment period.

Types of MRAs

Two-piece adjustable MRAs are the most popular types of oral appliances, since these enable an easy titration of the

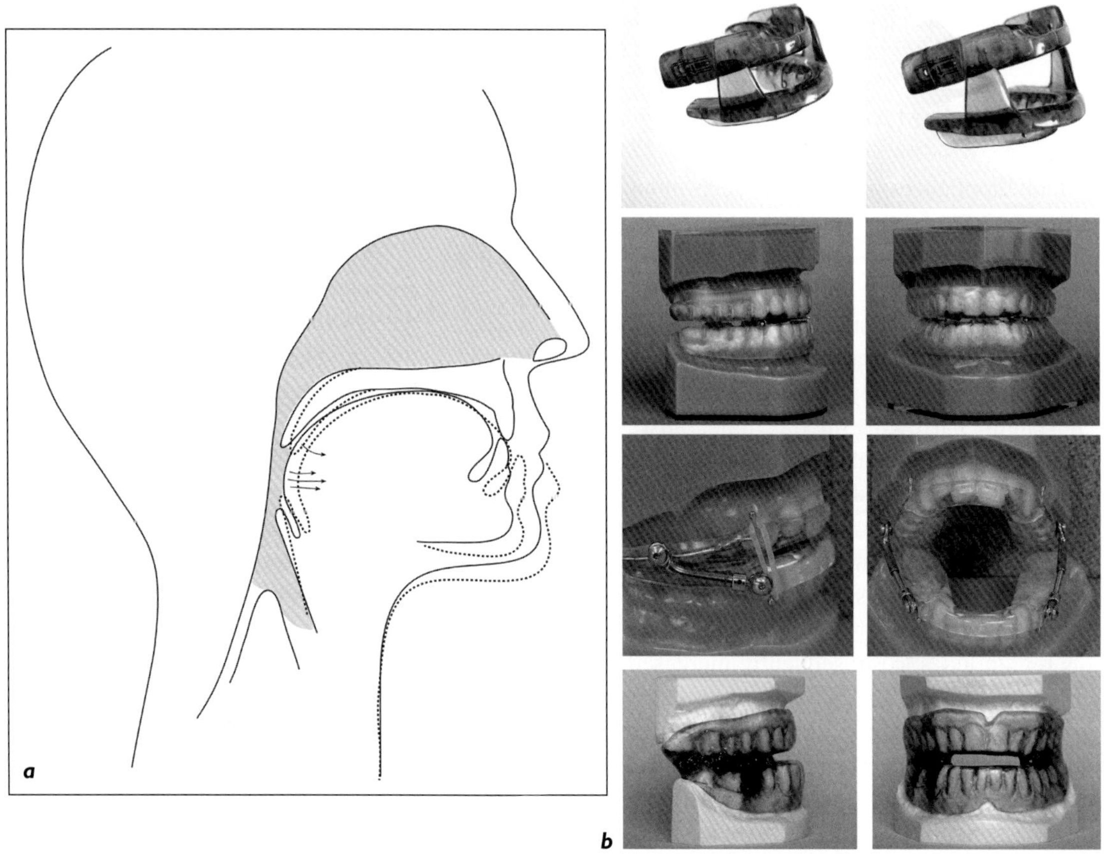

Fig. 1. ***a*** The intended effect of MRA on the soft palate and tongue. ***b*** From top: SomnoMed adjustable oral appliance (courtesy of SomnoMed), Klearway adjustable oral appliance (courtesy of Prof. Alan A. Lowe and Great Lakes Orthodontics, Ltd., Tonawanda, N.Y., USA), Herbst adjustable oral appliance (courtesy of Great Lakes Orthodontics, Ltd.), Monoblock elastomeric oral appliance.

optimal degree of mandibular advancement (fig. 1). A remotely controlled MRA may further facilitate the titration procedure [21]. One-piece, monoblock types of MRAs, in contrast, are made with the mandible in a fixed position (fig. 1). Adjustment of these devices has to be performed at a dental laboratory, where the upper and lower parts of the device are separated and thereafter fixated together in another position after a new bite registration from the patient. Custom-made MRAs are most common. These devices are made from individual plaster casts and a wax index, which determines the mandibular repositioning. There are also prefabricated MRAs, often of the boil-and-bite type. A prefabricated device has been found to be ineffective in reducing sleep apneas compared with the effects from a custom-made one [22]. This may be explained by a poorer fixation to the teeth of a prefabricated device compared with an MRA which is made to fit the individual dentition. Various designs of custom-made devices also differ in their effects on OSA. The adjustable Karwetzky activator produced a better apnea reduction than another adjustable device, the Silensor® [1, 2]. On the other hand, there were similar effects on sleep apneas from a monoblock MRA and the adjustable Herbst appliance with similar degrees of mandibular advancement, but the monoblock device produced better effects on symptoms, snoring, sleep arousals and slow wave sleep than the adjustable device [1, 2]. In yet another study, the Herbst appliance had a better effect on subjective sleepiness than the adjustable Twin Block appliance, although these two devices were equally effective against sleep apnea [23].

More comparisons of treatment effects on OSA and snoring between different designs of MRAs are essential in order to define golden standards for construction details for these appliances.

Definitions of Treatment Success

Different definitions of treatment success for MRAs have been used, such as a cut-off point of the total apnea/hypopnea index, with limits of below 5, 10 or 15. The percentage reduction of sleep apneas, with a cut-off point at 50% has also been used to define treatment success. The relief of pretreatment symptoms, mainly daytime sleepiness is often added to the above criteria.

Effects on OSA

Treatment success defined in various ways has varied from 19 to over 80% of selected OSA patients treated with MRAs [1] (table 1). A recent Cochrane review has stated that there are clear effects from MRAs on OSA with reductions of 11–15 apneas and hypopneas per hour of sleep compared with placebo treatment according to results from studies so far [5, 7, 8, 11, 12] (table 1). Arousals are reduced, and there are also indications that minimum oxygen desaturation increases with an active device compared with a placebo treatment [5, 7, 8, 11, 12]. CPAP has, however, a better effect on sleep apnea with further reductions of 8–13 apneas and hypopneas per hour of sleep compared with MRAs [3, 4, 6, 9–12]. There is also a larger increase in minimum oxygen desaturation and decrease in sleep arousals from CPAP compared with oral appliances [3, 4, 9–12]. These comparisons have primarily been derived from samples of patients within the milder range of disease severity with apnea/hypopnea indices of between 5 to 30, with only single cases above that level. Also among the mildest cases with an apnea/hypopnea index between 5 and 15, CPAP produced better effects on sleep apneas than MRA [11]. Still, symptoms were equally reduced by both treatments and the patients preferred MRAs [11].

A comparison between MRA and uvulopalatopharyngo plasty (UPPP), has shown that MRA more effectively reduces sleep apneas among patients who continue using the device [1, 2, 12]. The effects on sleepiness and vitality were similar between the two treatments, but the patients were more content with UPPP. Disadvantages from the two treatments include persistent swallowing problems in 10% of patients treated with UPPP and the discontinuation of treatment in about one third of MRA patients after 4 years. Many patients with insufficient positive effects from UPPP may, however, experience treatment success with MRAs.

MRAs are effective in selected patients with sleep apnea. CPAP should, however, be regarded as the first treatment of choice in patients with a more severe OSA.

Predictors of Treatment Success

Predictors of treatment success with MRAs are usually sought among the ethological factors in OSA, e.g. male gender, obesity, craniomandibular abnormalities and age, disease severity and the possibilities for these devices to counteract a pharyngeal collapse. In this way, the elimination of the pharyngeal obstruction during mandibular advancement and a concomitant Muller manoeuvre [24] or during sedation [25] observed by MRI imaging or nasendoscopy has predicted treatment success in OSA and snoring. New results suggest that awake flow-volume curves may predict the treatment response to MRAs [26]. Validation of these methods in larger samples may result in useful prediction methods.

In a large cohort of treated patients, the predictive strength of variables from the sleep apnea recording, MRA design and a number of background variables were tested [14]. There was a gender difference in treatment effect in favor of the women in that study. Among men, supine-dependent sleep apneas and a larger mandibular advancement favored success, while weight increase during treatment related to a poorer treatment outcome. Among women, it was favorable to have a milder disease and no symptoms of nasal congestion. The gender difference in treatment effect of MRAs may be explained by the longer and more collapsible airway in men compared with what has been found in women [14], with increasing difficulties to avoid upper airway collapse by the simple mandibular repositioning procedure in men. In addition, men more often have supine-dependent sleep apneas and they also reduce their upper airway dimensions more when they move their lower jaws backwards from a rest position compared with women [27]. This probably explains why position dependency and the degree of mandibular advancement were good predictors of treatment success in men only in that study [14].

A number of morphologic predictor variables for MRAs have also been proposed, but the value of these in the predictions of treatment success in clinical practice is uncertain. Consequently, a short soft palate, a narrow pharynx or a wide one and a high tongue position as well as a number of skeletal variables such as maxillar prognathia, mandibular retrognathia and either a large mandibular plane angle or a small one have been related to treatment success with MRAs [13]. Also younger and slimmer patients with thinner necks have been found to be more successful with the device compared with older and more obese patients [1]. In line with these results, a weight increase by more than 3–4 kg during treatment has been related to a reduced chance of treatment success with MRA in men with OSA [14]. In many studies, there is no association between obesity or age and MRA treatment effects. The continuum of craniofacial and pharyngeal abnormalities in relation to other factors such as the degree of obesity and age as well as difficulties in measuring the pharyngeal soft tissue morphology may explain the inconsistent results.

Sleep apnea recording and patient records contain useful prediction information. A milder disease, supine dependency in men, female gender, younger age and less obesity are related to treatment success. The benefits from additional diagnostic tools such as cephalometry or MRI have to be evaluated in more studies before the risks and costs related to these procedures can be considered. More research regarding predictors of treatment success for MRAs in OSA is needed.

Effects on Symptoms

Many snorers seek medical attention because of poor sleep quality and problems to keep awake during the daytime. The majority of OSA patients suffer from excessive daytime sleepiness [28, 29]. Snoring women are particularly affected by sleepiness. Frequent awakenings at night with sleep disruption and oxygenation dips are suggested to cause daytime sleepiness and cognitive deficits in patients with OSA [28]. Daytime sleepiness is, however, more common than cognitive deficits in sleep apnea patients [29]. This is compatible with the pathophysiological mechanism that cognitive impairment and effects on quality of life occur as a result of increased sleepiness rather than being a primary symptom [29]. A more severe disease is therefore related to poorer cognitive performance compared with a milder disease. Sleepiness may, however, exist together with a large variation in sleep apnea frequency [29]. Consequently, it may be difficult to evaluate treatment effects on symptoms in patients who have been selected mainly on the basis of laboratory measurements of sleep apneas rather than sleepiness or cognitive dysfunction.

Despite the frequent symptoms of OSA, there are few randomized controlled trials of effects of MRAs on sleepiness and cognitive function [4, 6–8, 10–12]. This probably reflects the fact that oral appliances are primarily recommended for patients with mild OSA and snoring, who have been regarded to suffer from less symptoms and consequences on everyday life than patients with a more severe disease. Also, CPAP has been found to produce less symptomatic effects in patients with milder sleep apnea than in patients with a more severe disease [29].

Slight reduction in subjective sleepiness, measured as 1- to 2-step decrease in the Epworth Sleepiness Scale score has been detected in patients treated with MRAs in comparison with patients treated with control devices [7, 8, 12] or a placebo tablet [11], but the results are inconsistent. The decrease in subjective sleepiness from MRAs has been suggested to be similar to that of CPAP or poorer, depending on factors such as the design of the oral appliance and patient's compliance [4, 6, 10–12]. The effect of MRA on objective sleepiness is variable [1, 11], although this may be an effect of the lack of objective sleepiness among cases with milder OSA. Despite the insufficient evidence for these devices regarding symptoms, clinical experience witnesses of patients who describe that they have got a 'new life' with their devices.

Inconsistent results regarding effects on cognitive performance, well-being and health have been found for both CPAP and MRAs, with equal effects in some studies and a better effect from CPAP than MRA in others [6, 10–12]. Placebo effects on tests of neuropsychological function, mood and quality of life [11] and risks for hang-over effects in crossover studies make the overall results of cognitive effects of MRAs difficult to interpret.

The evidence for symptomatic effects from MRAs is insufficient so far.

Effects on Snoring

An MRA has been found to reduce subjective and objective snoring in frequency and loudness compared with a control device in the short-term [1] (table 1). Snoring is, however, better controlled with CPAP than with MRA (table 1). Objective reduction of about half of the number of snores per hour of sleep has been calculated in combined results from studies of patients treated with MRAs [30]. One uncontrolled study has been performed on patients with upper airway resistance syndrome, who responded with reduced subjective and objective daytime sleepiness, a better sleep quality with less fragmentation and less snoring [13].

MRA reduces the frequency and loudness of snoring. There are no methods to predict the successful reduction in snoring, so far.

Effects on Blood Pressure

The short-term effects of MRAs on blood pressure have been evaluated in two studies [11, 31]. In one study, there was a decrease in the 24-hour diastolic blood pressure after 4-week treatment with MRAs compared with control devices in symptomatic OSA patients [31]. The blood pressure was particularly reduced in the early morning hours with an average of 3 mm Hg in patients treated with MRAs [31]. The authors concluded that the effect of oral appliance therapy on blood pressure was similar to that of CPAP according to previous reports. In the other study, the diastolic blood pressure decreased only during the night after 3 months of treatment with MRAs [11].

There are promising results regarding reductions in blood pressure from MRAs in a few studies. More studies including the knowledge of the underlying mechanism for the increase in blood pressure among OSA patients may lead to better understanding of treatment effects of MRAs on secondary effects from OSA.

Long-Term Effects

Patients who experience initial treatment success have about 80% chance to remain so, if they continue to use their MRAs for the following 2–5 years according to a few, long-term studied, small samples [13]. Increased snoring during treatment is common.

The follow-up of patients in the longer term is important, since factors such as weight gain, a worn out appliance and redevelopment of symptoms may require adjustment or replacement of the appliance, reassessment of the condition with a new sleep apnea recording or recommendations of another treatment.

Compliance

One quarter of patients who initiate treatment have been reported to discontinue during the first years [14] and more than two thirds may give up the treatment in the longer term [2]. Patients with pretreatment symptoms and the effective control of these [13], patients who do not experience side effects and nonobese patients have a higher compliance rate than others [14], which indicates that the compliance rate is highly related to the efficacy of the appliance.

Patient's Preference

Three studies so far have compared different types of MRAs regarding patient's preference, but there is no general consensus based on these results. In one study [1, 2], more patients preferred a monoblock MRA to the adjustable Herbst appliance, and in another study [23], more patients preferred the Herbst appliance to the adjustable Twin Block device. Finally, more patients preferred the adjustable hard acrylic Karwetzky activator to the Silensor, a soft elastomeric adjustable device [1, 2]. However, most patients who respond to treatment prefer MRA to CPAP, probably because the oral appliances are generally easier to use [1, 3, 4, 12].

No specific appliance has yet been identified to be best tolerated by the patients. The skills of the therapist in relation to a specific type of treatment most certainly also influence the patient's choice of appliance.

Contraindications

One third of patients who have been referred to a sleep laboratory for suspected sleep apnea have been found to have odontological contraindications, such as an insufficient number of teeth, periodontal disease or temporomandibular joint disorders [1, 2]. Another fifth of the patients may require close supervision of their dental conditions in order to avoid odontological complications during treatment with MRAs [1, 2]. Although oral health shows demographical, socioeconomical and age-related differences, these figures clearly demonstrate a restriction for this type of treatment.

Side Effects

Temporary short-term side effects from the introduction of a foreign body in the mouth are common. The nightly use of MRAs gives, however, more problems with excessive salivation or dryness, tenderness of teeth and jaws and the perception of an abnormal bite in the mornings than control devices [1, 2, 12, 13]. Exaggerated gag reflex, fracture of teeth and fillings or an aggravation of a temoporomandibular joint disorder may also complicate the treatment [1, 2]. These short-term adverse effects have been considered to be negligible among patients who continue treatment. On the other hand, patients with a poor treatment outcome report more dominating side effects compared with patients who use an efficient appliance.

In the longer term, most side effects disappear [1, 2, 13]. No permanent effects on the temoporomandibular joint [20] or masticatory muscles have been observed, but the development of abnormal bites becomes more common. The patients are seldom aware of any adverse effects on the dentition, except for the more extreme ones [13]. The prevention of upper airway collapse during sleep by the forward and vertical displacement of the mandible produces backward forces on the upper teeth and maxilla and forwardly directed forces on the lower dentition and the mandible when the lower jaw attempts to go back to its normal postural position. The expected orthodontic effects with a backward tipping of the upper front teeth, a forward movement of the lower front teeth and mandible are more or less clinically obvious, but may also be monitored on cephalograms. The distance between the incisors in the sagittal and vertical direction, the overjet and the overbite, diminishes [13]. Depending on the initial bite characteristics, this will have a different impact on various patients. A normal bite may change into a mesial occlusion, i.e. the lower dentition anterior to the upper dentition. In contrast, patients with distal occlusion may receive more normal bite conditions during treatment. After 2 years, about one fifth of the patients have been found to receive bite changes of more than 1 mm, and after 5 years this figure has increased to about one third of the patients [13]. Extreme bite changes have been reported in single patients, with 3–5 mm change in dental occlusion after about 2 years [13]. Unacceptable dental side effects result in recommendations for an alternative treatment. Even so, clinical experience suggests that many patients prefer to continue with their appliances, since the advantages from the treatment are more important for them than the problems with bite changes. Moreover, the bite changes often diminish in patients who discontinue with the appliance.

A deep bite with the upper incisors interlocking the lower ones with 3 mm or more diminishes the risk for long-term bite changes [15]. The use of a soft elastomeric appliance which extends over the alveolar processes or a smaller repositioning by the appliance have also been found to reduce the change in dental occlusion compared with the use of a hard acrylic appliance that is only fixed to the teeth or larger displacements of the lower jaw by the appliance. These prediction possibilities will be particularly useful in patients with initially normal bites.

Bite changes represent an increasing problem with the common use of MRAs during longer periods of time. The bite changes may be reduced by the individualization of appliance design, patient selection and more intense follow-up of patients who are at risk of dental side effects.

Interdisciplinary Collaboration

The interdisciplinary collaboration is of great importance to receive optimal treatment effects from MRAs. The physician at the sleep apnea clinic has the diagnostic, therapeutic and overall medical responsibility for the treatment. The dentist takes care of the more precise installation of MRAs including odontological concerns and the regular follow-ups of treatment in close collaboration with the sleep apnea clinic. A written referral including the results from the sleep apnea recording and a preliminary oral examination is sent by the physician to the dentist who is trained to treat sleep apnea and snoring. After a more detailed oral examination, the dentist determines if the patient is suitable for an oral appliance and informs the patient about the expected effects and side effects from the appliance before treatment starts. The patient is referred back to the sleep laboratory for a renewed sleep apnea recording with the appliance, after the dentist has evaluated the treatment regarding subjective effects and comfort. A follow-up sleep recording is recommended, since the improvement of symptoms is insufficient to predict a successful apnea reduction by the appliance. Twenty-five percent of patients who report reduced snoring with MRAs have been observed to have an insufficient apnea reduction by this type of treatment. The exact regimen for longer-term follow-up has to be individualized based on a number of factors such as sleep apnea severity, type of bite and oral health. During the follow-up visits, the dentist monitors the usage, side effects and other complications, the effectiveness of the appliance on snoring, sleepiness and sleep apneas and the condition of the appliance. The control of side effects at least every 2nd year and the replacement of the appliance with a new one within a period of 3–5 years are often necessary. The continuous contact with the sleep laboratory is important, since the treatment effects on OSA may vary over time, which may necessitate a renewed sleep apnea recording or the patient may desire another treatment for sleep apnea because of side effects or medical concerns.

Conclusions

MRAs are an established treatment for selected patients with OSA and snoring. More research is needed, however, to determine which patients will particularly benefit from the appliance, especially regarding symptomatic effects, long-term effects and the risk of side effects.

Continuous education and the exchange of knowledge between different areas of expertise in this new field of sleep medicine will be of particular importance for this highly interdisciplinary treatment modality.

References

1 Ferguson KA, Cartwright R, Rogers R, Schmidt-Nowara W: Oral appliances for snoring and obstructive sleep apnea: a review. Sleep 2006;29:244–262.

2 Hoekema A, Stegenga B, De Bont LG: Efficacy and co-morbidity of oral appliances in the treatment of obstructive sleep apnea-hypopnea: a systematic review. Crit Rev Oral Biol Med 2004;15:137–155.

3 Ferguson KA, Ono T, Lowe AA, Keenan SP, Fleetham JA: A randomized crossover study of an oral appliance vs. nasal continuous positive airway pressure in the treatment of mild-moderate obstructive sleep apnea. Chest 1996;109:1269–1275.

4 Ferguson KA, Ono T, Lowe AA, al-Majed S, Love LL, Fleetham JA: A short term controlled trial of an adjustable oral appliance for the treatment of mild to moderate obstructive sleep apnoea. Thorax 1997;52:362–368.

5 Mehta A, Qian J, Petocz P, Darendeliler MA, Cistulli PA: A randomized, controlled study of a mandibular advancement splint for obstructive sleep apnea. Am J Respir Crit Care Med 2001;163:1457–1461.

6 Engleman HM, McDonald JP, Graham D, Lello GE, Kingshott RN, Coleman EL, Mackay TW, Douglas NJ: Randomized crossover trial of two treatments for sleep apnea/hypopnea syndrome: continuous positive airway pressure and mandibular repositioning splint. Am J Respir Crit Care Med 2002;166:855–859.

7 Gotsopoulos H, Chen C, Qian J, Cistulli PA: Oral appliance therapy improves symptoms in obstructive sleep apnea: a randomized, controlled trial. Am J Respir Crit Care Med 2002;166:743–748.

8 Johnston CD, Gleadhill IC, Cinnamond MJ, Gabbey J, Burden DJ: Mandibular advancement appliances and obstructive sleep apnoea: a randomized clinical trial. Eur J Orthod 2002;24:251–262.

9 Randerath WJ, Heise M, Hinz R, Ruehle KH: An individually adjustable oral appliance vs. continuous positive airway pressure in mild-to-moderate obstructive sleep apnea syndrome. Chest 2002;122:569–575.

10 Tan YK, L'Estrange PR, Luo YM, Smith C, Grant HR, Simonds AK, Spiro SG, Battagel JM: Mandibular advancement splints and continuous positive airway pressure in patients with obstructive sleep apnoea: a randomized cross-over trial. Eur J Orthod 2002;24: 239–249.

11 Barnes M, McEvoy RD, Banks S, Tarquinio N, Murray CG, Vowles N, Pierce RJ: Efficacy of positive airway pressure and oral appliance in mild to moderate obstructive sleep apnea. Am J Respir Crit Care Med 2004;170:656–664.

12 Lim J, Lasserson TJ, Fleetham J, Wright J: Oral appliances for obstructive sleep apnoea. Cochrane Database Syst Rev 2006;1: CD004435.

13 Cistulli PA, Gotsopoulos H, Marklund M, Lowe AA: Treatment of snoring and obstructive sleep apnea with mandibular repositioning appliances. Sleep Med Rev 2004;8: 443–457.

14 Marklund M, Stenlund H, Franklin KA: Mandibular advancement devices in 630 men and women with obstructive sleep apnea and snoring: tolerability and predictors of treatment success. Chest 2004;125:1270–1278.

15 Marklund M: Predictors of long-term orthodontic side-effects from mandibular advancement devices in patients with snoring and obstructive sleep apnea. Am J Orthod Dentofacial Orthop 2006;29:214–221.

16 Schwab RJ, Kuna ST, Remmers JE: Anatomy and physiology of upper airway obstruction; in Kryger MH, Roth T, Dement WC (eds): Principles and Practice of Sleep Medicine, ed 4. Philadelphia, Elsevier Saunders, 2005, pp 983–1000.

17 Tsuiki S, Lowe AA, Almeida FR, Kawahata N, Fleetham JA: Effects of mandibular advancement on airway curvature and obstructive sleep apnoea severity. Eur Respir J 2004;23: 263–268.

18 Lorino AM, Maza M, d'Ortho MP, Coste A, Harf A, Lorino H: Effects of mandibular advancement on respiratory resistance. Eur Respir J 2000;16:928–932.

19 Battagel JM, Johal A, L'Estrange PR, Croft CB, Kotecha B: Changes in airway and hyoid position in response to mandibular protrusion in subjects with obstructive sleep apnoea (OSA). Eur J Orthod 1999;21:363–376.

20 de Almeida FR, Bittencourt LR, de Almeida CI, Tsuiki S, Lowe AA, Tufik S: Effects of mandibular posture on obstructive sleep apnea severity and the temporomandibular joint in patients fitted with an oral appliance. Sleep 2002;25;507–513.

21 Tsai WH, Vazquez JC, Oshima T, Dort L, Roycroft B, Lowe AA, Hajduk E, Remmers JE: Remotely controlled mandibular positioner predicts efficacy of oral appliances in sleep apnea. Am J Respir Crit Care Med 2004;170:366–370.

22 Vanderveken OM, Marklund M, Braem MJ, Devolder A, Boudewyns AN, Verbracken J, Franklin KA, De Backer WA, Van de Heyning PH: Comparison of a custom-made and a prefabricated mandibular advancement device for treatment of sleep-disordered breathing: a prospective, randomized cross-over trial. (Abstract, ATS 2005).

23 Lawton HM, Battagel JM, Kotecha B: A comparison of the Twin Block and Herbst mandibular advancement splints in the treatment of patients with obstructive sleep apnoea: a prospective study. Eur J Orthod 2005;27: 82–90.

24 Sanner BM, Heise M, Knoben B, Machnick M, Laufer U, Kikuth R, Zidek W, Hellmich B: MRI of the pharynx and treatment efficacy of a mandibular advancement device in obstructive sleep apnoea syndrome. Eur Respir J 2002;20:143–150.

25 Battagel JM, Johal A, Kotecha BT: Sleep nasendoscopy as a predictor of treatment success in snorers using mandibular advancement splints. J Laryngol Otol 2005;119:106–112.

26 Zeng B, Gotsopoulos H, Ng AT, Qian J, Darendeliler AM, Cistulli PA: Can flow-volume curves predict the outcome of mandibular advancement splint (MAS) treatment in OSA patients? (Abstract, ATS 2005).

27 Mohsenin V: Effects of gender on upper airway collapsibility and severity of obstructive sleep apnea. Sleep Med 2003;4:523–529.

28 Weaver TE, George CFP: Cognition and performance in patients with obstructive sleep apnea; in Kryger MH, Roth T, Dement WC (eds): Principles and Practice of Sleep Medicine, ed 4. Philadelphia, Elsevier Saunders, 2005, pp 1023–1033.

29 Engleman HM, Douglas NJ: Sleep 4: Sleepiness, cognitive function, and quality of life in obstructive sleep apnoea/hypopnoea syndrome. Thorax 2004;59:618–622.

30 Hoffstein V: Snoring and upper airway resistance; in Kryger MH, Roth T, Dement WC (eds): Principles and Practice of Sleep Medicine. ed 4. Philadelphia, Elsevier Saunders, 2005, pp 1001–1012.

31 Gotsopoulos H, Kelly JJ, Cistulli PA: Oral appliance therapy reduces blood pressure in obstructive sleep apnea: a randomized, controlled trial. Sleep 2004;27;934–941.

Marie Marklund
Department of Orthodontics
Umeå University
SE–901 87 Umeå (Sweden)
Tel. +46 907 856195
Fax +46 901 32578
E-Mail Marie.Marklund@odont.umu.se

Randerath WJ, Sanner BM, Somers VK (eds): Sleep Apnea.
Prog Respir Res. Basel, Karger, 2006, vol 35, pp 160–163

Electrical Stimulation of the Upper Airways Muscles

Winfried J. Randerath

Institute for Pneumology at the University Witten/Herdecke, Clinic for Pneumology and Allergology, Center of Sleep Medicine and Respiratory Care, Bethanien Hospital, Solingen, Germany

Abstract

The upper airway muscles are importantly affected in obstructive sleep apnea syndrome (OSAS). The most important dilator, the genioglossus, shows augmented activity during wakefulness which decreases during sleep. Moreover, it shows greater fatigue and structural changes such as abnormal fiber morphology, inflammation and increased connective tissue in OSAS. Because of the crucial role of the muscles in the upper airway patency there is interest if electrical stimulation can improve the efficacy of the muscles and lead to new therapeutic options for OSAS. Indeed, the upper airways resistance can experimentally be reduced in animals, healthy persons and patients with OSAS using surface and intraneural stimulation. To translate these results in clinical application, apnea-triggered stimulation during sleep has been studied. However, although there were some positive effects the results were inconsistent and relevant side effects, such as arousals, were found. Tongue muscle training is the most recent approach to improve the function of the upper airways muscles. However, although snoring significantly improved there was no relevant reduction of respiratory disturbances in general. In conclusion, neurostimulation cannot be recommended for clinical use at this time. However, the available data prove the importance of the muscles in the pathophysiology of OSAS and the partial positive effects in patients encourage to go forward with this approach.

Obstruction of the upper airways in obstructive sleep apnea syndrome (OSAS) is associated with diminished neuromuscular activity of the dilating muscles [1] that stiffen the pharyngeal airway during inspiration [2]. Several factors have been proposed to influence the muscle tone of the upper airways: The ineffective muscle response to hypercapnia, hypoxia or negative pressure may be a possible predisposing factor for OSAS [3]. Moreover, breathing through a narrowed airway generates a greater negative intraluminal pressure, which increases the collapsing force so that pharyngeal muscles must contract more forcefully [3]. The activity of the dilator muscles is dependent on the sleep state. With sleep onset, supraglottic resistance increases in healthy persons. This phenomenon is even more pronounced in snorers and sleep apnea patients. Recent findings indicate that topical receptor mechanisms in the nasopharynx importantly influence the dilator activity in OSAS [4]. However, at sleep onset, the activity decreases largely in most patients [5].

The genioglossus muscle is one of the major pharyngeal dilators which pulls the tongue forward, thereby enlarging the cross-section of the upper airways. It has been described that sleep apnea patients when compared with normal cases have augmented genioglossus activity during wakefulness [5]. This activity is thought to represent a neuromuscular compensatory mechanism of compromised upper airway patency [6]. However, significant decreases in activity are observed during sleep when compared to controls [5, 7]. In an in vitro study, Carrera et al. [8] recently found a greater genioglossus fatigability in OSAS than in control subjects. It has been shown that episodic hypoxia/asphyxia reduces upper airway muscle endurance and selectively impairs pharyngeal dilator responses to physiological stimulation [9]. Moreover, in an animal model Petrof et al. [10] found abnormal fiber morphology, inflammatory cell infiltrates and increased connective tissue in upper airways dilator muscles. The changes were consistent with muscle injury and were accompanied with changes to the proportions of the muscle fiber types. Series et al. [11] described similar increases of the cross-sectional area of muscle fiber and the number of fast-twitch fibers in patients with OSAS. Therefore, there is no evidence that the morphological changes in sleep apnea are beneficial.

In the light of these findings, the question arose if electrical stimulation of the muscles of the upper airways could improve the efficacy of the muscles and could be used as an alternative treatment for OSAS.

Acute Effects of Neuromuscular Stimulation on the Upper Airways Diameter

Most studies in this field applied electrical neurostimulation during sleep with the intention of illustrating acute modifications of airflow dynamics. These investigations provided contradictory results [12–23]. In 1989, Miki et al. [12] studied the stimulation of the genioglossus muscle in dogs. They found that the resistance of the upper airways increased while the negative tracheal pressure was continuously lowered in the experimental setting. Under electrical neurostimulation, the resistance of the upper airways was significantly reduced. It reached a plateau on a low level with stimulation frequencies of at least 50 Hz. Additionally, Yoo et al. [13] demonstrated in a canine model that nonselective hypoglossus stimulation yielded the greatest improvement in upper airways resistance as compared with that for selective activation of the geniohyoid, genioglossus, and hyoglossus/styloglossus muscles. Odeh et al. [14] performed electrical stimulation of the dilating muscles in dogs and measured flow and pressure profiles of the upper airways. Schnall et al. [15] studied the effects of transmucosal and transcutaneous stimulation in wake healthy persons. In both studies, only stimulation of the genioglossus significantly reduced the upper airways resistance. These results could be confirmed by Bishara et al. [16] who directly stimulated the genioglossus, the geniohyoideus, and the sternohyoideus in dogs. Only the stimulation of the genioglossus muscle was able to reopen a total obstruction.

In conclusion, experimental surface and intraneural stimulation has been shown to reduce upper airways resistance in animals, healthy persons and patients with OSAS. In particular, stimulation of the genioglossus muscles resulted in a significant reduction in airway resistance and an increase in the critical collapsing pressure. Genioglossus stimulation is most important to widen the shape of the upper airways.

Apnea-Induced Neurostimulation: Clinical Application

Investigations on the use of electrical stimulation in patients also provided heterogeneous results. Schwartz et al. [24] found that intraneural stimulation of the hypoglossal nerve significantly improved respiratory disturbances during sleep. Based on their results in dogs, Miki et al. [25] carried out a study on the influence of percutaneous submental electrostimulation of the genioglossus muscles in 6 patients with OSAS. Stimulation was performed during sleep and was triggered by apnea of more than 5 s duration. This resulted in a reduction in the apnea index and in the number of oxygen desaturations to under 85% [25]. Miki et al. [25] did not find any negative effects such as arousals, increased blood pressure or heart rate. In contrast, Guilleminault et al. [26] failed to observe an enlargement of the upper airways either under submental or intraoral stimulation. Moreover, they reported contractions of the platysma, undesired movements of the tongue, and induction of EEG arousals. Oliven et al. [27] studied the effect of stimulation with sublingual surface electrodes and found a reduction of the transpharyngeal resistance and an improvement of the airflow. However, they were not able to reopen obstructive apneas. Moreover, Decker et al. [28] using submental surface electrodes and implanted intraneural electrodes found only an inconsistent termination of the apneas.

Therefore, although neuromuscular stimulation triggered by apneas improves respiratory disturbances during sleep it is – by now – not sufficiently effective to treat the complex sleep apnea syndrome.

Tongue Muscle Training

Muscle training using electrical neurostimulation (ENS) has been found to effectively strengthen skeletal muscles in pathological or posttraumatic situations. In healthy muscles, ENS can induce the activity of motor units which are difficult to activate voluntarily [29]. It has been shown that ENS with a frequency of 50 Hz activates both muscle fiber types completely and homogeneously [30]. Moreover, in contrast to the structural changes of the upper airways muscles in the

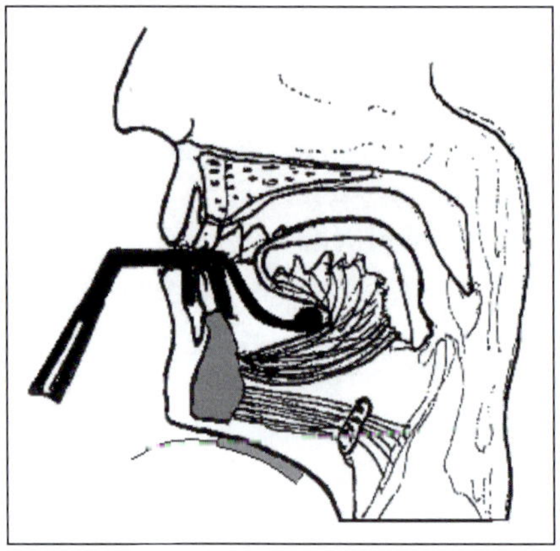

Fig. 1. Stimulation is performed using a chin electrode with both a positive and negative lead and an oral electrode which is placed as a ring on the teeth. The stimulating part of the oral electrode is placed beneath the tongue.

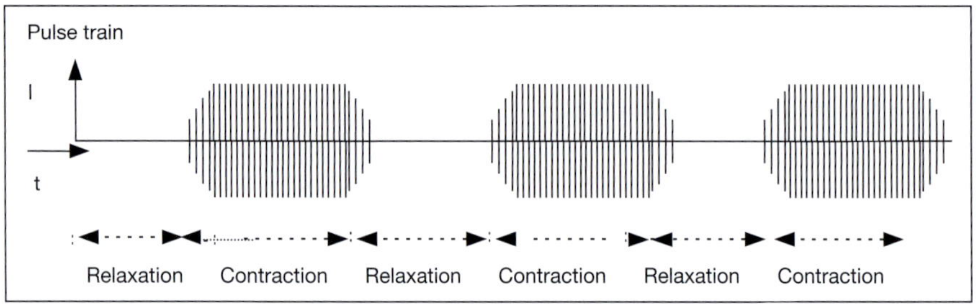

Fig. 2. Stimulation consists of a relaxation cycle and a contraction cycle. The contraction cycle consists of two parts, a ramp-up phase (1.5 s) and contraction phase. The relaxation cycle consists of a ramp down phase (1.0 s) followed by a phase of no stimulation. Only during the contraction cycle and ramp down phase are stimulation pulses transmitted in a pulse train between the electrodes.

course of sleep apnea, no inflammatory changes have been observed under electrical stimulation in skeletal muscles [31]. Neurostimulation of the upper airways muscles during sleep induces acute transient improvements in airflow dynamics but can be limited by side effects. Taking together the findings on the training of skeletal muscles and the effects of neurostimulation on the upper airways, the question arose whether training of the tongue muscles during the daytime might improve the strength of the dilator muscles and, therefore, reduce nocturnal respiratory disturbances without impairing sleep quality. The rationale of the tongue muscle training was to improve the maximum muscle activity by stimulating both the fast- and the slow-twitch fibers more homogeneously and to maintain a sufficient activity level in spite of the fall during sleep.

Only few data on the tongue muscle training from clinical trials are available. In a noncontrolled study, Wiltfang et al. [32] found an increase in tongue muscle power and reported sufficient training effects in a single case. However, controlled studies in large groups on daytime tongue muscle training comparing with either CPAP or placebo were needed. Therefore, a randomized, double-blind, placebo-controlled study to evaluate the efficacy and compliance of a tongue muscle training by electrical neurostimulation in patients was recently published [33]. The stimulating electrode was placed centrally below the tongue with the aim of achieving stimulation of the genioglossus muscles (fig. 1). The stimulation device produced a symmetric biphasic output. The net direct current delivered into the load was <0.1 mA (fig. 2). 57 patients with mild or moderate OSAS (apnea/hypopnea index (AHI) 10–40/h) practiced tongue muscle training for 20 min twice a day during the daytime for 8 weeks.

There was no significant change in the AHI or the sleep profile either under placebo or stimulation. However, snoring improved significantly under stimulation (baseline 63.6 ± 23.1 epochs/h, stimulation 47.5 ± 31.2, $p < 0.05$) but not under placebo. There was a small subgroup of patients with a baseline AHI <25/h whose AHI decreased significantly. The reduction of snoring was even more pronounced in this group of responders. In contrast, under placebo no responders were to be found. The conclusions of the study are limited by several aspects. It was not possible to take morphological factors such as anatomical differences in the shape of the upper airways, BMI, body position or variability in the upper airway function during sleep into account. As it is not known whether even weak pulses might have a stimulating effect, even applying minimal stimulation in the placebo group was avoided. However, the absence of sensation during training cannot be excluded as a reason for the larger number of drop-outs in the placebo group [33].

It is not clear how long the therapeutic effect in the responders persists and whether a longer duration of training beyond 8 weeks, or repetition of training after an interval, might be beneficial. However, at this time the results do not permit recommending tongue muscle training as an alternative treatment in patients with OSAS. Nevertheless, the partially positive results encourage further studies on methods which aim at influencing the muscle function [33].

References

1 Remmers JE, de Groot WJ, Sauerland EK, Anch AM: Pathogenesis of upper airways occlusion during sleep. J Appl Physiol 1978; 44:931–938.
2 Block AJ, Faulkner JA, Hughes RL, Remmers JE, Thach B: Factors influencing upper airways closure. Chest 1984;86:114–122.
3 Deegan PC, McNicholas WT: Pathophysiology of OSAS; in McNicholas WT (ed): Respiratory Disorders during Sleep. Sheffield, European Respiratory Society Journals, 1998, pp 28–62.
4 Fogel RB, Malhotra A, Shea SA, Edwards JK, White DP: Reduced genioglossal activity with upper airway anesthesia in awake patients with OSA. J Appl Physiol 2000;88:1346–1354.
5 Mezzanotte WS, Tangel DJ, White SC: Influence of sleep onset on upper-airway muscle activity in apnea patients versus normal controls. Am J Resp Crit Care Med 1996;153: 1880–1887.
6 Mezzanotte WS, Tangel DJ, White DP: Waking genioglossal EMG in sleep apnea patients vs. normal controls (a neuromuscular compensatory mechanism). J Clin Invest 1992;89:1571–1579.
7 Wiegand DA, Latz B, Zwillich CW, Wiegand L: Upper airway resistance and geniohyoid muscle activity in normal men during wakefulness and sleep. J Appl Physiol 1990;69: 1252–1261.
8 Carrera M, Barbe F, Sauleda J, Tomas M, Gomez C, Agusti AG: Patients with obstructive sleep apnea exhibit genioglossus dysfunction that is normalized after treatment with continuous positive airway pressure. Am J Respir Crit Care Med 1999;159:1960–1966.
9 Bradford A, McGuire M, O'Halloran KD: Does episodic hypoxia affect upper airway dilator muscle function? Implications for the pathophysiology of obstructive sleep apnoea. Respir Physiol Neurobiol 2005;147:223–234.
10 Petrof BJ, Pack AI, Kelly AM, Eby J, Hendricks JC: Pharyngeal myopathy of loaded upper airway in dogs with sleep apnea. J Appl Physiol 1994;76:1746–1752.
11 Series F, Cote C, Simoneau JA, Gelinas Y, St Pierre S, Leclerc J, Ferland R, Marc I: Physiologic, metabolic, and muscle fiber type characteristics of musculus uvulae in sleep apnea hypopnea syndrome in snorers. J Clin Invest 1995;95:20–25.
12 Miki H, Hida W, Shindoh C, Kikuchi Y, Chonan T, Taguchi O, Inoue H, Takishima T: Effects of electrical stimulation of the genioglossus on upper airway resistance in anesthetized dogs. Am Rev Resp Dis 1989;140: 1279–1284.
13 Yoo PB, Durand DM: Effects of selective hypoglossal nerve stimulation on canine upper airway mechanics. J Appl Physiol 2005;99: 937–943.
14 Odeh M, Schnall R, Gavriely N, Oliven A: Effect of upper airway muscle contraction on supraglottic resistance and stability. Respir Physiol 1993;92:139–150.
15 Schnall RP, Pillar G, Kelsen SG, Oliven A: Dilatory effects of upper airway muscle contraction induced by electrical stimulation in awake humans. J Appl Physiol 1995;78:1950–1956.
16 Bishara H, Odeh M, Schnall RP, Gavriely N, Oliven A: Electrically-activated dilator muscles reduce pharyngeal resistance in anaesthetized dogs with upper airway obstruction. Eur Respir J 1995;8:1537–1542.
17 Series F, Marc I: Influence of genioglossus tonic activity on upper airway dynamics assessed by phrenic nerve stimulation. J Appl Physiol 2002;92:418–423.
18 Isono S, Tanaka A, Nishino T: Effects of tongue electrical stimulation on pharyngeal mechanics in anaesthetized patients with obstructive sleep apnoea. Eur Respir J 1999;14: 1258–1265.
19 Eisele DW, Smith PL, Alam DS, Schwartz AR: Direct hypoglossal nerve stimulation in obstructive sleep apnea. Arch Otolaryngol Head Neck Surg 1997;123:57–61.
20 Smith PL, Eisele DW, Podszus T, Penzel T, Grote L, Peter JH, Schwartz AR: Electrical stimulation of upper airway musculature. Sleep 1996;19:S284–S287.
21 Schwartz AR, Eisele DW, Hari A, Testerman R, Erickson D, Smith PL: Electrical stimulation of the lingual musculature in obstructive sleep apnea. J Appl Physiol 1996;81:643–652.
22 Eisele DW, Schwartz AR, Hari A, Thut DC, Smith PL: The effects of selective nerve stimulation on upper airway airflow mechanics. Arch Otolaryngol Head Neck Surg 1995;121: 1361–1364.
23 Mann EA, Burnett T, Cornell S, Ludlow CL: The effect of neuromuscular stimulation of the genioglossus on the hypopharyngeal airway. Laryngoscope 2002;112:351–356.
24 Schwartz AR, Bennett ML, Smith PL, De Backer W, Hedner J, Boudewyns A, van de Heyning P, Ejnell H, Hochban W, Knaack L, Podszus T, Penzel T, Peter JH, Goding GS, rickson D, Testerman R, Ottenhoff F, Eisele DW: Therapeutic electrical stimulation of the hypoglossus nerve in obstructive sleep apnea. Arch Otolaryngol Head Neck Surg 2001;127:1216–1223.
25 Miki H, Hida W, Chonan T, Kikuchi Y, Takishima T: Effects of submental electrical stimulation during sleep on upper airway patency with obstructive sleep apnea. Am Rev Resp Dis 1989;140:1285–1289.
26 Guilleminault C, Powell N, Bowman B, Stoohs R: The effect of electrical stimulation on obstructive sleep apnea syndrome. Chest 1995;107:67–73.
27 Oliven A, Schnall RP, Pillar G, Gavriely N, Odeh M: Sublingual electrical stimulation of the tongue during wakefulness and sleep. Respir Physiol 2001;127:217–226.
28 Decker MJ, Haaga J, Arnold JL, Atzberger D, Strohl KP: Functional electrical stimulation and respiration during sleep. J Appl Physiol 1993;75:1053–1061.
29 Hainaut K, Duchateau J: Neuromuscular electrical stimulation and voluntary exercise. Sports Med 1992;14:100–113.
30 Cabric M, Appell HJ, Resic A: Effects of electrical stimulation of different frequencies on the myonuclei and fiber size in human muscle. Int J Sports Med 1987;8:323–326.
31 Wehrle U, Dusterhoft S, Pette D: Effects of chronic electrical stimulation on myosin heavy chain expression in satellite cell cultures derived from rat muscles of different fiber-type composition. Differentiation 1994;58:37–46.
32 Wiltfang J, Klotz S, Jordan W, Cohrs S, Engelke W, Ludwig A, Hajak G: Erste Ergebnisse zum Training der suprahyoidalen Muskulatur bei Probanden und einem Patienten mit obstruktiver Schlafapnoe. Somnologie 1997;1:160–164.
33 Randerath WJ, Galetke W, Domanski U, Weitkunat R, Ruhle KH: Tongue-muscle training by intraoral electrical neurostimulation in patients with obstructive sleep apnea. Sleep 2004;27:254–259.

Prof. Dr. Winfried J. Randerath
Institute for Pneumology at the University Witten/Herdecke
Clinic for Pneumology and Allergology
Center of Sleep Medicine and Respiratory Care, Bethanien Hospital
Aufderhöherstrasse 169–175
DE–42699 Solingen (Germany)
Tel. +49 212 63 6000, Fax +49 212 63 6005
E-Mail randerath@klinik-bethanien.de

Randerath WJ, Sanner BM, Somers VK (eds): Sleep Apnea.
Prog Respir Res. Basel, Karger, 2006, vol 35, pp 164–166

Cardiac Pacemaker Therapy in Sleep Apnea

Thomas Schichtl Michael Pfeifer

Klinik Donaustauf, Klinik und Poliklinik für Innere Medizin 2, Universität Regensburg, Regensburg, Germany

Abstract

Since sleep apnea and cardiac arrhythmia requiring pacemaker therapy are quite common, the idea of using pacemakers for the treatment of sleep apnea could be interesting. A review of the current literature regarding pacemaker therapy in sleep apnea was compiled using PubMed. Regarding central-sleep apnea with Cheyne-Stokes breathing (CSB) caused by heart failure, it could be shown that a pacemaker therapy especially used for cardiac resynchronization therapy could improve heart function and thus CSB. For obstructive sleep apnea (OSA), in 2002 one study attracted some attention while it showed significant improvement of OSA by nocturnal pacing with an implanted usual pacemaker. Atrial overdrive pacing was performed 15 bpm above mean nocturnal heart rate. Subsequent studies were done to assess these findings. In three well-performed and quite similar investigations, the results of the foregoing study could not be replicated. While in these studies CPAP was apparently effective in treating OSA, atrial overdrive pacing showed no effect. While pacemaker treatment used for resynchronization in heart failure therapy is effective in amending central sleep apnea with Cheyne-Stokes breathing, the majority of the current findings cannot confirm that pacemaker therapy in obstructive sleep apnea is useful.

Many patients suffer from obstructive sleep apnea. In addition, central sleep apnea with Cheyne-Stokes breathing is common, at least in patients with congestive heart failure. Cardiac arrhythmias, which require pacemaker therapy (e.g. bradyarrhythmias) also are quite frequent, especially in older people (i.e. 60 years of age and above). Furthermore, there is some evidence that sleep apnea, e.g. in inducing cardiac overload and provoking hypertension, could trigger cardiac arrhythmias [1, 2].

Considering this, it seems quite clear that a relevant number of people who suffer from sleep apnea also have implanted pacemakers. Thus, the idea of using these devices as a possible treatment option for sleep apnea came up.

Pacing and Central Sleep Apnea in Heart Failure

In the case of central sleep apnea with Cheyne-Stokes breathing (due to congestive heart failure), this approach appeared to be more promising: as heart failure results, e.g. by a diminished cardiac output and a prolonged circulation time, in Cheyne-Stokes breathing, a stabilization of heart function, e.g. resulting in improved stroke volume, could possibly abolish this form of central sleep apnea.

In this context, the mechanism of biventricular pacing is interesting: in patients with enlarged left ventricles and a desynchronized pattern of cardiac muscle contraction, beneficial effects of resynchronization therapy by biventricular pacing could be observed. In many cases, an augmentation of stroke volume and performance indices could be shown. Also, implantation of biventricular pacing devices in patients with heart failure and Cheyne-Stokes breathing led to a significant reduction of this pathologic breathing pattern [3, 4].

Obstructive Sleep Apnea

Besides ventricular stimulation pacing – and focusing on atrial pacing – some excitement arose, as in 2002 Garrigue et al. [5] published a work on atrial overdrive pacing in sleep apnea. They showed a detectable improvement in sleep-disordered breathing by modification of formerly implanted cardiac pacemakers. In this study, two-chamber pacemakers in DDD mode featuring a rest-rate algorithm were used. The pacemakers had been implanted because of symptomatic bradycardia. 15 patients were evaluated in a single-blinded, randomized, cross-over design trial. At baseline, the mean nocturnal heart rate was assessed. On two further nights, rest rate was elevated 15 beats above the mean nocturnal heart rate. By this, a reduction in the apnea/hypopnea index (central and obstructive together) from 28 ± 21/h to 11 ± 14/h ($p < 0.001$) was achieved. In controls, the pacemakers were set to a VVI mode with a constant base rate of 40 beats/min. Compared to the control group, in which no improvement of sleep-disordered breathing was noticed, the changes in the pacing group were significant. Although the effects were stronger in patients with Cheyne-Stokes breathing, they were also detectable and significant in obstructive sleep apnea.

Regarding the group of patients with central sleep apnea and considering the pathophysiologic insights mentioned above, the results seemed to be quite plausible.

As the pathophysiologic background of obstructive sleep apnea consists basically in an obstruction of the upper airways, it did not seem quite evident how a change in cardiac pacing patterns could be of any effect.

Yet, various considerations were made for how a higher heart beat could influence obstructive sleep apnea [6, 7]. For example, an enhanced respiratory drive due to cardiac pacing was discussed. Critics argued that a possible effect could coexist, e.g. in sympathetic activation and therefore in deranged quality of sleep. Perhaps sleep architecture was affected and fewer amounts of slow-wave and REM sleep led to a smaller number of apneas. Garrigue and his team unfortunately did not show detailed data of parameters describing sleep quality [5].

As the results of the Garrigue group seemed so astonishing, some study groups tried to repeat those findings. For example, in 2005, Lüthje et al. [8] examined (in a study design nearly analogue to that of the Garrigue group) 20 patients with predominantly obstructive sleep apnea by equal elevation of nocturnal heart rate. Regarding sleep-disordered breathing, nearly no significant effect could be shown.

In another recent study, pacing with a temporary lead (15 beats higher than the baseline heart rate) was compared to CPAP therapy in 10 patients with obstructive sleep apnea. While CPAP worked well, pacing showed no effect [9].

Another investigation dealing with this subject was conducted by Simantirakis et al. [10]. The study examined 16 patients with moderate-to-severe obstructive sleep apnea and normal left ventricular function in whom a dual-chamber pacemaker had been implanted. The eligible patients had a programmed backup pacing at a rate below 40 bpm. Atrial overdrive pacing was compared to CPAP therapy: after randomization, one group was assigned to atrial overdrive pacing at 15 bpm above the spontaneous mean nocturnal heart rate. In the other group, the original pacing rate was unchanged. The first group received overdrive pacing for 1 month and the second group received nCPAP for 1 month. After 1 month, the groups were switched in a crossover design. Polysomnographic recordings were done at baseline, after one night of pacing, after 1 month of pacing or CPAP and after 1 month subsequent to crossover. Short- and long-term overdrive pacing led to no reduction in AHI ($p = 0.82$ for short-term pacing/0.87 for long-term pacing), desaturation index ($p = 0.66/0.82$) and total sleep time ($p = 0.35/0.16$), while CPAP apparently was very effective (e.g. reduction in AHI from 49 to 2.7, with $p < 0.001$).

In conclusion, this study showed that atrial overdrive pacing after 1 night and after treatment during 1 month was not at all effective in treating obstructive sleep apnea.

Conclusions

Considering the majority of the current findings (fig. 1), the results of Garrigue et al. [5] could not be approved and, on the contrary, appear to be falsified [11]. Up to now, the inefficacy of a cardiac pacing therapy in obstructive sleep apnea could be shown regarding short- and long-term effects and in investigating slight, moderate and severe sleep apnea. Yet one bigger study initiated by St. Jude Medical ('BREATHE' – base rest rate elevation for apnea therapy) investigating this problem is still ongoing.

Furthermore, it is shown in animal models that overdrive pacing, at least in principle, could lead to increased mortality [12]. Therefore, discerning long-term observations of overdrive pacing therapy would be necessary anyway.

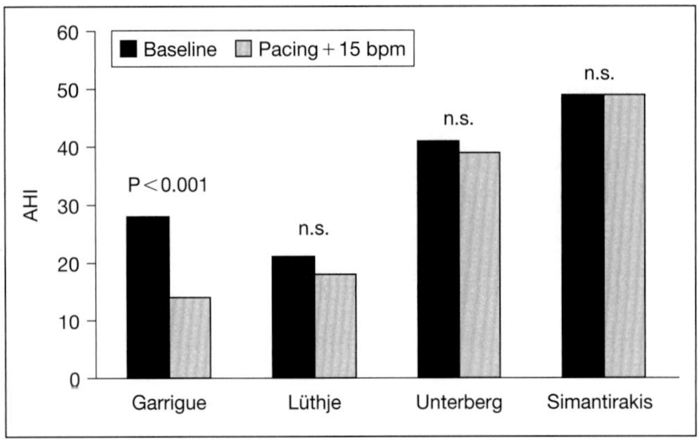

Fig. 1. Effect of atrial pacing on the apnea/hypopnea index (AHI) in patients with obstructive sleep apnea. Comparison of different controlled studies.

Away from biventricular pacemakers for resynchronization therapy in heart failure, Floras and Bradley [13] appear to be right in arguing that the 'door (for atrial overdrive pacing in sleep apnea) seems to be closed'.

References

1 Gami AS, Pressman G, Caples SM, Kanagala R, Gard JJ, Davison DE, Malouf JF, Ammash NM, Friedman PA, Somers VK: Association of atrial fibrillation and obstructive sleep apnea. Circulation 2004;110:364–367.

2 Roche F, Xuong AN, Court-Fortune I, Costes F, Pichot V, Duverney D, Vergnon JM, Gaspoz JM, Barthelemy JC: Relationship among the severity of sleep apnea syndrome, cardiac arrhythmias, and autonomic imbalance. Pacing Clin Electrophysiol 2003;26:669–677.

3 Sinha AM, Skobel EC, Breithardt OA, Norra C, Markus KU, Breuer C, Hanrath P, Stellbrink C: Cardiac resynchronization therapy improves central sleep apnea and Cheyne-Stokes respiration in patients with chronic heart failure. J Am Coll Cardiol 2004; 44:68–71.

4 Gabor JY, Newman DA, Barnard-Roberts V, Korley V, Mangat I, Dorian P, Hanly PJ: Improvement in Cheyne-Stokes respiration following cardiac resynchronisation therapy. Eur Respir J 2005;26:95–100.

5 Garrigue S, Bordier P, Jais P, Shah DC, Hocini M, Raherison C, Tunon De Lara M, Haissaguerre M, Clementy J: Benefit of atrial pacing in sleep apnea syndrome. N Engl J Med 2002;346:404–412.

6 Gottlieb DJ: Cardiac pacing: a novel therapy for sleep apnea? N Engl J Med 2002;346: 444–445.

7 Drazen JM: Sleep apnea syndrome. N Engl J Med 2002;346:390.

8 Lüthje L, Unterberg-Buchwald C, Dajani D, Vollmann D, Hasenfuss G, Andreas S: Atrial overdrive pacing in patients with sleep apnea with implanted pacemaker. Am J Respir Crit Care Med 2005;172:118–122.

9 Unterberg C, Lüthje L, Szych J, Vollmann D, Hasenfuss G, Andreas S: Atrial overdrive pacing compared to CPAP in patients with obstructive sleep apnoea syndrome. Eur Heart J 2005;26:2568–2575.

10 Simantirakis EN, Schiza SE, Chrysostomakis SI, Chlouverakis GI, Klapsinos NC, Siafakas NM, Vardas PE: Atrial overdrive pacing for the obstructive sleep apnea-hypopnea syndrome. N Engl J Med 2005;353:2568–2577.

11 Pepin JL, Defaye P, Garrigue S, Poezevara Y, Lévy P: Overdrive atrial pacing does not improve obstructive sleep apnoea syndrome. Eur Respir J 2005;25:343–347.

12 Wilson JR, Douglas P, Hickey WF, Lanoce V, Ferraro N, Muhammad A, Reichek N: Experimental congestive heart failure produced by rapid ventricular pacing in the dog: cardiac effects. Circulation 1987;75:857–867.

13 Floras JS, Bradley TD: Atrial overdrive pacing for sleep apnea: a door now closed? Am J Respir Crit Care Med 2005;172:1–3.

Prof. Dr. M. Pfeifer
Klinik Donaustauf, Klinik und Poliklinik für Innere Medizin 2
Universität Regensburg
Franz-Josef-Strauss-Allee 11
DE–93042 Regensburg (Germany)
Tel. +49 094 03 80215
Fax +49 094 03 80212
E-Mail michael.pfeifer@klinik.uni-regensburg.de

Randerath WJ, Sanner BM, Somers VK (eds): Sleep Apnea.
Prog Respir Res. Basel, Karger, 2006, vol 35, pp 167–173

Surgical Treatment for Obstructive Sleep Apnea

A.N. Boudewyns P.H. Van de Heyning

Department of Otorhinolaryngology, Head and Neck Surgery, Antwerp University Hospital, Edegem, Belgium

Abstract

Continuous positive airway pressure (CPAP) is the first-line treatment for obstructive sleep apnea (OSA) because of its proven beneficial effects upon associated morbidity, daytime symptoms and quality of life. Nevertheless, CPAP compliance is an important problem in a subgroup of patients. Surgery can be considered as a first-line treatment in mild OSA and in patients with moderate-to-severe disease for whom other noninvasive treatments have failed. Surgical treatment of OSA aims to correct anatomical abnormalities in the upper airway (UA), contributing to its collapse during sleep. The concept of a two-level (retropalatal and retrolingual) pharyngeal collapse seems overly simplified as recent investigations on the pattern of UA collapse during sleep indicate that most OSA patients have a diffuse pattern of UA collapse. This information resulted in the development of a 'multilevel surgical concept' dictated by the patient's anatomy. In this chapter, emphasis will be placed upon the rationale of this approach, the related anesthetic risks and the definition of outcome measures. In addition, the importance of ventilatory instability and collapse of the lateral wall in the development of new surgical modalities will be discussed.

Rationale of Obstructive Sleep Apnea Surgery

Snoring and obstructive sleep apnea (OSA) are caused by a partial or complete collapse of the upper airway (UA) during sleep. This collapse might be located anywhere between the choanae and the epiglottis. Several methods have been employed to identify the site of UA collapse in OSA patients. By means of UA pressure measurements during sleep, we have demonstrated that the majority of OSA patients have multiple sites of UA obstruction during sleep; that the site of obstruction may vary according to sleep stage and that extension of collapse to lower sites of the UA can occur during REM sleep [1]. The majority of patients were found to obstruct at the level of the naso- and oropharynx, a finding that has been confirmed by other investigators [2]. These observations are in accordance with the concept of 'disproportionate anatomy', i.e. unfavorable anatomic features of the surrounding soft tissues and underlying facial skeleton, predisposing to OSA. At present, there is a consensus among clinicians that OSA results from diffuse UA narrowing which includes the soft palate, lateral pharyngeal wall and tongue base. Only a minority (1–2%) of OSA patients have a specific space-occupying abnormality in the UA for which surgical removal is corrective.

Three major categories of UA surgery can be discerned: soft tissue surgery, skeletal framework surgery and tracheotomy. Soft tissue surgery aims to remove or reduce the volume of UA soft tissues such as the tonsils, uvula and soft palate or tongue base. The goal of skeletal framework surgery is to modify the facial skeleton from which the soft tissues are suspended. This results in a repositioning of UA soft tissues. Tracheotomy restores UA patency through bypassing the UA. For a detailed description of surgical techniques and their respective results, the reader is referred to some recent review papers on this subject [3, 4].

Interpretation of Surgical Results

Papers on UA surgery are frequently flawed by methodological and statistical errors, making correct interpretation of the presented data a difficult task. Bridgman et al. [5] recently reviewed the literature on surgery for OSA through the Cochrane Airways Group Sleep Apnea Randomized Controlled Trial Register. No randomized controlled trials could be identified by this search strategy comparing any surgical intervention for OSA with another surgical or non-surgical treatment modality. In addition, the reviewers emphasized the following methodological difficulties: (1) the lack of a consensus on the definition of OSA in descriptive studies, and (2) the effectiveness of the interventions was assessed by a variety of outcome measures (both subjective and objective) and long-term follow-up data were often lacking. The final conclusion of the Cochrane review was that, given the lack of good trial-based evidence, surgery for OSA should be restricted to surgery carried out as part of clinical trials and patients should be informed about the experimental nature of the surgical procedure. In daily practice, however, a less dogmatic approach might be adopted since considerable clinical experience with the various UA surgical procedures has been obtained over the past years. The lack of a consensus on the definition of OSA and 'surgical success' seriously hampers the interpretation of surgical results and comparisons among different treatment options. The criteria employed by Scher et al. [6] in their meta-analysis on surgical treatment for OSA, are a reduction of the respiratory disturbance index (RDI: number of apneas and hypopneas/hour of sleep) for at least 50% and a postoperative RDI $<$20/h or a reduction of the apnea index (AI: number of apneas/hour of sleep) for at least 50% and a postoperative AI $<$10/h. These criteria are frequently employed in the current literature on OSA surgery but their validity might be questioned given the recent data that even mild forms of OSA might be associated with cardiovascular morbidity [7]. Another subject of discussion and controversy in reporting surgical results is the definition of outcome measures. From our present understanding about the pathophysiological consequences of OSA, it can be inferred that the RDI or AI does not represent the ideal outcome variable. Other polysomnographic variables such as oxygen desaturations, the amount of sleep fragmentation, cardiac events and patient-based factors such as the degree of daytime sleepiness or obesity are probably better related to the long-term health consequences of OSA [8]. The American Academy of Otolaryngology, Head and Neck Surgery Sleep Apnea Treatment Outcomes Pilot study (OSATOPS), attempted to define a clinical-severity staging system for patients with OSA. This staging system incorporates both polysomnographic and patient-related factors and is based upon the Epworth Sleepiness Scale (ESS), Body Mass Index (BMI), presence of redundant pharyngeal tissue, RDI and minimum oxygen saturation during apneas [9]. Although further validation studies are required, this proposal might signify an important step forward towards a multidimensional approach including both subjective and objective parameters. The tendency among surgeons to perform multiple procedures in various combinations in a single operative session is another confounding factor in the interpretation of surgical results. This is certainly true when the associated procedures (especially nasal surgery or tonsillectomy) are not reported in detail in the methodology and the composite surgical results are assessed in 1 postoperative polysomnography (PSG). In line with the prevailing concepts about the pathophysiology of OSA, UA collapsibility as such might be used as an outcome parameter for surgical treatment. The critical closing pressure (P_{crit}) can be considered as a measure of UA collapsibility and varies along a continuum from health (low collapsibility, $P_{crit} <$ atmospheric pressure) to disease (high collapsibility, $P_{crit} >$ atmospheric pressure). Specific treatment strategies have been shown to result in a predictable decrease in P_{crit} [10]. Effective treatment of obstructive apnea and hypopnea can only be obtained when P_{crit} decreases to near -4 cm H_2O, thus converting patients from OSA to snorers. Knowledge of P_{crit} for a given patient prior to treatment and information about the magnitude of the P_{crit} change that can be obtained by a particular treatment can be used to select patients for a specific treatment or a combination of treatment strategies [10] (fig. 1a, b).

Surgical Failures

In the 1980s, Fujita et al. [11] introduced uvulopalatopharyngoplasty (UPPP) as a surgical procedure for OSA. For about 15 years, it has been the standard surgical treatment for this condition until, in 1996, a critical review was performed about the surgical results by Sher et al. [6]. In their meta-analysis of more than 500 cases from 37 papers, it was found that only 39% of unselected OSA patients met the success criterion defined as a postoperative reduction in RDI by $>$50% and a postoperative RDI $\leq$20/h. UPPP failures are usually attributed to a lack of modification at secondary sites of UA collapse located lower in the pharynx, to persistent retropalatal collapse due to an increased thickness of the soft palate after surgery, to postoperative weight gain and smoking. Data from UA

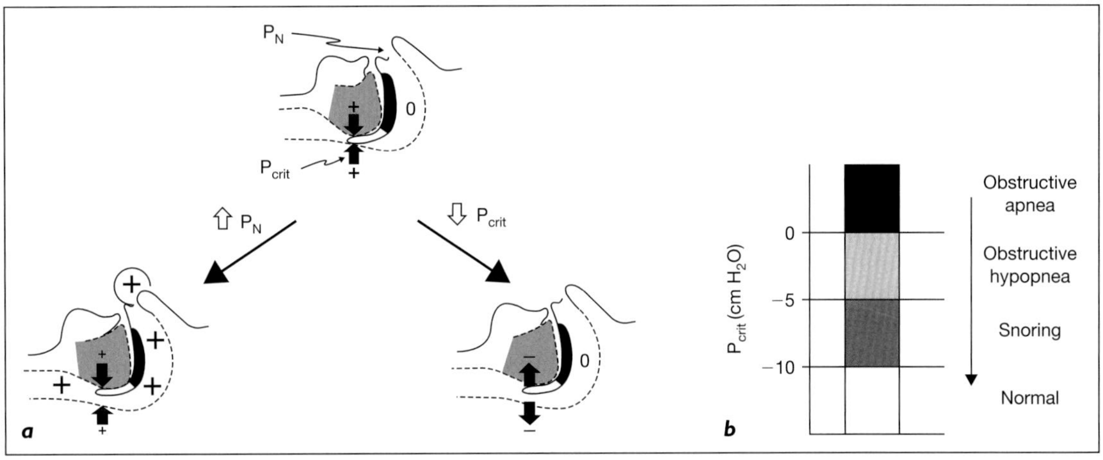

Fig. 1. ***a*** Upper airway patency can be restored by elevating the nasal pressure (left arrow) or by lowering P_{crit} (right arrow). ***b*** Discrete ranges of P_{crit} are illustrated for individuals with varying degrees of UA obstruction during sleep. The response to therapy is dependent upon the initial P_{crit} measurement and the magnitude of the fall in P_{crit} after (surgical) intervention. Reprinted with permission from Winakur et al. [35].

pressure measurements performed during sleep before and after UPPP confirmed the persistence of UA obstruction at the level of the tongue base and hypopharynx [12]. Upper airway surgical techniques involving the retrolingual region have been developed to address persistent or additional collapse in this region. In addition, surgical strategies have evolved towards a 'multiple sites of obstruction/multiple treatments' concept adapted to the individual UA anatomic features. Gupta et al. [13] performed a survey among Ear Nose and Throat surgeons regarding their workup and treatment of patients suspected of having OSA. Palatoplasty, septoplasty, tonsillectomy and turbinate reduction were among the most popular surgical procedures performed by the respondents. Only 28% used any procedure to address hypopharyngeal airway compromise such as genioglossus or hyoid advancement. The authors suggested that failure to address obstruction at the hypopharyngeal level could lead to inadequate treatment of OSA. The Stanford Protocol is one example of a staged surgical approach for UA reconstruction [14]. Clinical examination, fiberoptic endoscopy and cephalometry serve as a guidance to classify patients according to the type of pharyngeal obstruction as proposed by Fujita and Simmons [15]. Phase I surgical treatment consists of nasal reconstruction, UPPP for class I patients (retropalatal collapse), genioglossal advancement (GA) plus hyoid myotomy and suspension (MMS) for class III patients (retrolingual collapse) and a combination of these procedures in class II patients (retrolingual and retropalatal collapse). For those patients with significant persistent OSA and patients who are willing to undergo additional surgery, phase 2 of the protocol is performed consisting of maxillomandibular advancement (MMA). This approach has become under criticism and the generalizability of the surgical results has been questioned. Some investigators advocate that MMA be performed as the primary surgical treatment in some moderately overweight, skeletally deficient patients thereby avoiding the need for repeated anesthesia and surgery [16]. In addition, the significant morbidity associated with these procedures has a negative impact on patient acceptance (immediate surgical risks include tooth injury, wound infection, postoperative UA compromise; long-term risks are permanent anesthesia of the cheek, lips or chin). Alterations in the facial contour should be anticipated and it may take about 10 weeks before patients can resume their professional activities [16]. Another modality of phased UA surgery was proposed by Hessel et al. [17]. For patients with multilevel obstruction (as demonstrated during sleep endoscopy), the first approach is correction of obstruction at the nasal level. If improvement is insufficient, secondly, the retropalatal level (palate/uvula/tonsils) is approached, and, finally, if still necessary the retrolingual obstruction (tongue base/epiglottis) is corrected. Kao et al. [18] reported the results of such an anatomically based surgical approach. Forty-two patients who failed a trial of CPAP were included. A site-directed multistage surgical plan was outlined based upon clinical examination, fiberoptic nasopharyngoscopy with Mueller's maneuver, CT scan of the sinuses, and PSG.

Nasal surgery (septoplasty, turbinoplasty or endoscopic surgery) was performed in 85.6%; palatal surgery (UPPP/tonsillectomy) was performed in 92.8%, and 85.6% of the patients underwent radiofrequency volume reduction (RFVR) of the tongue base. Overall, RDI fell from 38.2 to 12.7/h and a 50% reduction in RDI or RDI <20/h could be obtained in 83.3%. Cure rates were better in patients with mild OSA as compared to those with severe disease.

A staged approach implies repeat anesthetic procedures and hospitalization and from a theoretical point of view, the results of each surgical step and thus the validation of the next step should be justified by a PSG examination since several studies have underlined the discrepancies between subjective reports and objective data. This is, however, impossible in clinical practice and further studies are required to delineate the most cost/effective approach.

In contrast with the staged approach, a variety of different surgical procedures might be combined in the same single treatment session. The application of radiofrequency energy (RFe) to obtain a volume reduction of specific UA tissues seems to lend itself to this approach although with modest success rates [19]. Stuck et al. [20] reported on the combined RFVR treatment of the tongue base and soft palate in 18 patients with moderately severe OSA. Treatment was performed under local anesthesia with a mean of 2.7 sessions/patient. Patients were selected upon clinical signs of both palatal and tongue base obstruction. Subjects with previous velopharyngeal surgery or with relevant enlargement of the uvula, tonsillar hypertrophy or webbing >1 cm were excluded. There was a significant subjective improvement in excessive daytime sleepiness and snoring but only 33% of the patients were cured (defined as a reduction in RDI >50% with a postoperative RDI <15/h). Overall postoperative morbidity and complication rate were low and did not seem to increase when soft palate RFVR was added to the tongue base approach. The authors therefore recommended to perform a combined approach (soft palate and tongue base RFVR) in patients with palatal and tongue base obstruction provided there is no relevant enlargement of the uvula, no tonsillar hypertrophy and if there is ≤1 cm of webbing. Long-term follow-up data >1 year after combined RFVR treatment of palate and tongue base for mild-to-moderate OSA indicate that OSA-related quality of life, daytime sleepiness and RDI all significantly improved at extended follow-up [21].

Nasal Obstruction and OSA

Whereas the nose represents the primary route of breathing, especially during sleep, the role of nasal breathing and the importance of nasal obstruction in the pathogenesis of OSA is incompletely understood and subject of much controversy. Theoretically, the presence of an increased nasal resistance might contribute to sleep-disordered breathing (SDB) through several mechanisms: (1) The passage of airflow through the nasal cavity has a stimulant effect on breathing, an effect that is mediated by nasal receptors sensitive to airflow. An increase in nasal resistance (NR) may cause a switch to mouth breathing during sleep and result in a decreased activation of nasal receptors with a negative impact on ventilation. (2) An increase of the NR generates an increased negative inspiratory pressure causing turbulence in the relaxed soft tissues and upper airway collapse. (3) Mouth breathing results in a posterior displacement of the tongue which might further compromise the UA. Data obtained with experimentally induced nasal obstruction in normal subjects showed a positive association between nasal obstruction and the occurrence of snoring, apnea and hypopnea [22]. Nasal obstruction is also an important factor contributing to CPAP intolerance reported by about 47% of the patients [23] and correction of nasal obstruction either medical or surgical, improves CPAP compliance. Several studies performed in patients with SDB failed to demonstrate a linear relationship between awake nasal resistance and apnea severity [24] and the effects of improving nasal obstruction (either medical or surgical) in this population are controversial. The results of isolated nasal surgery on OSA are often poor. Verse et al. [25] summarized the effects of nasal surgery for OSA based on a review of the available literature between 1983 and 2000 and found that the overall success rate of isolated nasal surgery in 57 OSA subjects was only 18%. Friedman et al. [26] performed a prospective study on 50 OSA patients undergoing isolated nasal surgery. In this study, the effect of nasal surgery on CPAP pressure was documented and a significant decrease of effective CPAP level was found in the severe OSA patients 10.1 vs. 7.4 cm H_2O postoperatively ($p < 0.01$). Based upon the available data, it can be concluded that there is clinical evidence to suggest a role of nasal obstruction in the pathogenesis of snoring and OSA and normalization of nasal resistance either by medical or surgical methods should be integrated in the therapeutic management of these patients. Realistic expectations must however be put forward and discussed with the patients before surgery. Isolated nasal surgery is likely to decrease the feeling of nasal obstruction, improve daytime sleepiness and feelings of unrefreshing sleep but is unlikely to cure OSA. In subjects with CPAP intolerance due to nasal obstruction, an improvement in mask tolerance can be expected after treatment of nasal obstruction.

Anesthetic Risk and OSA Surgery

OSA patients are at increased risk during surgical procedures under general anesthesia. These risks might relate either to their OSA and associated morbidities (hypoventilation, cardiovascular vulnerability) or to difficulties with airway control (due to obesity or UA anatomic features typically of OSA such as crowding of the oropharynx, a long thick soft palate, tonsillar hypertrophy, macroglossia and retrognathism). The incidence of perioperative complications in OSA patients undergoing surgery for other medical conditions is unknown. Guidelines for pre- to postoperative management of OSA patients were recently published by a Clinical Practice Review Committee of the American Academy of Sleep Medicine [27]. Surgical treatment for OSA is associated with an increased risk for postoperative UA edema with life-threatening hypoxemia. This is especially true for tongue base procedures, UPPP and maxillofacial surgery. Nasal packing might adversely affect the breathing pattern and worsen OSA and should therefore be avoided or removed as soon as possible. Keeping in mind the increased risk of OSA patients for procedures under general anesthesia and the present tendency to combine several procedures in 1 patient, the safety of this approach might be questioned. This issue was recently addressed in a study of 85 OSA patients undergoing a combination of extended uvulopalatal flap surgery and septomeatoplasty [28]. The study included middle aged subjects (<50 years) in otherwise good health, without morbid obesity and undergoing simultaneous (n = 55) (group 1) or staged surgery (n = 30) (group 2). Nasal surgery was performed after palatopharyngeal surgery (in the case of single treatment session), nasal packing was removed during the first postoperative day and patients received humidified oxygen via a nasal mask during the postoperative period. There were no intraoperative complications or incidents of UA compromise in the immediate postoperative period in either group. An analysis of cost-effectiveness demonstrated a major reduction in medical expenses in the simultaneous surgery group that could mainly be attributed to a shorter total length of hospitalization. Busaba et al. [29] retrospectively reviewed the charts of 91 OSA patients undergoing UPPP ± tonsillectomy and nasal airway surgery (n = 63) (group 1) or palatopharyngeal and nasal surgery in a staged fashion (n = 28) (group 2). One patient in group 1 and 2 subjects from group 2 had genoid advancement. Two patients in group 2 underwent RFVR of the tongue base. Patients had moderately severe OSA and both groups had various comorbidities. Airway problems did not occur in the immediate postoperative period and the postoperative complication rate was comparable for both groups at 4.8% and 3.6%, respectively. These studies show that combined nasal/palatopharyngeal surgery might be safe and more cost efficient in middle-aged, moderately severe OSA patients without morbid obesity. Whether this also applies to other OSA subgroups (morbidly obese, severe OSA, significant comorbidities) remains unknown and additional studies are necessary before any recommendations can be made on this subject. Unfortunately, none of these studies addressed the patient 's acceptance or the degree of discomfort (especially in combined surgical approaches).

New Developments in OSA Surgery

Adjuvant Medical Treatment with Acetazolamide (ACET)

Apart from anatomical factors and intrinsic collapsibility, the magnitude of ventilatory instability is considered as a determinant of pharyngeal obstruction. Considering the respiratory system, loop gain represents the gain or sensitivity of the negative feedback loop that controls ventilation. Extended circulation time, small lung volumes and an increased responsiveness to hypoxia, hypercapnia or both, tend to destabilize the respiratory control system and thus increase loop gain. Recent data indicate that OSA patients have a much higher loop gain than controls, suggesting an intrinsically less stable ventilatory control system. Wellman et al. [30] found a strong correlation between loop gain and RDI in patients with atmospheric P_{crit} values ($r = 0.88$, $p = 0.0016$) and suggested that this group of patients may be highly susceptible to changes in ventilatory instability. The effect of ACET on ventilatory instability has previously been demonstrated in patients with central sleep apnea. Taking into account the susceptibility for ventilatory instability of mainly hypopneic subjects (atmospheric P_{crit}) and the beneficial effects of ACET on ventilatory control, we investigated the adjuvant role of ACET administration after UPPP in mild OSA patients. Preliminary data of this double-blind, placebo-controlled, randomized trial suggest a beneficial effect on RDI after 3 months treatment with ACET following UPPP [31]. This opens new perspectives for a combined medical/surgical approach in OSA patients that addresses the key factors in the pathogenesis of this disease: pharmacological treatment to reduce ventilatory instability and surgery to decrease UA collapsibility.

Surgery of the Lateral Pharyngeal Walls: Hyoid Expansion

The tongue and soft palate are generally considered to be the most important soft tissue structures contributing to

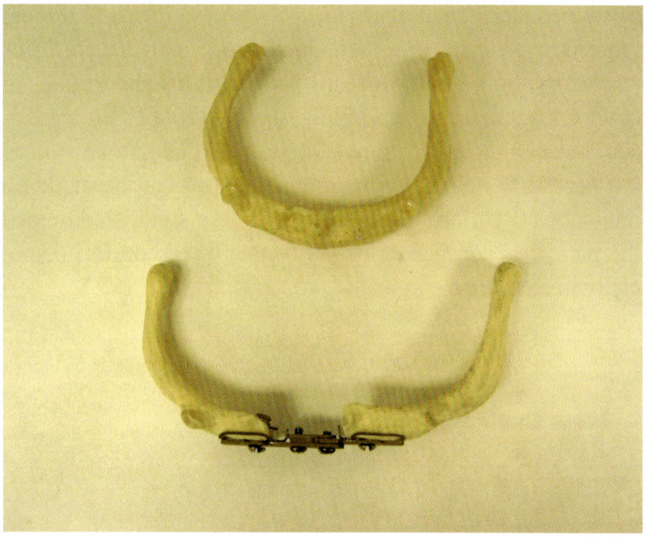

Fig. 2. Hyoid expansion on a cadaver specimen: the hyoid bone is transected at the midline and a titanium stent is secured to both parts, resulting in an increased distance between the major cornu. Reproduced with permission from Aspire Medical.

UA collapse. Based upon studies using volumetric magnetic resonance imaging (MRI), Schwab et al. [32] emphasized the importance of the lateral pharyngeal walls in controlling UA patency during sleep. The lateral walls are complex structures composed of several muscle groups (hyoglossus, styloglossus, stylohyoid, stylopharyngeus, palatoglossus, palatopharyngeus, the pharyngeal constrictors), lymphoid tissue (palatine tonsils) and pharyngeal mucosa. A beneficial effect of MMA on lateral wall collapse was observed in a study by Li et al. [33] using fiberoptic nasopharyngoscopy with the Müller maneuver. This effect might be mediated through the effect of skeletal surgery on the suprahyoid and velopharyngeal musculature [4] and on the constrictor muscles [32]. The efficacy and safety of less-invasive surgical techniques affecting lateral wall collapse is a subject of ongoing research. One of the possibilities under investigation is the use of hyoid expansion; a concept based upon experimental data obtained in dogs undergoing expansion hyoidplasty [34]. The hyoid bone is intimately related to UA structures that might contribute to UA collapse during sleep: the base of the tongue and the distal oropharyngeal and superior hypopharyngeal walls. If the hyoid bone is cut at the midline and expanded laterally through the insertion of a stent between both parts of the hyoid bone, the following anatomical changes could be expected: a lateral displacement of the greater cornu with the middle pharyngeal constrictor, the hyoglossus and stylopharyngeus (components of the lateral wall) and an anterior displacement of the base of the tongue [34] (fig. 2). The possibility of treating moderately severe OSA subjects with hyoid expansion by means of a titanium implant, is currently under investigation at 3 European Centers (Antwerp, Mannheim and Amsterdam).

Conclusions

Surgical treatment for OSA has evolved towards an individually tailored approach taking into account a variety of patient-related factors such as specific UA anatomic features, the degree of obesity, OSA severity, degree of maxillomandibular deficiency and co-morbidity. Careful patient selection, ability to perform varied surgical approaches, and willingness to utilize more than one procedure when necessary are the cornerstones of a successful management plan. Future research in this field should provide an answer to the following questions: (1) Which approach (single stage or multi-step) is the most cost-effective in a particular category of patients (taking into account OSA severity, comorbidity, anesthetic risks and economic costs)? (2) Which outcome parameters, other than RDI, are the most clinically useful to assess the effect of surgery on OSA severity, quality of life and long-term morbidity? (3) Which tools can provide more insight into the importance of nasal obstruction and its relationship and help to predict the outcome of nasal surgery? (4) What is the exact role of new treatment options such as hyoid expansion and combined pharmacological/surgical treatment of these subjects?

References

1 Boudewyns A, Van de Heyning PH, De Backer WA: Site of upper airway obstruction in obstructive sleep apnoea and influence of sleep stage. Eur Respir J 1997;10: 2566–2572.

2 Rama AN, Tekwani SH, Kushida CA: Sites of obstruction in obstructive sleep apnea. Chest 2002;122:1139–1147.

3 Sher AE: Upper airway surgery for obstructive sleep apnea. Sleep Med Rev 2002;6:195–212.

4 Li KK: Surgical therapy for adult obstructive sleep apnea. Sleep Med Rev 2005;9:201–209.

5 Bridgman SA, Dunn KM, Ducharme F: Surgery for obstructive sleep apnoea (Cochrane Review). The Cochrane Library, Issue 4. Chichester, Wiley, 2003.

6 Sher AE, Schechtman KB, Piccirillo JF: The efficacy of surgical modifications of the upper airway in adults with obstructive sleep apnea syndrome. Sleep 1996;19:156–177.

7 Shahar E, Whitney CW, Redline S, Lee ET, Newman AB, Nieto FJ, O' Connor GT, Boland LL, Schwartz JE, Samet JM: Sleep-disordered breathing and cardiovascular

disease: cross-sectional results of the Sleep Heart Health Study. Am J Respir Crit Care Med 2001;163:19–25.
8 Piccirillo JF: More information needed about the long-term health consequences of mild to moderate obstructive sleep apnea. Arch Otolaryngol Head Neck Surg 2001;127: 1400–1401.
9 Piccirillo JF: Outcomes research and obstructive sleep apnea. Laryngoscope 2000;110: 16–20.
10 Gold AR, Schwartz AR: The pharyngeal critical pressure: the whys and hows of using nasal continuous positive airway pressure diagnostically. Chest 1996;110:1077–1088.
11 Fujita S, Conway WA, Zorick FJ, Roth T: Surgical correction of anatomic abnormalities in obstructive sleep apnea syndrome: uvulopalatopharyngoplasty. Otolaryngol Head Neck Surg 1981;89:923–934.
12 Boudewyns A, De Backer WA, Van de Heyning P: Pattern of upper airway obstruction during sleep before and after uvulopalatopharyngoplasty in patients with obstructive sleep apnea. Sleep Med 2001;2:309–315.
13 Gupta VK, Reiter ER: Current treatment practices in obstructive sleep apnea and snoring. Am J Otolaryngol 2004;25:18–25.
14 Riley RW, Powell NB, Li KK, Guilleminault C: Surgical therapy of obstructive sleep apnea-hypopnea syndrome; in Kryger MH, Roth T, Dement WC (eds): Sleep Medicine. Philadelphia, Saunders, 2000, pp 913–928.
15 Fujita S, Simmons FB: Pharyngeal surgery for obstructive sleep apnea and snoring; in Fairbanks DNF, Fujita S, Ikematsu T (eds): Snoring and Obstructive Sleep Apnea. New York, Raven Press, 1987, pp 101–128.
16 Bettega G, Pépin JL, Veale D, Deschaux C, Raphaël B, Lévy P: Obstructive sleep apnea syndrome: fifty-one consecutive patients treated by maxillofacial surgery. Am J Resp Crit Care Med 2000;162:641–649.
17 Hessel NS, de Vries N: Results of uvulopalatopharyngoplasty after diagnostic work-up with polysomnography and sleep endoscopy: a report of 136 snoring patients. Eur Arch Otorhinolarygol 2003;260:91–95.
18 Kao YH, Shnayder Y, Lee KC: The efficacy of anatomically based multilevel surgery for obstructive sleep apnea. Otolaryngol Head Neck Surg 2003;129:327–335.
19 Fischer Y, Khan M, Mann WJ: Multilevel temperature-controlled radiofrequency therapy of soft palate, base of tongue, and tonsils in adults with obstructive sleep apnea. Laryngoscope 2003;113:1786–1791.
20 Stuck BA, Starzak K, Hein G, Verse T, Hörmann K, Maurer JT: Combined radiofrequency surgery of the tongue base and soft palate in obstructive sleep apnea. Acta Otolaryngol (Stockh) 2004;124:827–832.
21 Steward DL, Weaver EM, Woodson BT: Multilevel temperature-controlled radiofrequency for obstructive sleep apnea: extended follow-up. Otolaryngol Head Neck Surg 2005;132:630–635.
22 Rappai M, Collop NA, Kemp S, de Shazo R: The nose and sleep-disordered breathing. What we know and what we do not know. Chest 2003;124:2309–2323.
23 Kribbs NB, Pack AI, Kline LR, Getsy JE, Schuett JS, Henry JN, Maislin G, Dinges DF: Objective measurement of patterns of nasal CPAP use by patients with obstructive sleep apnea. Am Rev Respir Dis 1993;147:887–895.
24 Young TB, Finn L, Kim H: Nasal obstruction as a risk factor for sleep-disordered breathing. J Allergy Clin Immunol 1997;99: S757–S762.
25 Verse T, Maurer JT, Pirsig W: Effect of nasal surgery on sleep-related breathing disorders. Laryngoscope 2002;112:64–68.
26 Friedman M, Tanyeri H, Lim JW, Landsberg R, Vaidyanathan K, Caldarelli D. Effect of improved nasal breathing on obstructive sleep apnea. Otolaryngol Head Neck Surg 2000; 122:71–74.
27 Meoli AL, Rosen CL, Kristo D, Kohrman M, Gooneratne N, Aguillard RN, Fayle R, Troell R, Kramer R, Casey KR, Coleman J: Upper airway management of the adult patient with obstructive sleep apnea in the perioperative period-avoiding complications. Sleep 2003; 26:1060–1065.
28 Hsueh-Yu L, Pa-Chun W, Chung-Yao H, Shee-Wei L, Ning-Hung C, Shih-An L: Combined nasal-palatopharyngeal surgery for obstructive sleep apnea: simultaneous or staged? Acta Oto-Laryngol 2005;125:1–5.
29 Busaba NY: Same-stage nasal and palatopharyngeal surgery for obstructive sleep apnea: is it safe? Otolaryngol Head Neck Surg 2002;126:399–403.
30 Wellman A, Jordan AS, Malhotra A, Fogel RB, Schory K, Edwards JK, White DP: Ventilatory control and airway anatomy in obstructive sleep apnea. Am J Respir Care Med 2004; 170:1225–1232.
31 Vanderveken OM, Devolder A, Boudewyns AN, Hamans E, Verbraecken JA, Troosters F, Van de Heyning PH, De Backer WA: Acetazolamide administration following upper airway surgery for SDB: preliminary results of a randomized, double-blind, placebo-controlled study. Eur Respir J 2005;26(suppl 49):201S.
32 Schwab RJ, Gefter WB, Hoffman EA, Gupta KB, Pack AI: Dynamic upper airway imaging during awake respiration in normal subjects and patients with sleep-disordered breathing. Am Rev Respir Dis 1993;148:1385–1400.
33 Li KK, Guilleminault C, Riley RW, Powell NB: Obstructive sleep apnea and maxillomandibular advancement: an assessment of airway changes using radiographic and nasopharyngoscopic examinations. J Oral Maxillofac Surg 2002;60:526–530.
34 Thawley SE, Vandermeer PJ, Waters RC, Ogura JH: Expansion hyoidplasty: a potential surgical procedure designed for selected patients with obstructive sleep apnea syndrome: experimental canine results. Laryngoscope 1983;93:1387–1395.
35 Winakur SJ, Smith PL, Schwartz AL: Pathophysiology and risk factors for obstructive sleep apnea. Semin Respir Crit Care Med 1998;19:99–112.

A.N. Boudewyns, MD, PhD
Antwerp University Hospital
Department of Otorhinolaryngology
Head and Neck Surgery, Wilrijkstraat 10
BE–2650 Edegem (Belgium)
Tel. +32 03 821 33 85
Fax +32 03 821 35 06
E-Mail An.Boudewyns@uza.be

Randerath WJ, Sanner BM, Somers VK (eds): Sleep Apnea.
Prog Respir Res. Basel, Karger, 2006, vol 35, pp 174–179

Alternative Therapies for Obstructive Sleep Apnea Syndrome: Behavioral and Pharmacological Options

Ian E. Smith

Respiratory Support and Sleep Centre, Papworth Hospital, Cambridge, UK

Abstract

Many people with obstructive sleep apnea syndrome (OSAS) are treated well with continuous positive airway pressure (CPAP) but an important number cannot tolerate it or have ongoing symptoms despite good compliance. Alternative therapies are needed for these patients. Weight loss should be encouraged in all obese subjects since this may reduce or even cure the OSAS and the risks from associated disorders particularly diabetes. Bariatric surgery may be the most effective approach. In some patients OSAs are particularly prominent when they are in the supine position and position therapy can improve symptoms. Drug therapy for OSAS has a limited role although there are promising developments. OSAS associated with nasal obstruction may respond to topical steroids in adults and children. Drugs that increase ventilatory drive have proven to be ineffective or poorly tolerated. There are mixed results from trials of vasoactive compounds but antihypertensives are safe to prescribe to patients with both OSAS and hypertension. The role of serotonin (5HT) in controlling upper airway tone is complex. The mixed 5HT agonist/antagonist mirtazipine may be useful but data are limited. Cholinergic drugs (e.g. physostigmine) warrant further investigation particularly in nonobese individuals. Patients with ongoing daytime sleepiness despite compliance with otherwise effective CPAP therapy may benefit from modafanil to increase daytime alertness once other causes of hypersomnolence have been excluded.

The upper airway of individuals affected by obstructive sleep apnea syndrome (OSAS) can be narrowed but is patent during wakefulness at least when in an upright posture. Mass loading due to obesity, changes in the direction of forces on assuming a supine position, respiratory drive instability and the state-dependent fall in drive to the airway dilator muscles may all contribute to collapse of the upper airway during sleep. Each of these mechanisms is a potential target for therapies other than CPAP or upper airway surgery to ameliorate the impact of OSAS.

Weight Loss

The relationship between weight and sleep-disordered breathing was examined over 4 years in a Wisconsin cohort [1]. Compared to those with stable weight subjects who gained more than 10% of their body weight were at a 6-fold risk of developing moderate-to-severe OSAs. Those who lost 10% of their weight had a 26% fall in the apnea/hypopnea index (AHI). However, such weight loss is not easy to achieve or maintain and there is some doubt about the duration of any benefits. Some people develop recurrent OSAs despite maintaining weight loss [2].

Bariatric surgery may offer some patients a means of losing a considerable amount of weight where changes in diet and life style have failed. A recent systematic review and meta-analysis of the outcomes of this approach included 136 studies with data from 22,000 subjects [3]. The population was very obese with a mean BMI preoperatively of 47 and 19.6% of the subjects had sleep-disordered breathing. Irrespective of the surgical approach there were important reductions in sleep-disordered breathing with resolution in up to 86% of subjects. There were also dramatic reductions in the frequency of diabetes and hypertension and there is evidence of increased quality of life and longevity post-procedure.

Position Therapy

Some people may have apneas only when sleeping supine but even in those with apneas in all sleeping positions the severity of apneas is usually greater when supine and are more likely to lead to arousals [4]. It is possible to reduce the amount of sleeping time that is spent supine using pillows or a vest with a tennis ball sewn into the back. In a single-blind study, position therapy was compared with CPAP and although it was not as effective in reducing the AHI, position therapy improved sleep quality and daytime alertness to an equal extent [5]. It can also lead to a reduction in 24-hour blood pressure recordings [6].

Drug Treatments for OSAS

A large number of drugs have been trialed as treatments for OSAS. Many of the studies have been poorly designed with no control limb and very small numbers. In this section data from some of the better designed studies are presented and discussed.

Topical Therapy to the Upper Airway

In the balance of forces affecting the patency of the upper airway, the calibre of the lumen is an important factor. When subjects with both OSAS and rhinitis were randomised to either fluticasone or placebo, active treatment led to a lower AHI ($p < 0.05$) and an increase in subjective daytime alertness [7]. A reduction in AHI has also been shown in children with adenotonsillar hypertrophy treated with nasal fluticasone again with an improvement in symptoms [8].

It has been proposed that surface forces, influenced by pharyngeal secretions, contribute to the closure of the upper airway during apneas [9]. Jokic et al. [9] trialed a soft tissue lubricant (intranasal phosphocholinamin) in mild to moderate OSAS. In all 10 subjects the AHI was lower after the active preparation than after placebo (fig. 1). There were fewer arousals from sleep on the active treatment. Unfortunately, the compound is based on mineral oil making it unsafe for long-term use with a risk of lipoid pneumonia on repeated application.

Drugs Affecting Respiratory Drive

A number of compounds that increase respiratory drive have been tried in patients with OSAS. Increasing the suction pressure produced by the diaphragm could theoretically increase the number of apneas by increasing the transluminal pressure across the upper airway. Instability in drive may exacerbate OSAs by producing periodic respiratory effort [10] and so increasing the stability of the ventilatory drive should perhaps be the aim of such therapy.

Progestogens increase ventilatory drive but in a randomised controlled trial (RCT) in subjects with OSAS medroxyprogesterone had no positive effects [11]. Acetazolamide inhibits carbonic anhydrase producing a metabolic acidosis that increases ventilatory drive. In an uncontrolled study, it reduced apnea frequency in patients with OSAS by around a quarter [12]. In an RCT acetazolamide reduced the AHI by nearly half (fig. 1) [13]. However, there was no improvement in sleep quality and the subjects did not report any reduction in daytime somnolence, only 1 patient tolerated it long term. There have been several uncontrolled trials of theophylline in OSAS and 2 RCTs, 1 each with theophylline [14] and aminophylline [15]. In both of these studies there was a decrease in the total number of obstructive apneas but not their frequency during sleep. In the aminophylline study there was a 24% decrease in the time overnight spent asleep on the active drug compared to placebo [15].

Vasoactive Medication

Clonidine is an alpha-adrenergic agonist used to control hypertension, which suppresses REM sleep, when OSAs may be particularly prominent. In the only RCT describing its use in OSAS there was no significant reduction in AHI but REM sleep was only completely suppressed in 2 of 8 subjects [16]. In subjects where REM sleep was not suppressed, the AHI in REM sleep was paradoxically increased. In an uncontrolled trial metoprolol and the ACE inhibitor cilazapril were both shown to reduce apnea frequency by about a third but sleep quality and daytime

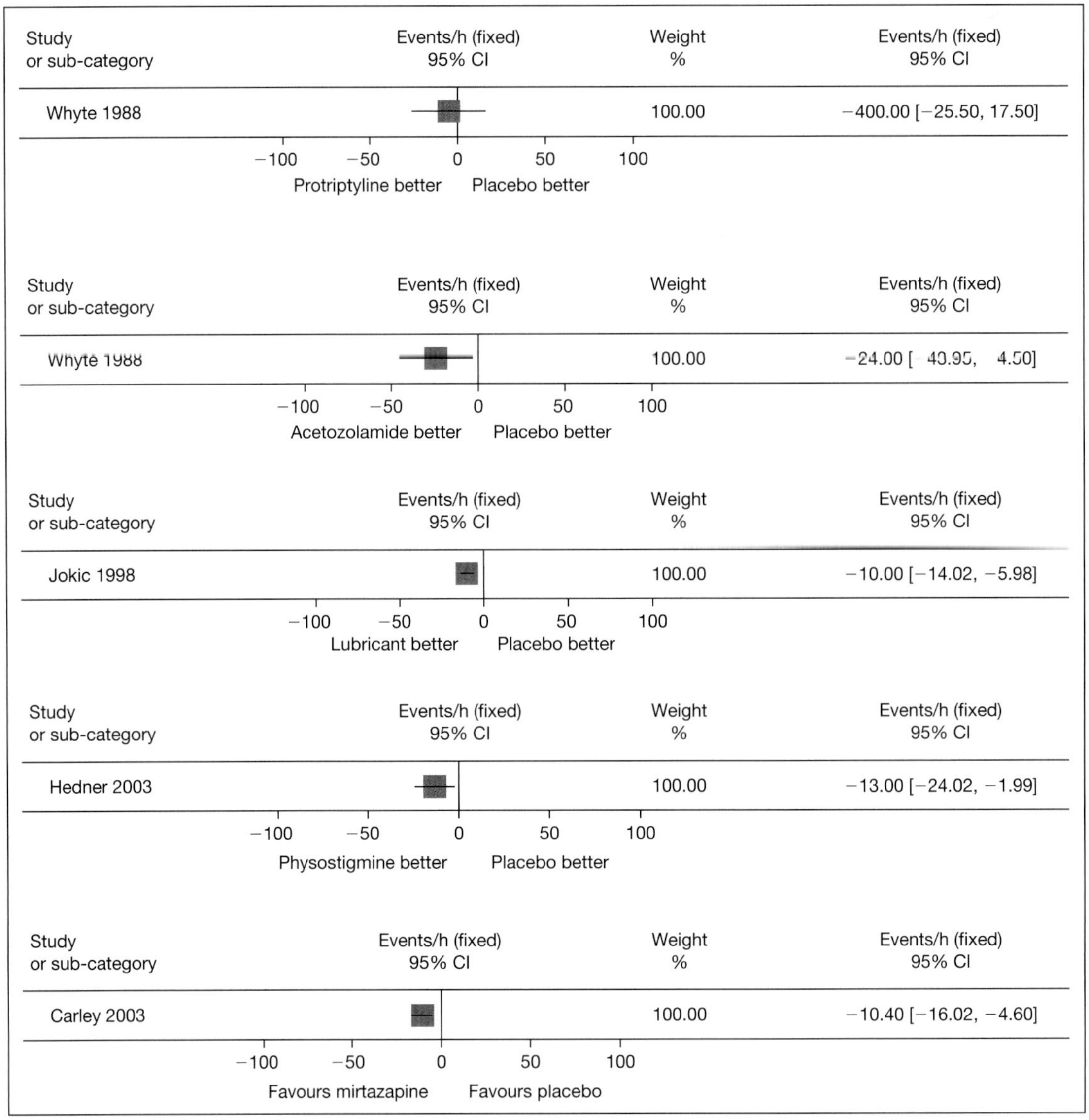

Fig. 1. Graphic representation of effectiveness of medication in reducing apnea/hypopnea index (events/h). Protriptyline the most studied drug is ineffective. Although acetazolamide reduces AHI by a half, it is poorly tolerated long term. Nasal lubricant reduced AHI in NREM sleep but there is no compound available for long-term use. Physostigmine and mirtazapine have been effective in reducing AHI on single night studies. No long-term data have yet been published. Reproduced with permission from The 2005 Cochrane Review [41]. The studies Whyte 1988, Jokic 1998, Hedner 2003 and Carley 2003 are referenced in the current text as [13, 9, 36 and 28], respectively.

symptoms were not reported [17]. In contrast, in an RCT cilazapril reduced blood pressure with only a minor reduction in OSA during NREM sleep [18]. Another study randomised patients with hypertension and OSAS to treatment with two of five agents to compare the effects of atenolol, amlodipine, enalapril, hydrochlorothiazide and losartan [19]. Atenolol was most effective in reducing blood pressure. None of the drugs reduced the AHI or daytime symptoms. Finally, celiprolol another beta-adrenergic blocking agent does not reduce OSAS severity [20]. While there is remaining doubt about whether anti-hypertensives can ameliorate OSAS they do not lead to deterioration and so treatment of hypertension can be recommended in OSAS patients.

Serotonin Agonists and Antagonists

There is tonic serotonergic input from the medullary raphe to the hypoglossal motor neurones which, acting through genioglossus, increases upper airway patency. This tonic input decreases from wakefulness to NREM to a minimum in REM sleep [21]. Increasing serotonin (5HT) levels, administering 5HT agonists or reducing negative feedback on pre-synaptic 5HT receptors with specific antagonists during sleep offer possible therapeutic approaches to OSAS. It should be noted, however, that animal models particularly employing vagotomy might have exaggerated the importance of 5HT in controlling airway tone [22].

The tricyclic antidepressant protriptyline reduces reuptake of 5HT and noradrenaline in the brain. It reduces REM sleep and in a cat model at least preferentially activates both hypoglossal and recurrent laryngeal nerve activity without altering phrenic nerve activity [23]. However, in three RCTs no difference was found in the frequency of apneas overnight or any other measure of a respiratory disturbance during sleep compared to placebo [13, 24, 25]. Side effects including dry mouth, urinary hesitance, impotence and visual disturbance were frequent. The specific serotonin reuptake inhibitor (SSRI) paroxetine has been shown to increase genioglossus activity in healthy volunteers during wakefulness, when the serotonergic medullary raphe nuclei are most active [26]. During sleep and in particular REM sleep these neurones are less active and since there are lower levels of 5HT released preventing reuptake is less likely to affect airway tone. In a study of paroxetine in OSAS patients there was only a modest improvement in the apnea frequency overall from 25 to 18/h [27]. There was a 35% drop in the number of apneas in NREM sleep but no change in the frequency in REM and no reduction in daytime symptoms.

Mirtazapine is an agonist at 5-HT1, and antagonist at 5-HT2 and 5-HT3 receptors. As a 5HT agonist it offers the possibility of affecting airway tone in REM sleep when SSRIs have been shown to be ineffective. In a controlled trial published in abstract form it decreased the mean AHI (fig. 1) but no long-term data were presented [28]. A case report of an individual intolerant of CPAP who was treated with mirtazapine has been published subsequently [29]. This man had a baseline AHI of 40.4 and on follow-up 3 months later had an AHI of 9.3 with a subjective improvement in well-being.

At different sites and in different animal models 5HT has been shown to decrease rather than increase genioglossus activity presumably through autoregulatory mechanisms acting at the pre-synaptic receptors. Possibly by blocking this action the 5HT antagonist and anti-emetic ondansetron decreases the frequency of apneas in adult bulldogs [30]. There has been one study of ondansetron in humans with OSAS, which showed no effect on sleep apnea possibly due to dosage issues [31].

Cholinergic Agents

Acetylcholine has effects on the upper airway dilators. In the rat the application of nicotinic agents to the hypoglossal motor neurones increases tone in genioglossus, while muscarinic agents reduce tone [32]. In one study, nicotine gum which has only a short half-life of action reduced the number of apneas in the first 2 h of sleep [33]. There was no apparent change in sleep structure. In an RCT, 20 non-smoking snorers were administered transdermal nicotine or placebo [34]. The intensity of snoring was decreased by the active treatment but the number of apneas was not and sleep quality deteriorated. Other nicotinic agonists might be more beneficial but there are no data available to date.

There is a relationship in patients with multi-system atrophy between reduced thalamic nerve terminal density and the frequency of OSAs [35]. It was postulated that this may be due to decreased pontine cholinergic projections and as a consequence physostigmine was trialed in patients with OSAS [36]. The overall AHI was reduced by 23% compared to placebo (fig. 1) with greater effects at the end of the night when it was thought that the drug concentration was optimised and in REM sleep. During REM sleep in the final third of the night the reduction in AHI was 67.5%. Only subjects with a body weight of <120% ideal were admitted to the trial and there was an inverse relationship between body weight and AHI reduction. It is interesting that physostigmine both decreased AHI in REM sleep and increased REM duration while REM-suppressing agents such as protriptyline and clonidine have been ineffective in reducing AHI [13, 16, 24, 25].

Persisting Daytime Sleepiness on CPAP Treatment

In some people even when abnormal respiratory events during sleep are normalised by CPAP therapy, disabling daytime somnolence persists. It is important in this situation to review the original diagnosis and consider alternative or co-existing reasons for sleepiness. If no other remediable cause is identified, then wakefulness-promoting drugs can be considered. Amphetamines improve daytime alertness in OSAS patients [37] but have considerable drawbacks including abuse potential and cardiovascular side effects. Modafinil is a wake-promoting agent, chemically unrelated to amphetamines. Its exact mechanism of action is not yet known but there is evidence that it reduces persistent sleepiness in patients complying with CPAP therapy [38]. Although there has been concern that it might reduce compliance with CPAP this was not demonstrated in two published series [38, 39]. In one smaller study there was a slight decrease in CPAP usage [40]. This is unlikely to be of clinical significance but the possibility of decreased CPAP usage should be borne in mind.

References

1 Peppard PE, Young T, Palta M, Dempsey J, Skatrud J: Longitudinal study of moderate weight change and sleep-disordered breathing. JAMA 2000;284:3015–3021.
2 Sampol G, Munoz X, Sagales MT, Marti S, Roca A, Dolors de la Calzada M, Lloberes P, Morell F: Long-term efficacy of dietary weight loss in sleep apnoea/hypopnoea syndrome. Eur Respir J 1998;12:1156–1159.
3 Buchwald H, Avidor Y, Braunwald E, Jensen MD, Pories W, Fahrback K, Schoelles K: Bariatric surgery: a systematic review and meta-analysis. JAMA 2004;292:1724–1737.
4 Oksenbert A, Khamaysi I, Siverbert DS, Tarasiuk A: Association of body position with severity of apneic events in patients with severe non-positional obstructive sleep apnea. Chest 2000;118:1018–1024.
5 Jokic R, Klimaszewski A, Crossley M, Sridhar G, Fitzpatrick MF: Positional treatment vs. continuous positive airway pressure in patients with positional obstructive sleep apnoea syndrome. Chest 1999;115:771–781.
6 Berger M, Oksenberg A, Silverberg DS, Arons E, Radwan H, Iaina A: Avoiding the supine position during sleep lowers 24 h blood pressure in obstructive sleep apnea (OSA) patients. J Hum Hypertens 1997;11:657–664.
7 Kiely JL, Nolan P, McNicholas WT: Intranasal corticosteroid therapy for obstructive sleep apnoea in patients with co-existing rhinitis. Thorax 2004;59:50–55.
8 Brouillette RT, Manoukian JJ, Ducharme FM, Oudjhane K, Earle LG, Ladan S, Merielli A: Efficacy of fluticasone nasal spray for pediatric obstructive sleep apnoea. J Pediatr 2001;138: 838–844.
9 Jokic R, Klimaszweski A, Mink J, Fitzpatrick MF: Surface tension forces in sleep apnea: the role of a soft tissue lubricant. Am J Respir Crit Care Med 1998;157:1522–1525.
10 Younes M: Contributions of upper airway mechanics and control mechanisms to severity of obstructive sleep apnea. Am J Respir Crit Care Med 2003;168:645–658.
11 Cook WR, Benich JJ, Wooten SA: Indices of severity of obstructive sleep apnea syndrome do not change during medroxyprogesterone acetate therapy. Chest 1989;96:262–266.
12 Tojima H, Kunitomo F, Kimura H, Tatsumi K, Kuriyama T, Honda Y: Effects of acetazolamide in patients with sleep apnoea syndrome. Thorax 1988;43:113–119.
13 Whyte K, Gould G, Airlie A, Shapiro CM, Douglas NJ: Role of protriptyline and acetazolamide in the sleep apnoea/hypopnoea syndrome. Sleep 1988;11:463–472.
14 Mulloy E, McNicholas WT, Theophylline in obstructive sleep apnoea: a double blind evaluation. Chest 1992;101:753–757.
15 Espinosa H, Antic R, Thornton AT, McEvoy RD: The effects of aminophylline on the sleep and sleep-disordered breathing in patients with obstructive sleep apnea syndrome. Am Rev Respir Dis 1987;136:80–84.
16 Issa F: Effect of clonidine in obstructive sleep apnoea. Am Rev Respir Dis 1992;145: 465–469.
17 Weichler U, Kerres-Mayer B, Mayer J, Weber K, Hoffman R, Peter JH: Influence of antihypertensive drug therapy on sleep pattern and sleep apnea activity. Cardiology 1991;78: 124–130.
18 Grote L, Wutkewicz K, Knaack L, Ploch T, Hedner J, Hermann JP: Association between blood pressure reduction with antihypertensive treatment and sleep apnea activity. Am J Hypertens 2000;13:1280–1287.
19 Kraiczi H, Hedner J, Peker Y, Grote L: Comparison of atenolol, amlodipine, enalapril, hydrochlorothiazide and losartan for antihypertensive treatment in obstructive sleep apnea. Am J Respir Crit Care Med 2000;161: 1423–1428.
20 Planes C, Foucher A, Leroy M, Dartois N, Juste K, Baillart O, Raffestin B: Effect of celiprolol treatment in hypertensive patients with sleep apnea. Sleep 1999;22: 507–513.
21 Jacobs BL, Azmitia EC: Structure and function of the brain serotonin system. Physiol Rev 1992;72:165–229.
22 Sood S, Morrison JL, Liu H, Horner RL: Role of endogenous serotonin in modulating genioglossus muscle activity in awake and sleeping rats. Am J Respir Crit Care Med 2005;72:1338–1347.
23 Bonora M, St John WM, Bledsoe TA: Differential elevation by Protriptyline and depression by diazepam of upper airway respiratory motor activity. Am Rev Respir Dis 1985;131:41–45.
24 Brownell LGP, West P, Sweatman P, Acres JC, Kryger MH: Protriptyline in obstructive sleep apnea: a double blind trial. N Engl J Med 1982;307:1037–1042.
25 Stepanski EJ, Conway WA, Young DK, Zorick FJ, Wittig RM, Roth T: A double blind trial of protriptyline in the treatment of sleep apnea syndrome. Henry Ford Hosp Med J 1988;36: 5–8.
26 Sunderram J, Parisi RA, Strobel RJ: Serotonergic stimulation of the genioglossus and the response to nasal continuous positive airway pressure. Am J Respir Crit Care Med 2000;162:925–929.
27 Kraiczi H, Hedner J, Dahlof P, Ejnell H, Carlson J: Effect of serotonin uptake inhibition on breathing during sleep and daytime symptoms in obstructive sleep apnea. Sleep 1999;22:61–67.
28 Carley DW, Olopade C, Seink S, Radulovacki M: Serotonin antagonist improves sleep apnea. Sleep Medicine 2003;4(suppl 1):S6.
29 Castillo JL, Menendez P, Segovia L, Guilleminault C: Effectiveness of mirtazapine in the treatment of sleep apnea/hypopnea syndrome (SAHS). Sleep Med 2004;5: 507–508.
30 Veasey SC, Chachkes J, Fenik P, Hendricks JC: The effects of ondansetron on sleep-disordered breathing in the English Bulldog. Sleep 2001;24:155–160.
31 Stradling J, Smith D, Radulovacki M, Carley C: Effect of ondansetron on moderate obstructive sleep apnoea, a single night, placebo-controlled trial. J Sleep Res 2003;12:169–170.
32 Liu X, Sood S, Liu H, Horner RL: Opposing muscarinic and nicotinic modulation of hypoglossal motor output to genioglossus muscle in rats in vivo. J Physiology 2005;565: 965–980.
33 Gothe B, Strohl KP, Levin S, Cherniack NS: Nicotine: a different approach to treatment of obstructive sleep apnea. Chest 1985;87:11–17.
34 Davila DG, Hunt RD, Offord KP, Harris CD, Sherard JW Jr: Acute effects of transdermal nicotine on sleep architecture, snoring, and sleep-disordered breathing in nonsmokers. Am J Respir Crit Care Med 1994;150:469–474.
35 Gilman S, Chervin RD, Koeppe RA, Consens FB, Little R, An H, Junck L, Heumann M: Obstructive sleep apnoea is related to a thalamic cholinergic deficit in MSA. Neurology 2003;61:35–36.
36 Hedner J, Kraiczi H, Peker Y, Murphy P: Reduction of sleep-disordered breathing after physostigmine. Am J Respir Crit Care Med 2003;168:1246–1251.

37 Guilleminault C, Philip P: Tiredness and somnolence despite initial treatment of obstructive sleep apnea syndrome (what to do when an OSAS patient stays hypersomnolent despite treatment). Sleep 1996;19(suppl 9):S117–S122.
38 Pack AI, Black JE, Schwartz JRL, Matheson JK: Modafinil as adjunct therapy for daytime sleepiness in obstructive sleep apnoea. Am J Respir Crit Care Med 2001;164:1675–1681.
39 Black JE, Douglas NJ, Earl CQ: Modafinil OSA Study Group. Efficacy and safety of modafinil as adjunctive therapy for excessive sleepiness associated with obstructive sleep apnea (abstract). Sleep 2002;25(suppl 1):A22.
40 Kingshott RN, Vennelle M, Coleman EL, Engleman HM, Mackay TW, Douglas NJ: Randomized, double-blind, placebo-controlled crossover trial of modafinil in the treatment of residual excessive daytime sleepiness in the sleep apnea/hypopnea syndrome. Am J Respir Crit Care Med. 2001;163: 918–923.
41 Smith IE, Lasserson T, Wright J: Drug therapy for OSA (Cochrane Review). The Cochrane Library, 2005, in press.

Dr. Ian E. Smith
Respiratory Support and Sleep Centre
Papworth Hospital, University of Cambridge
Cambridge CB3 8RE (UK)
Tel. +44 1480 830541, Fax +44 1480 36 4568
E-Mail ian.smith@papworth.nhs.uk

Randerath WJ, Sanner BM, Somers VK (eds): Sleep Apnea.
Prog Respir Res. Basel, Karger, 2006, vol 35, pp 180–191

Central Sleep Apnea, Hypoventilation Syndromes and Periodic Breathing Disorders

S.M. Caples[a] V.K. Somers[b]

Division of [a]Pulmonary and Critical Care Medicine, and [b]Cardiovascular Diseases, Department of Internal Medicine, Mayo Clinic and Mayo Foundation, Rochester, Minn., USA

Abstract

Central sleep apnea and hypoventilation syndromes are increasingly important clinical entities, in part because of their associations with pervasive conditions such as heart failure and obesity. While disruption of ventilatory control appears to contribute to these disorders, much remains unknown about pathophysiologic mechanisms and optimal treatment methods. This chapter explores some of these issues in the context of the most recent research data, and also discusses some less common disorders of ventilatory control that may be encountered by the sleep medicine specialist.

Definitions

A 1999 joint consensus statement [1] was prepared in an effort to standardize definitions of sleep-related breathing disorder syndromes as well as techniques for measurement to guide future research. While some of these recommendations will be referred to, it should be noted that an updated scoring manual is expected from the American Academy of Sleep Medicine (AASM) in 2006.

The nosology of the central sleep apnea (CSA) syndromes have lacked rigid standardization, probably owing to the relative infrequency with which some of the clinical disorders are encountered in clinical practice. The AASM published the Second Edition of the International Classification of Sleep Disorders (ICSD-2) in 2005 [2]. The reader is referred to that publication for details, but we will utilize this classification scheme whenever possible in describing clinical syndromes in this chapter.

In the broadest sense, CSA is characterized by episodes of apnea or hypopnea related to loss of ventilatory output from the central respiratory generator in the brainstem to the respiratory pump. During polysomnography (PSG), the scorable central event has been defined by an absent (apnea) or reduced (hypopnea) respiratory effort associated with decrements in airflow, lasting at least 10 s. It should be noted that centrally mediated pauses in breathing may be a natural occurrence, such as with a *sleep onset central apnea* during the transition from wakefulness to light sleep. While the esophageal balloon is considered the gold standard to confirm reductions or absence of respiratory effort, central apneas appear to be adequately scored by plethysmographic measurement of chest wall and abdominal motion, a technique with reasonable reliability that is unlikely to misclassify a patient's sleep-related breathing disorder [3, 4]. Cardiogenic oscillations noted in the airflow signal seen with a patent upper airway may further confirm that an apneic event is not obstructive [5].

Historically, CSA syndromes have been broadly divided into two general classes based upon the presence or absence of hypercapnia during wakefulness; this heterogeneity was described by Bradley et al. in 1986 [6]. As will be discussed later, those disorders associated with daytime hypercapnia (some hypoventilation syndromes) appear to result from global derangements in ventilation and ventilatory drive during both wakefulness and sleep. Disorders without hypercapnia, and importantly often associated with *hypo*capnia, include primary CSA syndrome, Cheyne-Stokes breathing pattern (also been referred to as periodic breathing) seen most commonly in the setting of heart failure (HF) or central neurologic disease, and high altitude periodic breathing (HAPB).

Control of Ventilation and the Influence of Sleep

Ventilation is broadly controlled by both chemical/ metabolic stimuli (PaO_2 and $PaCO_2$) as well as neurobehavioral factors. The latter are prominent during wakefulness, and include stimuli from higher cortical centers related to daily living behaviors, such as phonation and deglutition as well as visual and auditory cues thought to contribute to an overall increase in tonic output from the cerebral cortex to the respiratory centers in the brainstem. During sleep, with loss of this neurobehavioral input, ventilation is driven by an automatic system which integrates afferent signals from peripheral (primarily sensing PaO_2) and central (sensing $PaCO_2$) chemoreceptors as well as vagally mediated feedback from lung and chest wall mechanoreceptors [7].

The reduction in ventilation associated with sleep appears to be multifactorial in origin [8]. NREM sleep is associated with a twofold increase in upper airway resistance [9] which appears to be due in part to reduced neuromuscular input as demonstrated by electromyographic recordings of upper airway muscles. This reduction in neuromuscular control originates primarily from the tonic background, although decrements may be seen on phasic stimulation during inspiration [10]. These regional effects coupled with reductions in both the hypoxic and hypercapnic ventilatory response [8], result in modest hypoventilation associated with 2–4% reductions in oxyhemoglobin saturation and a 3–6 mm Hg increase in the partial pressure of carbon dioxide [11, 12]. Further decrements in the ventilatory response occur during REM sleep [13], despite the return of behavioral cortical activity which is characterized by an irregular breathing pattern thought to be associated with dreaming. There is some evidence to suggest that premenopausal women maintain ventilatory responsiveness during the state change from wakefulness to NREM sleep [14], a finding which may be important in explaining the reduced risk of sleep-disordered breathing (SDB) noted in the same population [15].

During both wakefulness and sleep, the most sensitive determinant of ventilation is $PaCO_2$, the level of which is linearly related to minute ventilation. Thus, small changes in arterial CO_2 tension actuate a change in ventilation. Oxygen tension also appears to play a role in the drive to breathe, but relatively large decrements ($PaO_2 < 60$ mm Hg) are required before an appreciable increase in minute ventilation is encountered (a hyperbolic response) [16]. Skatrud and Dempsey [17] were among the first to describe an apneic threshold, a $PaCO_2$ level below which was frequently associated with central apnea during NREM sleep in healthy individuals. Hypoxia appears to promote apnea indirectly by stimulating ventilation with resultant hypocapnia sufficient to cross the apneic threshold [17], a mechanism which is important in periodic breathing at high altitude (discussed later).

The goal of the ventilatory control system is to maintain homeostasis of blood gas tensions within a tightly controlled range. The determinants of this system have been modeled after an engineering concept known as loop gain [18, 19], which considers the overall gain of a system based upon feedback from multiple inputs. In its most simplistic terms, as outlined by Khoo et al. [18], the ventilatory system is under the influence of:

1. Respiratory pump and gas exchange capabilities of the lungs and body tissues ('plant gain')
2. Central and peripheral chemoreflexes ('controller gain')
3. Circulatory time (as determined by fluctuations in cardiac output and cerebral blood flow)

This homeostatic model has been applied to some of the fundamental pathophysiologic mechanisms related to SDB, including obstructive sleep apnea (OSA) [20, 21] (fig. 1). Those mechanisms as they relate to CSA will be discussed in this chapter.

The Association between Central and Obstructive SDB

There are features of OSA and CSA that are physiologically distinct. For example, obstructive apneas are most profound and frequent during REM sleep, as a result of muscle atonia during this stage. Central events, on the other hand, are rare during REM sleep, which probably relates to the relatively minor role of PCO_2 in driving ventilation during this stage [22] where behavioral influences become more prominent. Still, there appears to be considerable overlap between pathophysiologic mechanisms in OSA and CSA.

It is unusual to encounter pure CSA without discernible superimposed obstructive events either within an apnea (so-called 'mixed apnea') or co-existing during a single night. This coupling likely represents overlap of the pathophysiologic and neuromuscular mechanisms that govern aspects of both ventilatory control and upper airway patency. There are several lines of evidence to suggest OSA and CSA may share common pathophysiologic mechanisms. Central apneas during Cheyne-Stokes breathing

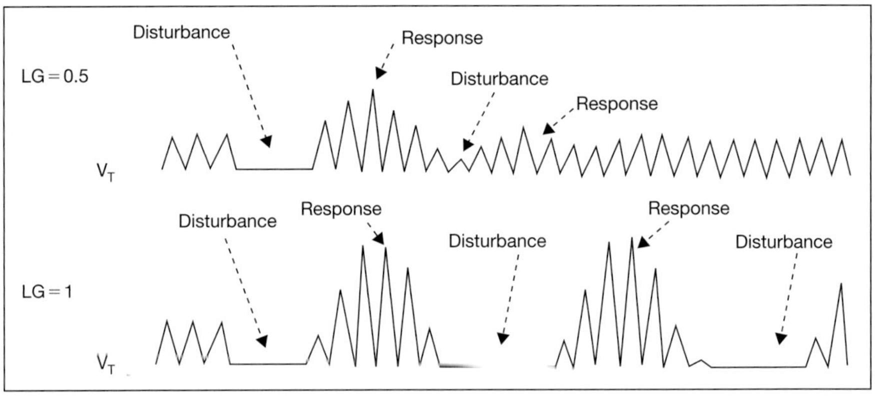

Fig. 1. Comparative ventilatory responses to apnea (the first disturbance) in 2 individuals with differing loop gain (LG). An LG of 0.5 produces a regular ventilatory pattern, while a heightened LG (LG = 1) results in an exaggerated response with subsequent oscillation. From White [21].

pattern have been found to be frequently accompanied by upper airway occlusion [23]. Induction of periodic breathing with hypoxic gas mixtures results in upper airway narrowing in both snorers [24] and normal volunteers [25], an effect confirmed by electromyographic recordings of upper airway muscles [26]. In HF, there is evidence for an overnight shift in predominance of obstructive apneas to central apneas, an effect which may be mediated by deteriorating cardiac function [27]. Further evidence of the association between upper airway narrowing and central events is derived from an observed increase in central apneas in the supine position [28] and a reduction in central events with the use of continuous positive airway pressure (CPAP) treatment [29, 30].

Primary CSA

Also referred as idiopathic CSA, this remains a relatively uncommon disorder and, as a result, the pathophysiology and natural history are not well understood. What does appear to be a consistent finding among these patients is an exaggerated ventilatory response to $PaCO_2$ during both wakefulness and sleep, representative of high loop gain predisposing to respiratory control system instability, as described in a series of papers by Bradley's group [6, 31, 32]. This increased sensitivity to blood carbon dioxide tensions results in lower baseline $PaCO_2$ (around 35 mm Hg), close to the apneic threshold, thereby predisposing to apnea. Associated arousals manifest with abrupt hyperventilation [32] and further propagation of ventilatory instability. That arousals and ventilatory pattern in CSA are not the cyclical waxing and waning as seen in Cheyne-Stokes respiration suggest additional or pathophysiologically distinct mechanisms at work. However, raising the $PaCO_2$ by inhaled CO_2 or increasing dead space was sufficient to nearly eradicate central apneas in a group of patients with CSA [33]. Polysomnographically, central apneic events are typically seen during NREM sleep, probably because the reduction in CO_2 sensitivity during REM sleep [13] renders the ventilatory response less capable of crossing the apneic threshold.

Given the uncommon occurrence of CSA, its epidemiology is not well described. Most, but not all [34] studies suggest a middle to older age male predominance. Evidence for heritability of chemosensitivity in other clinical settings, such as chronic obstructive pulmonary disease (COPD) [35] and neuromuscular disease [36], suggests a possible familial role in CSA, although this has not been confirmed.

Dominant clinical features of CSA include fragmented sleep with frequent awakenings which may lead to daytime hypersomnolence. Insomnia is often reported, and it is possible that each condition feeds the other, as the apneic threshold is frequently violated during wake-sleep transitions. According to the 1999 Guidelines, more than 5 central events per hour of sleep are required to make a diagnosis of CSA. However, absence of outcomes research does not allow severity grading of CSA based upon the apnea/hypopnea index (AHI) as has been applied to patients with OSA. Central apneas usually result in oxyhemoglobin desaturation but, on account of enhanced ventilatory drive and less obesity-related chest wall restriction, are often modest in comparison to those encountered during obstructive apneas in OSA. In general, cardiovascular sequelae of CSA are thought to be relatively mild [37], although systematic studies to confirm this are lacking.

As there are no high level clinical trials comparing treatment options and efficacy in CSA, the literature has been largely based upon clinical case reports or series. That said, there appears to be a number of viable treatment options for the CSA patient suffering from sleep disruption and/or resultant daytime functional sequelae. CPAP therapy has been shown to be effective in some patients with CSA [29, 30]. Given the pathophysiologic similarities between CSA and OSA previously outlined and evidence for dysfunctional upper airway mechanics in CSA, this finding is not surprising, although the effects of CPAP may be independent of upper airway closure and more related to influences on ventilatory drive. Furthermore, since OSA and CSA often co-exist, a trial of CPAP seems warranted in many instances, particularly in the somnolent, obese, and/or snoring patient with central apneas on PSG.

Very limited data suggest that supplemental oxygen may be effective in reducing central apneic events in CSA [38], although possibly at the risk of increasing the frequency of obstructive apneas in those with mixed disease [39]. Its mechanism of action is not completely clear but it probably acts to suppress ventilatory drive and hyperventilation, thus moving the $PaCO_2$ away from the apneic threshold.

The efficacy of acetazolamide in CSA has also been reported in two studies with treatment duration of 7–30 days [40, 41]. This carbonic anhydrase inhibitor is believed to act by inducing a mild metabolic acidosis, resulting in a widened gap between the prevailing $PaCO_2$ and the $PaCO_2$ associated with the apneic threshold [42]. A third study described emergence of obstructive apneas following acetazolamide therapy for mixed sleep apnea CSA [43], a finding possibly explained by heightened respiratory muscle force in response to metabolic acidosis, resulting in more negative upper airway intralumenal pressures.

Cheyne-Stokes Breathing Pattern (Cheyne-Stokes Respiration)

Cheyne-Stokes respiration (CSA-CSR), an increasingly common form of SDB most often encountered in the setting of HF, is a breathing pattern characterized by crescendo-decrescendo tidal volumes with intervening central apneas. This waxing and waning pattern has also been referred to as *periodic breathing*. In contrast to OSA, where arousals typically occur with apnea termination, arousals from sleep in CSA-CSR tend to occur at the height of the hyperpneic phase following apnea. Considering this propensity for sleep disruption, it is not clear why daytime symptoms in CSA-CSR may not be as prominent as in OSA [44, 45].

CSA-CSR in HF has been associated with increased mortality [46, 47]. The severity of CSA is thought to be, to some extent, a reflection of underlying cardiac dysfunction, which could partially explain the mortality association. However, multivariate analyses suggest that CSA-CSR may be an independent risk factor for mortality [47]. Potential mechanisms may relate to cardiac decompensation associated with apnea-induced hypoxemia, sympathetic activation, or repetitive arousals and sleep fragmentation [48]. Perhaps as a consequence, CSA in HF has been associated with cardiac pathologies that could further worsen prognosis, such as atrial fibrillation [49].

The characteristic waxing and waning pattern of alternating apneas and hyperpneas in CSA-CSR is readily recognized on PSG (fig. 2). The cycle length, found to approximate 60 s, is significantly longer than those encountered in primary CSA [50], and appears to correlate with circulatory delay. The 1999 Guidelines require 5 or more central apneas or hypopneas per hour of sleep as well as at least 10 consecutive minutes of cyclic crescendo and decrescendo changes in breathing amplitude [1]. There are scant outcome data upon which to base severity criteria in CSA-CSR. Reported variables include the central apnea index [51], the central AHI, and the quantity or percentage of sleep time with periodic breathing [47]. Lanfranchi et al. [47] found prognostic significance in the central AHI but not in the percentage of sleep time spent with periodic breathing.

Mechanisms of CSA-CSR in HF

Many of the pathophysiologic mechanisms in HF and CSA-CSR relate to abnormalities in ventilatory control as outlined in the model above, although integrated reflexes and pathways are undoubtedly more complex. Circulatory delay in association with reduced cardiac output in systolic HF is reproducible in models of CSA in animals [52] and usually is present in human patients with HF and CSA-CSR [53, 54]. Naughton et al. [55] showed that circulatory delay appears to play an important role in determining CSA-CSR cycle length.

On the other hand, interindividual variation in central and peripheral chemoreflex sensitivity ('controller gain') may explain why some patients with HF do not develop central apnea. HF patients with CSA-CSR have consistently been found to have heightened ventilatory responses to blood CO_2 tensions, as in primary CSA, often resulting in hypocapnia [31, 56, 57]. Javaheri and Corbett [58] reported that hypocapnia is often modest ($PaCO_2$ range of 32–34 mm Hg) and is not invariably present during wakefulness. Recalling that a stable ventilatory rhythm is maintained by a 3–6 mm Hg rise in PCO_2 associated with normal NREM sleep, small decrements in PCO_2 below the

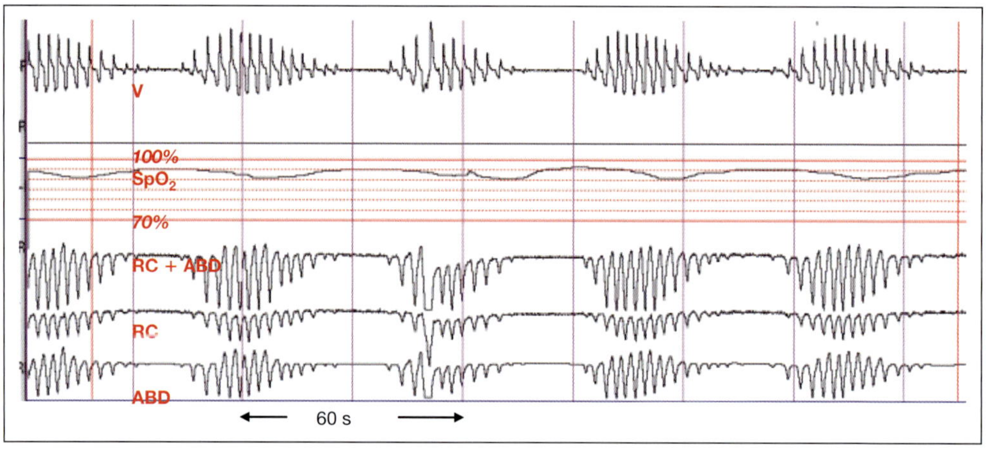

Fig. 2. Cheyne-Stokes respiration seen on PSG in an individual with HF (180 s of data). Note rhythmic oscillations in ventilation with an approximate cycle length of 60 s. Because of circulatory delay, oxyhemoglobin desaturations manifest on pulse oximetry near the end of the subsequent hyperpneic phase. V = Nasal airflow; SpO_2 = oxyhemoglobin saturation; RC = rib cage movements; ABD = abdominal movements. From the Mayo Clinic Sleep Disorders Center.

apneic threshold are often sufficient to destabilize the system, resulting in ventilatory oscillations manifesting as CSA-CSR [57, 58]. The intervening apneas perpetuate the vicious cycle as resulting hypercapnia elicits an exaggerated ventilatory response on subsequent cycles.

Sensitivity to CO_2 positively correlates with the severity of the CSA-CSR as determined by the AHI [57]. Furthermore, HF patients also have enhanced CO_2 sensitivity and relative hyperventilation *during exercise* (represented by the VE/VCO_2 slope), a finding that has been shown to be of prognostic importance [59, 60] and may be representative of global derangements in CO_2 metabolism in this population. A nonrandomized observation of CPAP compared with O_2 therapy in HF with CSA showed improvement of the VE/VCO_2 slope in the CPAP group but not in those treated with O_2 [61]. Further evidence for derangements in CO_2 processing in HF include a reduced cerebrovascular response to hypocapnia in those with CSA-CSR compared to those without [62]. Finally, very recent data suggest that hypocapnia-induced destabilization of ventilatory control appears to be specific to systolic dysfunction and circulatory delay in HF. A prospective evaluation of stroke patients showed that those with systolic dysfunction and hypocapnia had a higher prevalence of CSA independent of stroke type or brain location [63]. Despite the common occurrence of hypocapnia in hepatic cirrhotics, related to metabolic derangements and alterations in pulmonary hemodynamics [64, 65], cirrhotics with normal left ventricular (LV) function (ejection fraction 60%) matched with HF patients (ejection fraction 23%) for $PaCO_2$ levels showed little to no CSA compared with the high rate in the HF group [66].

Leptin, the protein product of the adipocyte *ob/ob* gene, may provide a mechanistic link between cardiac dysfunction and ventilatory control. Leptin is predominantly implicated in appetite, weight and metabolism regulation, but has also been linked to CO_2 sensitivity [67]. In a knockout model of obese mice, leptin infusions appeared to prevent respiratory depression, particularly during REM sleep [68]. Disturbed leptin metabolism in HF [59] may conceivably contribute to the heightened CO_2 sensitivity (controller gain) and predisposition to CSA-CSR in HF.

Increased cardiac filling pressures (pulmonary capillary wedge pressures) have been associated with worsening of CSA-CSR [69]. This may explain the increase in central apnea frequency as HF severity worsens, as well as when HF patients change from the upright to the supine posture [28]. While overt alveolar flooding is probably needed to stimulate ventilation on the basis of hypoxemia, subtle pulmonary interstitial edema commonly resulting from increases in cardiac filling pressures in HF can increase ventilation by stimulation of vagally mediated lung irritant receptors [36, 79], thereby leading to mild chronic hypocapnia. There may also be interactions between the respiratory control center and cardiac mechanoreceptors or other pressure-sensitive cardiac receptors that elicit reflex changes in ventilatory control.

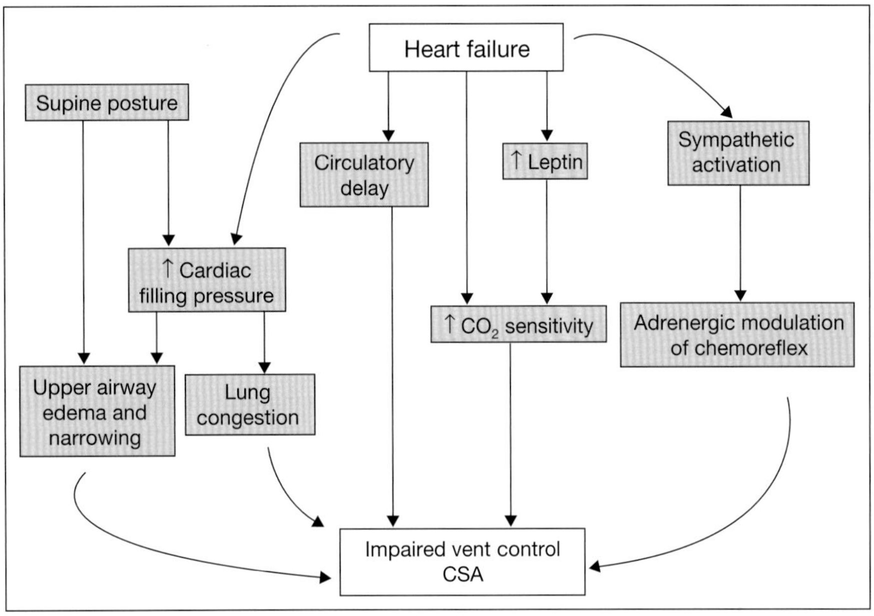

Fig. 3. Potential pathways linking HF to CSA. Instability of ventilatory control, a primary intermediary mechanism, may be induced by a number of tertiary pathways. See text for details. From Caples et al. [70].

Figure 3 summarizes possible pathophysiologic mechanisms in HF and CSA [70].

Further evidence from a recent interventional trial also implicates increased cardiac filling pressures and resultant instability of ventilatory control in the pathogenesis of CSA-CSR. Sinha et al. [71] found that in 14 patients with HF (LV ejection fraction 25 ± 5%), intraventricular conduction delays and CSA-CSR, cardiac resynchronization therapy (CRT) markedly reduced CSA-CSR at 17-week follow-up (mean AHI 19 ± 10 to 4.6 ± 4.4). LV ejection fraction increased to a mean of 35% and significant improvements were noted in quality of life. At baseline, CSA-CSR patients demonstrated increased ventilatory responses to exercise (VE/VCO_2 slope) in keeping with other studies showing abnormalities in CO_2 metabolism in these patients [59, 60]. However, CRT resulted in a reduction in this measure that was comparable to that of 10 other subjects without CSA-CSR who underwent CRT. While long-term outcome data are not yet available, it is possible, although not proven, that some of the survival benefit attributed to CRT in HF patients in recently published large-scale studies may be related to amelioration of central apnea in this patient population [72, 73]. It is likely that CRT-related stabilization of loop gain is at least partly responsible for the improvement in CSA-CSR, although further study will be needed to clarify other mechanisms, and if any further benefit is afforded those HF patients with co-existing OSA and CSA.

Treatment of CSA-CSR

Directed Treatment of Underlying HF

There are currently no defined criteria for treatment of CSA-CSR and, importantly, no high-level trials have been published to show an improvement in cardiovascular outcomes with directed treatment of CSA-CSR. Aggressive treatment of the underlying HF would be expected to improve CSA-CSR, although systematic data to confirm this are sparse. A single study, pre-dating the widespread use of β-blockers for HF, showed significant attenuation of breathing events in a minority of patients after 2 months of medical therapy following acute HF [74]. Clearly, further studies assessing the impact of medical therapy on CSA-CSR in larger populations of HF patients are needed. Case reports of surgical correction of cardiac valvular disease, particularly of the mitral valve, describe marked improvement in CSA-CSR [75]. CSA-CSR was eradicated in 7 of 13 patients following heart transplantation for HF, but persisted in another 4 patients postoperatively [76]. As discussed previously, CRT seems to reverse CSA-CSR in those carefully selected candidate patients, although the benefit over and above those related to enhancing cardiac function, if any, is not clear.

Positive Airway Pressure and Adaptive Servo-Ventilation

Aside from its reversal of apnea as described in the setting of primary CSA, CPAP has salutary effects on cardiac function on account of inspiratory muscle unloading and reduction of cardiac afterload related to increasing intrathoracic pressure [77]. A controlled trial of CPAP or usual care followed those with HF with and without CSA. CPAP was associated with an increase in ejection fraction and reduced risk of heart transplant only in those with CSA [78]. The multicenter CANPAP trial also showed slight improvements in ejection fraction and reduced sympathetic activity but failed to show a survival benefit in those with HF and CSA-CSR randomized to CPAP therapy [79]. The authors hypothesized that improvements in medical therapy over the course of the multi-year study (use of β-blockers in particular) reduced mortality in all subjects to the point of irreversibly underpowering the study, but it is also noteworthy that the AHI was reduced by only about 50% in the treatment group. Thus, while there is ample evidence to consider a trial of CPAP in the HF patient with symptoms referable to poor sleep quality, such data not only call into question the adequacy of treatment but also the incompletely understood role, if any, of CSA-CSR in the morbidity and mortality of HF patients [80].

Adaptive servo-ventilation (ASV) utilizes an algorithm to analyze a patient's ventilatory rhythm and estimates a minute ventilation with which to target support. While providing support during apneas and hypopneas, ASV is designed to avoid overventilation during the hyperpneic phase, promoting more uniform ventilation and reducing arousals from sleep. Previously available only outside of the U.S., the ASV mode recently received FDA approval and is targeted for U.S. distribution in 2006. ASV has been shown to effectively suppress CSA-CSR and may be preferred over CPAP by patients [51, 81]. A 1-month randomized trial comparing therapeutic ASV with subtherapeutic ASV showed significant improvements in daytime sleepiness and reductions in neurohormonal activity associated with active treatment in patients with stable HF and CSR-CSA [82]. A recent randomized crossover trial has demonstrated superiority of ASV over CPAP and NPPV in normalizing breathing and sleep parameters in patients with CSA syndromes with and without HF [Morgenthaler et al., unpubl. data].

Supplemental Oxygen

Supplemental O_2 has also been a popular treatment choice for CSA. As mentioned previously, it is believed to suppress ventilatory drive thereby buffering the apneic threshold, but it is also conceivable that the O_2 improves cardiac function, thereby indirectly reducing periodic breathing. A two-night randomized controlled trial yielded a greatly reduced AHI in men with severe HF and nocturnal hypoxemia [83].

Inhaled CO_2

Since hypocapnia, as mentioned earlier, appears to be intimately related to the pathogenesis of CSA-CSR, it would follow that increasing $PaCO_2$ by inhalation of CO_2 or by enhancing dead space may ameliorate ventilatory instability, as has been demonstrated in primary CSA [33]. In fact, one night of inhaled CO_2 administered to 6 patients with severe stable HF resulted in virtual eradication of CSA-CSR [84]. However, the long-term effects are unknown and there is evidence for worsened sleep quality and fragmented sleep architecture associated with CO_2 treatment. Moreover, there is evidence that a single night of treatment may be harmful in those with HF, as demonstrated by an increase in measured sympathetic activity [85].

Theophylline

Theophylline, a phosphodiesterase inhibitor with bronchodilatory properties, has also been shown to be a central respiratory stimulant [86], possibly by antagonizing adenosine in the brainstem [87]. Use of theophylline for asthma and other bronchospastic diseases fell out of favor, in part because other anti-inflammatory therapies were found to be more effective, but also because of the risk of neuroexcitatory adverse effects such as tachycardia, which were found to be coupled to serum concentrations above the therapeutic range of 10–20 ug/ml). Five-day oral administration of theophylline, resulting in modest serum concentrations (11 μg/ml) reduced the frequency of central apneas and hypopneas as well as the duration of arterial oxyhemoglobin desaturation in a controlled trial of 15 men with stable CHF (LVEF $< 45\%$) [88]. The lack of improvement in ventricular function, as well as a case report of efficacy in treating CSA-CSR in the setting of normal ventricular function [89] suggests the central mechanism of action noted above, which may have a stabilizing effect on ventilatory output. Safety concerns related to theophylline use and arrhythmogenesis in HF patients, a population with sympathetic overactivity, may be tempered by these findings related to relatively low serum concentrations. Furthermore, a recent study showed that similarly modest serum theophylline levels do not increase sympathetic activity or heart rate in HF patients as is seen in healthy individuals [90]. Nevertheless, a cautious approach is warranted since long-term use of another phosphodiesterase inhibitor, milrinone, was shown to increase mortality in patients with HF [91].

Acetazolamide

Javaheri [92] recently published results of a randomized placebo controlled trial of 6 nights of single-dose acetazolamide in a small group of men with stable HF and CSA. Acetazolamide significantly improved the central apnea index (mean 44 to 23 per hour) as well as the nadir saturation value compared with placebo. That blood gas analysis found the $PaCO_2$ to be lower in the treatment group confirms the importance of the *difference* between the prevailing $PaCO_2$ and the $PaCO_2$ associated with the apneic threshold, rather than the absolute values, in triggering ventilatory instability. It should be noted that while the effects on CSA are presumably due to alterations in $PaCO_2$, diuretic effects with subsequent reductions in pulmonary edema cannot be excluded as an added mechanism of action.

High Altitude Periodic Breathing (HAPB)

Nearly anyone ascending to elevations greater than 7,500 meters will experience HAPB, characterized by cyclic central apneas and hyperpneas associated with repetitive arousals, fragmented sleep of poor quality and occasional dyspnea [93]. Significant symptoms can also occur at lesser elevations, as low as 3,500 meters [94]. Such a prevalence suggests that HAPB is a normal response to altitude rather than a pathologic finding per se. The onset of HAPB is co-incident with ascension and usually occurs the first night at elevation. The pathophysiologic mechanism appears to be heightened sensitivity to hypoxia with an exaggerated ventilatory response to reduced ambient oxygen levels leading to hypocapnia, followed by a similar cascade during sleep as seen in CSA-CSR [95]. Lack of potentiation of this peripheral chemoreflex in Himalayan Sherpas who do not manifest HAPB at altitude suggest accommodation of the hypoxic ventilatory response over time, although after 32 days at elevation, Caucasian lowlanders continued to demonstrate ventilatory instability [96]. Those who also develop pulmonary edema related to high altitude have more frequent central apneic events thought to result from worsened hypoxemia related to ventilation-perfusion mismatching [97]. As in primary CSA, HAPB is most common during NREM sleep with the dampened peripheral chemoreflex having a protective effect during REM sleep.

If available, supplemental oxygen is effective at reversing HAPB, while inhaled CO_2 may reduce apneas but appears to have no effect on the periodicity of ventilation [96]. Both acetazolamide and theophylline were found to significantly reduce the central AHI in a placebo-controlled trial of HAPB conducted at 3,500 meters [94]. Notably, as in Javaheri's trial in HF patients with CSA-CSR [88], measured serum theophylline levels were relatively low (4–6 μg/ml in this study), underscoring an incomplete understanding of mechanisms of action of theophylline or other phosphodiesterase inhibitors.

Sleep Hypoventilation Syndromes

The most frequently encountered hypoventilation syndromes during sleep are those associated with another medical condition. Most notable among these are pulmonary disorders such as COPD as well as restrictive lung diseases related to neuromuscular impairment. According to ICSD-2, these secondary sleep hypoventilation syndromes share similar polysomnographic features, of which one or more should be present to confirm the diagnosis:

1. An oxygen saturation during sleep of <90% for more than 5 min with a nadir of at least 85%
2. More than 30% of total sleep time at an oxygen saturation of <90%
3. Sleeping arterial blood gas with $PaCO_2$ that is abnormally high or disproportionately increased relative to levels during wakefulness

Obstructive or central disordered breathing events may or may not be an associated feature. Treatment should be directed at the underlying disorder but noninvasive positive pressure ventilation should be considered in those with associated pulmonary hypertension, cor pulmonale or polycythemia.

Congenital Central Alveolar Hypoventilation Syndrome

Congenital central alveolar hypoventilation syndrome (CCHS, also referred to as Ondine's curse) is a very rare disorder (<1,000 cases worldwide) characterized by failure of central ventilatory mechanisms and hypoventilation often beginning in infancy [98]. Not uncommonly, clinical attention comes with an episode of acute respiratory failure with failure to wean from mechanical ventilation in an otherwise healthy-appearing infant. Other cases characterized by chronic sleep-related hypoventilation manifest later in childhood with overt hypercapnic and hypoxemic respiratory failure accompanied by cor pulmonale and polycythemia. Despite reaching early developmental milestones, patients with progressive untreated respiratory failure may develop cognitive delay or growth retardation [98]. Associated clinical features include Hirschsprung's disease and autonomic dysfunction as manifested by reduced heart rate variability and blood pressure irregularities [99].

The pathophysiology of CCHS appears related to dysfunctional integration of respiratory afferents in the brainstem, which, despite a radiographically normal appearance, results in blunted chemoreflexes and lack of subjective

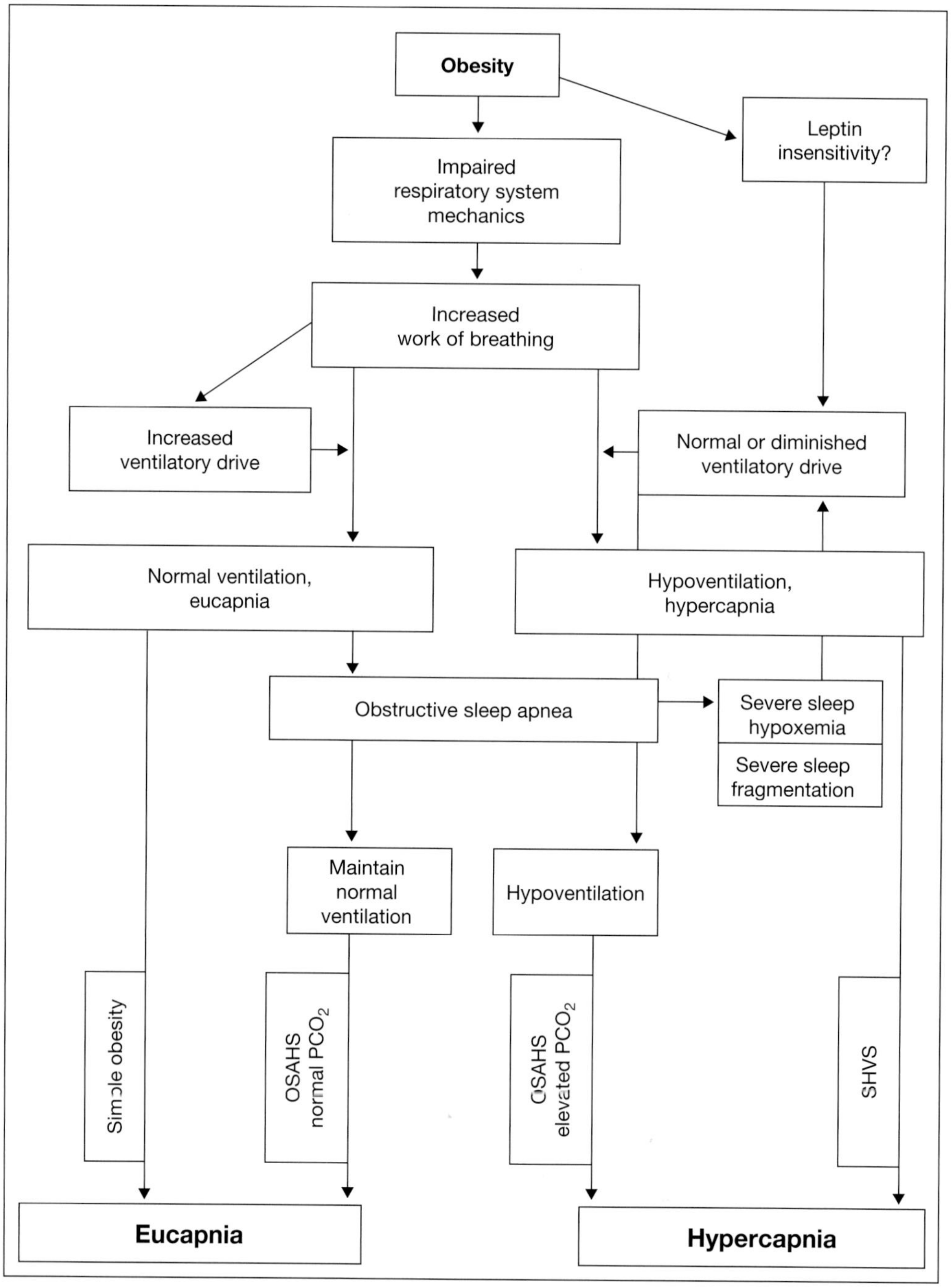

Fig. 4. Possible pathophysiologic mechanisms and interactions which may lead to hypercapnia during wakefulness in the obesity-hypoventilation syndrome. OSAHS = Obstructive sleep apnea/hypopnea syndrome; SHVS = sleep hypoventilation syndrome. From Olson and Zwillich [104].

dyspnea despite obvious gas exchange abnormalities. Hypoventilation, often without accompanying apneas, is the dominant finding on PSG. Recent data have implicated mutations in *PHOX2B*, a gene associated with central and peripheral autonomic nervous control [100]. Although expression of the disease in siblings and monozygotic twins has been reported, current evidence suggests that CCHS is the result of de novo gene mutations [101].

Treatment consists of assisted ventilation either by noninvasive means or by tracheotomy. In many instances, ventilation is required only during sleep, although more advanced cases may require continuous support day and night. While some patients have aged into early adulthood, treatment is likely to be a lifelong requirement [98].

Obesity Hypoventilation Syndrome (Encompassed by the ICSD-2 Sleep-Related Hypoventilation/Hypoxemia due to Neuromuscular and Chest Wall Disorders)

Previously referred to as the Pickwickian syndrome, derived from a character in Dickens' novel *The Posthumous Papers of the Pickwick Club*, the obesity hypoventilation syndrome (OHS) is an increasingly recognized disorder. The epidemiology of OHS is not well described, and it is likely that the disorder remains underappreciated or misdiagnosed as asthma or COPD. Nearly one third of hospitalized patients with a BMI ≥ 35 kg/m^2 demonstrated otherwise unexplained daytime hypoventilation [102] with the prevalence increasing to nearly half of patients with a BMI ≥ 50 kg/m^2.

Daytime hypercapnia ($PaCO_2 > 45$ mm Hg) is a cardinal sign of OHS, reflecting reduced ventilation during wakefulness as well as sleep. While the pathophysiology of OHS has not been completely elucidated, it is believed to result from a combination of mechanical load imposed by obesity and alterations in both hypoxic and hypercapnic ventilatory drive, as reported by Zwillich et al. in 1975 [103, 104]. Obesity is associated with reduced chest wall compliance [105], decreased total lung volume and expiratory reserve volume [106], and elevated airway resistance [107]. Ventilation-perfusion abnormalities result from reduced effective volumes in the lung bases which are preferentially perfused (via gravitational effects) by an expanded lung blood volume (fig. 4).

Knockout mice studies describe important effects of the hormone leptin on ventilation in obesity [68]. Leptin acts, among other sites, in the hypothalamus to induce satiety, and serum levels closely correlate with total body fat content. Patients with OSA have even higher than expected leptin levels for their degree of obesity [108], suggesting resistance to the appetite-suppressing effects, and perhaps other physiologic effects, of leptin. CPAP therapy has been shown to reduce leptin levels in the absence of weight loss [109].

It may seem implicit that all obese persons with hypoventilation would manifest SDB and OSA. Indeed, the majority of a select group of OHS patients demonstrated SDB during nocturnal monitoring [110]. CPAP has been shown to ameliorate blood gas abnormalities and daytime symptoms in a group of OHS patients not known to have OSA [111]. However, not all patients with OHS demonstrate SDB on nocturnal monitoring, so the contribution of SDB to the cardiopulmonary pathophysiology of OHS is not entirely clear. Furthermore, sleep-related hypoventilation and hypoxemia may prove resistant to CPAP, which may necessitate the addition of supplemental oxygen or alternative treatment with noninvasive positive pressure (bilevel) ventilation. Clinical trials comparing different treatment options are currently lacking, although weight loss should be universally recommended.

Available evidence suggests that cardiopulmonary morbidity in OHS is striking. Autopsy data show biventricular failure as a frequent cause of death, with marked changes in the pulmonary vasculature consistent with pulmonary hypertension [112]. The independent contribution of OSA in the genesis of cardiopulmonary abnormalities in OHS is not clear, and it may be that obesity itself is a more important risk factor [113]. In the absence of substantial weight loss, however, directed treatment of SDB may help prevent cardiovascular complications. Alternatively, more radical weight loss options, such as bariatric surgery, could be considered in OHS patients, given their high cardiopulmonary morbidity.

Occasionally, a patient may demonstrate evidence for sleep-related hypoventilation/hypoxemia without obesity, sleep apnea or any predisposing comorbid condition, in which case an ICSD-2 diagnosis of idiopathic sleep related nonobstructive alveolar hypoventilation could be made. This disorder is thought to result from reduced chemoreflex sensitivity with or without alterations in medullary ventilatory drive. Treatment may include supplemental oxygen or positive pressure ventilation.

References

1 Flemons WW, et al: Sleep-related breathing disorders in adults: recommendations for syndrome definition and measurement techniques in clinical research. Sleep 1999;22:667–689.
2 American Academy of Sleep Medicine: The International Classification of Sleep Disorders, ed 2. Westchester, American Academy of Sleep Medicine, 2005.
3 Staats BA, et al: Chest wall motion in sleep apnea. Am Rev Respir Dis 1984;130:59–63.
4 Boudewyns A, et al: Assessment of respiratory effort by means of strain gauges and esophageal pressure swings: a comparative study. Sleep 1997;20:168–170.
5 Morrell MJ, et al: The assessment of upper airway patency during apnea using cardiogenic oscillations in the airflow signal. Sleep 1995; 18:651–658.
6 Bradley TD, et al: Clinical and physiologic heterogeneity of the central sleep apnea syndrome. Am Rev Respir Dis 1986;134:217–221.
7 Sullivan CE, et al: Primary role of respiratory afferents in sustaining breathing rhythm. J Appl Physiol 1978;45:11–17.

8 White DP: Occlusion pressure and ventilation during sleep in normal humans. J Appl Physiol 1986;61:1279–1287.
9 Lopes JM, et al: Total airway resistance and respiratory muscle activity during sleep. J Appl Physiol 1983;54:773–777.
10 Mezzanotte WS, Tangel DJ, White DP: Waking genioglossal electromyogram in sleep apnea patients versus normal controls (a neuromuscular compensatory mechanism). J Clin Invest 1992;89:1571–1579.
11 Gothe B, et al: Effect of progressive hypoxia on breathing during sleep. Am Rev Respir Dis 1982;126:97–102.
12 Birchfield RI, Sieker HO, Heyman A: Alterations in blood gases during natural sleep and narcolepsy; a correlation with the electroencephalographic stages of sleep. Neurology 1958;8:107–112.
13 Douglas NJ, et al: Hypercapnic ventilatory response in sleeping adults. Am Rev Respir Dis 1982;126:758–762.
14 White DP, et al: Hypoxic ventilatory response during sleep in normal premenopausal women. Am Rev Respir Dis 1982;126:530–533.
15 Young T, Peppard PE, Gottlieb DJ: Epidemiology of obstructive sleep apnea: a population health perspective. Am J Respir Crit Care Med 2002;165:1217–1239.
16 Douglas NJ: Control of ventilation during sleep. Clin Chest Med 1985;6:563–575.
17 Skatrud JB, Dempsey JA: Interaction of sleep state and chemical stimuli in sustaining rhythmic ventilation. J Appl Physiol 1983;55: 813–822.
18 Khoo MC, et al: Factors inducing periodic breathing in humans: a general model. J Appl Physiol 1982;53:644–659.
19 Khoo MCK: Determinants of ventilatory instability and variability. Respir Physiol 2000;122:167–182.
20 Younes M, et al: Chemical control stability in patients with obstructive sleep apnea. Am J Respir Crit Care Med 2001;163:1181–1190.
21 White DP: Pathogenesis of obstructive and central sleep apnea. Am J Respir Crit Care Med 2005;172:1363–1370.
22 Dempsey JA, et al: The ventilatory responsiveness to CO2 below eupnoea as a determinant of ventilatory stability in sleep. J Physiol 2004;560:1–11.
23 Alex CG, Onal E, Lopata M: Upper airway occlusion during sleep in patients with Cheyne-Stokes respiration. Am Rev Respir Dis 1986;133:42–45.
24 Warner G, Skatrud JB, Dempsey JA: Effect of hypoxia-induced periodic breathing on upper airway obstruction during sleep. J Appl Physiol 1987;62:2201–2211.
25 Onal E, et al: Induction of periodic breathing during sleep causes upper airway obstruction in humans. J Appl Physiol 1986;61: 1438–1443.
26 Hudgel DW, et al: Changes in inspiratory muscle electrical activity and upper airway resistance during periodic breathing induced by hypoxia during sleep. Am Rev Respir Dis 1987; 135:899–906.
27 Tkacova R, et al: Overnight shift from obstructive to central apneas in patients with heart failure: role of PCO2 and circulatory delay. Circulation 2001;103:238–243.
28 Sahlin C, et al: Cheyne-Stokes respiration and supine dependency. Eur Respir J 2005;25: 829–833.
29 Issa FG, Sullivan CE: Reversal of central sleep apnea using nasal CPAP. Chest 1986;90: 165–171.
30 Hoffstein V, Slutsky AS: Central sleep apnea reversed by continuous positive airway pressure. Am Rev Respir Dis 1987;135: 1210–1212.
31 Xie A, et al: Hypocapnia and increased ventilatory responsiveness in patients with idiopathic central sleep apnea. Am J Respir Crit Care Med 1995;152:1950–1955.
32 Xie A, et al: Interaction of hyperventilation and arousal in the pathogenesis of idiopathic central sleep apnea. Am J Respir Crit Care Med 1994;150:489–495.
33 Xie A, et al: Effects of inhaled CO2 and added dead space on idiopathic central sleep apnea. J Appl Physiol 1997;82:918–926.
34 Roehrs T, et al: Sleep-wake complaints in patients with sleep-related respiratory disturbances. Am Rev Respir Dis 1985;132: 520–523.
35 Fleetham JA, Arnup ME, Anthonisen NR: Familial aspects of ventilatory control in patients with chronic obstructive pulmonary disease. Am Rev Respir Dis 1984;129:3–7.
36 Wilson DO, Sanders MH, Dauber JH: Abnormal ventilatory chemosensitivity and congenital myopathy. Arch Intern Med 1987; 147:1773–1777.
37 Bradley TD, Phillipson EA: Central sleep apnea. Clin Chest Med 1992;13:493–505.
38 Martin RJ, et al: Acute and long-term ventilatory effects of hyperoxia in the adult sleep apnea syndrome. Am Rev Respir Dis 1982; 125:175–180.
39 Gold AR, Bleecker ER, Smith PL: A shift from central and mixed sleep apnea to obstructive sleep apnea resulting from low-flow oxygen. Am Rev Respir Dis 1985;132:220–223.
40 White DP, et al: Central sleep apnea. Improvement with acetazolamide therapy. Arch Intern Med 1982;142:1816–1819.
41 DeBacker WA, et al: Central apnea index decreases after prolonged treatment with acetazolamide. Am J Respir Crit Care Med 1995;151:87–91.
42 Nakayama H, et al: Effect of ventilatory drive on carbon dioxide sensitivity below eupnea during sleep. Am J Respir Crit Care Med 2002;165:1251–1260.
43 Sharp JT, et al: Effect of metabolic acidosis upon sleep apnea. Chest 1985;87:619–624.
44 Kaneko Y, et al: Cardiovascular effects of continuous positive airway pressure in patients with heart failure and obstructive sleep apnea. N Engl J Med 2003;348:1233–1241.
45 Mansfield DR, et al: Controlled trial of continuous positive airway pressure in obstructive sleep apnea and heart failure. Am J Respir Crit Care Med 2004;169:361–366.
46 Hanly P, Zuberi-Khokhar N: Increased mortality associated with Cheyne-Stokes respiration in patients with congestive heart failure. Am J Respir Crit Care Med 1996;153:272–276.
47 Lanfranchi PA, et al: Prognostic value of nocturnal Cheyne-Stokes respiration in chronic heart failure. Circulation 1999;99:1435–1440.
48 Lanfranchi PA, Somers VK: Sleep-disordered breathing in heart failure: characteristics and implications. Respir Physiol Neurobiol 2003;136:153–165.
49 Sin DD, et al: Risk factors for central and obstructive sleep apnea in 450 men and women with congestive heart failure. Am J Respir Crit Care Med 1999;160:1101–1106.
50 Hall M, et al: Cycle length of periodic breathing in patients with and without heart failure. Am J Respir Crit Care Med 1996;154: 376–381.
51 Teschler H, et al: Adaptive pressure support servo-ventilation: a novel treatment for Cheyne-Stokes respiration in heart failure. Am J Respir Crit Care Med 2001;164:614–619.
52 Crowell JW, Guyton AC, Moore JW: Basic oscillating mechanism of Cheyne-Stokes breathing. Am J Physiol 1956;187:395–398.
53 Cherniack NS, Longobardo GS: Cheyne-Stokes breathing. An instability in physiologic control. N Engl J Med 1973;288:952–957.
54 Khoo MC, Gottschalk A, Pack AI: Sleep-induced periodic breathing and apnea: a theoretical study. J Appl Physiol 1991;70: 2014–2024.
55 Naughton M, et al: Role of hyperventilation in the pathogenesis of central sleep apneas in patients with congestive heart failure. Am Rev Respir Dis 1993;148:330–338.
56 Solin P, et al: Peripheral and central ventilatory responses in central sleep apnea with and without congestive heart failure. Am J Respir Crit Care Med 2000;162:2194–2200.
57 Javaheri S: A mechanism of central sleep apnea in patients with heart failure. N Engl J Med 1999;341:949–954.
58 Javaheri S, Corbett WS: Association of low $PaCO_2$ with central sleep apnea and ventricular arrhythmias in ambulatory patients with stable heart failure. Ann Intern Med 1998;128: 204–207.
59 Wolk R, Johnson BD, Somers VK: Leptin and the ventilatory response to exercise in heart failure. J Am Coll Cardiol 2003;42: 1644–1649.
60 Chua TP, et al: Clinical correlates and prognostic significance of the ventilatory response to exercise in chronic heart failure. J Am Coll Cardiol 1997;29:1585–1590.
61 Arzt M, et al: Nocturnal continuous positive airway pressure improves ventilatory efficiency during exercise in patients with chronic heart failure. Chest 2005;127:794–802.
62 Xie A, et al: Cerebrovascular response to carbon dioxide in patients with congestive heart failure. Am J Respir Crit Care Med 2005;172: 371–378.
63 Nopmaneejumruslers C, et al: Cheyne-Stokes respiration in stroke: relationship to hypocapnia and occult cardiac dysfunction. Am J Respir Crit Care Med 2005;171:1048–1052.
64 Moreau R, et al: Arterial and mixed venous acid-base status in patients with cirrhosis. Influence of liver failure. Liver 1993;13:20–24.
65 Rodriguez-Roisin R, et al: Gas exchange and pulmonary vascular reactivity in patients with

liver cirrhosis. Am Rev Respir Dis 1987;135: 1085–1092.
66 Javaheri S, et al: Hypocapnia is not a predictor of central sleep apnea in patients with cirrhosis. Am J Respir Crit Care Med 2005;171: 908–911.
67 Tankersley C, et al: Modified control of breathing in genetically obese (ob/ob) mice. J Appl Physiol 1996;81:716–723.
68 O'donnell CP, et al: Leptin prevents respiratory depression in obesity. Am J Respir Crit Care Med 1999;159:1477–1484.
69 Solin P, et al: Influence of pulmonary capillary wedge pressure on central apnea in heart failure. Circulation 1999;99:1574–1579.
70 Caples SM, Wolk R, Somers VK: Influence of cardiac function and failure on sleep-disordered breathing: evidence for a causative role. 10.1152/japplphysiol.00676.2005. J Appl Physiol 2005;99:2433–2439.
71 Sinha A-M, et al: Cardiac resynchronization therapy improves central sleep apnea and Cheyne-Stokes respiration in patients with chronic heart failure. J Am Coll Cardiol 2004; 44:68–71.
72 Bristow MR, et al: Cardiac-resynchronization therapy with or without an implantable defibrillator in advanced chronic heart failure. N Engl J Med 2004;350:2140–2150.
73 Cleland JGF, et al: The effect of cardiac resynchronization on morbidity and mortality in heart failure. N Engl J Med 2005;352: 1539–1549.
74 Tremel F, et al: High prevalence and persistence of sleep apnoea in patients referred for acute left ventricular failure and medically treated over 2 months. Eur Heart J 1999;20: 1201–1209.
75 Rubin AE, et al: Elimination of central sleep apnoea by mitral valvuloplasty: the role of feedback delay in periodic breathing. Thorax 2004;59:174–176.
76 Mansfield DR, et al: The effect of successful heart transplant treatment of heart failure on central sleep apnea. Chest 2003;124: 1675–1681.
77 Naughton MT, et al: Effect of continuous positive airway pressure on intrathoracic and left ventricular transmural pressures in patients with congestive heart failure. Circulation 1995;91:1725–1731.
78 Sin DD, et al: Effects of continuous positive airway pressure on cardiovascular outcomes in heart failure patients with and without Cheyne-Stokes respiration. Circulation 2000; 102:61–66.
79 Bradley TD, et al: Continuous positive airway pressure for central sleep apnea and heart failure. N Engl J Med 2005;353: 2025–2033.
80 Somers VK: Sleep – a new cardiovascular frontier. 10.1056/NEJMe058229. N Engl J Med 2005;353:2070–2073.
81 Philippe C, et al: Compliance with and efficacy of adaptive servo-ventilation (ASV) versus continuous positive airway pressure (CPAP) in the treatment of Cheyne-Stokes respiration in heart failure over a six month period. 10.1136/hrt.2005.060038. Heart, 2005:p. hrt.2005.060038.
82 Pepperell JC, et al: A randomized controlled trial of adaptive ventilation for Cheyne-Stokes breathing in heart failure. Am J Respir Crit Care Med 2003;168:1109–1114.
83 Hanly PJ, et al: The effect of oxygen on respiration and sleep in patients with congestive heart failure. Ann Intern Med 1989;111: 777–782.
84 Steens RD, et al: Effect of inhaled 3% CO2 on Cheyne-Stokes respiration in congestive heart failure. Sleep 1994;17:61–68.
85 Andreas S, et al: Treatment of Cheyne-Stokes respiration with nasal oxygen and carbon dioxide. Eur Respir J 1998;12:414–419.
86 Eldridge FL, et al: Mechanism of respiratory effects of methylxanthines. Respir Physiol 1983;53:239–261.
87 Eldridge FL, Millhorn DE, Kiley JP: Antagonism by theophylline of respiratory inhibition induced by adenosine. J Appl Physiol 1985; 59:1428–1433.
88 Javaheri S, et al: Effect of theophylline on sleep-disordered breathing in heart failure. N Engl J Med 1996;335:562–567.
89 Pesek CA, et al: Theophylline therapy for near-fatal Cheyne-Stokes respiration. A case report. Ann Intern Med 1999;130:427–430.
90 Andreas S, et al: Differential effects of theophylline on sympathetic excitation, hemodynamics, and breathing in congestive heart failure. Circulation 2004;110:2157–2162.
91 Packer M, et al: Effect of oral milrinone on mortality in severe chronic heart failure. The Promise Study Research Group. N Engl J Med 1991;325:1468–1475.
92 Javaheri S: Acetazolamide improves central sleep apnea in heart failure: a double-blind, prospective study. 10.1164/rccm.200507-1035OC. Am J Respir Crit Care Med 2006; 173:234–237.
93 Anholm JD, et al: Operation Everest II: arterial oxygen saturation and sleep at extreme simulated altitude. Am Rev Respir Dis 1992; 145:817–826.
94 Fischer R, et al: Theophylline and acetazolamide reduce sleep-disordered breathing at high altitude. 10.1183/09031936.03.00113102. Eur Respir J 2004;23:47–52.
95 Xie A, Skatrud JB, Dempsey JA: Effect of hypoxia on the hypopnoeic and apnoeic threshold for CO2 in sleeping humans. J Physiol 2001;535:269–278.
96 Lahiri S, Maret K, Sherpa MG: Dependence of high altitude sleep apnea on ventilatory sensitivity to hypoxia. Respir Physiol 1983;52: 281–301.
97 Eichenberger U, et al: Nocturnal periodic breathing and the development of acute high altitude illness. Am J Respir Crit Care Med 1996;154:1748–1754.
98 American Thoracic Society: Idiopathic Congenital Central Hypoventilation Syndrome – Diagnosis and Management. Am J Respir Crit Care Med 1999;160: 368–373.
99 Weese-Mayer DE, et al: Congenital central hypoventilation syndrome: diagnosis, management, and long-term outcome in thirty-two children. J Pediatr 1992;120:381–387.
100 Amiel J, et al: Polyalanine expansion and frameshift mutations of the paired-like homeobox gene PHOX2B in congenital central hypoventilation syndrome. Nat Genet 2003;33:459–461.
101 O'Brien LM, et al: Autonomic function in children with congenital central hypoventilation syndrome and their families. 10.1378/chest. 128.4.2478. Chest 2005;128: 2478–2484.
102 Nowbar S, et al: Obesity-associated hypoventilation in hospitalized patients: prevalence, effects, and outcome. Am J Med 2004;116: 1–7.
103 Zwillich CW, et al: Decreased hypoxic ventilatory drive in the obesity-hypoventilation syndrome. Am J Med 1975;59:343–348.
104 Olson AL, Zwillich C: The obesity hypoventilation syndrome. Am J Med 2005;118: 948–956.
105 Suratt PM, et al: Compliance of chest wall in obese subjects. J Appl Physiol 1984;57: 403–407.
106 Koenig S: Pulmonary complications of obesity. Am J Med Sci 2001;321:249–279.
107 Zerah F, et al: Effects of obesity on respiratory resistance. Chest 1993;103:1470–1476.
108 Phillips BG, et al: Increases in leptin levels, sympathetic drive, and weight gain in obstructive sleep apnea. Am J Physiol Heart Circ Physiol 2000; 279:H234–H237.
109 Harsch IA, et al: Leptin and ghrelin levels in patients with obstructive sleep apnoea: effect of CPAP treatment. Eur Respir J 2003;22: 251–257.
110 Jones JB, et al: Oxyhemoglobin saturation during sleep in subjects with and without the obesity-hypoventilation syndrome. Chest 1985;88:9–15.
111 Sullivan CE, Berthon-Jones M, Issa FG: Remission of severe obesity-hypoventilation syndrome after short-term treatment during sleep with nasal continuous positive airway pressure. Am Rev Respir Dis 1983;128: 177–181.
112 Ahmed Q, Chung-Park M, Tomashefski JF Jr: Cardiopulmonary pathology in patients with sleep apnea/obesity hypoventilation syndrome. Hum Pathol 1997;28:264–269.
113 Otto MEB, Bijoy MB, Gregory Gilman K: Anna Svatikova, Carolyn Fieseler, Virend K. Somers: tissue doppler ecocardiography in obesity – selective changes in right but not left ventricular function. Circulation 2003; 108:IV:440.

Virend K. Somers
Division of Cardiovascular Diseases
Department of Internal Medicine
Mayo Clinic and Mayo Foundation
200 1st Street SW
Rochester, MN 55901 (USA)
Tel. +1 507 255 1144
Fax +1 507 255 7070
E-Mail somers.virend@mayo.edu

Randerath WJ, Sanner BM, Somers VK (eds): Sleep Apnea.
Prog Respir Res. Basel, Karger, 2006, vol 35, pp 192–203

Cardiovascular Complications of Sleep-Related Breathing Disorders

M.T. Naughton[a] B.M. Sanner[b]

[a]General Respiratory and Sleep Medicine, Department of Allergy, Immunology and Respiratory Medicine, Monash University, The Alfred Hospital, Melbourne, Vic., Australia; [b]Department of Internal Medicine, Bethesda Krankenhaus, Ruhr University Bochum, Wuppertal, Germany

Abstract

Obstructive sleep apnea is associated with an increased risk of cardiovascular disease and stroke. Three pathophysiological mechanisms characterize sleep-related breathing disorders: (1) upper airway instability; (2) respiratory control instability, and (3) respiratory pump disorders. Especially the intrathoracic pressure swings during obstructed breathing, hypoxemia as a result from apneic events, and arousals from sleep (terminating the apneas) are responsible for the cardiovascular consequences. Obstructive sleep apnea is an independent risk factor for systemic hypertension and has also been implicated in the pathogenesis of pulmonary hypertension, arrhythmias, atherosclerosis, coronary artery disease and myocardial infarction, stroke, and congestive heart failure. Treatment of obstructive sleep apnea – especially with CPAP – improves breathing and eliminates the acute hemodynamic effects during sleep. In addition, long-term treatment with CPAP has a beneficial influence on the cardiovascular consequences: left ventricular function, systemic and daytime pulmonary hypertension improve, and there is also evidence that the otherwise increased cardiovascular morbidity and mortality can be normalized.

Pathophysiology

Sleep-related breathing disorders are intertwined with cardiovascular disease by virtue of their shared real estate (i.e. the thorax) and common interacting physiology. Three pathophysiological mechanisms characterize sleep related breathing disorders, namely: (a) upper airway instability (e.g. sleep related loss of muscle tone leading to snoring and 'obstructive' hypopneas and apneas); (b) respiratory control instability (e.g. hyperventilation with circulatory delay causing periodic drive to breathe), and (c) respiratory pump disorders (e.g. chest wall abnormalities or 'restrictive' ventilatory defects). Each mechanism impacts upon the development of obstructive sleep apnea hypopnea syndrome (OSAHS) (fig. 1), central sleep apnea with Cheyne-Stokes respiration (CSA-CSR) (fig. 2) and sleep-related hypoventilation. Each mechanism may be influenced by, or has an effect upon, the cardiovascular system.

Upper Airway Instability

Upper airway instability and collapse occurs either during inspiration, where negative intraluminal forces predominate and the so-called collapsing pressure (P_{crit}) is negative, or during expiration, when the intraluminal collapsing pressure is positive [1]. The former usually occurring in patients with skeletal or soft tissue anatomic abnormalities (e.g. narrow high-arched palate, retrognathia, nasal obstruction) whereas the later occurs in patients with obesity or drugs affecting upper airway tone (sedatives, alcohol [2]).

In either case, upper airway occlusion occurs for periods of 10–90 s during which time, vigorous respiratory drive occurs resulting in numerous futile efforts to inspire. Each effort being associated with increasing large negative intrathoracic pressure whilst hypoxia and hypercapnia become progressively greater, heart rate slows down (diving

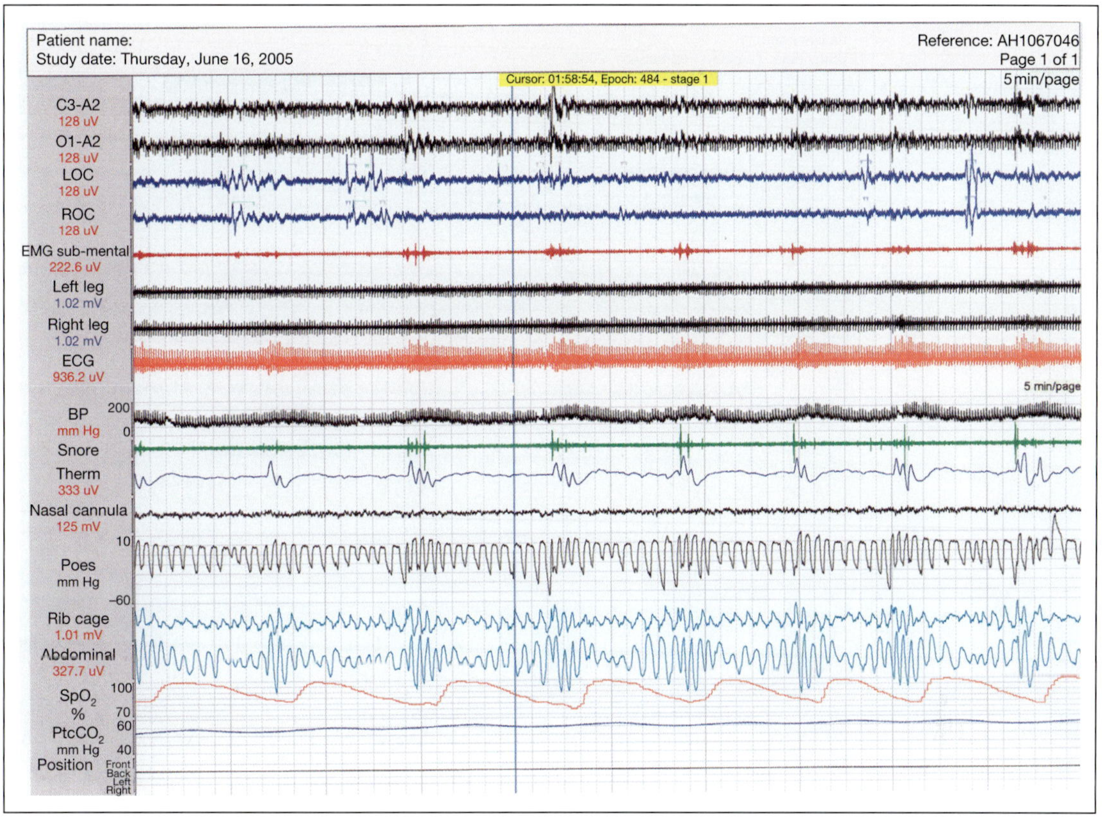

Fig. 1. A 5-minute polysomnograph of a patient with obesity and idiopathic cardiomyopathy (LVEF 40%). Note esophageal pressure swings to –55 mm Hg during apneas associated with falls in SpO_2 from 95 to 75%, a $PtcCO_2$ ranging between 52 and 57 mm Hg, BP peak of 170/90 mm Hg and an apnea/hyperpnea cycle length of 43 s. Also note lack of nasal cannulae signal, yet intermittent oronasal thermistor flow indicating nasal obstruction and oral breathing.

reflex) until an arousal occurs (precipitated by hypercapnia, hypoxemia, work of breathing) at which time airway patency returns. Following the apnea, the arousal related return of airway patency may be partial (in which snoring persists), or complete (in which ventilation occurs without snoring) for the 3–5 breaths before deep sleep returns. Systemic blood pressure oscillates with each inspiratory effort during the apnea, then surges up with the arousal, and later returns to baseline with the onset of sleep and the next apnea.

Sleep is characterized by a unique autonomic state and this can be disturbed by upper airway instability. If one considers a 4-step change from (1) quiet wakefulness, to (2) stages 1 and 2 NREM sleep, to (3) stages 3 and 4 NREM sleep or slow wave sleep and finally to (4) REM sleep, sympathetic tone falls from wakefulness to stages 1 + 2, and further reduces in slow wave sleep, and rises in REM sleep to levels seen in wakefulness [3]. Thus, sleep has a powerful effect on SNS activity.

Parasympathetic or vagal tone however rises with state change from wakefulness to stages 1 + 2 and further to SWS and REM sleep. Parasympathetic activity appears to be influenced, not just by sleep, but also by circadian timing, such that PNS activity may be increased during the night in subjects who remain awake [4].

Upper airway instability during sleep resulting in snoring, hypopneas or apneas result in changes in autonomic control. During the apnea, whilst airflow is absent and hypoxia is occurring, there is an acute reduction in sympathetic activity. When each apnea is terminated, sympathetic activity surges up, in parallel with rise in heart rate and systemic and pulmonary artery blood pressure. With recurrent apneas, the overall net sympathetic activity, as measured awake or asleep, increases [3, 5].

Respiratory Control Instability

Under normal circumstances, respiratory control is influenced by several factors whilst awake: cortical factors (to

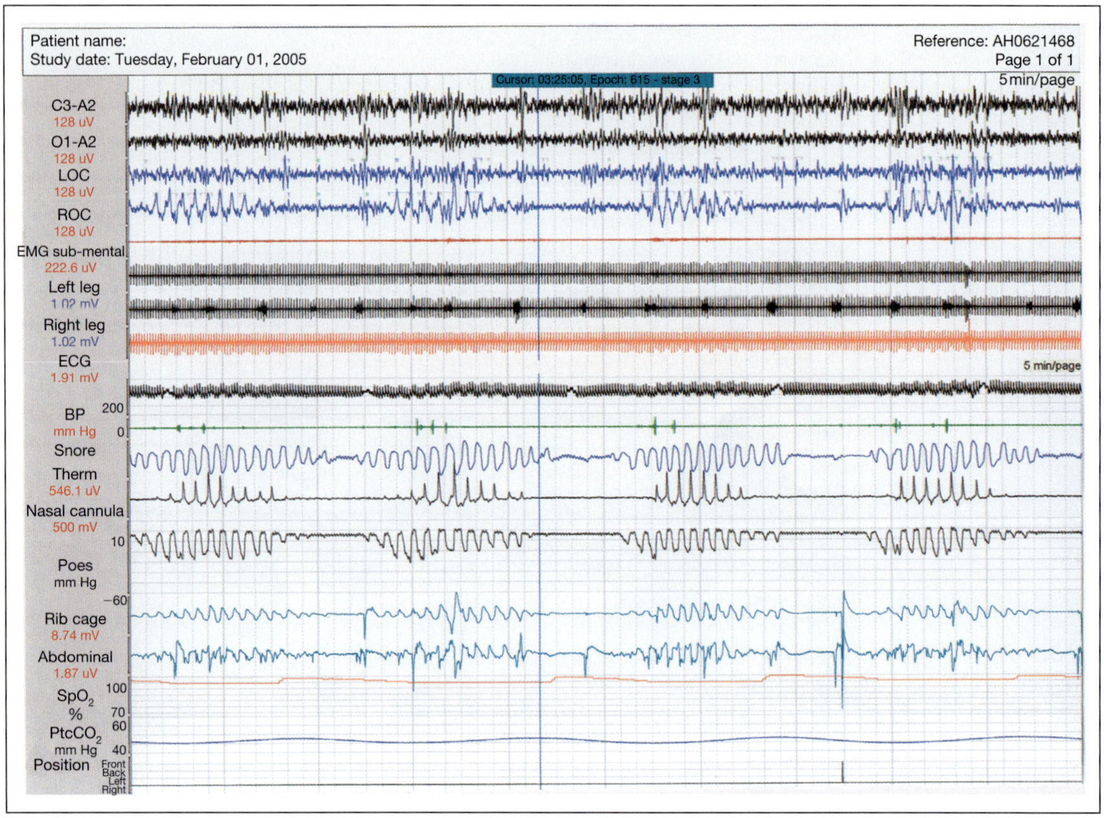

Fig. 2. A 5-minute polysomnograph of a patient with advanced ischemic cardiomyopathy (LVEF 15%). Note absent esophageal pressure swings during the apneas followed by swings to –30 mm Hg during the peak of ventilation associated with falls in SpO_2 from 98 to 94%, $PtcCO_2$ oscillating from 44 to 48 mm Hg, periodic limb movements in right leg, and an apnea hyperpnea cycle length of ~75 s. Also note the cardiac oscillations on the thermistor trace on apneas 1, 2 half of 3 and 4: these represent an open upper airway, which closes mid apnea in the 3rd apnea. Also note some snoring during the peak of ventilation. Finally, note difference in airflow between oronasal thermistor and nasal pressure cannulae, indicating intermittent oral airflow, possibly due to nasal obstruction.

allow respiration to synchronize with speech, swallowing, laughter, etc.), a waking neural drive and finally a metabolic drive [6].

Whilst asleep, there is loss of cortical control and the waking neural drive. The metabolic threshold required to stimulate ventilation is raised and the overall drive to ventilate is diminished by ~20%. Thus, during sleep, ventilation is under a negative feedback system, where metabolic factors (reflecting the efficiency of ventilation) are sensed centrally by two neurologically distinct chemoreceptors: a rapidly responsive carotid body and a more slowly responsive pons. The speed at which messages from the lung are sensed by the brain is the afferent loop of the feedback system and is usually ~10 s (time it takes blood leaving the pulmonary vein to reach the peripheral chemoreceptors). This time can become prolonged in the setting of impaired cardiac output (slow rate or reduced stroke volume) to values of 20–30 s [7].

Respiratory Pump

Significant lung volume changes occur with changes in posture and sleep/wake state. These changes are exaggerated in diseases of the nervous, cardiac or pulmonary systems which may result in exaggerated loss of oxygen stores or greater ventilation perfusion (VQ) matching.

Under normal conditions, the change in posture from seated to supine induces a ~20% reduction in end-expiratory lung volume [8], and a further reduction in lung volume occurs with transition from wake to sleep. Respiratory pump muscle activity also alters with sleep with a progressive reduction in accessory and intercostals muscle activity with sleep, and a greater dependence upon diaphragm activity.

Reduced pump activity in patients with cardiovascular disease may occur in the settings of massive obesity, diaphragmatic palsy post-thoractomy for cardiac surgery, heart failure related myopathy, effusions and cardiomegaly. Reductions in lung volume will exaggerate the hypoxemia related to a disturbance to ventilation, thus exaggerating the 'plant gain' of periodic breathing.

Systemic Hypertension

During sleep, and parallel to apneas, there is a gradual increase of systemic blood pressure, the maximum taking place during the postapneic hyperventilation period. The amount of blood pressure increase at the end of the apnea correlates with the degree of the arousal that terminates the apnea [9]. As a result, patients with obstructive sleep apnea (OSA) are often nondippers during 24-hour blood pressure monitoring. This is of importance because the presence of a disturbed circadian blood pressure profile might constitute a further risk factor with regard to cardiovascular sequelae. It could be shown that the percentage of nondippers was higher in patients with moderate to severe OSA compared to those with mild OSA [10].

While the causal association between OSA and nighttime hypertension is well accepted, the relation to daytime hypertension is less clear. This is due to the fact that patients with hypertension and patients with OSA have common risk factors like obesity (and its pattern of distribution), alcohol consumption, age, male gender, and decreased physical activity. Approximately 50% of OSA patients are hypertensive – both nocturnal and daytime blood pressure are raised – whereas one third of hypertensive patients have disturbed breathing patterns during the night. Furthermore, there is an association between the degree of breathing disturbance during the night and the height of blood pressure during the day. The first direct evidence of a cause and effect relationship between OSA and the development of systemic hypertension came from an animal model in 1997 [11]. Meanwhile several well-conducted, large population-based studies have also been able to prove an independent association with a dose-response relationship between these two conditions in man [12] indicating that OSA constitutes a risk factor for hypertension and subsequent cardiovascular morbidity [13]. Interestingly, in the Sleep Heart Health Study, sleep-disordered breathing was associated only with systolic/diastolic hypertension (and not with isolated systolic hypertension) in those aged $<$60 years. No association was found between sleep-disordered breathing and hypertension in those aged $\geq$60 years [14].

These results induced the National High Blood Pressure Education Program (NHBPEP) of the National Heart, Lung, and Blood Institute to publish updated consensus recommendations for the prevention and treatment of hypertension and to declare OSA as an identifiable cause of hypertension in their JNC 7 report [15]. Given the high prevalence of OSA, this causal association could explain a substantial number of cases of hypertension and its sequelae, such as cardiovascular and cerebrovascular morbidity and mortality. Furthermore, OSA could be the most frequent cause of hypertension.

How can the relationship between OSA and hypertension be explained? It has been shown that OSA patients have an increased sympathetic activity not only during the night but also during the day [3]. Furthermore, they have a higher norepinephrine-release rate to hypoxia than controls, increased endothelin-1 levels, and a reduced endothelium-dependent vascular relaxation [16].

The standard treatment for OSA – continuous positive airway pressure (CPAP) – reduces blood pressure [17]. This reduction is seen in both systolic and diastolic blood pressure, and during both wake and sleep, suggesting that the fall is associated with a general change in vascular pressure regulation and is not attributable solely to the correction of the acute hemodynamic effects during the night. The reduction in blood pressure is similar in magnitude or even higher to that seen in pharmacological intervention studies. The influence on blood pressure depends on the severity of OSA. Patients with more severe disease show a larger fall in blood pressure with CPAP than those with less severe disease. It is of great importance to emphasize that effective treatment is necessary to achieve success. An even 50% reduction in the apnea-hypopnea index (AHI) with subtherapeutic CPAP did not result in a decrease in blood pressure [18].

The drop in mean blood pressure by 3.3–10 mm Hg would be predicted to reduce coronary heart disease event risk by 15–37% and stroke risk by 20–56%. CPAP might also improve other vascular risk factors – like cholesterol levels, leptin regulation, and platelet aggregability [19] – and therefore produce a risk benefit greater than might be expected from the blood pressure changes alone [17].

Not only CPAP, but also effective oral appliance therapy for OSA results in a reduction in blood pressure, similar to that reported with CPAP therapy [20].

So far, there are only limited data available to predict the blood pressure-lowering effect of CPAP therapy. The available data suggest that OSA patients with a high pulse pressure or elevated heart rates at baseline (indicative of an increased sympathetic activity) [21], with nondipping during 24-hour blood pressure monitoring [22], and without blood pressure lowering medication [23], are more likely to experience lower blood pressure values with effective treatment.

Furthermore, the polymorphism of the β_1-adrenoceptor appears to have an impact on heart rate and blood pressure response to CPAP therapy [24].

Pulmonary Hypertension

Changes in pulmonary artery pressure within an obstructive apnea during NREM sleep are well known. Usually intravascular pulmonary artery pressure decreases during the apnea and increases at the resumption of breathing. Transmural pulmonary artery pressure (i.e. corrected for intrathoracic pressure swings) increases progressively throughout the apnea with a maximum during the final occluded efforts and sustained during the early phase of hyperventilation. It could be shown that the increase of transmural pulmonary artery pressure during an obstructive apnea is associated with both the degree of hypoxemia – as a result of the apnea – and the height of intrathoracic pressure swings [25]. Hypoxia raises endothelin concentrations and influences the NO-dependent vasodilation; this results in pulmonary vasoconstriction. Intrathoracic pressure swings induce an increased venous reflow to the right ventricle, thereby augmenting right ventricular stroke volume (and pulmonary artery pressure). Furthermore, a right-left shift of the septum increases left ventricular end-diastolic pressure and capillary wedge pressure.

Mild daytime pulmonary hypertension is a common complication in patients with OSA syndrome, with a prevalence of approximately 20% [26]. Pulmonary hypertension in these patients is often associated with obesity or chronic obstructive lung disease, but it can occur even in the absence of lung or heart disease [27]. In this situation, pulmonary hypertension is related to the severity of OSA.

The potential mechanisms of daytime pulmonary hypertension in OSA are still under debate. Serum levels of vascular endothelial growth factor – a hypoxia-sensitive glycoprotein stimulating neoangiogenesis – are elevated in patients with OSA [28]. It is assumed that the postcapillary component of daytime pulmonary hypertension is due to diastolic dysfunction and that the precapillary component results from repetitive hypoxia-reoxygenation during the night, leading to both pulmonary vasoconstriction and vascular endothelial remodeling. It is also suggested that genetic factors determine the link between hypoxia and the manifestation of pulmonary hypertension.

Treatment of OSA with CPAP improves daytime pulmonary hypertension and total pulmonary vascular resistance. The greatest improvement could be shown in patients with sustained daytime pulmonary hypertension [29].

Given the association between daytime pulmonary hypertension and OSA, sleep-disordered breathing should be ruled out in patients with pulmonary hypertension of unknown etiology.

Arrhythmias

Sinus arrhythmia is the commonest ECG rhythm noted in patients with OSAHS. Although not strictly a pathological arrhythmia, it is a cardiac rhythm marker of the cardiac autonomic response to OSAHS. During the obstructive apnea, whilst hypoxemia occurs with an absence of airflow, a vagal or 'diving reflex' response occurs which results in bradycardia. At the apnea termination, hypoxemia with airflow occurs resulting in a transient tachycardia which subsides once the coinciding surge in system blood pressure is registered by the baroreflex system which prompts a relative slowing of the heart rate towards normality or until the next apnea begins. As such a typical tachy-bradycardia, with a cycle length of 30–90 s during sleep of a snorer, is often indicative of moderate to severe OSAHS in a patient with intact autonomic control. Indeed, analysis of heart rate variability may provide an additional diagnostic tool for OSAHS.

The loss of tachy-bradycardia response, replaced with a fixed heart rate (in which there is a lack of heart rate variability), indicates failed autonomic responses. Specifically, it may indicate a loss of baroreflex (vagal) control and excessive sympathetic activity, a forerunner to the development of systemic hypertension.

Importantly the recognition of sinus tachycardia during sleep at night may represent the side effects of therapeutic, illicit or social drugs. Alternatively anxiety or medical conditions (thyrotoxicosis, anemia or failure of heart, lungs or liver) may contribute. In 1968, the Framingham study identified the importance of tachycardia being a marker of greater mortality and the sleep study provides an opportunity to identify this adverse risk factor [30].

The recognition of bradycardia also may represent normality (extreme fitness) or pathology, namely hypothyroidism, heart block or side effect of medication (e.g. beta blockers). Sinus pause of up to 2–3 s duration are not infrequently seen in severe OSAHS and are a normal physiological response to apnea without airflow. Transient heart block may also occur and has been reported in up to 10% of patients with OSA [31]. Those most at risk have pre-existing conduction disturbances or are taking negatively chronotropic medications. Sinus pause (up to 13 s) is not uncommonly observed in polysomnograms (fig. 3). Reports of sinus pause

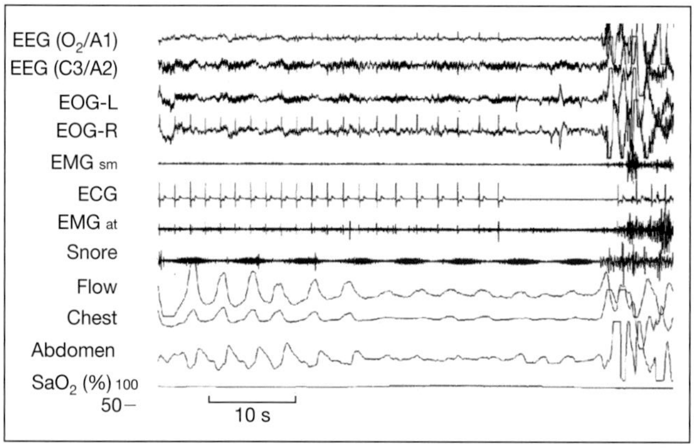

Fig. 3. A polysomnograph showing a 13 s sinus pause associated with an obstructive hypopnea. Reprinted with permission [48].

>13 s have not been reported to the best of our knowledge. This may be explained by the reports that asystole is associated with loss of consciousness at about 7 s with overt seizures at 15 s [32]. Indeed, careful reading of the description of acute arrest to cerebral circulation studies [32] indicate eye twitching at ~7 s which may indicate the onset of seizure activity, an appearance noted on polysomnography (fig. 3) [33]. In the situation of sinus arrest with OSASH, there is resumption of ventilation prior to the 13 s which may represent a response to hypotension rather than the usual triggers for arousal (hypoxia, hypercapnia and upper airway irritation).

Approximately 25% of patients with moderately severe OSA will have brief supraventricular arrhythmias, or rate dependent bundle branch block, which relate to degree of nocturnal hypoxemia. Moreover, ~50% of patients with established atrial fibrillation (AF) have symptoms of OSA, compared with ~3% of a general population [34]. The AF may initially only be transient during sleep and most commonly in REM sleep when there is excessive background sympathetic activity similar to wakefulness [3]. Mooe et al. [35] reported that OSAHS was an independent predictor for the development of AF post-coronary artery bypass surgery. Treatment of OSAHS can halve the re-occurrence rate of AF post-cardioversion [36].

Possible factors related to OSAHS that might contribute to AF include (a) sympathetic hyperactivity related to hypoxemia, hypercapnia and arousals; (b) impaired and reset parasympathetic and baroreceptor activity secondary to large negative intrathoracic pressure swings; (c) myocardial ischemia related to hypoxemia and increased myocardial work related to surges in systemic blood pressure upon a background of coronary artery disease, and (d) atrial chamber dilatation related to large negative intrathoracic pressure swings.

AF is important to recognize as it carries significant mortality, morbidity and economic costs [34, 36]. The age-adjusted prevalence of AF has tripled from the 1960s to the 1980s. Obesity, a major risk factor for OSA, has reached endemic proportions. These facts coupled, and based upon current scientific knowledge, questioning for OSA should be considered in all patients with AF. Recognition of this subgroup of AF patients is important as the AF-associated stroke rate is likely to remain high. In addition, there is a theoretical risk that CPAP treatment of OSA with AF, may result in reversion from AF to SR, and expulsion of a mural thrombus.

Ventricular ectopy is common, as is transient ventricular tachycardia, usually self terminating. Development of ST change and broadening of the QRS complex during sleep may also indicate cardiac decompensation during sleep. In addition, a high frequency of ventricular ectopic beats has been observed in patients with OSA and heart failure [37]. Treatment with nocturnal CPAP has been shown to abolish the majority of these bradyarrhythmias and ectopic beats [31].

Coronary Artery Disease and Myocardial Infarction

OSAHS may be a potential cause of coronary artery disease (CAD). On a mechanistic level, there is now evidence that OSAHS causes endothelial damage and dysfunction, and thus may be a cause of generalized atherosclerosis. Vascular wall damage can occur with recurrent hypoxemia and hyperoxia, altered autonomic control, and production of oxygen free radicals. Altered endothelial function (loss of naturally occurring nitric oxide) [38], greater blood coagulability [19], elevated fibrinogen levels [39], impaired vasodilatation [40] and the development or association with type 1 [41] and 2 [42] diabetes mellitus all will contribute to the development of premature vascular disease.

Epidemiological evidence has shown OSAHS to be common amongst patients with myocardial infarction: Hung et al. [43] showed an apnea index >5 events/h being associated with a 23 odds ratio of myocardial infarction, greater than that seen with smoking. Recently, this was confirmed with a Spanish 12-year follow-up study of 1,651 patients with varying degrees of OSAHS, indicating that the presence of untreated OSA was associated with a sevenfold incidence of mortality and non-fatal cardiovascular events, a risk factor greater than that of systemic blood pressure and smoking history [44].

Peker et al. [45] have published data from a 7-year follow up of a sleep clinic population. In this group, those with OSAHS at baseline had a 4.9 times greater chance of developing cardiovascular disease during the follow-up period, independent of age, BMI and blood pressure. The Sleep Heart Health Study [46] showed only a modest association between OSAHS and IHD in its recent cross sectional analysis. Those in the highest quartile of AHI (AHI >11 events/h) had only a 1.3 increased risk of self reported IHD compared to those in the lowest quartile of AHI. However, the small number of patients in the analysis with very severe OSAHS may attenuate this effect.

A separate issue is the prognosis of patients with both CAD and OSAHS. Possible reasons for a worse prognosis due to OSAHS include the precipitation of nocturnal ischemia/infarction and arrhythmias, or the acceleration of pre-existing atherosclerosis. Nocturnal ischemia is common in patients with both OSAHS and CAD, and, similarly, OSAHS has been found to be very common in patients with nocturnal ischaemia. A study with a 5-year follow-up of patients known to have CAD, revealed mortality to be significantly higher in those with OSAHS, independent of confounding factors [47].

Another interesting observation is the circadian pattern of myocardial infarcts and death. It has been well accepted that the peak time of onset of myocardial infarction ~8:00 a.m. occurs between 6:00 a.m. and 12 midday – a time that includes the final hours of sleep and the transition from sleep to wakefulness [48]. Recently, a study of 112 patients who had undergone polysomnography who had died suddenly from cardiovascular causes over a 6-year period reported that the majority of deaths occurring during the hours 00:00 and 06:00 were in patients with an OSAHS [49]. Specifically, 46% of the patients dying in this 6-hour block of time had OSAHS.

Stroke

There is increasing clinical data supporting an independent association between OSAHS and stroke. Snoring carries a 1.3- to 10-fold greater odds ratio of lifetime stroke [50]. OSAHS occurs in 30–80% of patients with acute stroke [50], whilst there is a spontaneous resolution over 3–12 months in up to 50% of patients [51]. Patients with recurrent stroke are more likely to have OSAHS than first-stroke patients [52]. The Sleep Heart Health Study demonstrated that those community dwellers with an AHI >11 events/h were 1.6 times more likely to have reported a history of stroke compared to those with an AHI <1.4 events/h [46].

It has been controversial whether OSAHS is a cause or consequence of stroke. OSAHS may be a cause of stroke through the mechanisms of (a) AF and mural thrombus; (b) vibration injury to carotid endothelium and potential to develop thrombus; (c) swings in blood pressure with impaired cerebrovascular blood flow autoregulation; (d) greater coagulability, and (e) paradoxical emboli via a patent foramen ovale. Alternatively, OSAHS may result from stroke-related alterations in upper airway tone and collapsibility.

Treatment of the OSAHS with CPAP appears to reduce mortality and hospital length of stay, and improve markers of stroke severity (e.g. Barthel Index) [53]. However, less than 50% of patients with a stroke and OSAHS tolerate CPAP treatment [54]. Unfortunately, no controlled trials are available to assess the effect of CPAP on stroke outcome.

In contrast to OSAHS, a small proportion (<20%) of stroke survivors have CSA-CSR. It has been unclear whether CSA-CSR occurs primarily due to the stroke or represents subtle or occult congestive heart failure (CHF). Unfortunately, most studies in which CSA-CSR was attributed to stroke did not report the objective cardiac examination or investigations in full. This has been seen to be problematic, given that >25% of stroke patients have underlying cardiovascular disease. A recent report addresses this issue [55]. These investigators prospectively performed polysomnography in 93 consecutive patients recovering from an acute stroke and observed CSA-CSR in 19%. In such patients, CSA-CSR was related to hypocapnia secondary to cardiac impairment (often occult) and not to the site of the stroke.

Congestive Heart Failure

Congestive heart failure (CHF) has emerged as the most expensive medical condition in the western world. An increasing prevalence and incidence of CHF, frequent hospitalizations plus increasing variety of medical therapies, many of which are costly (e.g. left ventricular assist devices and biventricular pacers) have contributed to an annual estimate of USD 50 billion which is spent per annum in USA on patients with CHF [56]. The mortality of CHF ranges from 20 to 50% at 2 years, which equates with many malignancies.

Current understanding of pathophysiology suggests that CHF is due to either systolic (failure of contraction) and/or diastolic left ventricular failure (failure of relaxation) (fig. 4–8) and/or conduction abnormalities (e.g. sick sinus syndrome, AF). It is estimated that systolic and diastolic

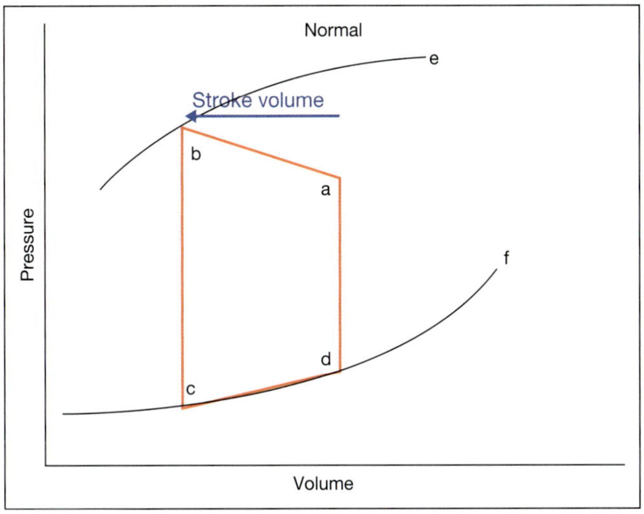

Fig. 4. Pressure-volume (V) curve of left ventricle indicating (a) initiation of systole; (b) end of systole; (c) beginning of diastole, and (d) end of diastole. Line (e) is the isovolumic pressure line and (f) the line of constant preload. The horizontal arrow indicates stroke volume.

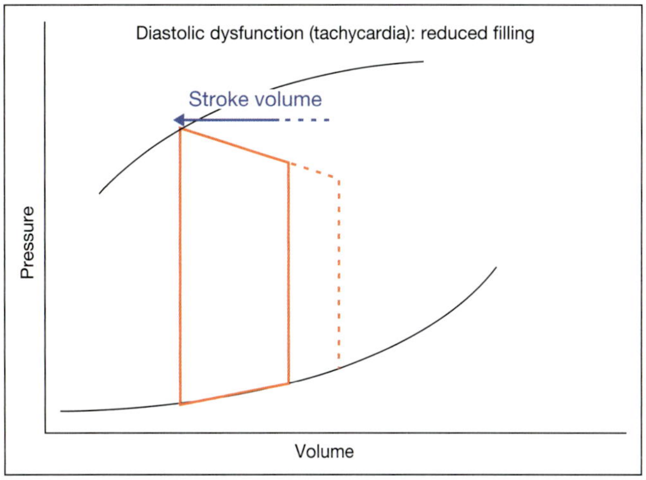

Fig. 6. Pressure-volume curve of left ventricle change from normal (dotted lines) to tachycardia and decompensated diastolic dysfunction with reduced stroke volume (continuous line). Note a reduced diastolic filling time, and thus diastolic filling and corresponding reduced stroke volume.

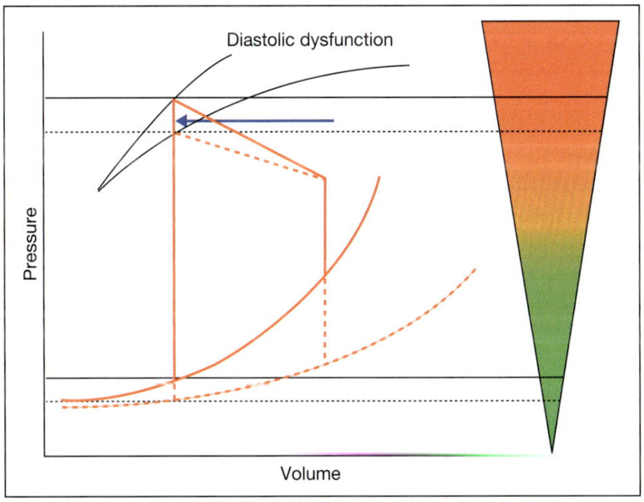

Fig. 5. Pressure-volume curve of left ventricle indicating early compensated diastolic dysfunction. Note an increase from normal (dotted line) to elevated (continuous line) systolic and diastolic blood pressures indicating an increase in cardiac work (as indicated by a more red appearance within the colored inverted triangle) with no change in stroke volume.

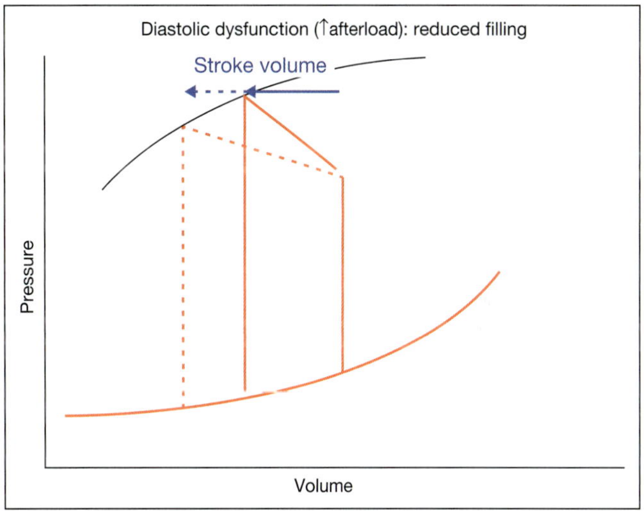

Fig. 7. Pressure-volume curve of left ventricle change from normal (dotted line) to one of increased afterload without the ability to increase the isovolumic pressure line (e.g. elevated blood pressure in CHF) with associated fall in stroke volume (continuous line). Further example of decompensated diastolic dysfunction.

left ventricular dysfunction occurs in up to 6% and 21% of community dwellers aged 45 years or older, respectively [57].

Patients with CHF can be staged into four (A–D) categories: stage A identifies the patient who is at high risk for developing CHF but has no structural disorder of the heart; stage B refers to a patient with a structural disorder of the heart but who has never developed symptoms of CHF; stage C denotes the patient with past or current symptoms of CHF associated with underlying structural heart disease, and stage D designates the patient with end-stage disease

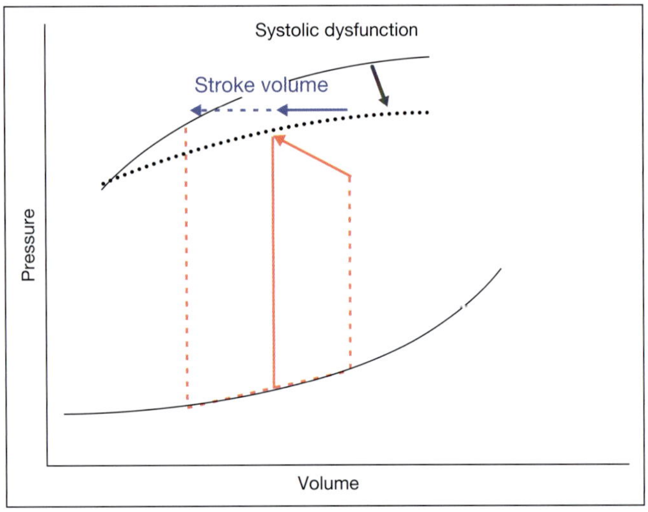

Fig. 8. Pressure-volume curve of left ventricle change from normal (dotted line) to one of systolic dysfunction with reduction in isovolumic line (black arrow), an increase in end diastolic volume and associated reduced stroke volume (continuous line). Example of systolic dysfunction.

who requires specialized treatment strategies such as mechanical circulatory support, continuous inotropic infusions, cardiac transplantation, or hospice care [56].

Treatment strategies have been well defined for CHF due to systolic or conduction abnormalities, where survival has been positively influenced by treatment. In contrast, diastolic dysfunction remains unknown territory in terms of cause and optimal management.

OSAHS is likely to be an important cause of diastolic dysfunction (table 1), due to hypoxemia, tachycardia, elevated left ventricular transmural pressure and vascular injury, which left unrecognized may lead to systolic dysfunction and conduction abnormalities. Whereas, CSA-CSR (table 2) may be a secondary response to severe CHF (of any cause) (table 3) due to hyperventilation, circulatory delay and plant gain (wet lungs) (table 4).

Under normal conditions, cardiac output falls during normal sleep, by approximately 20%, via the mechanisms of a drop in heart rate and stroke volume. Normal pressure volume curves are shown in figure 4. With upper airway instability, and the development of obstructive sleep disordered breathing, cardiac output may fall further for several reasons. First, the left ventricular transmural pressure will increase (due to large negative intrathoracic pressures during the apnea and elevated systolic pressures during the arousal). Elevated transmural pressure (akin to elevated afterload) will impede stroke volume mildly in healthy individuals, and to a greater degree in patients with impaired

Table 1. Mechanisms responsible for OSAHS contributing to vascular disease

Hypoxemia and hypercapnia
Increased sympathetic activity and respiratory drive
Negative intrathoracic pressure
Increased left ventricular afterload
Increased venous return
Endothelial damage due to hypoxia/hyperoxia
Loss of nitric oxide production
Arousal
Sympathetic activation
Increased heart rate
Systemic hypertension
Pulmonary hypertension
Patent foramen ovale
Shunting right to left
Stroke
Profound hypoxemia

Table 2. Clinical features which assist distinguishing OSAHS from CSA-CSR in CHF population

	OSAHS	CSA-CSR
Gender	Male + female	Male
Age	Younger	Older
Snoring history	Yes	Occasionally
Atrial fibrillation	Occasionally	More frequent
Obesity	Yes	Less common
Carbon dioxide	Normal/high	Low/normal
CHF severity	Mild-moderate	Moderate-severe
Hypoxemia	Moderate	Mild
Intrathoracic swings	Large	Mild
Sleep stage	REM	Stage 1+2

Table 3. Signs and symptoms of CHF: two major or one major and two minor are considered necessary to make a diagnosis

Major	Minor
Paroxysmal nocturnal dyspnea	Peripheral edema
Orthopnea	Night cough
Elevated JVP	Dyspnea on exertion
3rd heart sound	Hepatomegaly
Cardiomegaly on CXR	Pleural effusion
Pulmonary edema on CXR	Tachycardia (>120 bpm)
	Weight loss >4.5 kg in 5 days

Table 4. Mechanisms of positive airway pressure in heart failure

A Upper airway stability
B Intrathoracic
Increase end-expiratory lung volume
Increase alveolar pressure
Assist inspiratory muscles
Reduce left ventricular transmural pressure
Reduce preload
Reduce cardiac chamber size
Reduce cardiac mechanical work
Increase dead space and thereby increase CO_2
Attenuate sympathetic activity

baseline cardiac contractility. Second, inspiratory efforts will raise intrathoracic blood volume, a right ventricular dilatation may occur shifting the intraventricular septum towards the left ventricle. Third, stroke volume may fall with obstructive sleep disordered breathing, due directly to hypoxia (during the apnea) and tachycardia (at arousal), which have the capacity to precipitate impaired cardiac relaxation, thus reduced filling during diastole and the development of diastolic dysfunction (fig. 5, 6). Fourth, structural changes to the low pressure left atrium, due to the large negative intrathoracic pressure and impaired relaxation, may lead to left atrial dilatation and then to atrial fibrillation which will further reduce cardiac output. Fifth, with venous engorgement of the pulmonary vascular tree, alveolar leak may occur, leading in extreme situations to the development of pulmonary edema. Impaired systolic contraction follows (fig. 7) and later cardiac dilatation (fig. 8). Finally, elevations of right-sided pressures may lead to transient opening of foramen ovale [58].

There is now experimental and clinical evidence to support the hypothesis that OSAHS is deleterious to cardiac function. Firstly, studies in dogs have shown that 1–3 months of repetitive apneas can lead to impaired left ventricular ejection function (LVEF) and hypertension [59]. OSA is also strongly associated with systolic heart failure in human studies [60, 61]. In the Sleep Heart Health Study [46], the largest cardiovascular risk from OSA was seen for a history of cardiac failure. Those with an AHI >11 events/h had a relative risk of 2.4 for reporting a history of CHF compared to those with an AHI <1.4 events/h.

OSA and Diastolic Heart Failure

The apnea-induced hemodynamic changes cause acute reductions in left ventricular (LV) diastolic function. Negative intrathoracic pressure causes increased right ventricular filling with a subsequent shift of the intraventricular septum into the LV cavity. This reduces LV diastolic compliance. Hypoxemia leads to delays in ventricular relaxation and tachycardia, both of which also impair diastolic function. Chronically, OSA is associated with hypertension and increased LV wall thickness, which may lead to LV diastolic dysfunction [59, 62]. However, it remains controversial whether the change in LV muscle bulk occurs independently of associated hypertension, as evidence to this point in time has been conflicting. Recently [62], a report described reversible left ventricular diastolic dysfunction in a group of OSA patients using a randomized controlled cross-over design. Patients with diastolic dysfunction do not appear to have predisposition to hyperventilation or hypocapnia and thus do not develop CSA-CSR [63].

OSA and Systolic Heart Failure

If OSA adversely affects LVEF then one would expect improvement in cardiac performance following its treatment. Strong evidence supporting a beneficial effect of CPAP has now begun to emerge. A recent randomized controlled trial has shown improvements in LVEF from 25 to 34% with 1 month's CPAP treatment of OSA in patients (n = 24) with systolic heart failure in addition to reductions in chamber size [60]. In a larger (n = 40) and longer (3 month) randomized controlled Australian study LVEF increased from 38 to 43% with CPAP in addition to significant improvements in quality of life and autonomic activity [61].

References

1 Wellman A, Jordan AS, Malhotra A, Fogel RB, Katz ES, Schory K, Edwards JK, White DP: Ventilatory control and airway anatomy in obstructive sleep apnea. Am J Respir Crit Care Med 2004;170:1225–1232.

2 Scanlan MF, Roebuck T, Little PJ, Redman JR, Naughton MT: Effect of moderate alcohol upon sleep, breathing and sympathetic activity. Eur Resp J 2000;16:909–913.

3 Somers VK, Dyken ME, Clary MP, Abboud FM: Sympathetic activity neural mechanisms in obstructive sleep apnea. J Clin Invest 1995; 96:1897–1904.

4 Burgess HJ, Trinder J, Kim Y, Luke D: Sleep and circadian influences on cardiac autonomic nervous system activity. Am J Physiol 1997;273: H1761–H1768.

5 Solin P, Kaye DM, Little PHJ, Bergin P, Richardson M, Naughton MT: Impact of sleep apnea on sympathetic nervous system activity in heart failure. Chest 2003;123:1119–1126.

6 Dempsey JA, Smith CA, Przybylowski T, Chenuel B, Xie A, Nakayama H, Skatrud JB: The ventilatory responsiveness to CO2 below eupnoea as a determinant of ventilatory stability in sleep. J Physiol 2004;560:1–11.

7 Solin P, Roebuck T, Swieca J, Walters EH, Naughton MT: Effects of cardiac dysfunction upon non-hypercapnic central sleep apnea. Chest 1998;113:104–110.

8 Yap JCH, Moore DM, Cleland JGF, Pride NB: Effect of supine posture on respiratory mechanics in chronic left ventricular failure. Am J Respir Crit Care Med 2000;162: 1285–1291.

9 Lofaso F, Goldenberg F, D'Ortho MP, Coste A, Harf A: Arterial blood pressure response to transient arousals from NREM sleep in nonapneic snorers with sleep fragmentation. Chest 1998;113:985–991.

10 Pankow W, Nabe B, Lies A, Becker H, Köhler U, Kohl FV, Lohmann FW: Influence of sleep apnea on 24-hour blood pressure. Chest 1997;112:1253–1258.

11 Brooks D, Horner RL, Kozar LF, Render-Teixeira CL, Phillipson EA: Obstructive sleep apnea as a cause of systemic hypertension: evidence from a canine model. J Clin Invest 1997;99:106–109.

12 Nieto FJ, Young TB, Lind BK, Shahar E, Samet JM, Redline S, D'Agostino RB, Newman AB, Lebowitz MD, Pickering TG: Association of sleep-disordered breathing, sleep apnea, and hypertension in a large community-based study. JAMA 2000;283: 1829–1836.

13 Peppard PE, Young T, Palta M, Skatrud J: Prospective study of the association between sleep-disordered breathing and hypertension. N Engl J Med 2000;342:1378–1384.

14 Haas DC, Foster GL, Nieto FJ, Redline S, Resnick HE, Robbins JA, Young T, Pickering TG: Age-dependent associations between sleep-disordered breathing and hypertension. Circulation 2005;111:614–621.

15 Chobanian AV, Bakris GL, Black HR, Cushman WC, Green LA, Green LA, Izzo JL Jr, Jones DW: The seventh report of the Joint National Committee on Prevention, Detection, Evaluation, and Treatment of High Blood Pressure. JAMA 2003;289:2560–2572.

16 Duchna HW, Guilleminault C, Stoohs RA, Faul JL, Moreno H, Hoffr BB, Blaschke TF: Vascular reactivity in obstructive sleep apnea syndrome. Am J Respir Crit Care Med 2000;161:187–191.

17 Pepperell J, Ramdassingh-Dow S, Crosthwaite N, Mullins R, Jenkinson C, Stradling JR, Davies RJO: Ambulatory blood pressure after therapeutic and subtherapeutic nasal continuous positive airway pressure for obstructive sleep apnoea: a randomised parallel trial. Lancet 2002;359:204–210.

18 Becker HF, Jerrentrup A, Ploch T, Grote L, Penzel T, Sullivan CE, Peter JH: Effect of nasal continuous positive airway pressure treatment on blood pressure in patients with obstructive sleep apnea. Circulation 2003; 107:68–73.

19 Sanner B, Konermann M, Tepel M, Groetz J, Mummenhoff C, Zidek W: Platelet function in patients with obstructive sleep apnoea syndrome. Eur Respir J 2000;16:648–652.

20 Gotsopoulos H, Kelly JJ, Cistulli PA: Oral appliance therapy reduces blood pressure in obstructive sleep apnea: a randomized, controlled trial. Sleep 2004;27:934–941.

21 Sanner BM, Tepel M, Markmann A, Zidek W: Effect of continuous positive airway pressure therapy on 24-hour blood pressure in patients with obstructive sleep apnea syndrome. Am J Hypertens 2002;15:251–257.

22 Engleman HM, Gough K, Martin SE, Kingshott RN, Padfield PL, Douglas NJ: Ambulatory blood pressure on and off continuous positive airway pressure therapy for the sleep apnea/hypopnea syndrome: effects in 'non-dippers'. Sleep 1996;19:378–381.

23 Boergel J, Sanner BM, Keskin F, Bittlinsky A, Bartels NK, Buechner N, Huesing A, Rump LC, Muegge A: Obstructive sleep apnea and blood pressure. Interaction between the blood pressure-lowering effects of positive airway pressure therapy and antihypertensive drugs. Am J Hypertens 2004:17:1081–1087.

24 Boergel J, Schulz T, Bartels N, Epplen J, Buechner N, Rump LC, Huesing A, Sanner B, Muegge A: Modifying effects of the R389G ß1-adrenoceptor polymorphism on resting heart rate and blood pressure in patients with obstructive sleep apnea. Clin Science 2006;110:117–123.

25 Schafer H, Hasper E, Ewig S, Koehler U, Latzelsberger J, Tasci S, Luderitz B: Pulmonary haemodynamics in obstructive sleep apnoea: time course and associated factors. Eur Respir J 1998;12:679–684.

26 Chaouat A, Weitzenblum E, Krieger J, Oswald M, Kessler R: Pulmonary hemodynamics in the obstructive sleep apnea syndrome: results in 220 consecutive patients. Chest 1996;109: 380–386.

27 Sanner B, Doberauer C, Konermann M, Sturm A, Zidek W: Pulmonary hypertension in patients with obstructive sleep apnea syndrome. Arch Intern Med 1997;157: 2483–2487.

28 Schulz R, Hummel C, Heinemann S, Seeger W, Grimminger F: Serum levels of vascular endothelial growth factor are elevated in patients with obstructive sleep apnea and severe nighttime hypoxia. Am J Respir Crit Care Med 2002;165:67–70.

29 Sajkov D, Wang T, Saunders NA, Bune AJ, McEvoy RD: Continuous positive airway pressure treatment improves pulmonary hemodynamics in patients with obstructive sleep apnea. Am J Respir Crit Care Med 2002;165: 152–158.

30 Kannel WB, Kannel C, Paffenbarger RS, Cupples PH, Cupples LA: Heart rate and cardiovascular mortality: the Framingham study. Am Heart J 1987;113:1489–1494.

31 Harbison J, O'Reilly P, McNicholas WT: Cardiac rhythm disturbances in the obstructive sleep apnea syndrome: effects of nasal positive airway pressure therapy. Chest 2000;118: 591–595.

32 Rossen R, Kabat H, Anderson JP: Acute arrest of cerebral circulation in man. Arch Neurol Psychiat 1943;50:510–528.

33 Naughton MT: Cardiopulmonary interaction during sleep; in Donner CF, Ambrosino N, Goldstein RS (eds): Pulmonary Rehabilitation. London, Hodder Arnold, 2005, pp 98–111.

34 Gami AS, Pressman G, Caples SM, Kanagala R, Gard JJ, Davison DE, Malouf JF, Ammash NM, Friedman PA, Somers VK: Association of atrial fibrillation and sleep apnea. Circulation 2004;110:364–367.

35 Mooe T, Gullsby S, Rabben T, Eriksson P: Sleep-disordered breathing: a novel predictor of atrial fibrillation after coronary artery bypass surgery. Coron Artery Dis 1996;7: 475–478.

36 Kanagala R, Murali NS, Friedman PA, Ammash NM, Gersh BJ, Ballman KV, Shamsuzzaman AS, Somers VK: Obstructive sleep apnea and recurrence of atrial fibrillation. Circulation 2003;107:2589–2594.

37 Lanfranchi PA, Somers VK, Braghiroli A, Corra U, Eleuteri E, Giannuzzi P: Central sleep apnea in left ventricular dysfunction: prevalence and implications for arrhythmic risk. Circulation 2003;107:727–732.

38 Ip MSM, Tse HF, Lam B, Tsang KWT, Lam WK: Endothelial function in obstructive sleep apnea and response to treatment. Am J Respir Crit Care Med 2004;169:348–353.

39 Chin K, Ohi M, Kita H, Noguchi T, Otsuka N, Tsuboi T, Mishima M, Kuno K: Effects of NCPAP therapy on fibrinogen levels in obstructive sleep apnea syndrome. Am J Respir Crit Care Med 1996;153:1972–1976.

40 Kato M, Roberts-Thomson P, Phillips BG, Haynes WG, Winnicki M, Accurso V, Somers VK: Impairment of endothelium-dependent vasodilation of resistance vessels in patients with obstructive sleep apnea. Circulation 2000; 102:2607–2610.

41 Rees PJ, Prior JG, Cochrane GM, Clark TJ: Sleep apnea in diabetic patients with neuropathy. J R Soc Med 1981;74:192–195.

42 Babu AR, Herdegen J, Fogelfeld L, Shott S, Mazzone T: Type 2 diabetes, glycemic control

and continuous positive airway pressure in obstructive sleep apnea. Arch Intern Med 2005;165:447–452.
43 Hung J, Whitford EG, Parsons RW, Hillman DR: Association of sleep apnoea with myocardial infarction in men. Lancet 1990;336: 261–264.
44 Marin JM, Carrizo SJ, Vicente E, Agusti AG: Long-term cardiovascular outcomes in men with obstructive sleep apnoea-hypopnea with or without treatment with continuous positive airway pressure: an observational study. Lancet 2005;365:1046–1053.
45 Peker Y, Hedner J, Norum J, Kraiczi H, Carlson J: Increased incidence of cardiovascular disease in middle-aged men with obstructive sleep apnea: a 7-year follow-up. Am J Respir Crit Care Med 2002;166:159–165.
46 Shahar E, Whitney CW, Redline S, Lee ET, Newman AB, Javier Nieto F, O'Connor GT, Boland LL, Schwartz JE, Samet JM: Sleep-disordered breathing and cardiovascular disease: cross-sectional results of the Sleep Heart Health Study. Am J Respir Crit Care Med 2001;163:19–25.
47 Mooe T, Franklin KA, Holmstrom K, Rabben T, Wiklund U: Sleep-disordered breathing and coronary artery disease: long term prognosis. Am J Respir Crit Care Med 2001;164: 1910–1913.
48 Muller JE, Stone PH, Turi ZG, Rutherford JD, Czeisler CA, Parker C, Poole WK, Passamani E, Roberts R, Robertson T: Circadian variation in the frequency of onset of acute myocardial infarction. N Engl J Med 1985;313: 1315–1322.
49 Gami AS, Howard DE, Olson EJ, Somers VK: Day-night pattern of sudden death in obstructive sleep apnea. N Engl J Med 2005;352: 1206–1214.
50 Mohsenin V: Is sleep apnea a risk factor for stroke? A critical analysis. Minerva Med 2004;95:291–305.
51 Parra O, Arboix A, Bechich S, Garcia-Eroles L, Montserrat JM, Lopez JA, Ballester E, Guerra JM, Sopena JJ: Time course of sleep-related breathing disorders in first-ever stroke or transient ischemic attack. Am J Respir Crit Care Med 2000;161:375–380.
52 Dziewas R, Humpert R, Hopmann B, Kloska S, Ludemann P, Ritter M, Dittrich R, Ringelstein EB, Young P, Nabavi DG: Increased prevalence of sleep apnea in patients with recurring ischemic stroke compared with first stroke victims. J Neurol 2005;252:1394–1398.
53 Kaneko Y, Hajek VE, Zivanovic V, Raboud J, Bradley TD: Relationship of sleep apnea to functional capacity and length of hospitalization following stroke. Sleep 2003;26: 293–297.
54 Sandberg O, Franklin KA, Bucht G, Eriksson S, Gustafson Y: Nasal continuous positive airway pressure in stroke patients with sleep apnoea: a randomized treatment study. Eur Respir J 2001;18:630–634.
55 Nopmaneejumruslers C, Kaneko Y, Hajek V, Zivanovic V, Bradley TD: Cheyne-Stokes respiration in stroke: relationship to hypocapnia and occult cardiac dysfunction. Am J Respir Crit Care Med 2005;171:1048–1052.
56 Hunt SA, Baker DW, Chin MG, Cinquegrani MP, Feldman AM, Francis GS, Ganiats TG, Goldstein S, Gregoratos G, Jessup ML, Noble RJ, Packer M, Silver MA, Stevenson LW, Gibbons RJ, Antman EM, Alpert JS, Faxon DP, Fuster V, Gregoratos G, Jacobs AK, Hiratzka LF, Russell RO, Smith SC Jr, American College of Cardiology/American Heart Association Task Force on Practice Guidelines (Committee to Revise the 1995 Guidelines for the Evaluation and Management of Heart Failure), International Society for Heart and Lung Transplantation, Heart Failure Society of America: Guidelines for the Evaluation and Management of Chronic Heart Failure in the Adult: Executive Summary Circulation, 2001, vol 104, pp 2996–3007.
57 Redfield MM, Jacobsen SJ, Burnatt JC, Mahoney DW, Bailey KR, Rodeheffer RJ: Burden of systolic and diastolic ventricular dysfunction in the community. JAMA 2003; 289:194–202.
58 Shanoudy H, Soliman A, Raggi P, Liu JW, Russell DC, Jarmukli NF: Prevalence of patent foramen ovale and its contribution to hypoxemia in patients with obstructive sleep apnea. Chest 1998;113:91–96.
59 Parker JD, Brooks D, Kozar LF, Render-Teixeira CL, Horner RL, Bradley TD, Phillipson EA: Acute and chronic effects of airway obstruction on canine left ventricular performance. Am J Respir Crit Care Med 1999;160:1888–1896.
60 Kaneko Y, Floras JS, Usui K, Plante J, Tkacova R, Kubo T, Ando S, Bradley TD: Cardiovascular effects of continuous positive airway pressure in patients with heart failure and obstructive sleep apnea. N Engl J Med 2003;348:1233–1241.
61 Mansfield DR, Gollogly NC, Richardson M, Bergin P, Kaye DM, Naughton MT: Randomized trial of continuous positive airway treatment of obstructive sleep apnea in heart failure. Am J Respir Crit Care Med 2004;169:1–6.
62 Arias MA, Garcia-Rio F, Alonso-Fernandez A, Mediano O, Martinez I, Villamor J: Obstructive sleep apnea syndrome affects left ventricular diastolic function: effects of nasal continuous positive airway pressure in men. Circulation 2005;112:375–383.
63 Solin P, Roebuck T, Naughton MT: Cardiac diastolic function and hypercapnic ventilatory responses in central sleep apnoea. Eur Respir J 2002;20:717–723.

Matthew T. Naughton, MD
Department of Respiratory Medicine
Alfred Hospital
Commercial Road
Melbourne, Victoria, 3004 (Australia)
Fax +61 3 9276 3601
E-Mail m.naughton@alfred.org.au

Randerath WJ, Sanner BM, Somers VK (eds): Sleep Apnea.
Prog Respir Res. Basel, Karger, 2006, vol 35, pp 204–214

Sleep-Related Breathing Disorders in Children

R.S. Amin[a] L.F. Donnelly[b] D. Beebe[c] B.A. Chini[a]

[a]Division of Pulmonary Medicine, [b]Department of Radiology, [c]Division of Psychology, Cincinnati Children's Hospital Medical Center, Cincinnati, Ohio, USA

Abstract

Multiple genetic, metabolic and neuromuscular disorders in children are associated with abnormal control of breathing during sleep. More commonly are the breathing disorders associated with hypertrophy of the tonsils and adenoids. Removal of hypertrophied tonsils leads to transient and sometimes permanent resolution of the disorder. Persistence of breathing disorders during sleep after adenotonsillectomy requires evaluation of the anatomy and dynamics of the upper airway. Such an evaluation could shed light on the contribution of pharyngeal structures and dynamics to airway obstruction. Specifically the contribution of hypertrophied lingual tonsils, macroglossia or glossoptosis to airway obstruction could only be recognized through direct visualization of the airway during sleep. Such an approach could assist in designing an optimum management of a multifactorial disorder.

Childhood sleep-disordered breathing (SDB) encompasses children with obstructive sleep apnea syndrome (OSAS), the syndromes of central hypoventilation, and children with disorders of respiratory muscles.

As in adults, OSAS in children refers to a breathing disorder characterized by recurrent partial or complete episodes of upper airway obstruction, commonly associated with intermittent hypoxemia and sleep fragmentation. This definition, however, does not encompass the spectrum of severity of upper airway obstruction and increased airway resistance associated with sleep. The current definition of obstructive SDB is increasingly challenged by the recent evidence showing that children with prolonged periods during sleep of increased upper airway resistance but without obstructive sleep apnea (OSA) might exhibit neurocognitive deficits similar to those with intermittent upper airway obstruction. A broader definition of obstructive SDB in children has been proposed by Carroll [1]: 'Childhood obstructive SDB may be defined as a disorder of breathing during sleep characterized by prolonged increased upper airway resistance, partial upper airway obstruction, or complete obstruction that disrupts pulmonary ventilation, oxygenation, or sleep quality. Nighttime manifestations include some combination of snoring, increased respiratory effort, episodic hypoxemia, CO_2 retention, restless sleep, and increased numbers of arousals and awakenings from sleep. Daytime symptoms include excessive daytime sleepiness, daytime tiredness, fatigue, poor school performance, inattention, hyperactivity, oppositional behavior, and other subtle behavioral disturbances.'

While this definition encompasses childhood OSA, obstructive hypoventilation, and increased upper airway resistance syndrome (UARS), it imposes significant limitations as to the value of the available diagnostic methods in providing an accurate diagnosis across the entire spectrum of the syndrome and reliably identifying those at risk for adverse outcome from the disorder.

Epidemiology

At present, a minimum prevalence of childhood OSAS is estimated to be 2–3%, and the prevalence of habitual snoring may be as high as 20%. The peak incidence of OSAS occurs between 3 and 6 years of age, consistent with snoring prevalence. These epidemiological observations correspond to the findings in a longitudinal study by the group of Jeans which demonstrated that the soft tissues appear to grow more rapidly from 3 to 5 years of age than does the nasopharynx, leading to a relative decrease in the size of the airway at this period. Beyond the age of 5 years, the soft tissue area remains relatively constant whilst the nasopharynx increases in size. In contrast to the male predominance of OSAS in adults, epidemiologic studies and case series find a similar prevalence of snoring and OSAS in boys and girls.

Craniofacial anomalies, altered soft tissue size and neurologic disorders place infants and children at risk for OSAS.

Nasal and Oropharyngeal Pathologies

The most common type of childhood OSAS occurs in children between 2 and 8 years of age and is associated with adenotonsillary hypertrophy in most cases. Children without distinct craniofacial anomalies have subtle craniofacial morphometric features associated with OSA. Guilleminault found that children with the highest scores on a orocraniofacial clinical scale had SDB in the form of OSA or UARS. The orocraniofacial scale identified a subgroup of children with common craniofacial features: small chin, steep mandibular plane, retroposition of the mandible, long face, high hard palate and elongated soft palate. These features did not distinguish between children with OSAS and UARS, and absence of these features did not rule out SDB.

Soft tissues, particularly the adenoid and palatine tonsils, can also narrow the pharynx. These tissues grow progressively during childhood, and are maximal in the prepubertal years, coinciding with the peak incidence of childhood OSAS. In most children, without underlying medical conditions, surgical removal of enlarged tonsils and/or adenoid, cures or ameliorates the disorder. However, it is estimated that in 10–15% of otherwise normal children with OSAS, this disorder is not resolved by removal of the tonsils and adenoid, and only a weak relationship has been found between the severity of OSAS and the size of these tissues. This suggests that the pathogenesis of OSAS is more complex, involving other mechanisms, such as those leading to altered upper airway neuromotor tone during sleep.

Arens found that the overall volume of the tongue in normal children with OSAS did not differ from controls. Using magnetic resonance imaging (MRI), Arens also noted a 30% increase in the volume of the soft palate of children with mild to moderate OSAS compared to controls, thought due to edema and inflammatory changes secondary to chronic snoring as described in adults.

Atopy is strongly associated with habitual snoring. A study evaluating the prevalence and factors associated with snoring and habitual snoring in preschool and primary school children demonstrated that habitual snoring was significantly associated with allergic rhinitis (OR 2.90) and atopic dermatitis (OR 1.8). The odds ratio of children with all three atopic diseases, (asthma, allergic rhinitis, and atopic dermatitis), to have habitual snoring was 7.45, greater than obesity (OR 3.75). The association between snoring and rhinitis has been demonstrated in several other studies.

Neuromuscular Disorders

Effect of Sleep on the Respiratory System

Several changes in ventilatory control and respiratory muscle function occur with sleep onset, and familiarity with these changes provides a framework for understanding the pathophysiology of the early stages of chronic respiratory failure manifesting during sleep. These changes are presented below.

Reduction in Muscle Tone

There is a sleep-stage-related fall in postural muscle tone that reaches its nadir during REM sleep. Muscle hypotonia is attributed to supraspinal suppression of the gamma motor neuron drive and presynaptic inhibition of skeletal muscle spindle afferents. This muscle hypotonia clearly involves the intercostal and dilator muscles of the upper airway. In contrast, the diaphragm muscle with its scant muscle spindles is less subject to central inhibition and is therefore crucial in maintaining respiration during REM sleep. As such, the degree of alveolar hypoventilation during sleep and the accompanying hypoxemia and hypercapnia are dependent on diaphragmatic function.

Restrictive Ventilatory Defect

During normal sleep there is a fall in the functional residual capacity and a consequent reduction in O_2 storage. In patients with neuromuscular disorders, these changes are often exaggerated during sleep.

Upper Airway Resistance

Muscular hypotonia during sleep involves the dilator muscles of the upper airway, which leads to loss of tonic activity in the musculature of the tongue, pharynx, and larynx. A fall in the functional residual capacity further reduces the cross-sectional area of the upper airway and contributes to further increase in upper airway resistance. Some patients with neuromuscular disorders experience a rapid weight gain as the result of loss of ambulation. This weight gain leads to a significant degree of airway obstruction and possibly to OSA or obstructive hypoventilation during sleep. With the rise in upper airway resistance during sleep, patients with significant diaphragmatic weakness are sometimes unable to generate sufficient force to overcome the physiological changes of the upper airway caliber. As a result, they are unable to generate inspiratory flow.

Central Respiratory Drive

In normal sleep, the hypercapnic and hypoxic responses are diminished. This occurs because of an increase in upper airway resistance, as well as a decrease in the sensitivity of the chemoreceptors. This decline in chemosensitivity can contribute to sleep apnea in patients with neuromuscular diseases. Arousal from sleep during OSA is in part due to an increase in respiratory effort, which stimulates the chest mechanoreceptors. Prolonged OSA is frequently caused both by the inability of weak respiratory muscles to trigger an arousal response from the mechanoreceptor and the blunted central respiratory response to chemoreceptor input.

Stages of Respiratory Failure in Neuromuscular Disorders

Early evidence of respiratory muscle dysfunction is noted when muscles perform their function under conditions of stress, such as respiratory infection, recovery from general anesthesia, exercise, and sleep. In many instances, the onset of early respiratory insufficiency develops after the patient has lost ambulation. Detecting respiratory muscle dysfunction during exercise thus becomes unfeasible. In these patients, evaluation of breathing during sleep might then allow the identification of the early stages of respiratory muscle dysfunction. In slowly progressive neuromuscular disorders, respiratory failure advances in three stages. Alveolar hypoventilation during REM sleep, REM and NREM sleep and during wakefulness and sleep corresponds to stage 1, 2 and 3, respectively. The gradual transition from stage 1 to stage 3 respiratory failure is characteristic of Duchenne muscular dystrophy, in which there is a gradual progression of respiratory muscle weakness over two decades. In some disorders, such as congenital muscular dystrophy, if respiratory insufficiency is present, it might not progress beyond stage 1 or 2. In other disorders, respiratory muscle weakness is extremely severe, with patients presenting in stage 3 respiratory failure.

Risk Factors for SDB

Overweight

In adults, obesity is a major risk factor for OSAS. Earlier descriptions of childhood OSAS rarely described obese patients. Failure to thrive was a common complication in the earliest case reports of childhood OSAS. However, obesity now affects almost 1 in 5 children. The current pediatric literature suggests that obesity increases the risk for OSAS in all ages. In an epidemiologic study of 399 children, obesity was found to be the most significant risk factor for OSAS, with an odds ratio of 4.5. The group of Marcus studied obese children who did not present with symptoms of OSAS and found that 46% had abnormal polysomnography (PSG) and 27% had moderate to severe abnormalities. There was a positive correlation between obesity and the apnea index and an inverse relationship between obesity and oxygen saturation nadir.

Childhood obesity is on the rise, with the highest prevalence seen in adolescent children between 12 and 19 years of age. Recent data suggest that obesity may be a leading cause for OSAS during adolescent years. This form of OSAS shares much with the adult form of OSAS.

Exposure to Smoke

A 1989 study from Italy [2], found that 118 of 1,615 children aged 6–13 years were habitual snorers. Of these, 82 were exposed to passive parental smoking (69%). Children of smoking parents were more likely to be snorers than children whose parents never smoked (OR 1.85). Furthermore, they demonstrated a dose-effect relationship of smoking and snoring. The prevalence of habitual snoring increased significantly with the number of cigarettes smoked by parents.

A study from Singapore of over 11,000 children found that maternal smoking was significantly associated with habitual snoring, with an odds ratio of 2.22. Snoring is thought to reflect enhanced proliferation of lymphoid tissue induced by chemical irritation of the upper respiratory tract at an age when tonsils and adenoids are in a period of accelerated growth.

A study of over 3,600 Greek children found an odds ratio of 1.4 associated with passive smoking and habitual snoring.

Kahn studied 115 newborns within 1 week of birth and 394 infants at 11 weeks of life by overnight PSG. Prenatal smoking by mothers correlated with an increase in frequency and length of OSAs (relative risk 2.76) and a decrease in birth weight of their infants. Paternal smoking during pregnancy increased the risk of obstructive apneas only in the infants of smoking mothers.

Genetic Disorders

Common craniofacial anomalies affecting upper airway size and associated with OSAS include: Crouzon, Pfeiffer, Apert, Treacher-Collins, Nager, Hallerman-Streiff, Goldenhar, Rubinstein-Taybi, Doen, Beckwith-Wiedemann, Klippel-Feil, and Marfan syndromes, Robin sequence, choanal stenosis, and mucopolysaccharidosis. Some craniofacial syndromes, such as Down syndrome, are also associated with hypotonia, which can contribute to upper airway obstruction.

Macroglossia can significantly reduce upper airway size and commonly occurs in infants and children with Down syndrome, mucopolysaccharidosis and Beckwith-Wiedemann syndrome. In patients with glossoptosis, the tongue may prolapse posteriorly and occlude the airway, and is commonly seen in patients with a small and retrognothic mandible as in Robin sequence or in conditions with poor upper airway muscle tone, such as Down syndrome. Surgical correction of soft palate anomalies, such as cleft palate and velopharyngeal insufficiency, can be associated with OSAS. This includes patients who have had pharyngeal flap placement, which can lead to nasopharyngeal or oropharyngeal stenosis.

Down syndrome is the most common genetic disorder associated with craniofacial anomalies. OSAS is present in 30–60% of these patients. Midface and mandibular hypoplasia, glossoptosis, adenoid and tonsillar hypertrophy, laryngotracheal anomalies and obesity are the most common anatomic causes for OSAS in Down syndrome.

A pilot study of 19 young children with Down syndrome demonstrated a high prevalence of OSA. In this consecutively encountered, nonselected patient population, OSA was found in 79% of the subjects. More severe OSA was associated with a higher body mass index, older age, higher movement arousal index, and more sleep-related complaints. The investigators also found a significant inverse relationship between age and lowest SaO_2.

Inadequate Central Drive

The most common causes of inadequate central drive leading to chronic respiratory failure in children are related to congenital or acquired central hypoventilation syndromes. Congenital syndromes may present as isolated hypoventilation or may be associated with various genetic and metabolic abnormalities. Acquired hypoventilation occurs secondary to central nervous system infection, tumor, or trauma.

Congenital Central Hypoventilation Syndrome

Congenital central hypoventilation syndrome (CCHS) is defined as the failure of the automatic control of breathing; its etiology is unknown. This condition involves an integration abnormality of chemoreceptor input to the central controllers of respiration. Since breathing during NREM sleep is almost entirely controlled by the automatic system, ventilation is most compromised during NREM stages of sleep. The clinical presentation of CCHS varies depending on the degree of severity of the disorder. Infants with severe CCHS do not breathe spontaneously and require ventilatory assistance. Those with milder forms of the disorder often remain undiagnosed until they present with pulmonary hypertension and heart failure. Since more severely affected children hypoventilate both during wakefulness and sleep, they are diagnosed at an earlier age. During sleep, children with CCHS have absent or negligible ventilatory sensitivity both to hypercarbia and hypoxemia. This abnormal chemoreceptor response is also observed in patients with adequate daytime ventilation.

Patients with CCHS often have other abnormalities of autonomic nervous system functioning. Several reports have described the presence of decreased heart rate variability, decreased nocturnal blood pressure dipping, and diminished pupillary light response. There are also reports of esophageal achalasia. Recent studies describing the genetics of isolated CCHS found that 40–96% of children with this syndrome were found to have mutations of the *PHOX2b* gene, with the large majority occurring as de novo mutation.

A wide spectrum of genetic syndromes can be associated with central hypoventilation. These include myelomeningocele with Arnold Chiari malformation, skeletal dysplasia, Möbius syndrome, Prader-Willi syndromes, and inborn errors of metabolism such as pyruvate dehydrogenase complex deficiency, Leigh's disease, and carnitine deficiency.

Acquired Central Hypoventilation Syndrome

Abnormal central control of breathing can develop secondary to chronic respiratory failure caused by chronic lung disease. Persistent hypercapnia could blunt the ventilatory response to CO_2 in the presence of chronic lung disease. A similar effect could also develop from metabolic alkalosis and hypochloremia associated with diuretic therapy.

Clinical Features

While history of nocturnal symptoms could be a valuable tool in differentiating central from obstructive SDB, many studies have demonstrated the limited ability in distinguishing the degree of severity of obstructive SDB. Despite this limitation, clinical practice remains dependent on parental report as to the need for evaluation or treatment of SDB. History of snoring is the most common nighttime symptom of OSAS in children. Children with SDB may have obviously increased respiratory effort, which is often manifested as paradoxical inward rib cage motion. It is essential to recognize that paradoxical breathing during infancy and early childhood may represent a normal breathing pattern especially during REM sleep. Excessive nocturnal sweating and enuresis have been observed in children with SDB.

Neurocognitive Functions in Children with SDB

In adults, excessive daytime sleepiness associated with abnormal polysomnogram has become an important diagnostic criterion for SDB. Such a manifestation in children with SDB is very rare in the preadolescent age. However, daytime cognitive dysfunction and behavioral disorders are recognized at higher prevalence in children with SDB.

The cognitive and behavioral effects of OSA, commonly called 'neurobehavioral' because they are presumed to be mediated by the brain, were highlighted in some of the earliest reports in the published literature, and remain the focus of intense investigation. In 1889, Hill published a clinical description of children who snore, are sleepy during the day, and show academic underperformance. When the topic of pediatric OSA resurfaced in the published English literature nearly a century later, again academic and behavioral difficulties were highlighted in early case series. Interest in the neurobehavioral effects of pediatric OSA has since accelerated rapidly. A Medline search found over 60 relevant articles published from 2000 through mid-2005, more than had been cumulatively published since Hill's first observations a century earlier. The emerging picture is that pediatric OSA is associated with considerable neurobehavioral morbidity.

Excessive daytime sleepiness can occur in children with OSA, but it is far less frequent than in adults. Rather, in epidemiological studies, parent-reported snoring, a hallmark but nonspecific symptom of OSA, has been linked to poor academic performance, inattentiveness and hyperactivity in preschool and grade school children. Consistent with these findings, children who have been referred for adenotonsillectomy because of suspected OSA also display elevated rates of hyperactivity, rebelliousness, and aggression. Of note, however, a key limitation of most of these studies has been that both the independent variable (symptoms of OSA) and dependent variables (neurobehavioral functioning) have been gathered by parent report, raising concerns about potential reporter bias and what psychologists have termed 'method variance' – the tendency for spurious or inflated correlations between two variables that are gathered using the same methods. This limitation has been overcome by using independent sources of information regarding sleep and neurobehavioral functioning. With respect to the sleep, PSG techniques have been applied to show that preschool and grade school children with PSG-verified OSA display inattention, poor academic achievement, aggression, and overall behavioral maladjustment more often than their peers [3, 4]. Although two recent studies failed to find such associations, the samples a priori excluded children who had attention or behavioral disorders. Because such disorders are defined by the very behaviors suspected to be impacted by OSA – e.g. there is no medical 'test' for attention deficit/hyperactivity disorder (ADHD) – the a priori exclusion of such children may effectively 'control away' a meaningful effect. Recent data suggest that, among children with OSA, problems with impulse control, behavior regulation, and emotion regulation may be more prominent than difficulties with sustained attention or mood. Interestingly, one small but well-controlled study suggested that while parent-reported symptoms of snoring and restlessness each related in a unidirectional (monotonic) manner with ADHD symptoms, only children with mildly elevated ADHD symptoms showed PSG evidence of OSA; children with more severe ADHD symptoms were at no higher risk for OSA than non-hyperactive controls. To our knowledge, no published research from other groups has confirmed or refuted this finding but, as noted below, some have questioned whether conventional PSG indexes are adequately sensitive to SDB in children.

Another approach has been to obtain objective assessments of neurobehavioral functioning, most commonly office-based cognitive tests. Intellectual (IQ) tests have yielded conflicting findings. Several reports suggest the presence of lowered IQ scores among grade school children with SDB compared to controls. However, in each study, the controls were of above-average intelligence, while the children with SDB obtained scores in the average range. This may have been due to the use of volunteer control groups, which are often 'super-healthy' from a cognitive and behavioral standpoint [3]. Others who have used more representative sampling techniques or have covaried for potential confounding variables (e.g. family income) have found no intellectual deficits in grade-school children with OSA compared to controls. Interestingly, younger children may fare worse; three recent well-controlled studies found IQ deficits in preschool and 1st grade students with SDB [5]. These developmental discrepancies in IQ findings may reflect differences in measurement as different tests have been used with preschool children than with school-aged children. Compared to the IQ tests used with older children, those used with the younger children have placed greater emphasis on drawing abilities and auditory attention, two skills that have been found to be deficient among adults with OSA. Alternatively, there may be a moderating effect of age, in which young children are at greater risk of morbidity.

Children with OSA have been reported to show impairments on office-based tests of attention and executive functioning [3, 6], although the variety of tests that have been used across studies makes it difficult to integrate the findings. Studies that have used formal memory tests have yielded mixed results, with morbidity reported by some, but not others. These heterogeneous findings, which largely parallel the state of research into adult OSA, highlight the fact that attention, executive functioning, and memory are each heterogeneous domains, with fairly ambiguous boundaries conceptually and neuroanatomically. One challenge facing future researchers is to better define which aspects of attention, executive functioning, and memory, if any, are particularly vulnerable to OSA. A second challenge involves balancing the rigors of scientific control with applicability to daily life ('ecological validity'). Particularly with tests of attention and executive functioning, the well-structured, controlled office-based testing environment may prevent the expression of deficits that are better seen in more complex, less predictable natural (ecological) settings. To strike an optimal balance, we recommend gathering information from multiple sources, perhaps moving beyond office-based tests and parent report to include classroom observations and teacher reports. As of this writing, only one published study had presented data on teacher-reported outcome among a group of children with PSG-verified OSA. In 2004, we found evidence of teacher-reported deficits in behavior and emotion regulation using one data analytic approach, but not another – the meaning of this discrepancy was not immediately clear, but it appeared to be due at least in part to a small sample size.

Purported Mechanisms

The mechanisms that have been implicated in the development of vascular pathology in OSA have also been applied to neurobehavioral morbidity. Indeed, some have suggested that the primary mechanisms that underlie neurobehavioral deficits in adults with OSA are cerebrovascular in origin. It is unclear whether such a pathway, which is presumably most applicable to adults with long-standing disease sufficient to cause considerable vasculopathy, applies to children. Even so, there is evidence from animal research of a second, more direct path to neuropathology. In a rodent model, intermittent hypoxia has been demonstrated to increase oxidative stress, to upregulate proinflammatory cytokines, and to induce excessive nitric oxide levels, which collectively lead to cortical and hippocampal neuronal apoptosis and reduced hippocampal long-term potentiation (LTP) and associated spatial learning deficits. Further, genetic mutations that result in reduced free radical or nitric oxide production, as well as administration of antioxidant agents, appear to protect against apoptosis and learning deficits after intermittent hypoxia in rodent models. Translation of these findings to humans is bolstered by findings of elevated inflammatory markers, as well as precursors of such inflammation (e.g. changes in sympathetic-parasympathetic balance) in adults and children with OSA.

Others have focused less on cell death, and more on possible neurochemical aberrations among individuals with OSA. Intermittent hypoxia administered to neonatal rat pups results in long-term alterations in dopamine and behavioral evidence of overactivity and poor working memory. Although it is tempting to note parallels with psychiatric findings of aberrations in the dopaminergic system among children who have difficulties regulating attention and behavior, much research is needed to fill the gap between findings on intermittent hypoxia among neonatal rats and observations of the effects of OSA among human children.

As impressive as findings from these intermittent hypoxia models have been, hypoxia may not be the necessary precipitant of OSA-induced neurobehavioral deficits. Experimental sleep deprivation results in elevated peripheral markers for inflammation in otherwise healthy humans as well as inflammatory cytokine production and inhibition of hippocampal LTP and related learning deficits in sleep-deprived rodents. Indeed, children who are sleep deprived or have poor quality sleep, even in the absence of evidence of SDB, show at least some of the behavioral deficits that have been reported among children with OSA. Thus, poor quality sleep may act independently or synergistically with intermittent hypoxia to induce neurobehavioral morbidity in children with OSA. Conventional PSG indexes of hypoxia and sleep disruption provide little insight into their relative contribution to neurobehavioral deficits because these indexes are often strongly correlated and have moreover proven to be poor and inconsistent correlates of neurobehavioral outcome. Indeed, several recent studies have indicated that parent-reported chronic snoring in children, even in the absence of PSG-defined OSA, is associated with diminished neurobehavioral outcome. There have been attempts to develop more sensitive PSG-based indexes, such as the 'sleep pressure score' and respiratory cycle-related changes in EEG spectral power, but these require independent replication before they are widely accepted by the field.

Given that neurobehavioral deficits are presumed to be mediated by the brain, it is surprising that no neuroimaging findings on children with OSA had been published as of this writing. Among adults with OSA, structural MRI has yielded inconsistent and sometimes null findings. In contrast, magnetic resonance spectroscopy studies have consistently yielded significant results, pointing towards abnormalities in the hippocampus and frontal white matter, but not the prefrontal cortex or parietal white matter. Early functional MRI data suggest poor activation of dorsolateral prefrontal cortex in untreated adults with OSA when faced with a working memory task, a functional abnormality which appears to persist even after treatment. These data offer intriguing clues into the possible neural systems most implicated in the neurobehavioral deficits of adult OSA and, perhaps, pediatric OSA as well.

The nature, reversibility, and mechanisms by which neurobehavioral morbidity occurs in children with pediatric OSA are areas of active investigation. In this research, it will be important to take into consideration the potential impact of non-sleep-related variables, such as sociodemographic factors, which may account for considerable 'error variance' in analyses, providing a clearer picture of how OSA relates to daytime functioning. It will also be important to identify potential risk and resilience factors that increase or decrease a child's vulnerability to the neurobehavioral effects of OSA, such as age/development, sex, socioeconomic status, and cognitive 'reserve'. There is evidence that intermittent hypoxia results in the greatest neuronal damage in rats of an age roughly analogous to human childhood [7] and that, in other animals, sleep deprivation can derail neural and skill progression at critical points in development. Because many cognitive skills, including behavior and emotion regulation, show rapid progression throughout childhood, the neurodevelopmental insult presented by OSA may be particularly potent during these years. Although much work on this and other issues remains to be done, research findings to date clearly suggest that OSA can have considerable neurobehavioral consequences in children, and highlight the importance of early identification and intervention.

Cardiovascular Complications of SDB

Effect of OSAS on Pulmonary Artery Pressure

The relationship between OSAS and pulmonary hypertension in children has been described in single case reports and small case series. The prevalence and severity of pulmonary hypertension in children with SDB seems to be greater in children with co-morbid conditions. Studies which examined the presence of pulmonary hypertension in children without co-morbid conditions have revealed conflicting results. While one study found that all participants had pulmonary hypertension, two other studies found no evidence of abnormal elevation of pulmonary artery pressure. The reversibility of pulmonary hypertension in children with SDB was described in cases where SDB was treated with adenotonsillectomy, and with oxygen supplementation.

Effect of OSAS on Systemic Blood Pressure

While systemic hypertension is well described in adults with SDB, it has been described in only few cases of severe SDB in children. However, in several cross-sectional studies, a trend towards higher BP was observed in children with SDB [8–11]. None of the cross sectional studies found a higher prevalence of hypertension in children with SDB compared to controls. Evidence of blood pressure dysregulation in children with SDB in the form of increased blood pressure variability during wakefulness and sleep and smaller nocturnal blood pressure dipping was described in a study which examined 24-hour ambulatory blood pressure recording [12].

Evidence exists that SDB in children is associated with biventricular dysfunction. Changes in left ventricular geometry have been described in small case series [13–16]. A case control study showed that left ventricular mass and relative wall thickness were significantly greater in normotensive children with PSG-proven OSA compared to children with primary snoring and that an apnea/hypopnea index greater than 10/h increased the risk for left ventricular hypertrophy by 6 folds [17]. There is also evidence that left ventricular functions improve after treatment of SDB [18].

Diagnosis of SBD

In clinical practice, the diagnosis of SDB in children relies on the history of snoring and symptoms of obstructive breathing during sleep. This practice is in contradiction to the evidence provided in the literature, suggesting that history has significant limitations in discerning between SDB and snoring.

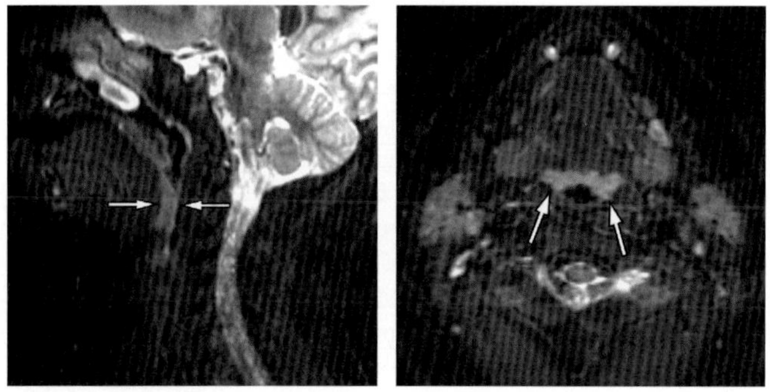

a b

Fig. 1. Enlarged lingual tonsils in a 5-year-old girl with Down syndrome and persistent OSA despite previous tonsillectomy and adenoidectomy. ***a*** Sagittal T_2-weighted MR image shows enlarged lingual tonsils (arrows) obstructing pharynx at level of base of tongue. ***b*** Axial T_2-weighted MR image again shows enlarged lingual tonsils (arrows).

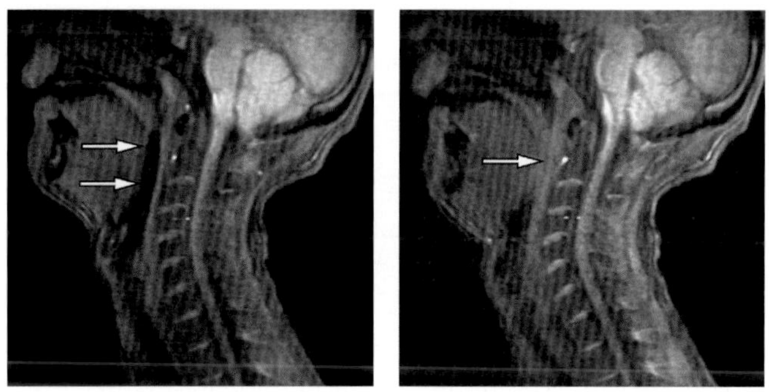

a b

Fig. 2. Hypopharyngeal collapse in an obese 5-year-old patient with persistent OSA despite previous tonsillectomy and adenoidectomy. ***a*** Sagittal cine MR image at time during respiratory cycle when hypopharynx at level of posterior tongue (arrows) is patent. ***b*** Sagittal cine MR image moment later shows collapse of hypopharynx (arrow).

More objective methods of diagnosis include PSG and radiographic airway evaluation, evaluation of central control of breathing and respiratory muscle strength.

Polysomnography

The technology used in the diagnosis of SDB in adults is applied to children. Whether PSG is sensitive enough to identify the whole spectrum of severity of SDB in children remains uncertain. The lack of strong association between the index of severity of SDB, namely the frequency of obstructive events during sleep, and neurocognitive functions suggest that PSG in children might underestimate the degree of severity of the disorder. Pediatric sleep laboratories choose threshold values, usually based on the ATS standards for cardiorespiratory sleep studies in children, that they consider to be diagnostic or strongly suggestive of significant childhood SDB. Abnormal values on pediatric PSG include: (1) obstructive apnea index > 1/h, (2) apnea/hypopnea index > 5/h, (3) peak end-tidal $CO_2 > 53$ mm Hg, (4) end-tidal $CO_2 > 50$ mm Hg for $>10\%$ of total sleep time and minimum $SpO_2 < 92\%$.

Airway Imaging

Radiographic evaluation of the airway of children with SDB is not routinely obtained. Evaluation of these children typically includes physical examination with direct inspection of the size of the palatine tonsils. In some cases, a lateral radiograph of the airway is obtained to evaluate the size of the adenoid tonsils and whether they encroach on the nasopharynx.

A subgroup of patients with OSA has more complex problems. This subgroup includes children with syndromes that predispose them to obstruction at multiple sites. Such conditions include Down syndrome, patients with craniofacial anomalies such as micrognathia, and children who have failed prior surgery directed at the elimination of OSA [19–23].

In such patients, MRI with cine sequences has become a useful tool to help determine the anatomic and dynamic causes of persistent OSA [19–23]. Dynamic imaging studies, such as MRI or cine MR studies, have been shown to affect management decisions in over 50% of cases of complex OSA [19–23]. The advantage of cine MR sleep studies is that both static anatomy as well as dynamic abnormalities that lead to functional collapse of the airway are depicted.

Once asleep, the patient is placed in the appropriate size and shaped coil. With this coil, the airway from the superior aspect of the nasal passage to the level of the trachea can typically be imaged. In small patients, the entire airway can be visualized from its superior to its inferior extent (carina). In large adult-sized patients, the inferior aspect of the trachea may not be positioned in the imaging field of view. The patient is imaged with the cervical spine in neutral position. Cine MR sequences are performed in the midline sagittal location, as well as in the transverse plane, at the level of the middle portion of the tongue. The sequence used to create the cine MR images is a fast gradient-echo sequence (8,200/3,600, 80° flip angle, 12-mm section thickness). Approximately 128 consecutive images are obtained in the same location during an imaging time of approximately 2 min. Therefore, each image correlates with approximately 1 s. The sagittal or axial images are then displayed in cine format and create a real-time 'movie' of airway motion. Cine MRI is helpful in depicting both anatomic causes of OSA and dynamic patterns of airway collapse, data that can be helpful in surgical decision making. Examples of different

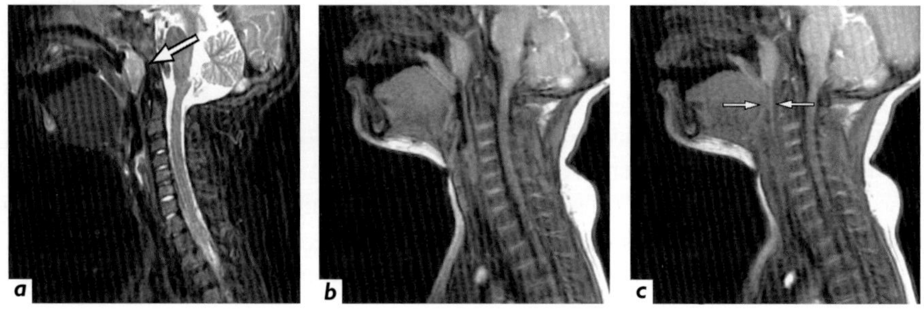

Fig. 3. Recurrent adenoid tonsil enlargement in a 5-year-old girl with persistent OSA despite previous tonsillectomy and adenoidectomy. ***a*** Sagittal T_2-weighted MR image shows recurrent adenoid tonsils as high signal tissue (arrow) in posterior nasopharynx. ***b*** Sagittal cine MR image at time during respiratory cycle when hypopharynx at level of posterior tongue is patent. ***c*** Sagittal cine MR image moment later shows collapse of hypopharynx (arrows) secondary to negative pressure generated at level of obstruction from adenoids.

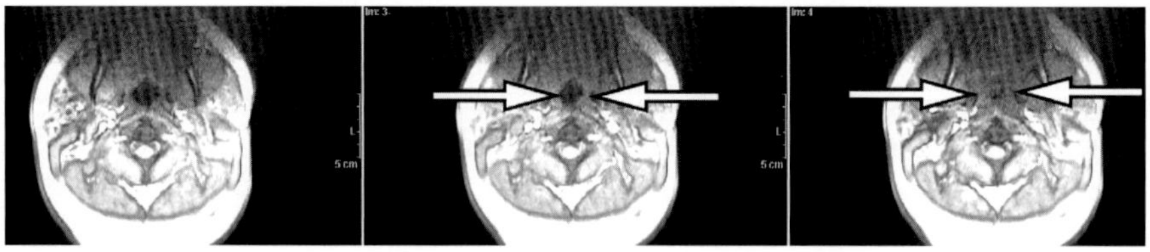

Fig. 4. Hypopharyngeal collapse in an obese 18-year-old patient with persistent OSA despite previous tonsillectomy and adenoidectomy. Consecutive cine axial images over time show progressive cylindrical collapse of the hypopharynx (arrows) from left to right.

anatomical causes for persistent upper airway obstruction are shown in figures 1–4.

Methods of Evaluation of SDB in Patients with Central Hypoventilation

Evaluation of the Chemical Control of Breathing

The primary function of breathing is to supply O_2 and remove CO_2 from the body in response to changes in arterial blood gas values. The negative feedback chemical control system is considered the fundamental mechanism of respiratory regulation. Chemical control of breathing is evaluated by the ventilatory responses to hypercapnia and hypoxia. The changes in PaO_2 are sensed by the peripheral chemoreceptors. The carotid body plays a predominant role in regulating PaO_2. Changes in PCO_2 are sensed by the central chemoreceptors and the carotid body. The stimulus to the central chemoreceptor is most closely approximated by the hydrogen ion concentration in the cerebral spinal fluid rather than in the arterial blood. The input from the chemoreceptors is integrated at the respiratory centers in the brain stem.

Hypercapnic Ventilatory Response

A linear relationship exists between $PaCO_2$ and alveolar ventilation. A hypercapnic ventilatory response is measured by the slope of the relationship between $PaCO_2$ and minute ventilation. Two standardized tests for hypercapnic response have been described. The first test, which is no longer used, involves a steady-state method in which subjects breathe several different concentrations of mixed CO_2, each for 5–15 min, until the ventilation becomes stable. In the commonly used rebreathing method, the subject rebreathes from a bag that contains a gas mixture consisting of 7% CO_2 and 93% O_2. Equilibration is achieved between mixed venous, arterial, and alveolar CO_2 and that inside the bag soon after rebreathing. After this initial period of equilibration, the changes in end-tidal CO_2 reflect the changes in PCO_2 at the chemoreceptor level. The hypercapnic ventilatory response is obtained by measuring minute ventilation simultaneously with end-tidal CO_2. The test is usually completed in 4–5 min, when the end-tidal CO_2 reaches 74. The relationship between end-tidal CO_2 and minute ventilation is linear and the hypercapnic ventilatory response curve is a straight line in the physiologic range. The slope S of the regression line and its intercept B on the end-tidal CO_2 axis are obtained from the following equation: VE = S (end-tidal CO_2 – B). S is expressed as the change in minute ventilation per change in end-tidal CO_2. This equation provides an index of respiratory chemosensitivity to hypercapnia. Normal values for the hypercapnic ventilatory response have been reported in children.

Hypoxic Ventilatory Response

In contrast to the ventilatory response to PCO_2, minute ventilation does not change until PaO_2 decreases to 50–60 Torr.

The difference in the shapes of the hypoxic and hypercapnic ventilatory response explains why the alveolar ventilation and arterial blood gases are determined by hypercapnic rather than by hypoxic chemosensitivity. Two methods have been described for the measurement of ventilatory response to isocapnic hypoxia. The first relies on end-tidal O_2 as the stimulus parameter. The second relies on O_2 saturation as the stimulus parameter. A linear regression can be applied to express the hypoxic chemosensitivity. Reported normal values for the hypoxic ventilatory response have also been described.

Tests of Respiratory Muscle Strength

The force generated by the respiratory muscles leads to displacement of the chest wall structures and ultimately to increasing or decreasing lung volume. This force is estimated as changes in pressure, and the shortening of muscle fibers is estimated as changes in lung volume. To test respiratory muscle strength, pressure can be measured either during a voluntary maneuver or during involuntary contractions, particularly in response to phrenic nerve stimulation.

The volitional tests of respiratory muscle strength include:

- Maximum static inspiratory and expiratory pressures
- Maximum static transdiaphragmatic pressure
- Maximum sniff pressure
- Maximum cough pressure

The nonvolitional tests of respiratory muscle strength include:

- Electrical phrenic nerve stimulation
- Magnetic phrenic nerve stimulation
- Twitch transdiaphragmatic pressure
- Abdominal muscle stimulation

Treatment of OSA

Adenotonsillectomy

The reversibility and long-term implications of OSA-linked neurobehavioral deficits are not fully known, but there is cause for both optimism and concern. Adenotonsillectomy is often effective in treating OSA and seems to contribute to subsequent academic, intellectual, and behavioral improvements. However, most adenotonsillectomy research has lacked longitudinal control groups, raising questions about whether parental expectancies or practice effects might account for findings. Moreover, treatments are unsuccessful in a substantial minority of cases [24] and it is likely that most children with OSA are not detected in the first place. This raises the possibility that OSA-related morbidity may worsen over time through disease progression, the accumulation of functional/adaptive failures, or inefficient neural development. What little evidence we have on long-term outcome suggests the development of a long-term delay or deficit. Several years ago, Gozal and Pope reported retrospectively-collected sleep data on nonsnoring middle-school students, and found evidence for long-term scholastic deficits among those who had snored as young children [7]. Recent prospectively-collected data further indicate that childhood snoring predicts the development of ADHD symptoms 4 years later, even after controlling for baseline hyperactivity and reported snoring at follow-up. The reversibility of cor-pulmonale and left ventricular dysfunction has been shown in small cross-sectional studies.

Continuous positive airway pressure is the second line of treatment of SDB in children. Several studies have shown a large degree of success in using this modality of treating children with the disorder [25].

References

1 Carroll JL: Obstructive sleep-disordered breathing in children: new controversies, new directions. Clin Chest Med 2003;24:261–282.

2 Corbo GM, Forastiere F, Agabiti N, et al: Snoring in 9- to 15-year-old children: risk factors and clinical relevance. Pediatrics 2001;108:1149–1154.

3 Beebe DW, Wells CT, Jeffries J, et al: Neuropsychological effects of pediatric obstructive sleep apnea. J Int Neuropsychol Soc 2004;10:962–975.

4 Rosen CL, Storfer-Isser A, Taylor HG, et al: Increased behavioral morbidity in school-aged children with sleep-disordered breathing. Pediatrics 2004;114:1640–1648.

5 Gozal D, O'Brien LM: Snoring and obstructive sleep apnoea in children: why should we treat? Paediatr Respir Rev 2004;5 Suppl A:S371–S376.

6 O'Brien LM, Ivanenko A, Crabtree VM, et al: Sleep disturbances in children with attention deficit hyperactivity disorder. Pediatr Res 2003;54:237–243.

7 Gozal E, Gozal D: Respiratory plasticity following intermittent hypoxia: developmental interactions. J Appl Physiol 2001;90:1995–1999.

8 Marcus CL, Greene MG, Carroll JL: Blood pressure in children with obstructive sleep apnea. Am J Respir Crit Care Med 1998;157:1098–1103.

9 Kohyama J, Ohinata JS, Hasegawa T: Blood pressure in sleep disordered breathing. Arch Dis Child 2003;88:139–142.

10 Kwok KL, Ng DK, Cheung YF: BP and arterial distensibility in children with primary snoring. Chest 2003;123:1561–1566.

11 Enright PL, Goodwin JL, Sherrill DL, et al: Blood pressure elevation associated with sleep-related breathing disorder in a community sample of white and Hispanic children: the Tucson Children's Assessment of Sleep Apnea study. Arch Pediatr Adolesc Med 2003;157:901–904.

12 Amin RS, Carroll JL, Jeffries JL, et al: Twenty-four-hour ambulatory blood pressure in children with sleep-disordered breathing. Am J Respir Crit Care Med 2004;169:950–956.

13 Appierto L, Cori M, Bianchi R, et al: Home care for chronic respiratory failure in children:

15 years experience. Paediatr Anaesth 2002;12: 345–350.
14 Rakela J, Perkins JD, Gross JB Jr, et al: Acute hepatic failure: the emerging role of orthotopic liver transplantation. Mayo Clin Proc 1989;64:424–428.
15 Adams N, Bestall JM, Jones PW: Inhaled beclomethasone versus budesonide for chronic asthma. Cochrane Database Syst Rev 2002:CD003530.
16 Gorur K, Doven O, Unal M, et al: Preoperative and postoperative cardiac and clinical findings of patients with adenotonsillar hypertrophy. Int J Pediatr Otorhinolaryngol 2001;59: 41–46.
17 Amin RS, Kimball TR, Bean JA, et al: Left ventricular hypertrophy and abnormal ventricular geometry in children and adolescents with obstructive sleep apnea. Am J Respir Crit Care Med 2002;165:1395–1399.
18 Amin R, Kimball T, Kalra M, et al: Left ventricular function in children with sleep-disordered breathing. Am J Cardiol 2005;95: 801–804.
19 Gibson SE, Myer CM, 3rd, Strife JL, et al: Sleep fluoroscopy for localization of upper airway obstruction in children. Ann Otol Rhinol Laryngol 1996;105:678–683.
20 Donnelly L, Strife JL, Myer CM: Dynamic sleep fluoroscopy in children with obstructive sleep apnea. Appl Radiol 2001;30:30–34.
21 Donnelly LF, Strife JL, Myer CM, 3rd: Glossoptosis (posterior displacement of the tongue) during sleep: a frequent cause of sleep apnea in pediatric patients referred for dynamic sleep fluoroscopy. AJR Am J Roentgenol 2000; 175:1557–1560.
22 Donnelly LF, Jones BV, Strife JL: Imaging of pediatric tongue abnormalities. AJR Am J Roentgenol 2000;175:489–493.
23 Donnelly LF, Surdulescu V, Chini BA, et al: Upper airway motion depicted at cine MR imaging performed during sleep: comparison between young Patients with and those without obstructive sleep apnea. Radiology 2003; 227:239–245.
24 National Center for Sleep Disorders Research. *2003 National Sleep Disorders Research Plan*. Bethesda, MD: National Institutes of Health, 2003.
25 Marcus CL, Ward SL, Mallory GB, et al: Use of nasal continuous positive airway pressure as treatment of childhood obstructive sleep apnea. J Pediatr 1995;127:88–94.

Raouf S. Amin, MD
Professor of Pediatrics
Director of Pulmonary Medicine
Children's Hospital Medical Center
Cincinnati, OH 45229 (USA)
Tel. +1 513 636 6771, Fax +1 513 636 4615
E-Mail raouf.amin@cchmc.org

Randerath WJ, Sanner BM, Somers VK (eds): Sleep Apnea.
Prog Respir Res. Basel, Karger, 2006, vol 35, pp 215–223

Sleep-Related Breathing Disorders in the Elderly

Jana R. Cooke[a] Sonia Ancoli-Israel[b]

Departments of [a]Medicine and [b]Psychiatry, University of California San Diego and Veterans Affairs San Diego Healthcare System, San Diego, Calif., USA

Abstract

Sleep-disordered breathing (SDB) is common in elderly with reported prevalence rates of 20–81%. Snoring and excessive daytime sleepiness (EDS) are the two principal symptoms of SDB, with insomnia, nocturnal confusion, and daytime cognitive impairment being less common presentations. The mortality and morbidity associated with SDB remain unclear in the elderly. In evaluating an elderly patient with questionable SDB a thorough sleep history needs to be taken, if possible in the presence of a bed partner or caregiver, focusing on symptoms of SDB and other sleep disorders. Unintentional napping may be a clue that a patient has SDB. If history is suggestive of SDB, an overnight sleep recording should be obtained. Initiation of treatment in older patients should be guided by the significance of the patient's symptoms and the severity of the SDB. Patients with more severe SDB deserve a trial of treatment. For those with milder levels of SDB, treatment should be considered if co-morbid conditions are present, such as hypertension, cognitive dysfunction, or EDS. Age alone, or assumed treatment noncompliance, should never be reasons to withhold treatment.

With aging, sleep disruption becomes a common problem with reports of 50% of adults over the age of 65 years complaining of difficulty sleeping [1]. There are a variety of causes of sleep disturbances in this population including underlying medical and psychiatric illness, medication use, shifting of the circadian rhythm and specific sleep disorders [2]. An increasingly recognized and important factor is the presence of sleep-disordered breathing (SDB) which has a reported prevalence of 20–81% in the elderly [3–5].

SDB is an umbrella term which includes a spectrum of breathing disorders ranging from benign snoring to obstructive apneas. In general, SDB is characterized by the complete cessation of respiration (apneas) and partial or reduced respiration (hypopneas) during sleep. Each event must last a minimum of 10 s and recur throughout the night, resulting in repeated arousals from sleep as well as nocturnal hypoxemia. The apnea index (AI) is the number of apneas per hour of sleep; the hypopnea index is the number of hypopneas per hour of sleep. The total number of apneas plus hypopneas per hour of sleep is called the apnea/hypopnea index (AHI) or respiratory disturbance index (RDI). Depending on the laboratory, an AHI or RDI $\geq$ 5–10 is required for the diagnosis of SDB.

Epidemiology

SDB has been shown to be more common in the elderly than in younger adults and more common in men than in women, although this gender difference is less pronounced in the elderly. Young et al. [6] reported the estimated prevalence of SDB among middle-aged adults 30–60 years of age, defined by an RDI $\geq$ 5 and the presence of excessive daytime sleepiness (EDS), to be 4% of men and 2% of women. In comparison, Ancoli-Israel [3] reviewed epidemiological studies on SDB in healthy elderly subjects and reported the prevalence rates for elderly women ranged from 19.5 to 60% and for elderly men from 28 to 62%. Combined prevalence rates for men and women range from 5.6 to 45%. SDB appears to be more prevalent in postmenopausal than premenopausal women, although it remains unclear if estrogen and progesterone are directly protective against the development of SDB [7].

Longitudinal and cross-sectional studies have both shown that the prevalence of SDB increases or stabilizes with increasing age [4, 8–10]. Hoch et al. [10] found that the median RDI and prevalence of SDB both increased significantly from age 60 to 90 years, with 2.9% of those age 60–69, 33.3% of those age 70–79, and 39.5% of those age 80–89 having an AHI ≥ 5.

In the largest series of randomly selected community-dwelling elderly, 65–95 years of age, Ancoli-Israel et al. [4], using objective measurements of SDB, reported that 24% had an AI ≥ 5 with an average AI of 13. In addition, 81% of the study subjects had an RDI ≥ 5, with an average RDI of 38. Using more stringent criteria, the prevalence rates were 62% for an RDI ≥ 10, 44% for an RDI ≥ 20, and 24% for an RDI ≥ 40. These rates were higher than had previously been reported, most likely because objective sleep recordings were used rather than subjective measurements such as self-reported snoring with observed apneas [11].

The Sleep Heart Health Study, a study of a community-based cohort of over 6,400 individuals (mean age 63.5 years with an age range of 40–98 years), reported prevalence rates of SDB by 10-year age groups [12]. For those subjects age 60–69, 32% had an AHI 5–14 and 19% had an AHI ≥ 15. For those age 70–79, 33% had an AHI 5–14 and 21% had an AHI ≥ 15. For those age 80–98, 36% had an AHI 5–14 and 20% had an AHI ≥ 15. When they focused only on those subjects with an AHI ≥ 15, they found a small increase in SDB prevalence with increasing 10-year age groups (fig. 1).

Elderly nursing home patients have been shown to have higher prevalence rates of SDB than those who live independently [13–15]. Ancoli-Israel et al. [14, 15] studied 235 nursing home patients and found that 70–90% had an RDI ≥ 5 and 50% had an RDI ≥ 20. Hoch and Reynolds [16] reported that over 40% of Alzheimer disease (AD) patients had SDB, significantly higher than age-matched depressed or healthy elderly subjects. Other studies have reported similar results [e.g. 17, 18]. In a review of seven different studies examining the prevalence in those elderly with vs. those elderly without dementia, Ancoli-Israel [3] reported prevalence rates of SDB ranging from 33 to 70% in demented subjects, compared with the reported 5.6–45% rate found in the nondemented elderly. Several studies found that the severity of the dementia was positively correlated with the severity of the SDB [14, 16].

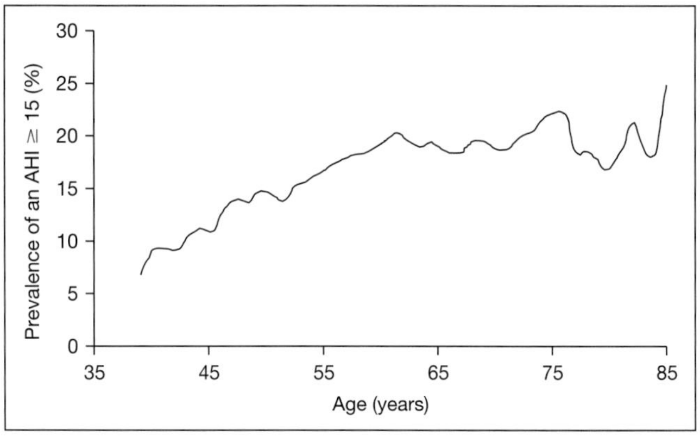

Fig. 1. Smoothed plot (5-year moving average) showing an increase in SDB prevalence with increasing 10-year age groups in those with AHI ≥ 15. Reprinted with permission from Arch Intern Med, April 22, 2002;162(8):895. Copyright© (2002), American Medical Association. All rights reserved.

Risk Factors

Established risk factors for SDB in the elderly include increasing age, gender, obesity, and symptomatic status [19]. Central obesity, in particular a body mass index (BMI) of ≥28, is the most predictive physical finding of SDB in the younger adult [19] with approximately 40% of those with a BMI over 40 and 50% of those with a BMI over 50 having SDB [20]. In the older adult, obesity and an elevated BMI are still strong predictors of the presence of SDB [4, 19, 21].

Other conditions that increase the risk of developing SDB include the use of sedating medications, alcohol consumption, family history, race, smoking, and upper airway configuration [19]. In general, few studies have explored the association between race and SDB. There is some evidence to suggest that SDB may be more severe but not more prevalent in older African-Americans than in older Caucasians [22, 23].

Clinical Features

The symptoms and clinical presentations of SDB may not differ from those of younger adults. Snoring and EDS are the two principal symptoms of SDB in the elderly. The snoring of patients with SDB, caused by airway collapse, can be loud enough to disrupt the bed partner and cause him/her to sleep in another room. In subjects 65 years and older, Enright et al. [11] reported a negative correlation between self-reported snoring and age, and loud snoring in this study was independently associated with BMI, diabetes, and arthritis in elderly women and alcohol use in elderly men. Approximately 50% of patients with habitual snoring have some degree of SDB, and snoring has been identified as an early predictor of SDB [24]. It should be noted, however, that not all patients who snore have SDB and not all patients with SDB snore. As many elderly live alone, this symptom may be difficult to identify.

EDS is a major feature of SDB in the elderly and is likely a result of the recurrent nighttime arousals and sleep fragmentation. The presence of EDS can have a profoundly detrimental effect on an elderly patient's quality of life as he/she may often fall asleep at inappropriate times during the day. This unintentional napping may manifest as falling asleep while watching television or movies, reading, attending meetings, working, driving and during conversations. EDS can cause occupational and social difficulties, reduced vigilance, and, most important in the elderly, is associated with cognitive deficits [25].

Other less common presentations in the elderly include insomnia, nocturnal confusion, and daytime cognitive impairment including difficulties with concentration and attention, and short-term memory loss [25].

Morbidity Associated with SDB

Cardiovascular Consequences

SDB is an established risk factor for hypertension in younger adults [26–28]. Lavie et al. [26] demonstrated a 'dose-response' relationship between apnea severity and elevations in blood pressure with each additional apneic event per hour of sleep increasing the odds of hypertension by 1%, and each oxygen desaturation of 10% increasing the odds by 13%. Even minimal amounts of SDB (AHI 0.1–4.9), considered by most to be nonpathologic, have been shown to increase the risk of developing hypertension compared to an AHI of zero [28].

In the older adult, however, the relationship between SDB and hypertension remains unclear. Earlier studies reported an association between hypertension and SDB in the older adult [29, 30], but more recent data from the Sleep Heart Health Study suggested that there was no association between SDB and systolic/diastolic hypertension in those aged ≥60 years [31].

Cardiac arrhythmia, myocardial infarction, hypercoagulable state, and sudden death have all been associated with the presence of SDB in adults [32, 33]. The relationship between SDB and cardiovascular events in the elderly is less clear as most studies have been performed in middle-age adults.

Some of the strongest evidence supporting the association between SDB and ischemic heart disease has emerged from the Sleep Heart Health Study which showed a positive association between the severity of SDB (based on overnight polysomnography) and the risk of developing cardiovascular disease including coronary artery disease and stroke [32]. In this study, even mild to moderate SDB was associated with the development of ischemic heart disease, independent of known cardiovascular risk factors. Cardiac patients with severe SDB are at extreme risk of suffering a myocardial infarction, almost 25 times that of patients with mild SDB [34]. Snoring itself has been reported to increase the risk of ischemic heart disease in both men and women [35].

A number of studies have also found a high prevalence of SDB in patients with congestive heart failure (CHF) [e.g. 36, 37]. Many speculate that SDB and CHF are an adverse combination in which SDB causes or exacerbates the heart failure. Central and obstructive sleep apnea as well as Cheyne-Stokes respiration (CSR) are all recognized as occurring commonly in patients with heart failure. These conditions represent a spectrum of severity from intermittent periodic respiration without apneas to cycles of hyperventilation and apneas during sleep. The hyperventilation that occurs after apnea is recognized clinically as paroxysmal nocturnal dyspnea. Javaheri et al. [37] reported that 40–50% of outpatients, predominantly male, with stable, mild, medically treated CHF had SDB, and AHI has been shown to be a powerful predictor of poor prognosis in this group of patients [38]. The Sleep Heart Health Study found that the severity of SDB was positively associated with the development of CHF and like ischemic disease, even mild to moderate SDB was associated with its development [32].

There is a growing body of literature that suggests a direct relationship between cerebrovascular accidents and SDB in adults. Studies have found an independent association between self-reported snoring and stroke, an association similar in strength to traditional risk factors for stroke such as hypertension, smoking, and hyperlipidemia [35, 39]. A number of studies, generally case-control and descriptive in design, have reported a high prevalence of SDB in patients who have suffered a cerebrovascular accident when compared to age- and gender-matched controls [35, 40]. Furthermore, the SDB persisted despite resolution of many of the stroke-related symptoms, strengthening the argument that the SDB preceded the development of cerebrovascular disease [35]. For those patients who have suffered a stroke, the presence of SDB has been found to be an independent prognostic factor related to mortality, with an implied 5% increase in mortality risk for each additional unit of AHI [41].

Some of the strongest prospective epidemiological evidence to date of the association between cerebrovascular accidents and SDB again comes from the Sleep Heart

Health Study [32]. This study has found an association between the severity of SDB and the risk of developing cerebrovascular disease, and has also reported that even mild to moderate SDB increases this risk [32]. Although the exact nature of the relationship between SDB and cerebrovascular disease in adults and the elderly remains unclear, most researchers appear to be embracing the idea that SDB precedes the development of stroke and may in fact be a modifiable risk factor [35].

Cognitive Impairment and Dementia

Cognitive dysfunction is another potentially harmful consequence of SDB. The negative effect of severe SDB (AHI $\geq$ 30) on cognitive dysfunction is well established, with consistent reports of impairment on attentional tasks, immediate and delayed recall of verbal and visual material, executive tasks, planning and sequential thinking, and manual dexterity [25, 42, 43]. In addition to the cognitive deficits that may occur as a result of SDB, there is evidence that many of the progressive dementias involve degenerative pathologies in brainstem regions, areas that are responsible for regulating respiration and other autonomic functions relevant to sleep maintenance. Therefore, sleep disorders such as SDB may be more likely to occur in this group of patients.

Studies examining the relationship between milder SDB and cognition are less clear-cut. Some studies have found that milder SDB (AHI 10–20) does not cause cognitive dysfunction in the absence of sleepiness [42]. However, some of these studies selected otherwise healthy elderly subjects to avoid possible confounding [44]. In addition, it is likely that SDB does not affect all areas of cognitive functioning equally, and therefore, it is possible that if a study only examined a small number of cognitive tasks, the findings could be negative.

There are two proposed explanations for the cognitive deficits found in patients with SDB. The first theory is that hypoxia resulting from SDB causes impairment in cognitive functioning. Studies have found that for patients with continuous hypoxia, there is a correlation between the severity of cognitive dysfunction and nocturnal oxygen saturation [45, 46]. As the oxygen saturation decreases, performance on various neuropsychological testing worsens. This relationship becomes less clear when patients have more intermittent hypoxia. One important consideration, however, is the wide variability in the severity of SDB from night to night. Depending on the severity of SDB and hypoxia the night prior to testing, the same patient may perform significantly better (or worse) from one day to the next. This variability may in fact partially explain the inconsistencies reported in the literature in regard to the effects of SDB on cognitive functioning. It remains unclear whether these hypoxia-related cognitive deficits are reversible with treatment.

The second possible reason cited for the cognitive impairment found in patients with SDB is EDS. EDS has been shown to interfere with attention and concentration abilities and to cause inconsistent performances on neuropsychological tests [47]. Therefore, it is plausible that the effect of SDB on cognitive functioning could simply be an effect of being excessively sleepy.

The relationship between SDB and cognitive impairment in demented elderly is becoming more clear. In institutionalized elderly, it has been found that those with severe dementia based on the Dementia Rating Scale (DRS) had more severe SDB compared to those with mild-moderate or no dementia [14]. Furthermore, those with more severe SDB performed worse on the DRS, suggesting that more severe SDB was associated with more severe dementia [14]. Another study estimated that an AHI = 15 is equivalent to the decrement of psychomotor efficiency associated with an additional 5 years of age [48]. In addition, some researchers speculate that SDB could actually be a cause of vascular dementia [49], as there are data to suggest that the hypertension, arrhythmias, decreased cardiac output, stroke volume, and cerebral perfusion associated with SDB may lead to a greater likelihood of cerebral ischemia and/or localized infarcts [50].

In our own laboratory, we have studied the relationship between SDB and cognitive impairment in both institutionalized and community-dwelling patients with AD [3, 14, 15, 51]. In both populations, SDB was highly prevalent. In the institutionalized AD patients, as RDI increased, cognitive functioning worsened, even when controlling for age [14]. There is also evidence to suggest that the severity of sleep disruptions in AD parallels the decline in cognitive functioning. Anatomically, the brainstem regions and neuronal pathways that regulate sleep/wake patterns are affected by the degenerative changes in AD [52]. We are currently completing a study that examines whether treatment of SDB in patients with AD would result in improvement in cognitive abilities.

Patients with Parkinson's disease (PD) have also been reported to have a higher prevalence rate of SDB when compared to age-matched controls [53, 54]. In addition, a great majority of PD patients have some subtle changes in cognition, and some 40% will progress to PD dementia [55]. As PD patients commonly experience alterations in respiratory function while awake, there are compelling reasons to think that patients with PD may be at risk of nocturnal hypoxemia and SDB. Anatomically, there is degeneration of the neurons in the reticular activating system as well as degeneration of the pathways arising from the dorsal raphe and locus coeruleus in PD, all of which likely contribute to sleep disturbances and daytime sleepiness in these patients [56]. The role that SDB plays in the cognitive dysfunction and eventual development of dementia experienced by the majority of PD patients remains unknown.

Mortality

Some research has suggested that patients with SDB are at increased risk of death compared to those without SDB. In many studies, patients with heart failure who develop SDB in combination with CSR experience an increased mortality [e.g. 57, 58]. Most of the studies on mortality have focused on younger adults, however, with few studies exclusively examining this aspect in the elderly.

In general, the risk of sudden death from cardiac causes is highest from 6 a.m. to noon and lowest from midnight to 6 a.m. [59]. In a study that reviewed death certificates and polysomnograms of patients, mostly in their 60–70s, who had suffered a sudden cardiac death, the authors found that those who had died from midnight to 6 a.m. had a significantly higher AHI than those who died during other time intervals during the day. This study reported that for patients with SDB, the relative risk of sudden death from cardiac causes from midnight to 6 a.m. was 2.57 [33].

Much of the data about SDB and overall mortality, however, suggest that there is an indirect relationship between the two. One study followed a cohort of noninstitutionalized older subjects (mean age 66) for 12 years and reported a mortality ratio of 2.7 for those with an RDI $\geq$10 [60]. Hoch et al. [61] reported that SDB was associated with an excess mortality rate of 450% in elderly patients with depression and cognitive impairment. Ancoli-Israel et al. [62] found that those community-dwelling elderly with more SDB (defined as an RDI $\geq$ 30) had significantly shorter survivals than those with mild-moderate or no SDB.

However, in other studies of community-dwelling elderly, RDI was not found to be an independent predictor of mortality [62, 63]. Rather, these studies found that cardiovascular and pulmonary conditions, including hypertension, were independent predictors of death, although there is evidence to suggest that these factors may be secondary to or associated with SDB. Therefore, it is possible that in elderly, SDB is one of several predisposing factors for cardiopulmonary disease, which, in combination, leads to increased mortality. This hypothesis is strengthened by a study by Ancoli-Israel et al. [64] which reported that elderly men with CHF had more severe SDB than those with no heart disease and men with both conditions, heart failure and SDB, had shortened life spans compared to those with just CHF, just SDB or neither.

More studies need to be undertaken to further elicit the exact nature of the relationship of SDB and mortality in the elderly, specifically in older women as most of the studies completed in this age category have involved predominantly men.

Clinical Assessment and Management of SDB

Presentation and Diagnosis

As discussed previously, EDS and snoring are the two main clinical features of SDB in the elderly. However, both aspects are common in the general elderly population. If an older adult complains of snoring or EDS, clinicians should not assume that this is due to normal aging nor should they assume that this is due to SDB – a complete evaluation is warranted.

Despite the commonality of EDS and snoring in the elderly, several features may guide the clinician toward the possibility of SDB. Daytime sleepiness and difficulty maintaining wakefulness during daily activities, such as holding conversations, driving, or unintentional napping should not be assumed to be normal. Although not usually associated with SDB, insomnia may also be a presenting complaint. Fragmented or restless sleep due to frequent nocturnal awakenings related to the apneas results in the subjective complaint of difficulty sleeping, often labeled as 'insomnia'. SDB may present as nocturnal confusion and/or daytime cognitive impairment, particularly in the areas of concentration, attention, and memory. Elderly patients with hypertension, especially hypertension that is difficult to treat despite appropriate medications, should be further evaluated for the presence of SDB.

As mentioned above, napping, specifically unintentional napping may be a clue that a patient has disrupted or insufficient sleep, possibly secondary to SDB. Elderly patients tend to nap more frequently than younger adults, and regular napping has been reported to be common in the elderly [65]. It is imperative that the clinician discern whether these naps are planned or unintentional, as the latter may indicate the inability to maintain wakefulness, and thus may suggest the presence of SDB. It is also important to bear in mind that there are a variety of other potential etiologies for EDS and unintentional napping, including other medical conditions (PD, abnormal thyroid function, malignancies, depression, nocturia related to benign prostatic hypertrophy) and medications (hypnotics, antidepressants, antihistamines, dopaminergics). Any of these may potentially contribute to daytime somnolence and unintentional napping.

To accurately assess the presence of SDB in the elderly, a stepwise process should be undertaken. A complete sleep history should be obtained, focusing on symptoms of SDB, symptoms of other sleep disorders (i.e. restless leg syndrome), and sleep-related habits and routines, if possible, with a bed partner, room mate or caregiver. The patient's medical history, including psychiatric and medical records should be thoroughly reviewed, paying particular attention to associated medical conditions and medications, the use of alcohol, and evidence of cognitive impairment. Lastly, when the above is suggestive of SDB, an overnight sleep recording should be obtained.

As with younger adults, the diagnosis of SDB in the elderly requires an overnight sleep recording. There are several potential challenges in obtaining sleep studies in the elderly including difficulties with transportation, management of technical equipment, and understanding complicated instructions. Furthermore, some may be resistant to spending the night in an unfamiliar environment. Involving the patient's spouse or caregiver and simple anticipation of the potential difficulties may solve some of these issues. In addition, if the clinician has a high index of suspicion of SDB, an unattended overnight sleep study may be sufficient for diagnosis. However, it should be noted that at the current time, Medicare will only reimburse attended sleep studies.

Treatment of SDB in the Elderly

Older patients who present with symptoms of SDB and who have daytime consequences should be considered for treatment. Several factors should be considered when deciding if an older patient should be treated for SDB. The significance of the patient's symptoms and the severity of the SDB should be the main guides in initiating treatment [66]. Patients with more severe SDB (RDI $\geq$ 20) deserve a trial of treatment. For those with milder levels of SDB (RDI $<$ 20), treatment should be considered if co morbid conditions are present, such as hypertension, cognitive dysfunction, or EDS. Age alone, or assumed noncompliance, should never be a reason to withhold treatment.

Treatment of SDB in the elderly is similar to that in younger adults. All patients should be counseled on weight loss and smoking cessation if indicated. For those with positional-related SDB, i.e. with more events typically occurring in the supine position, avoidance of this position and attempting to sleep in the lateral decubitus position may be somewhat effective. Long-acting sedating benzodiazepines should generally be avoided in the elderly with SDB as most of these medications are respiratory depressants and may actually increase the number and duration of apneas. Alcohol, even in small amounts, can also exacerbate SDB, and therefore, elderly patients with SDB should be encouraged to abstain completely from its consumption.

The gold standard for treatment is continuous positive airway pressure (CPAP), a device that provides continuous positive pressure via the nasal passages or oral airway, creating a pneumatic splint to keep the airway open during inspiration. If used appropriately, CPAP has been shown to safely and effectively manage SDB at night with minimal side effects [67].

Beneficial effects have been shown in older adults who are able to tolerate CPAP. Guilleminault et al. [68] reported that in older male subjects, treatment of SDB with CPAP resulted in improved nocturia, daytime somnolence, depression ratings, and quality of life scores. Another study found that treatment of SDB in older adults resulted in normalization of prethrombotic states, as with a reported lengthening of prothrombin time and increased fibrinogen levels [69]. Three months of compliant CPAP use in older adults has been reported to improve cognition, particularly in the areas of attention, psychomotor speed, executive functioning, and nonverbal delayed recall [43].

In a study of demented elderly with SDB, CPAP compliance was adequate, with the majority of patients using CPAP for about 5 h a night. The only factor that was associated with poor compliance was the presence of depression – not age, severity of dementia, or severity of SDB [70].

For those patients who have difficulty tolerating CPAP, there are two alternative treatments that should be considered: oral appliances and surgery. Oral appliances should generally be reserved and considered for those thinner patients with milder levels of SDB [71]. Reported effectiveness ranges from 50 to 100%. Patients with dentures are generally not candidates for this device although newer models can be fitted with dentures.

Surgical treatment, more popular a decade or so ago, involves correcting the anatomic abnormalities most responsible for the airway obstruction. There are several possible procedures, the most common being uvulopalatopharyngoplasty which involves excision of the soft palate and uvula [72]. It requires general anesthesia with its inherent risks and is only successful in approximately 50% of cases, with age $>$50 associated with poorer surgical outcome [73]. Surgical treatments are not often recommended in the older adults.

For those patients who cannot tolerate CPAP or an oral appliance and are poor surgical candidates, nocturnal oxygen supplementation may be considered. However, studies of its efficacy in the treatment of SDB are limited. In general, it has been demonstrated that oxygen does not reduce apneas or improve EDS as well as CPAP [74]. Studies have shown that when administered for one night, supplemental oxygen does improve the nadir saturation but may worsen respiratory acidosis associated with apneas [75]. There is evidence that oxygen supplementation during sleep in patients with SDB may cause a slight prolongation of the mean obstructive apnea duration [75]. Studies showing clinical objective improvement in SDB with the use of chronic supplemental oxygen administration are inconclusive. Patients who meet these criteria should undergo a full attended polysomnogram with oxygen supplementation to ensure that there is minimal increase in apnea duration and no worsening of cardiac arrhythmias prior to being prescribed oxygen for home use.

SDB in the Elderly – What Does It Mean?

There is a growing body of literature exploring SDB in the elderly. However, there is also an ongoing debate in the field as to whether SDB in the elderly is a distinct pathologic condition, different than that of middle-age adults. If SDB in the elderly is indeed a different disorder, to what degree does it differ? What does the presence of SDB in the elderly mean?

Researchers are attempting to answer some of these questions as most of the literature about SDB is based on middle-aged male adults which may not be applicable to the elderly (or to women of all ages). Levy et al. [40] studied a population of nearly 400 patients with suspected SDB, with ages ranging from <20 to >85 years old, all of whom were referred to a sleep center. The severity of SDB based on RDI and oxygen saturation did not differ in those subjects ≥65 years of age when compared to those subjects <65 years of age. However, the symptomatology and sequelae related to SDB were not reported, and therefore the consequences of SDB, regardless of severity, may indeed be different among the two groups of patients.

The natural history of SDB in the elderly remains relatively unknown although studies are underway. Young [76] points out that the natural history of any disease or condition in the elderly is complicated by several factors including the physiology of aging itself, other comorbid diseases, and differential survival. She proposes that a distinction should be made between age-dependent conditions, in which aging causes the pathology, and age-related conditions, in which the disease only occurs during a particular age period. Whether SDB is an age-dependent or an age-related condition remains unknown. The prevalence of SDB increases with age, and therefore SDB may be thought of as a condition that is age-dependent [4, 8–10]. If this is the case and SDB in older adults is the same condition with the same outcomes, then the elderly would need to be treated as aggressively as younger adults. However, while the prevalence of SDB in the elderly may be age-dependent, the severity of the SDB and its clinical significance in the elderly may be age-related. For example, Bixler et al. [9] reported that the prevalence of SDB increased in a sample of older men but that after controlling for BMI, the severity based on number of events and oxygen saturation actually decreased with age. Ancoli-Israel et al. [21] showed in an 18-year follow-up study of over 400 elderly patients with SDB that RDI did not continue to increase with age. Rather, if the patient's BMI remained stable, so did the RDI.

In addition, controversy exists regarding the effect of SDB on morbidity and mortality in the elderly. Results from clinical populations suggest the SDB in the elderly has minimal effect but population-based studies argue otherwise. As discussed previously, Ancoli-Israel et al. [62] followed a population of community-dwelling elderly for nearly 10 years and found that those elderly subjects with more severe SDB had significantly shorter survival, dying as much as 2 years earlier, than those with mild to moderate or no SDB. Others have reported an increased mortality as well [61]. On the other hand, Mant et al. [63] found that an RDI ≥15 did not predict death in nondemented, independent-living elderly. He et al. [77] reported that an AHI ≥ 20 predicted increased mortality in those under 50 but not those over 50. Similarly, others have reported that the survival rate in middle-aged patients with SDB is reduced when compared to age- and sex-matched controls, but that this pattern was not seen among older patients [78, 79].

Conclusion

Although not yet clearly established, there is some pathologic level of SDB above which treatment is both beneficial and acceptable. Therefore, clinicians need to use their best clinical judgment in first deciding which elderly should be treated for SDB and then how to most appropriately treat them. This needs to be done on an individual, case-by-case basis. In deciding whom to treat for SDB, treatment should be based on the total clinical picture and not on age.

Acknowledgement

This study was supported by grants NIA AG08415, NIA AG15301, NCI CA85264, NIH M01 RR00827, the Department of Veterans Affairs VISN-22 Mental Illness Research, Education and Clinical Center (MIRECC), and the Research Service of the Veterans Affairs San Diego Healthcare System.

References

1 Foley DJ, Monjan AA, Brown SL, Simonsick EM, Wallace RB, Blazer DG: Sleep complaints among elderly persons: an epidemiologic study of three communities. Sleep 1995;18:425–432.

2 Ancoli-Israel S: Insomnia in the elderly: a review for the primary care practitioner. Sleep 2000;23:S23–S30.

3 Ancoli-Israel S: Epidemiology of sleep disorders; in Roth T, Roehrs TA (eds): Clinics in Geriatric Medicine. Philadelphia, Saunders, 1989, pp 347–362.

4 Ancoli-Israel S, Kripke DF, Klauber MR, Mason WJ, Fell R, Kaplan O: Sleep disordered breathing in community-dwelling elderly. Sleep 1991;14:486–495.

5 Redline S, Kirchner L, Quan SF, Gottlieb DJ, Kapur V, Newman A: The effects of age, sex, ethnicity, and sleep-disordered breathing on sleep architecture. Arch Intern Med 2004;164:406–418.

6 Young T, Palta M, Dempsey J, Skatrud J, Weber S, Badr S: The occurrence of sleep disordered breathing among middle-aged adults. N Engl J Med 1993;328:1230–1235.

7 Young T, Rabago D, Zgierska A, Austin D, Laurel F: Objective and subjective sleep quality in premenopausal, perimenopausal, and postmenopausal women in the Wisconsin Sleep Cohort Study. Sleep 2003;26: 667–672.

8 Bliwise DL, Carskadon MA, Carey E, Dement WC: Longitudinal development of sleep-related respiratory disturbance in adult humans. J Gerontol 1984;39:290–293.

9 Bixler EO, Vgontzas AN, Ten Have T, Tyson K, Kales A: Effects of age on sleep apnea in men. Am J Res Crit Care Med 1998;157: 144–148.

10 Hoch CC, Reynolds CFI, Monk TH, Buysse DJ, Yeager AL, Houck PR, Kupfer DJ: Comparison of sleep-disordered breathing among healthy elderly in the seventh, eighth, and ninth decades of life. Sleep 1990;13: 502–511.

11 Enright PL, Newman AB, Wahl PW, Manolio TA, Haponik EF, Boyle P: Prevalence and correlates of snoring and observed apneas in 5,201 older adults. Sleep 1996;19:531–538.

12 Young T, Shahar E, Nieto FJ, Redline S, Newman AB, Gottlieb DJ, Walsleben JA, Finn L, Enright P, Samet JM: Predictors of sleep-disordered breathing in community-dwelling adults: the Sleep Heart Health Study. Arch Intern Med 2002;162:893–900.

13 Ancoli-Israel S, Parker L, Sinaee R, Fell R, Kripke DF: Sleep fragmentation in patients from a nursing home. J Gerontol 1989;44: M18–M21.

14 Ancoli-Israel S, Klauber MR, Butters N, Parker L, Kripke DF: Dementia in institutionalized elderly: relation to sleep apnea. J Am Geriatr Soc 1991;39:258–263.

15 Gehrman PR, Martin JL, Shochat T, Nolan S, Corey-Bloom J, Ancoli-Israel S: Sleep disordered breathing and agitation in institutionalized adults with Alzheimer's disease. Am J Geriatr Psychiatry 2003;11:426–433.

16 Hoch CC, Reynolds CFI: Cognitive function and sleep disordered breathing in dementia: the Pittsburg Experience; in Kuna ST, Suratt PM, Remmers JE (eds): Sleep and Respiration in Aging Adults. New York, Elsevier, 1991, pp 245–250.

17 Erkinjuntti T, Partinen M, Sulkava R, Telakivi T, Salmi T, Tilvis R: Sleep apnea in multiinfarct dementia and Alzheimer's disease. Sleep 1987;10:419–425.

18 Taylor W, Phillipson EA, Moldofsky H: Cognitive function and sleep disorderd breathing in normal elderly and patients with Alzheimer's disease; in Kuna ST, Suratt PM, Remmers JE (eds): Sleep and Respiration in Aging Adults. New York, Elsevier, 1991, pp 251–258.

19 Phillips B and Ancoli-Israel S: Sleep disorders in the elderly. Sleep Med 2001;2:99–114.

20 Kripke DF, Ancoli-Israel S, Klauber MR, Wingard DL, Mason WJ, Mullaney DJ: Prevalence of sleep disordered-breathing in ages 40–64 years: a population-based survey. Sleep 1997;20:65–76.

21 Ancoli-Israel S, Gehrman P, Kripke DF, Stepnowsky C, Mason W, Cohen-Zion M, Marler M: Long-term follow-up of sleep disordered breathing in older adults. Sleep Med 2001;2:511–516.

22 Ancoli-Israel S, Klauber MR, Stepnowsky C, Estline E, Chinn A, Fell R: Sleep-disordered breathing in African-American elderly. Am J Resp Crit Care Med 1995;152:1946–1949.

23 Redline S, Tishler PV, Hans MG, Tosteson T, Strohl KP, Spry K: Racial differences in sleep-disordered breathing in African-American and Caucasians. Am J Res Crit Care Med 1997;155:186–192.

24 Collop NA, Cassell DK: Snoring and sleep-disordered breathing; in Lee-Chiong TL, Sateia MJ, Carskadon MA (eds): Sleep Medicine. Philadelphia, Hanley & Belfus, 2002, pp 349–355.

25 Martin J, Stepnowsky C, Ancoli-Israel S: Sleep apnea in the elderly; in McNicholas WT and Phillipson EA (eds): Breathing Disorders During Sleep. London, W.B. Saunders Company, Lmt, 2002, pp 278–287.

26 Lavie P, Herer P, Hoffstein V: Obstructive sleep apnoea syndrome as a risk factor for hypertension: population study. BMJ 2000;320:479–482.

27 Nieto FJ, Young T, Lind B, Shahar E, Samet JM, Redline S, D'Agostino RB, Newman AB, Lebowitz MD, Pickering TG: Association of sleep-disordered breathing, sleep apnea, and hypertension in a large community-based study. JAMA 2000;283:1829–1836.

28 Peppard P, Young T, Palta M, Skatrud J: Prospective study of the association between sleep-disordered breathing and hypertension. New Eng J Med 2000;342:1378–1384.

29 Berry DTR, Phillips BA, Cook YR, Schmitt FA, Honeycutt NA, Edwards CL, Lamb DG, Magan LK, Allen RS: Sleep-disordered breathing in healthy aged persons: one-year follow-up of daytime sequelae. Sleep 1989;12: 211–215.

30 Stoohs RA, Gingold J, Cohrs S, Harter R, Finlayson E, Guilleminault C: Sleep-disordered breathing and systemic hypertension in the older male. J Am Geriatr Soc 1996;44: 1295–1300.

31 Haas DC, Foster GL, Nieto FJ, Redline S, Resnick HE, Robbins JA, Young T, Pickering TG: Age-dependent associations between sleep-disordered breathing and hypertension: importance of discriminating between systolic/diastolic hypertension and isolated systolic hypertension in the Sleep Heart Health Study. Circulation 2005;111:614–621.

32 Shahar E, Whitney CW, Redline S, Lee ET, Newman AB, Javier NF, O'Connor GT, Boland LL, Schwartz JE, Samet JM: Sleep-disordered breathing and cardiovascular disease: cross sectional results of the Sleep Heart Health Study. Am J Respir Crit Care Med 2001;163:19–25.

33 Gami AS, Howard DE, Olson EJ, Somers VK: Day-night pattern of sudden death in obstructive sleep apnea. New Eng J Med 2005;352: 1206–1214.

34 Hung J, Whitford EG, Parsons RW, Hillman DR: Association of sleep apnoea with myocardial infarction in men. Lancet 1990;336: 261–264.

35 Yaggi H, Mohsenin V: Obstructive sleep apnoea and stroke. Lancet Neurol 2004;3: 333–342.

36 Chan J, Sanderson J, Chan JW, Lai C, Choy D, Ho A, Leung R: Prevalence of sleep-disordered breathing in diastolic heart failure. Chest 1997;111:1488–1493.

37 Javaheri S, Parker TJ, Liming JD, Corbett WS, Nishiyama H, Wexler L, Roselle GA: Sleep apnea in 81 ambulatory male patients with stable heart failure types and their prevalences, consequences, and presentations. Circulation 1998;97:2154–2159.

38 Verrier RL: Cardiovascular disorders and sleep; in Lee-Chiong TL, Sateia MJ, Carskadon MA (eds): Sleep Medicine. Philadelphia, Hanley & Belfus, Inc, 2002, pp 447–453.

39 Jennum P, Schultz-Larsen K, Davidsen M, Christensen NJ: Snoring and risk of stroke and ischemic heart disease in a 70 year old population. A 6-year follow-up study. Int J Epidemiol 1994;23:1159–1164.

40 Levy P, Pepin JL, Malauzat D, Emeriau JP, Leger JM: Is sleep apnea syndrome in the elderly a specific entity? Sleep 1996;19:S29–S38.

41 Parra O, Arboix A, Montserrat JM, Quinto L, Bechich S, Garcia-Eroles L: Sleep-related breathing disorders: impact on mortality of cerebrovascular disease. Eur Respir J 2004;24: 267–272.

42 Redline S, Strauss ME, Adams N, Winters M, Roebuck T, Spry K, Rosenberg C, Adams K: Neuropsychological function in mild sleep-disordered breathing. Sleep 1997;20:160–167.

43 Aloia MS, Ilniczky N, Di Dio P, Perlis ML, Greenblatt DW, Giles DE: Neuropsychological changes and treatment compliance in older adults with sleep apnea. J Psychosom Res 2003;54:71–76.

44 Berry DTR, Phillips BA, Cook YR, Schmitt FA, Gilmore RL, Patel R, Keener TM, Tyre E: Sleep-disordered breathing in healthy aged persons: possible daytime sequelae. J Gerontol 1987;42:620–626.
45 Bedard MA, Montplaisir J, Richer F, Malo J: Nocturnal hypoxemia as a determinant of vigilance impairment in sleep apnea syndrome. Chest 1991;100:367–370.
46 Findley LJ, Barth JT, Powers DC, Wilhoit SC, Boyd DG, Suratt PM: Cognitive impairment in patients with obstructive sleep apnea and associated hypoxemia. Chest 1986;90: 686–690.
47 Lojander J, Kajaste S, Maasilta P, Partinen M: Cognitive functioning and treatment of obstructive sleep apnea syndrome. J Sleep Res 1999;8:71–76.
48 Kim HC, Young T, Matthews CG, Weber SM, Woodward AR, Palta M: Sleep-disordered breathing and neuropsychological deficits. A population-based study. Am J Respir Crit Care Med 1997;156:1813–1819.
49 Bliwise DL: Review: Sleep in normal aging and dementia. Sleep 1993;16:40–81.
50 Bliwise DL: Cognitive function and sleep disordered breathing in aging adults; in Kuna ST, Remmers JE, Suratt PM (eds). Sleep and Respiration in Aging Adults. New York, Elsevier, 1991, pp 237–244.
51 Ancoli-Israel S, Klauber MR, Gillin JC, Campbell SS, Hofstetter CR: Sleep in noninstitutionalized Alzheimer's disease patients. Aging Clin Exp Res 1994;6:451–458.
52 Prinz PN, Vitaliano PP, Vitiello MV, Bokan JA, Raskind M, Peskind E, Gerber C: Sleep, EEG and mental function changes in senile dementia of the Alzheimer's type. Neurobiol Aging 1982;3:361–370.
53 Maria B, Sophia S, Michalis M, Charalampos L, Andreas P, John ME, Nikolaos SM: Sleep breathing disorders in patients with idiopathic Parkinson's disease. Respir Med 2003;97: 1151–1157.
54 Arnulf I, Konofal E, Merino-Andreu M, Houeto JL, Mesnage V, Welter ML, Lacomblez L, Golmard JL, Derenne JP, Agid Y: Parkinson's disease and sleepiness: an integral part of PD. Neurology 2002;58:1019–1024.
55 Emre M: Dementia associated with Parkinson's disease. Lancet Neurol 2003;2: 229–237.
56 Schapira AH: Excessive daytime sleepiness in Parkinson's disease. Neurology 2004;63 (suppl 3):S24–S27.
57 Findley LJ, Zwillich CW, Ancoli-Israel S, Kripke DF, Tisi G, Moser KM: Cheyne-Stokes breathing during sleep in patients with left ventricular heart failure. South Med J 1985;78:11–15.
58 Hanly PJ, Zuberi-Khokhar NS: Increased mortality associated with Cheyne-Stokes respiration in patients with congestive heart failure. Am J Respir Crit Care Med 1996;153: 272–276.
59 Cohen MC, Rohtla KM, Lavery CE, Muller JE, Mittleman MA: Meta-analysis of the morning excess of acute myocardial infarction and sudden cardiac death. Am J Cardiol 1997;79:1512–1516.
60 Bliwise DL, Bliwise NG, Partinen M, Pursley AM, Dement WC: Sleep apnea and mortality in an aged cohort. Am J Public Health 1988;78:544–547.
61 Hoch CC, Reynolds CFI, Houck PR, Hall F, Berman SR, Buysse DJ, Dahl RE, Kupfer DJ: Predicting mortality in mixed depression and dementia using EEG sleep variables. J Neuropsychiatry Clin Neurosci 1989;1: 366–371.
62 Ancoli-Israel S, Kripke DF, Klauber MR, Fell R, Stepnowsky C, Estline E, Khazeni N, Chinn A: Morbidity, mortality and sleep disordered breathing in community dwelling elderly. Sleep 1996;19:277–282.
63 Mant A, King M, Saunders NA, Pond CD, Goode E, Hewitt H: Four-year follow-up of mortality and sleep-related respiratory disturbance in non-demented seniors. Sleep 1995; 18:433–438.
64 Ancoli-Israel S, DuHamel ER, Stepnowsky C, Engler R, Cohen-Zion M, Marler M: The relationship between congestive heart failure, sleep disordered breathing and mortality in older men. Chest 2003;124:1400–1405.
65 Wauquier A, Van Sweden B, Lagaay AM, Kemp B, Kamphuisen HAC: Ambulatory monitoring of sleep-wakefulness patterns in healthy elderly males and females (>88 years): the 'Senieur' protocol. J Am Geriatr Soc 1992;40:109–114.
66 Ancoli-Israel S, Coy TV: Are breathing disturbances in elderly equivalent to sleep apnea syndrome? Sleep 1994;17:77–83.
67 Grunstein R: Continuous positive airway pressure treatment for obstructive sleep apnea-hypopnea syndrome; in Kryger MH, Roth T, Dement WC (eds): Principles and Practice of Sleep Medicine. Philadelphia, Pa, Elsevier, 2005, pp 1066–1080.
68 Guilleminault C, Lin CM, Goncalves MA, Ramos E: A prospective study of nocturia and the quality of life of elderly patients with obstructive sleep apnea or sleep onset insomnia. J Psychosom Res 2004;56:511–515.
69 Zhang X, Yin K, Wang H, Su M, Yang Y: Effect of continuous positive airway pressure treatment on elderly Chinese patients with obstructive sleep apnea in the prethrombotic state. Chin Med J 2003;116:1426–1428.
70 Ayalon L, Ancoli-Israel S, Stepnowsky C, Palmer BW, Liu L, Loredo JS, Corey-Bloom J, Greenfield D, Cooke JR: Treatment adherence in patients with Alzheimer's disease and obstructive sleep apnea. Am J Geriatr Psychiatry 2006; in press.
71 Ferguson KA, Lowe AA: Oral appliances for sleep disordered breathing; in Kryger MH, Roth T, Dement WC (eds): Principles and Practice of Sleep Medicine. Philadelphia, Pa, Elsevier, 2005, pp 1098–1108.
72 Powell NB, Riley R, Guilleminault C: Surgical management of sleep disordered breathing; in Kryger MH, Roth T, Dement WC (eds): Principls and Practice of Sleep Medicine. Philadelphia, Pa, Elsevier, 2005, pp 1081–1097.
73 Sher AE, Schechtman KB, Piccirillo JF: The efficacy of surgical modifications of the upper airway in adults with obstructive sleep apnea syndrome. Sleep 1996;19:156–177.
74 Phillips BA, Schmitt FA, Berry DT, Lamb DG, Amin M, Cook YR: Treatment of obstructive sleep apnea. A preliminary report comparing nasal CPAP to nasal oxygen in patients with mild OSA. Chest 1990;98:325–330.
75 Fletcher EC, Munafo D: Role of nocturnal oxygen therapy in obstructive sleep apnea: when should it be used? Chest 1990;98: 1497–1504.
76 Young T: Sleep-disordered breathing in older adults: is it a condition distinct from that of middle-aged adults? Sleep 1996;19:529–530.
77 He J, Kryger MH, Zorick FJ, Conway W, Roth T: Mortality and apnea index in obstructive sleep apnea: experience in 385 male patients. Chest 1988;94:9–14.
78 Lavie P, Lavie L, Herer P: All-cause mortality in males with sleep apnoea syndrome: declining mortality rates with age. Eur Respir J 2005;25:514–520.
79 Noda A, Okada T, Yasuma F, Sobue T, Nakashima N, Yokota M: Prognosis of the middle-aged and aged patients with obstructive sleep apnea syndrome. Psychiatry Clin Neurosci 1998;52:79–85.

Sonia Ancoli-Israel, PhD
Department of Psychiatry 0603
University of California San Diego
La Jolla, CA 92093–0603 (USA)
Tel. +1 858 642 3828
Fax +1 858 552 7536
E-Mail sancoliisrael@ucsd.edu

Randerath WJ, Sanner BM, Somers VK (eds): Sleep Apnea.
Prog Respir Res. Basel, Karger, 2006, vol 35, pp 224–237

Sleep-Disordered Breathing in Pregnancy

Colin E. Sullivan Natalie Edwards

David Read Laboratory, Medicine, University of Sydney, Sydney, Australia

Abstract

Complaints of sleep disturbance are common during pregnancy, and there are many factors that are likely contributors. Hormonal and biochemical changes and the physical effect of the enlarging uterus are all probable mechanisms. Emerging evidence suggests that sleep disordered breathing (SDB) is particularly prevalent during pregnancy, chiefly late pregnancy, and this may be a significant factor contributing to sleep disruption. Both the prevalence and severity of snoring increase progressively throughout pregnancy, with reported snoring being as high as 46% during the last trimester of pregnancy, and estimated prevalence of clinically significant SDB greater than 10%. Both epidemiological data and case reports of obstructive sleep apnoea (OSA) suggest that SDB in pregnancy has adverse effects on maternal health and fetal development. Upper airway flow limitation, which is the characteristic pattern of SDB in women with preeclampsia, leads to marked vascular reactivity, with associated increments in peripheral vascular resistance and systemic arterial blood pressure and suppression of maternal cardiac output. Sleep-induced maternal hemodynamic compromise in preeclampsia is associated with adverse fetal consequences. The use of low levels of nasal continuous positive airway pressure (nasal CPAP) during maternal sleep in preeclampsia effectively reverses the sleep-induced maternal hemodynamic consequences and may also improve fetal outcome.

The prevalence of disorders of breathing in sleep is very high, with obstructive sleep apnoea (OSA) being among the commonest of chronic disorders. Obstructive apnoea has much co-morbidity, including obesity, the metabolic syndrome and type II diabetes, hypertension, cardiac arrhythmias and other vascular disorders. Although sleep apnoea has been the focus of clinical practice for pulmonologists, the fact that as many as 30% of general cardiology patients and more than 50% of stroke victims may have undiagnosed sleep apnoea underpins the need for sleep apnoea to be diagnosed and managed by all clinicians. Early in the understanding of sleep apnoea, the general notion of the disorder was that it was essentially limited to males. While it is true that many more men suffer from snoring and sleep apnoea than women, it is equally true that it is also a common disorder in women [1]. Although it was clearly described in women at the beginning of the period of wider clinical recognition of sleep apnoea in the 1980s, it is only now appreciated that we have systematically missed sleep-disordered breathing (SDB) in women because of our assumption that it was exclusively a male disorder; the prototype 'model' of a sleep apnoea patient for most clinicians is a heavy middle-aged male snorer, with excessive sleepiness. Women may have a delayed onset of snoring and sleep apnoea, have a different symptom spectrum, and often have a pattern of SDB involving partial upper airway obstruction (the high upper airway resistance syndrome). The focus on the presence of complete obstructive events in the polysomnogram has distracted us from recognising the importance of SDB with upper airway flow limitation and an absence of frank obstructive events. Importantly, there is evidence that where women have SDB they are at a higher risk of the cardiovascular consequences. This observation first emerged from the earliest epidemiological data of Lugaresi et al. [2], but has recently become more evident [3]. The hormonal changes of the menstrual cycle which produce periodically enhanced pressor responses to the type of blood gas changes that occur in obstructive apnoea [4] may be one potential mechanism of this association.

A new part of the SDB spectrum in women is emerging: The role of high upper airway resistance in sleep as a pathophysiologic mechanism in the commonest of clinical disorders of pregnancy, preeclampsia. The most important finding in this area is not so much that there is SDB, but that given the pathological state of the endothelial system in preeclampsia, otherwise 'mild' upper airway flow limitation provokes a major pathological change in the circulatory system. The consequences of this otherwise mild SDB in preeclampsia are not respiratory; they are squarely in the cardiovascular domain. An important message from this new understanding is that it is not so much the apnoea index, apnoea duration, or even the extent of hypoxaemia, but how the system responds to those challenges. An individual with a predisposed abnormality (or risk factor), such as endothelial cell dysfunction in the case of preeclampsia, has resultant dangerous levels of hypertension in sleep, whereas someone not predisposed would have minimal changes in systemic blood pressure with a similar level of challenge.

The second part of the new understanding is that OSA in pregnancy appears to be more common than previously considered. In fact, more correctly, no one would consider sleep apnoea to be an issue in pregnant women, with young women representing the antithesis of the sleep apnoea phenotype, despite well-reported individual cases of obstructive apnoea in women. Yet it is now emerging that as pregnancy evolves, snoring becomes more prevalent. Importantly, as obesity becomes more prevalent in young people, the likelihood of a significant number of pregnant women developing clinically important SDB is increasing. Some estimates of the potential level of this prevalence could be as high as 10% in the third trimester. A final part of this picture relates to the methods that we use to diagnose SDB. The standard polysomnogram mostly systematically misses the type of problem that dominates the pattern of sleep disorders in pregnancy. Unless some measure of upper airway flow limitation is used, the significance of the respiratory sleep disturbance will be missed. Even more importantly, for preeclampsia (and pregnancy in general) the standard polysomnogram does not measure the variables of interest. It is only because we could measure systemic arterial blood pressure continuously during sleep that we could demonstrate the major pathological changes occurring during sleep (i.e., cardiovascular and haemodynamic); the important variables in this clinical circumstance are cardiovascular.

The purpose of this chapter is to provide an overview of sleep and breathing in pregnancy, and our goal is to generate ideas for new directions in research.

Changes in Sleep Architecture during Pregnancy

Normal pregnancy has a major impact on sleep architecture. These changes stem predominantly from biochemical and hormonal changes during the first and second trimesters of pregnancy; however, physical changes associated with the developing fetus predominate in the last trimester of pregnancy. While a number of studies have investigated sleep in pregnancy, most have concentrated on late pregnancy. Data from those in which sleep was investigated early in pregnancy indicate that total sleep time is significantly increased during the first trimester of pregnancy [5, 6]. Nonetheless, the overriding impact of pregnancy on maternal sleep throughout gestation is to generally reduce sleep quality and quantity. The second and third trimesters of pregnancy are associated with significant decreases in sleep quantity and quality when compared with the non-pregnant state [5–11]. There are a number of factors during pregnancy that determine these changes. Progesterone concentration rises sharply from the moment of implantation, produced predominantly by placental tissue. Changes in progesterone appear to override other hormonal changes during the first trimester of pregnancy, with its soporific properties predominating [12]. Progesterone metabolites appear to act as agonists on the gamma amino butyric acid subtype A receptor [13], thereby mimicking many of the effects that benzodiazepines have on sleep architecture, including decreased sleep latency, increased sleep time, marginally decreased time spent in REM sleep and increased REM sleep latency, increased power in the 11–16 Hz frequency range (the sleep spindle frequency range) and decreased power in the low frequency range (≤7 Hz). Oestrogen also undoubtedly plays a role in altering sleep architecture during pregnancy, predominantly by its inhibitory effect on REM sleep [14].

While the first trimester of pregnancy is associated with an increase in TST, on objective measures, the remainder of pregnancy tends to be associated with a reduction in sleep efficiency and TST [5, 6, 10, 11], although women tend to perceive that they spend more time sleeping [7]. Most studies agree that SWS is reduced during pregnancy, particularly late pregnancy [6, 11, 15].

Thus, while progesterone appears to dominate the impact of sleep on pregnancy during the first trimester of pregnancy, increasing the TST and decreasing the relative amount of SWS, the changes in sleep architecture that are associated with the latter half of pregnancy tend to be dominated by other factors. The decrease in percentage of SWS during the latter half of pregnancy may be attributed to increased progesterone concentration, while the decreased sleep efficiency may be due predominantly to the physical discomfort that is associated with pregnancy; factors including nocturia, fetal movement, uterine contractions, gastroesophageal reflux and backaches all contribute to physical discomfort and thereby, sleep disruption, during the latter stages of pregnancy. Although prolactin, a slow wave sleep stimulant, is increased during pregnancy, this has little impact on SWS during pregnancy for two reasons; primarily, both oestrogen and progesterone effectively block prolactin receptors, thereby reducing the activity of circulating prolactin. Additionally, the predominant form of prolactin prior to delivery is the glycosylated form (g-prolactin), which is less biologically active [16], and therefore has little impact on SWS. It should be noted that no study has adequately addressed the issue of upper airway flow limitation as a cause of disturbed sleep in late pregnancy, so it is possible, concurrent with the increase in snoring, that there is an increase in respiratory-induced arousals in late pregnancy.

Restless legs syndrome (RLS) is an important factor associated with sleep disruption in pregnancy. The prevalence of RLS during pregnancy increases in association with increasing gestational age, from between 0 to 10% prior to pregnancy to 15% during the second trimester, and further, to between 23 and 27% during the third trimester [17, 18]. The increased prevalence of RLS during pregnancy is almost certainly related to altered haematology and blood biochemistry, including reduced mean corpuscular volume and haemoglobin [18] and reduced serum folate and ferritin concentrations [17]. Once again, there are no studies seeking a potential link between respiratory sleep disturbance and myoclonus, both of which are known to develop in parallel in other subject groups.

While biochemical factors play an important role in determining sleep patterns, of equal importance to sleep initiation and maintenance during pregnancy are the physical changes that are associated with pregnancy. The enlarging uterus has many effects on maternal anatomical and physiological function. Nocturia is an important factor causing sleep disruption; increased urinary frequency is related to compression of the urinary bladder by the gravid uterus. Although fetal sleep patterns tend to correlate well with maternal sleep patterns, thereby reducing the number of large movements that are associated with periods of wakefulness in the fetus, maternal sleep is still often markedly disrupted by fetal movements during the second and third trimesters of pregnancy. The fetus begins uncoordinated movements at approximately the 16th week of pregnancy, and these movements become steadily more coordinated and larger as the pregnancy progresses. Fetal movements tend to be clustered towards the latter stages of maternal sleep, and there is some evidence to suggest that fetal and maternal REM sleep states coincide [19]. This is of significance to maternal sleep as fetal REM sleep induces movements that may be associated with maternal sleep disturbance. Aside from the importance of sleep and its disorders in pregnancy, this is an important observation as it adds further evidence to the hypothesis that the circadian sleep rhythm is entrained to maternal rhythms from early in fetal life.

While sleep disruption is commonplace in pregnancy, normal circadian sleep and hormonal rhythms are maintained during pregnancy [20]. Actigraphy during late pregnancy has demonstrated maintenance of relatively consolidated nocturnal sleep with some daytime napping noted [15]. It is notable that maternal cortisol concentration (as indicated by salivary cortisol measurements) is markedly augmented in pregnancy, averaging approximately twice non-pregnant levels [21]; however, the normal circadian pattern is preserved, with nadirs typically occurring around midnight and persistence of early morning peaks [22]. While placental growth hormone concentration is increased in the maternal circulation during pregnancy, secretion of human growth hormone (HGH) from the maternal pituitary is suppressed throughout pregnancy [23]. Little is known about the circadian and/or ultradian patterns of pituitary HGH during pregnancy, although studies in sheep suggest that peaks in maternal pituitary secretion of growth hormone occur from 21:00 to 01:00, which is similar to the pattern in non-pregnant ewes [24].

The circadian rhythmicity of serum melatonin concentrations appears to be unaltered by pregnancy, although there is some evidence that the relative levels when compared to serum cortisol concentrations may be altered in association with poor sleep in pregnancy [25].

Although many of the normal hormonal secretory patterns that are associated with sleep are maintained during pregnancy, there are also a number of hormones that do not maintain this normal circadian secretory pattern. Notably, maternal pituitary secretion of the hormone prolactin shows a pulsatile secretory pattern that is dissimilar to the normal circadian rhythm of prolactin secretion noted to occur in normal non-pregnant subjects [22], suggesting an absence of a relationship between maternal slow wave sleep and pituitary secretion of prolactin.

Sleep-Related Symptoms in Pregnancy

While insomnia and excessive daytime sleepiness (EDS) occur commonly in pregnancy, The International Classification of Sleep Disorders suggest that both of these conditions be recognised as sleep disorders and term them 'pregnancy-associated sleep disorders' [26].

Insomnia

Complaints of disturbed sleep are common in pregnancy. The many factors described above lead to a large proportion of women complaining of broken sleep and insomnia. Clearly, adherence to the standard sleep hygiene recommendations is an important basic management approach, but the major reality of an enlarging gravid uterus and its mechanical effects, uterine contractions and hormonally mediated sleep disruptions will have an impact in the majority of women. The sensible approach is to support the woman in living with this natural phenomenon without the request or need for drugs. There are a number of medications that are considered safe for use in pregnancy (in pregnancy category A, indicating that a large number of pregnant women have taken the medication without increasing the frequency of malformations of harmful effects on the fetus), including diphenhydramine hydrochloride, doxylamine succinate, chloral hydrate; none of the benzodiazepine agonists that are commonly used as sleep aids are recommended for use during pregnancy [27].

Daytime Sleepiness

The complaint of daytime sleepiness during pregnancy is common. While approximately a third of non-pregnant women report daytime sleepiness of varying degrees, a study of a large cohort of women during the 6th month of pregnancy report daytime sleepiness [28]. The reasons for increased daytime sleepiness during pregnancy are varied, but include increased sleep disruption stemming from urinary frequency and RLS, and also from the neurological impact of progesterone, which is soporific [13]. It is also important to consider the probability that some of this excess sleepiness may be the result of unrecognised SDB. Notably, there is a paucity of objective data on daytime sleepiness in pregnancy. Given the potential fetal risks, the use of stimulants should be avoided. There are no clear guidelines for the management of severe, abnormal sleepiness in pregnancy, including where it precedes the pregnancy, as in the case of narcolepsy. Discontinuation of stimulant use in this situation is advisable. Although newer stimulants are promising in terms of side effects in the non-pregnant patient, there are currently no data available regarding fetal safety.

Respiratory Changes and Their Association with Sleep in Pregnancy

It is now widely held that the incidence of snoring is increased during pregnancy [28–30, 79–81]. The incidence of the full spectrum of sleep breathing disorders is, however, less clear. During the late 80s and early 90s, most researchers suggested that pregnancy, and the associated high progesterone concentrations were effective protection against SDB, and indeed, progesterone was trialled as a treatment for SDB, but proved ineffective at substantially reducing the respiratory disturbance index, although it did improve oxygenation in patients with obesity hypoventilation syndrome [31]. Most now suggest that pregnancy may be an independent risk factor for SDB [32–35]. This has been unsubstantiated to date by robust data sets. Small clinical data sets to date of women predisposed to SDB are certainly highly suggestive of exacerbation or precipitation of this disease during pregnancy [36].

The maternal respiratory system undergoes marked changes throughout pregnancy. From the moment of conception, increasing circulating progesterone concentrations incrementally increase ventilatory drive. The respiratory centre in the ventrolateral medulla, which is bathed in cerebrospinal fluid, is extraordinarily sensitive to fluctuations in hydrogen ion concentration (H^+). It has long been known that progesterone is a powerful respiratory stimulant, and that increased circulating progesterone concentrations further increase sensitivity to (H^+) [37]. However, for progesterone to be an effective respiratory stimulant, prior exposure of the brainstem to oestrogen and consequent development of progesterone receptors is required. In the absence of prior exposure to oestrogen, progesterone has little impact on centrally mediated respiratory drive [38].

As a consequence of upregulation of ventilatory drive during pregnancy, increased minute ventilation, decreased arterial pCO_2 (30–32 Torr) and relative respiratory alkalosis at rest (pH 7.44) persist throughout pregnancy [39]. This has a number of effects that have the potential to impact upon sleep and ventilatory control. Primarily, with increasing ventilatory drive, diaphragmatic efforts become relatively enhanced – leading to increasingly negative upper airway pressures. The state of maternal sleep, particularly maternal REM sleep, is associated with reduced upper airway muscle tone; this leads to an increased propensity for collapse of the upper airway as the walls of the upper airway, and subsequent upper airway induced hypoventilation. Furthermore, increased pH and respiratory alkalosis lead to increased respiratory instability at sleep onset [40] as there is an increased gradient between apnoeic threshold during wakefulness and that during sleep when compared with the normal non-pregnant state. This may induce increased respiratory instability during the transition from sleep to wakefulness and during the lighter stages of NREM sleep. We have recently identified a greater prevalence of respiratory instability during maternal sleep, as evidenced by a greater number of centrally mediated respiratory events as pregnancy progresses in a small number of subjects studied sequentially [unpubl. data], suggesting increased instability as pregnancy advances.

Changes in maternal blood biochemistry also mediate changes in the affinity of haemoglobin for oxygen molecules. Relative alkalosis is associated with a shift in the oxyhaemoglobin desaturation curve to the right [41]. The physiological outcome of this is for the maternal haemoglobin to have a lower binding capacity for oxygen molecules. In practical terms, this means that for any given level of maternal arterial oxygen partial pressure (pO2) the saturation of the haemoglobin is lower. This is advantageous for the developing fetus as the available oxygen is relatively less tightly bound to maternal haemoglobin and therefore more readily available to the growing fetus. This also allows for improved maternal peripheral oxygenation, although it does have the disadvantage that uptake of oxygen molecules from the maternal pulmonary capillary system is marginally impaired. While this effect is offset during late pregnancy by an increase in maternal arterial oxygen partial pressure (PaO_2) during wakefulness (increasing to approximately 99 Torr) [42], this protection is lost during sleep so that mean PaO_2 during sleep in pregnancy is reduced to approximately 90 Torr. These data are substantiated by a study in the early 90s during which arterial oxyhaemoglobin saturation was significantly reduced during sleep in pregnant women when compared with the same women during the postpartum period [11]. However, this needs to be viewed in relationship to the increased cardiac output (see below) that occurs in pregnancy, so that the overall tissue oxygen delivery is likely to be increased.

In addition to the generation of greater negative upper airway pressures as a result of increased circulating progesterone concentrations, the calibre of the upper airway, particularly the oropharyngeal airway, is also reduced in pregnancy [43, 81]. This stems from a combination of increased circulating progesterone and oestrogen. Under normal circumstances, progesterone in combination with oestrogen partially disrupts the integrity of the vascular endothelial layer, leading to leakage of fluid from the intra- to the extravascular space [44] – resulting in oedema. The internal lumen of the upper airway during pregnancy is thus subject to narrowing as a result of accumulation of fluid in the extravascular space. Additionally, oestrogen is a potent vascular dilator and often induces vasomotor rhinitis during pregnancy [45]. Rhinitis narrows the nasal airway and thereby induces more negative upper airway pressures during inspiration, increasing the propensity for upper airway collapse (fig. 1).

Relaxin is a central hormone of pregnancy; it is produced by the corpus luteum and secreted in a continuous fashion throughout pregnancy. Its first identification was as a substance that promotes ligament relaxation and softening of the cervix in preparation for delivery [46]. Relaxin has a large number of diverse physiological roles [reviewed in 47] undoubtedly many of which have not yet been identified, and others that are not completely understood. With reference to sleep, and particularly the upper airway in sleep, relaxin is responsible for relaxation of soft tissue throughout the body, including the upper airway. Of interest, too, are the insulin-like properties that may promote insulin resistance and gestational diabetes mellitus, a disorder of pregnancy that may be linked with sleep.

Pulmonary mechanics are markedly altered during pregnancy. While changes in parameters including reductions in functional residual capacity and expiratory reserve volume and increases in the alveolar-arterial oxygen difference occur as a result of the gravid uterus impinging into the pulmonary space, a number of other respiratory dynamics are altered as a result of biochemical changes that are associated with pregnancy. Reduced resting lung volume [48] and hypocapnia [49] are both associated with increased airway resistance; however, total pulmonary resistance is decreased by 50% during pregnancy [49]. Of these changes, probably the most important in terms of SDB and the impact on maternal oxygenation is the reduction in expiratory reserve volume, as this may be associated with accelerated oxygen loss in the event of either centrally mediated or obstructive hypoventilation that may be induced by sleep.

Snoring and SDB in Pregnancy

Although the biochemical and physiological changes that are associated with pregnancy are likely to promote SDB, our current knowledge of the range of SDB during

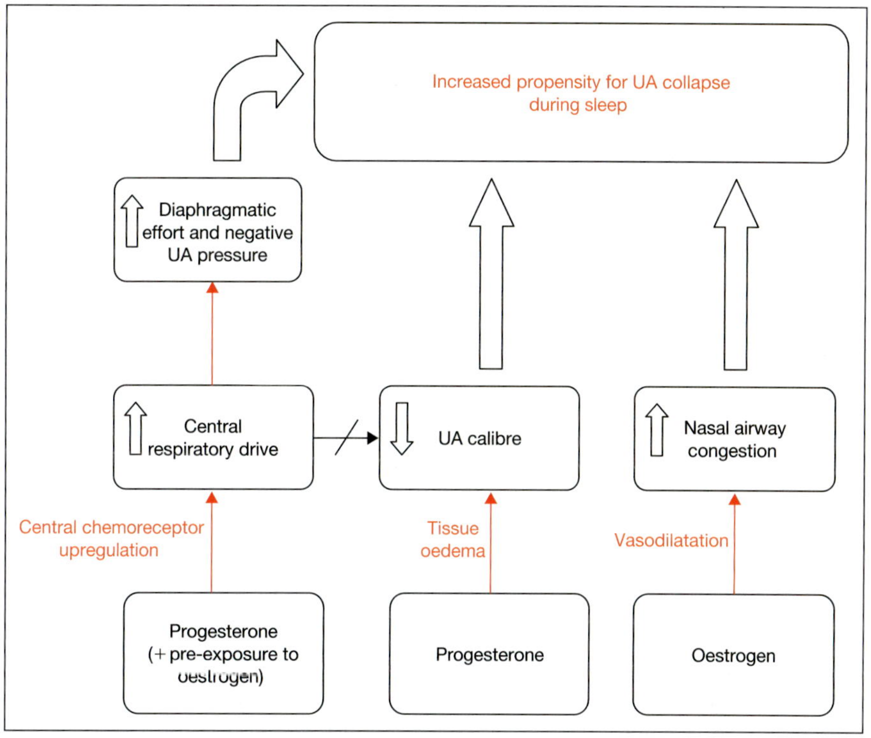

Fig. 1. Diagram of the interactions between progesterone and oestrogen during pregnancy that may predispose the pregnant patient to an increased risk of SDB. UA = Upper airway.

pregnancy is still minimal. While there is agreement that the prevalence of snoring is increased in pregnancy, the true occurrence is somewhat unclear. The largest systematic study of snoring in pregnancy that also included an objective measure of SDB [28] documented a sharp increase in snoring from 4% of the cohort prior to pregnancy to 12%; the increase in snoring during pregnancy is confirmed by a number of other questionnaire-based studies that report similar rates of snoring in the pregnant population, although the absolute magnitude is somewhat variable, ranging from 14 [30] to 23% [29]. While these studies confirm an increase in snoring during pregnancy, there are few studies that have systematically investigated the occurrence of SDB in pregnancy using objective physiological recordings; with the exception of studies of obesity in pregnancy [50] and preeclampsia [51] the few studies that have been conducted systematically tend to have focused on normal pregnancy [11, 42, 52]. Conversely, there are a number of case reports in which pregnancy is suggested to be responsible for precipitation or exacerbation of pre-existing SDB [32, 35, 53, 54]. A recent study from our laboratory, which investigated SDB during late pregnancy and then again following delivery, demonstrated marked improvement or complete resolution of SDB within 6 months postpartum in a group of women who had moderate to severe OSA during late pregnancy [36]. Notably, these patients were otherwise normal, having presented to their respective physicians with complaints of EDS. We have also consistently demonstrated the presence of SDB during pregnancy in women with preeclampsia [51]. However, it is important to note that the characteristic abnormality is upper airway flow limitation in the absence of complete obstructive apnoeas.

Given the currently available data and assessing the multitude of factors that may contribute to SDB, it is likely that the prevalence of SDB is higher during pregnancy than in non-pregnant women. Considering that the estimated prevalence of sleep apnoea (as indicated by an apnoea/hypopnoea index of greater than 5 per hour of sleep) in women of child-bearing age is in the order of 6.5–8.5% of the population [1], it is likely that the prevalence of SDB in pregnancy, particularly late pregnancy, exceeds 10%. A number of studies support this estimate [79–81].

Cardiovascular Function in Pregnancy

Pregnancy is associated with a range of haemodynamic and cardiovascular changes that have the potential to impact on the way that the maternal system reacts to sleep and sleep disorders. The maternal vasculature is adjusted such that in normal pregnancy, it allows for relatively high flow and low resistance when compared with the non-pregnant vascular system. Similarly, the placenta, under normal conditions allows a high flow rate and offers remarkably low resistances to impede blood flow.

Following implantation of the embryo, the maternal cardiovascular system undergoes substantial adjustments that continue throughout the pregnancy. The first notable change in maternal cardiovascular and haemodynamic control is peripheral vasodilatation; the predominant factor responsible for initiating and maintaining pregnancy-induced vasodilatation is increments in circulating oestrogen concentrations, which is a marked vasodilator through both endothelium-mediated vascular relaxation [reviewed in 55], and through other cellular mechanisms [reviewed in 56]. Relaxin is also a vasodilator that contributes to the reduction in peripheral vascular tone during pregnancy [47]. Although peripheral vascular tone is reduced during pregnancy, the normal circadian rhythm is maintained, with a reduction in peripheral vascular tone that is specifically associated with sleep [57]. The mechanism of reduced peripheral vascular tone during sleep in pregnancy is undoubtedly similar to that in the non-pregnant subject, i.e. a relative shift in autonomic tone from sympathetic to parasympathetic predominance; this sleep-induced reduction in peripheral vascular tone is reversed in preeclampsia such that sleep is associated with increments in peripheral vascular tone [57].

Intravascular volume increases markedly during pregnancy, which is attributable predominantly to an increase in plasma volume. Little is known about the circadian rhythmicity of intravascular volume in pregnancy, but studies of cardiac output and stroke volume from our laboratory [57] would lead us to suggest that in normal pregnancy it remains relatively stable during sleep. While maternal cardiac output is reduced marginally during sleep in normal pregnancy, this is attributable predominantly to reductions in heart rate, while stroke volume changes little, suggesting that venous return does not change substantially during sleep in pregnancy, which would lead to the conclusion that intravascular volume also remains relatively stable during the shift from wakefulness to sleep in normal pregnancy.

One of the most important maternal cardiovascular adjustments for the fetus is the increase in maternal cardiac output. Cardiac output begins to increase from the first trimester of pregnancy, with a 22% increase by the 8th week of pregnancy, and continues to increase until approximately the 36th week of pregnancy, at which time it reaches a maximum of 40% above pre-pregnancy levels. Increments in cardiac output during pregnancy occur as a result of the combination of increased stroke volume (which dominates) and increased heart rate. There have been few studies of the association between sleep and cardiac output in pregnancy, although we have recently shown small decrements that are associated with sleep, particularly NREM sleep in normal pregnancy [57]. The marginal reduction in cardiac output that is associated with sleep in normal pregnancy occurs as a result of the combination of reduced heart rate, which is associated with a sleep-related shift in autonomic tone to the predominance of parasympathetic activity, and a marginal reduction in stroke volume. It is important to note the marked decrease in cardiac output that can occur when the pregnant subject assumes the supine position, occurring as a result of partial occlusion of the vena cava and resultant reduction in venous return from the lower body. Although most pregnant women are aware that the supine posture is not an ideal position, the supine posture is occasionally assumed during sleep. For example, approximately 8% of the total sleep time was spent in the supine posture in a group of 10 women with OSA during pregnancy [36]. Given the potentially lethal combination of apnoea-induced hypoxaemia and reduced cardiac output, this mechanism, occurring during maternal sleep may be a possible cause of late fetal death.

The combination of increased cardiac output and decreased total peripheral resistance in pregnancy results in a marginal reduction in maternal blood pressure under normal circumstances. While there is a reduction in maternal blood pressure that is associated with pregnancy, the normal circadian blood pressure rhythm is maintained in normal pregnancy; thus maternal blood pressure may reach nadirs as low as 80/40 mm Hg (systolic/diastolic blood pressure) during the sleep period.

Pathophysiology of Cardiorespiratory Adjustments during Sleep in Preeclampsia

In contrast to normal pregnancy, in hypertensive disorders of pregnancy, the circadian blood pressure rhythm is flattened or reversed such that nocturnal blood pressure is as high or higher than daytime blood pressure values [58] (fig. 2). Thus, nocturnal blood pressure in women with preeclampsia may reach peaks as high as 180–200 systolic and 90–110 diastolic [51, 58]. There is evidence from epidemiological studies that maternal SDB interacts with the maternal cardiovascular system to increase the risk of hypertensive diseases of pregnancy, including essential hypertension and preeclampsia [29].

We have demonstrated that episodes of maternal hypertension during sleep are specifically associated with episodes of upper airway dysfunction in women with preeclampsia. Furthermore, incremental increases in blood pressure associated with maternal sleep in preeclampsia can be reduced

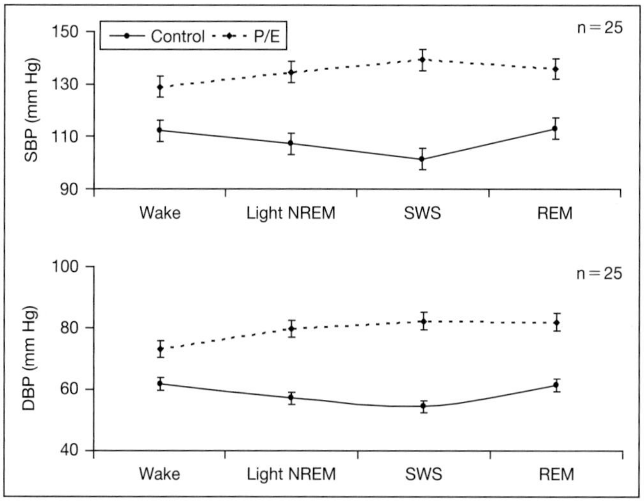

Fig. 2. The blood pressure during wakefulness and different sleep stages in normal women and in women with preeclampsia, demonstrating a link between sleep and increasing blood pressure in women with preeclampsia.

or reversed with the use of nocturnal nasal continuous positive airway pressure (CPAP) treatment, titrated to control sleep-induced upper airway dysfunction [51].

Preeclampsia is predominantly a disease of the maternal vascular endothelium; its origins are from the first trimester of pregnancy with abnormally shallow invasion of placental trophoblasts into the maternal endometrium [reviewed in 59]. This leads to abnormal flow characteristics within the placental vessels such that the normal circumstance of high flow, low resistance to blood flow is reversed, with decreased flow and increased placental vascular resistance [60]. As a result an inflammatory process is set into place whereby the placenta produces large quantities of inflammatory mediators that have effects throughout the maternal circulation. The vascular endothelium, which is particularly responsive to these inflammatory mediators, then becomes highly susceptible to pressor-inducing stimuli, mediating peripheral vascular constriction, while also sustaining damage resulting in an increased loss of intravascular fluid into the interstitial space [61]. These processes lead to hypertension, oedema and end organ damage. The clinical effects of preeclampsia, though initiated at the time of implantation, do not become apparent until the third trimester of pregnancy. At this time, the dominant clinical picture is one of hypertension associated with proteinuria (evidence of renal damage), oedema both peripherally and in the central nervous system and other widespread inflammatory processes. However, abnormal vascular endothelial function can be identified early in the second trimester, prior to the occurrence of clinical symptoms.

We have recently shown that upper airway dysfunction during sleep is common in preeclampsia [51], and the pathological processes that are involved in preeclampsia may be exacerbated as a result of a cascade of events triggered by obstructed breathing during sleep. Importantly, the degree of upper airway dysfunction found in pre-eclamptic patients would be regarded as clinically insignificant in other patients. We rarely observed apnoeic events that would meet current criteria to be defined as apnoeas or hypopnoeas in this group, and oxyhaemoglobin desaturation was also uncommon. However, this apparently minor degree of upper airway flow limitation markedly increases blood pressure during sleep. In association with this marked degree of hypertension that is associated with sleep in preeclampsia, there is also substantial peripheral vasoconstriction, and also marked reductions in maternal cardiac output [57] (fig. 3). Our findings of upper airway dysfunction in preeclampsia have recently been confirmed by others [82].

In contrast to normal pregnancy, preeclamptic pregnancy is associated with reduced intravascular volume, which is almost certainly potentiated during sleep. We have demonstrated reduced stroke volume that is specifically associated with sleep in women with preeclampsia; restricted venous return resulting from reduced intravascular volume may be implicated in the aetiology of reduced stroke volume both during sleep, and during wakefulness, in women with preeclampsia. The underlying endothelial cell abnormality with leakage of intravascular fluid into the interstitial space is the predominant mechanism. One additional mechanism that may contribute to reductions in intravascular volume in preeclampsia may be increased upper airway resistance during sleep. As already discussed, increased upper airway resistance during sleep is common in women with preeclampsia. From studies in male apnoeic subjects, it is well known that increasingly negative intrathoracic pressures are associated with increased release of atrial natriuretic peptide (ANP) [62]; ANP is a potent diuretic hormone and may contribute substantially to intravascular depletion in women with preeclampsia. Studies have demonstrated elevated blood levels of ANP in women with preeclampsia [63].

That the proximate cause for the rise in blood pressure in sleep is the mild upper airway obstruction was clearly demonstrated by the ease with which low levels of nasal CPAP, titrated to reverse the upper airway flow limitation, inhibited the sleep-linked rise of arterial blood pressure [51]. It is of major significance that the rise in blood pressure in these subjects is not the result of apnoea-induced oxyhaemoglobin desaturation, the process most favoured as the mediator of the vascular consequences of sleep apnoea. Although nasal CPAP might have some unidentified

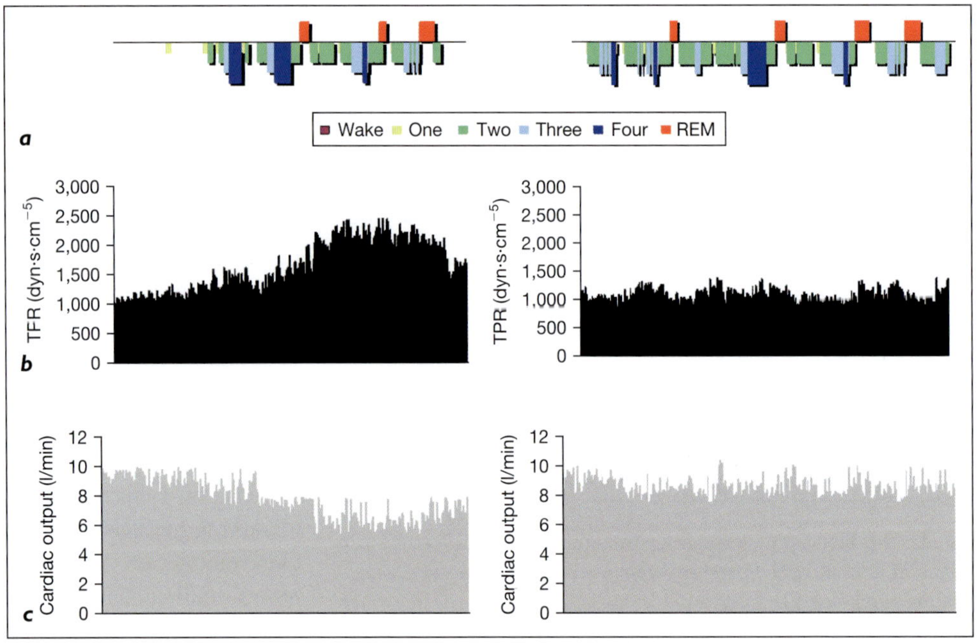

Fig. 3. Maternal sleep stage (***a***), total peripheral resistance (***b***) and cardiac output (***c***) in a patient with preeclampsia and SDB before (left) and during (right) nocturnal nasal CPAP treatment, showing marked peripheral vasoconstriction and reductions in maternal cardiac output and their reversal with nasal CPAP treatment.

beneficial therapeutic effects, we have proposed that the way in which it treats the sleep-induced hypertensive episodes is by preventing otherwise minor increments in arterial CO_2 associated with the upper airway flow limitation. Hypercapnia is a well-documented source of centrally mediated vasoconstriction. It is notable that few studies have attempted to evaluate the potential role of hypercapnia on cellular mechanisms that might be involved in the adverse outcomes of sleep apnoea. However, hypercapnia has potent effects on pathways that lead to free radical production and has been implicated as an amplifier of oxidative inflammatory lung disease [64]. Arterial CO_2 levels are not routinely measured as part of the polysomnogram and potentially represent yet another 'blind' spot in our understanding of the pathophysiology of SDB.

Although the reasons for the development of upper airway flow limitation in preeclampsia are unknown, recent findings suggest that the upper airway in preeclampsia becomes particularly vulnerable because of the development of oedema and narrowing of the internal lumen [43]. The changes that occur lead to a long segment of narrowing of the upper airway, and in part explain the nature of the flow limitation, which is characterised by relatively slow oscillations in flow during inspiration, in contrast to the 30–50 Hz that characterises palatal snoring. This also probably accounts for the fact that the form of upper airway flow limitation in preeclampsia may not be associated with loud audible snoring, a major reason why the prevalence of upper airway dysfunction during sleep in preeclampsia may be underestimated in questionnaire studies that enquire about audible snoring.

Our current hypothesis is that partial obstruction during sleep is associated with a marginal relative hypercapnia. Increased arterial, and subsequently CSF, pCO_2 stimulates the ventrolateral medulla to increase peripheral sympathetic activity. While under normal circumstances the system can adequately cope with these changes, in preeclampsia the damaged endothelium is hyper-responsive to this otherwise insignificant pressor stimulus, leading to exacerbation of peripheral vasoconstriction. Reversal of this sequence of events with the use of nasal CPAP leads to suppression of the marked hypertensive episodes that are associated with sleep in preeclampsia [51]. However, it is possible that direct effects of CO_2/pH changes on vascular endothelial function contribute to the sleep-linked pressor response in preeclampsia.

Preeclampsia also appears to have a striking impact on maternal sleep architecture, with marked increments in amount of slow wave sleep evident during the nocturnal sleep period [51]. The pathophysiology leading to these changes is likely a combination of increased circulating inflammatory mediators, especially TNF-α, which are associated with augmentation of SWS [65], and increased intracranial pressure associated with cerebral oedema, which is also associated with pathological high voltage low frequency EEG activity [66]. There is a great need for further investigation in this area.

Maternal Sleep and the Initiation of Labour

While we have thus far considered the impact of pregnancy on sleep, the interaction of sleep and labour is another important area, and may provide considerable insight into both the normal physiology of sleep, and also the interactions of maternal physiology and labour.

Although the notion that maternal sleep is important for normal fetal development is a 'received truth', there is very little data to support or illuminate the issue. However, there are a number of outstanding studies that do provide strong support for this general notion. Clearly, maternal fetal interaction is basic to normal pregnancy, and issues such as maternal nutrition and maternal health are critical to normal fetal development and the delivery of a normal healthy infant. In turn, normal sleep is known to be critical to development, and to be important to normal health.

Important physiological-sleep links such as the coupling of growth hormone secretion to SWS, and the likely feed forward role of sleep in growth and development provide strong evidence for a key role of sleep itself in overall development and well-being. Sleep as the conduit through which major physiological events during development occur is underpinned in the research that indicates the onset of puberty is first heralded by an increase in sleep and in particular SWS in adolescence [67], and by the marked increase in secretion of pituitary sex hormone triggered by SWS (or at least co-ordinated by SWS) prior to the physical changes that characterise sexual maturity. It is therefore not a great leap of understanding to propose that maternal sleep in pregnancy has an important role in fetal development; however, there is a paucity of data linking maternal sleep-wake behaviour with fetal development. Undoubtedly, a key reason for this is that it is very hard to study. Thus, most of our understanding comes from animal studies, particularly the sheep model. Sterman [19] performed an early study of human fetal movements and their association with maternal state in 1967. This pioneering work showed a diurnal linkage between increasing numbers of fetal movements (which are highly indicative of fetal correlates of REM sleep) and maternal REM sleep. We have recently undertaken a series of studies on a cohort of 21 normal pregnant women in the last trimester of pregnancy and have also demonstrated a strong link between maternal REM sleep and increased fetal movements [unpubl. data].

It is unclear whether the links between maternal and fetal behaviour involve a direct role of sleep itself, or an indirect role, such as may be mediated through maternal hormonal systems, or whether it is simply a result of synchronisation of the fetal and maternal circadian clocks. The fetus is known to have a functioning central circadian clock in the suprachiasmatic nucleus by the 30th week of pregnancy [68], so it is not unreasonable to suggest that some form of synchronisation of maternal and fetal sleep rhythms occurs. Our recognition and understanding of this area is rudimentary at best, but given the now well-known critical role that sleep plays in development after birth, there is a high probability that similar links exist between maternal sleep and fetal development that remain to be revealed. One well-documented link between maternal and fetal behavioural states is mediated through maternal food intake, and in particular carbohydrate load. There is a marked increase in fetal movements following maternal feeding, and it is possible that such a mechanism is the dominant source of maternal fetal synchronisation.

One remarkable observation suggests that both maternal and fetal sleep have an important role in timing the onset and progression of labour. In the primate, labour is initiated during nocturnal hours. In a primate model, the pattern of uterine contraction shifts from regular 'contractures' (equivalent to Braxton-Hicks contractions) to 'contractions', which are characterised by shorter, more intense myometrial muscular forces, over a 5- to 7-day period, signalling the onset of fully established labour. This shift in the type and intensity of contractions was specifically linked to maternal sleep in this model [69]. The initiation of labour is triggered by the fetal release of cortisol in the sheep, and by androgens in other mammalian species. Clearly our understanding of this area is cursory, but it is possible that a better understanding might provide important clinical outcomes in determining the timing of delivery and may provide important clues as to the causes and management of postmaturity.

The association between maternal sleep and labour is further evidenced by a study in which poor maternal sleep (both disrupted maternal sleep and short duration of maternal sleep) during late pregnancy is associated with longer labour times and substantial increases in the rate of caesarean delivery [20].

Finally, in reviewing maternal sleep and its association with labour, the study of Driver and Shapiro [10] provides some insight into the interaction between the two. They performed a longitudinal study of sleep architecture from early pregnancy until the postpartum period and coincidentally found a marked increase in SWS that was specifically associated with the onset of labour in one subject. The significance of this is unclear, however, it may reflect either the release of factors during sleep that are involved in the initiation of labour, or alternatively, may reflect the labour-induced release of substances that coincidentally have an impact on sleep architecture. One of these may be prolactin, the secretion of which is increased during labour [70].

While this review has to this point focused on maternal sleep and its impact on maternal physiology and pathophysiology, we have not yet considered the impact that maternal sleep has on fetal outcome. In reviewing the impact of pregnancy on maternal sleep, the impact of maternal sleep in both normal and abnormal pregnancy on the developing fetus must be considered.

The Interaction of Maternal and Fetal Sleep and Breathing

The fetus has a functional circadian rhythm generator early in gestation but the mother generates most of the timing cues. This area is reviewed in [71]. Maternal feeding plays an important role in entraining the fetal rest/activity cycle. However, there are number of interesting observations that suggest that maternal and fetal sleep states interact.

The fetus develops a period cycle of rest/activity, states which broadly equate to NREM and REM sleep states, and this cycle is well established by the third trimester, with a periodicity of about 40 min during the earlier half of pregnancy, and 60 min near term. Barcroft and Barron [72] were first to show that the fetus could make breathing movements. The latter were easy to elicit by cutaneous stimulation early in fetal development; breathing movements became harder to provoke later in gestation, which they attributed to the development of a powerful central inhibition. Subsequently, Dawes et al. [73] found that fetal breathing occurred regularly throughout gestation. They also identified three sleep states in the fetal lamb; quiet (or inactive) sleep that occurred for 55% of the time, 'active' sleep (REM sleep) characterised by movements, REMs, and a characteristic electrocorticography that lasted about 40% of time. The third state they defined as 'apparently' awake lasted only 5% of the recording time. Fetal breathing movements were almost entirely confined to the periods of REM sleep.

It is likely that the phenomenon of REM state-linked fetal breathing movements is representative of the way in which the brain plays a critical role in overall development; internally generated neural activity, in the case of fetal breathing, is playing a driving role in the development of the overall respiratory system. This centrally generated activity likely drives the development of the medullary automatic control centres, neural programs, neurochemical patterning, neural paths, respiratory muscles and lung growth.

Remarkably, maternal breathing disturbances, such as sleep apnoea, are powerful inhibitors of fetal breathing movements [unpubl. data] and fetal body movements (fig. 3, 4), which is, likely, indicative of its impact on fetal REM sleep. Thus, SDB in the pregnant woman in turn induces a disturbance of fetal sleep-wake patterning and inhibition of the normal breathing patterning; maternal SDB induces fetal SDB. Suppression of fetal breathing movements in the compromised fetus was demonstrated many years ago. In this interesting study increased maternal inspired oxygen to a level of 50% led to a large increase in fetal breathing movements where there was intrauterine growth retardation (IUGR), but had no effect on the breathing of the normal fetus [74]. Although a number of explanations were discussed, including the possibility of an increased fetal carbon dioxide level, the likely explanation was an improvement in fetal oxygenation, and removal of the powerful pontine suppression of fetal movements and breathing movements that hypoxemia induces. These old results are consistent with our new findings of the effects of maternal CPAP in preeclampsia, and suggest that sleep breathing disorders, and sleep-induced cardiovascular compromises should be routinely investigated in pregnancies with IUGR.

Maternal SDB is also associated with IUGR [29]. Under normal circumstances the interaction of sleep and the cardiovascular system in pregnancy is favourable to fetal growth and development. The circadian blood pressure profile is retained, with further reductions in total peripheral resistance [57], allowing the maintenance of low resistance, high flow through the placental vasculature. However, in pregnancy that is associated with SDB, the fetus may become markedly compromised. An early study of fetal behaviour during maternal apnoeic episodes has established a marked impact on fetal physiology, with episodes of marked bradycardia, which is highly indicative of fetal distress [75]. We have recently shown a significant correlation between maternal cardiac output specifically during the maternal sleep period and fetal birth weight in women

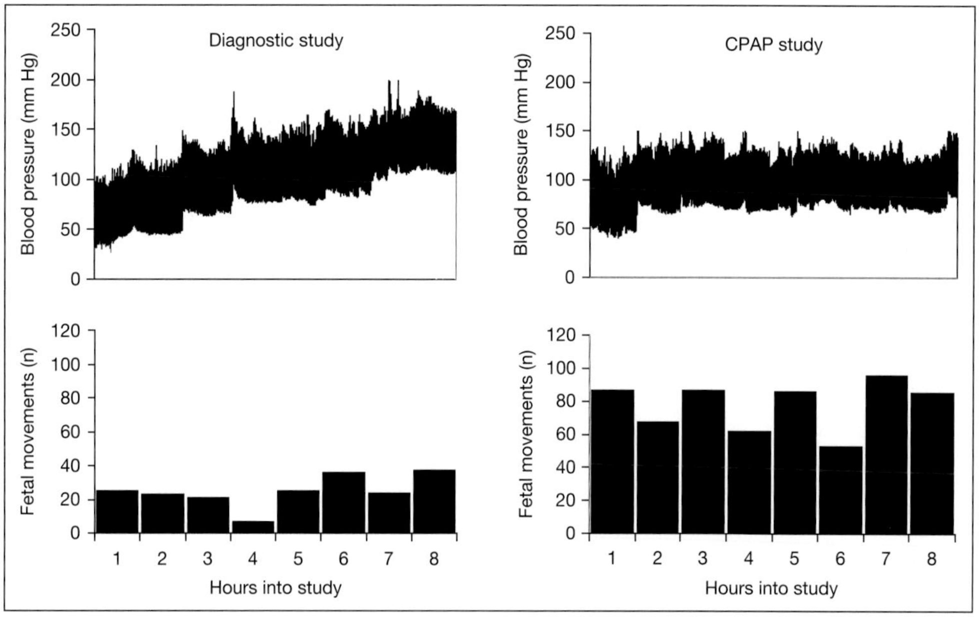

Fig. 4. A comparison of the number of fetal movements per hour of maternal sleep in association with maternal blood pressure in a patient with preeclampsia and SDB. The first panel indicates marked suppression of fetal movement in association with maternal blood pressure increments, while fetal movements are partially restored during treatment with nocturnal nasal CPAP. The reduced fetal movements included a marked suppression of fetal breathing movements, and a clear rebound of fetal breathing on the CPAP treatment night.

with coexisting preeclampsia and SDB [57], leading us to suggest that altered maternal haemodynamics during sleep have a marked impact on fetal outcome. Further epidemiological evidence to suggest a marked interaction between maternal SDB and fetal compromise is provided by a study of 502 singleton pregnancies in which fetal growth restriction and reduced Apgar scores were found to be significantly associated with maternal SDB as assessed by a questionnaire [29].

The finding that maternal sleep apnoea, and SDB in preeclampsia are likely causes of IUGR brings about another potentially interesting link. Barker [76] proposed that many adult diseases had their origins in the fetus and infant and in particular provide evidence that fetal growth retardation is a risk factor for subsequent adult obesity and vascular disease. This hypothesis has been the subject of extensive recent research and cannot be reviewed adequately here. However, IUGR is indeed a risk factor for the development of the metabolic syndrome [77]. Given the now established link between sleep apnoea and the metabolic syndrome, the remarkable further link is that snoring and sleep apnoea in pregnancy may play a role in the development of the metabolic syndrome, and in parallel sleep apnoea in later life by causing fetal growth retardation.

Sleep in the Postnatal Period

Most studies of sleep in the postnatal period suggest that marked sleep disruption occurs, predominantly as a result of the need to tend to the infant; this is magnified in new mothers [5]. However, while wake after sleep onset is magnified in new mothers, in those that are breastfeeding, there appears to be a marked physiological increase in the amount of time spent in SWS [10, 78], which is not reflected in mothers who do not breastfeed their infants [78]. The increase in SWS during the postnatal period in breastfeeding mothers is almost certainly associated with increments in circulating prolactin concentrations. This is an area of potentially fruitful research. As noted above, if sleep apnoea is present in later pregnancy, it mostly improves after delivery, although the long-term outcome of pregnancy-induced sleep apnoea, and the high upper airway resistance pattern of sleep breathing disorder in preeclampsia are unknown. It is probable that these subjects will develop SDB in later life.

In conclusion, the period of pregnancy and the postpartum period are both times of extensive fluctuation in sleep physiology. Maternal sleep is a time of particular vulnerability for both the mother and fetus, as well as an important time during which marked physiological changes may occur. SDB is part of preeclampsia and may play an important role in causing IUGR. OSA occurs in pregnancy, and is also a potentially reversible cause of IUGR and possibly unexpected late fetal death. This is going to be a more significant problem as the prevalence of obesity in young women increases, and the estimates of the extent on sleep apnoea could place it as high as 10% of pregnancies. The major impact of SDB in pregnancy is through its effects on the cardiovascular system. The current methods of diagnosing SDB are inadequate for evaluating pregnant patients, as they do not measure the relevant physiological variables. Our knowledge of this area to date is cursory and much more study in the area needs to be undertaken before we can have a clearer understanding of the role of maternal sleep in both normal and abnormal pregnancy.

References

1 Young T, Palta M, Dempsey J, Skatrud J, Weber S, Badr S: The occurrence of sleep-disordered breathing among middle-aged adults. N Engl J Med 1993;328:1230–1235.

2 Lugaresi E, Cirignotta F, Coccagna G, Piana C: Some epidemiological data on snoring and cardiocirculatory disturbances. Sleep 1980;3: 221–224.

3 Mooe T, Rabben T, Wiklund U, Franklin KA, Eriksson P: Sleep-disordered breathing in women: occurrence and association with coronary artery disease. Am J Med 1996;101: 251–256.

4 Edwards N, Wilcox I, Polo OJ, Sullivan CE: Hypercapnic blood pressure response is greater during the luteal phase of the menstrual cycle. J Appl Physiol 1996;81: 2142–2146.

5 Lee KA, Zaffke ME, McEnany G: Parity and sleep patterns during and after pregnancy. Obstet Gynecol 2000;95:14–18.

6 Hedman C, Pohjasvaara T, Tolonen U, Suhonen-Malm AS, Myllyla VV: Effects of pregnancy on mothers' sleep. Sleep Med 2002;3:37–42.

7 Mindell JA, Jacobson BJ: Sleep disturbances during pregnancy. J Obstet Gynecol Neonatal Nurs 2000;29:590–597.

8 Karacan I, Wayne H, Harman AW, Williams R, Webb W, Ross JJ: Characteristics of sleep patterns during late pregnancy and the postpartum periods. Am J Obstet Gynecol 1968;101: 579–586.

9 Nishihara K, Horiuchi S: Changes in sleep patterns of young women from late pregnancy to postpartum: relationships to their infants' movements. Percept Mot Skills 1998;87: 1043–1056.

10 Driver HS, Shapiro CM: A longitudinal study of sleep stages in young women during pregnancy and postpartum. Sleep 1992;15: 449–453.

11 Hertz G, Fast A, Feinsilver SH, Albertario CL, Schulman H, Fein AM: Sleep in normal late pregnancy. Sleep 1992;15:246–251.

12 Brunner DP, Munch M, Biedermann K, Huch R, Huch A, Borbely AA: Changes in sleep and sleep electroencephalogram during pregnancy. Sleep 1994;17:576–582.

13 Lancel M, Faulhaber J, Holsboer F, Rupprecht R: Progesterone induces changes in sleep comparable to those of agonistic $GABA_A$ receptor modulators. Am J Physiol 1996;271: E763–E772.

14 Fang J, Fishbein W: Sex differences in paradoxical sleep: influences of estrus cycle and ovariectomy. Brain Res 1996;734:275–285.

15 Shinkoda H, Matsumoto K, Park YM: Changes in sleep-wake cycle during the period from late pregnancy to puerperium identified through the wrist actigraph and sleep logs. Psychiatry Clin Neurosci 1999;53: 133–135.

16 Markoff E, Lee DW, Hollingsworth DR: Glycosylated and nonglycosylated prolactin in serum during pregnancy. J Clin Endocrinol Metab 1988;67:519–523.

17 Lee KA, Zaffke ME, Baratte-Beebe K: Restless legs syndrome and sleep disturbance during pregnancy: the role of folate and iron. J Womens Health Gend Based Med 2001;10: 335–341.

18 Manconi M, Govoni V, De Vito A, Economou NT, Cesnik E, Casetta I, Mollica G, Ferini-Strambi L, Granieri E: Restless legs syndrome and pregnancy. Neurology 2004;63: 1065–1069.

19 Sterman MB: Relationship of intrauterine fetal activity to maternal sleep stage. Exp Neurol 1967;19:98–106.

20 Lee KA, Gay CL: Sleep in late pregnancy predicts length of labor and type of delivery. Am J Obstet Gynecol 2004;191:2041–2046.

21 Allolio B, Hoffmann J, Linton EA, Winkelmann W, Kusche M, Schulte HM: Diurnal salivary cortisol patterns during pregnancy and after delivery: relationship to plasma corticotrophin-releasing-hormone. Clin Endocrinol 1990;33:279–289.

22 Eriksson L, Eden S, Holst J, Lindstedt G, von Schoultz B: Diurnal variations in thyrotropin, prolactin and cortisol during human pregnancy. Gynecol Obstet Invest 1989;27:78–83.

23 De Leo V, la Marca A, Lanzetta D, Pasqui L, Morgante G: Thyroid function in early pregnancy. II: Paradoxical growth hormone response to thyrotropin-releasing hormone. Gynecol Endocrinol 1998;12:197–201.

24 McMillen IC, Thorburn GD, Walker DW: Diurnal variations in plasma concentrations of cortisol, prolactin, growth hormone and glucose in the fetal sheep and pregnant ewe during late gestation. J Endocrinol 1987;114: 65–72.

25 Suzuki S, Dennerstein L, Greenwood KM, Armstrong SM, Sano T, Satohisa E: Melatonin and hormonal changes in disturbed sleep during late pregnancy. J Pineal Res 1993;15: 191–198.

26 American Academy of Sleep Medicine: International classification of sleep disorders, revised: Diagnostic and coding manual; in Chicago, Illinois, American Academy of Sleep Medicine, 2001.

27 MIMS: MIMS online; St Leonards, Medical Publishers Association of Australia, 2006.

28 Guilleminault C, Querra-Salva M, Chowdhuri S, Poyares D: Normal pregnancy, daytime sleeping, snoring and blood pressure. Sleep Med 2000;1:289–297.

29 Franklin KA, Holmgren PA, Jonsson F, Poromaa N, Stenlund H, Svanborg E: Snoring, pregnancy-induced hypertension, and growth retardation of the fetus. Chest 2000;117: 137–141.

30 Loube DI, Poceta JS, Morales MC, Peacock MD, Mitler MM: Self-reported snoring in pregnancy. Association with fetal outcome [see comments]. Chest 1996;109:885–889.

31 Strohl KP, Hensley MJ, Saunders NA, Scharf S, Brown R, Ingram RH: Progesterone administration and progressive sleep apneas. JAMA 1981;1230–1232.

32 Kowall J, Clark G, Nino Murcia G, Powell N: Precipitation of obstructive sleep apnea during pregnancy. Obstet Gynecol 1989;74: 453–455.

33 Lefcourt LA, Rodis JF: Obstructive sleep apnea in pregnancy. Obstet Gynecol Surv 1996;51:503–506.

34 Charbonneau M, Falcone T, Cosio MG, Levy RD: Obstructive sleep apnea during pregnancy. Therapy and implications for fetal health. Am Rev Respir Dis 1991;144:461–463.

35 Lewis DF, Chesson AL, Edwards MS, Weeks JW, Adair CD: Obstructive sleep apnea during pregnancy resulting in pulmonary hypertension. South Med J 1998;91:761–762.

36 Edwards N, Blyton D, Hennessy A, Sullivan C: Severity of sleep-disordered breathing improves following parturition. Sleep 2005; 28:737–741.

37 Zwillich CW, Natalino MR, Sutton FD, Weil JV: Effects of progesterone on chemosensitivity in normal men. J Clin Lab Med 1978;92: 262–269.

38 Hannhart B, Pickett CK, Moore LG: Effects of estrogen and progesterone on carotid body neural output responsiveness to hypoxia. J Appl Physiol 1990;68:1909–1916.
39 Lim VS, Katz AI, Lindheimer MD: Acid-base regulation in pregnancy. Am J Physiol 1976;231: 1764–1769.
40 Dempsey JA, Skatrud JB: A sleep-induced apneic threshold and its consequences. Am Rev Respir Dis 1986;133:1163–1170.
41 Kambam JR, Handte RE, Brown WU, Smith BE: Effect of normal and preeclamptic pregnancies on the oxyhemoglobin dissociation curve. Anesthesiology 1986;65:426–427.
42 Prodromakis E, Trakada G, Tsapanos V, Spiropoulos K: Arterial oxygen tension during sleep in the third trimester of pregnancy. Acta Obstet Gynecol Scand 2004;83:159–164.
43 Izci B, Riha RL, Martin SE, Vennelle M, Liston WA, Dundas KC, Calder AA, Douglas NJ: The upper airway in pregnancy and preeclampsia. Am J Respir Crit Care Med 2002;167:137–140.
44 Stachenfeld NS, Taylor HS: Effects of estrogen and progesterone administration on extracellular fluid. J Appl Physiol 2004;96: 1011–1018.
45 Mabry RL: Rhinitis of pregnancy. South Med J 1986;79:965–971.
46 Hisaw F: Experimental relaxation of the pubic ligament of the guinea pig. Proc Soc Exp Biol Med 1926;23:661–663.
47 Sherwood OD: Relaxin's physiological roles and other diverse actions. Endocr Rev 2004; 25:205–234.
48 Dubois A: Resistance to breathing; in Fenn WO, Rahn H (eds): Handbook of Physiology, Sec 3, Respiration. Baltimore, Waverly, 1964, pp 451–452.
49 Newhouse M, Becklake M, Macklem P, McGregor M: Effect of alterations in end-tidal CO2 tension on flow resistance. J Appl Physiol 1964;19:745–749.
50 Maasilta P, Bachour A, Terama K, Polo O, Laitinen LA: Sleep-related disordered breathing during pregnancy in obese women. Chest 2001;120:1448–1454.
51 Edwards N, Blyton DM, Kirjavainen T, Kesby GJ, Sullivan CE: Nasal continuous positive airway pressure reduces sleep-induced blood pressure increments in preeclampsia. Am J Respir Crit Care Med 2000;162:252–257.
52 Brownell LG, West P, Kryger MH: Breathing during sleep in normal pregnant women. Am J Respir Crit Care Med 1986;133:38–41.
53 Conti M, Izzo V, Muggiasca ML, Tiengo M: Sleep apnoea syndrome in pregnancy: a case report. Eur J Anaesthesiol 1988;151–154.
54 Hastie SJ, Prowse K, Perks WH, Atkins J, Blunt VAW: Obstructive sleep apnoea during pregnancy requiring tracheostomy. Aust N Z J Obstet Gynaecol 1989;3:365–367.
55 Rubanyi GM, Johns A, Kauser K: Effect of estrogen on endothelial function and angiogenesis. Vascul Pharmacol 2002;38:89–98.
56 White MM, Zamudio S, Stevens T, Tyler R, Lindenfeld J, Leslie K, Moore LG: Estrogen, progesterone, and vascular reactivity: potential cellular mechanisms. Endocr Rev 1995;16: 739–751.
57 Blyton DM, Sullivan CE, Edwards N: Reduced nocturnal cardiac output associated with preeclampsia is minimized with the use of nocturnal nasal CPAP. Sleep 2004;27: 79–84.
58 Redman CW, Beilin LJ, Bonnar J: Reversed diurnal blood pressure rhythm in hypertensive pregnancies. Clin Sci Mol Med Suppl 1976;3: 687S–689S.
59 Kaufman S: Control of intravascular volume during pregnancy. Clin Exp Pharmacol Physiol 1995;22:157–163.
60 Howie PW, Prentice CR, McNicol GP: Coagulation, fibrinolysis and platelet function in pre-eclampsia, essential hypertension and placental insufficiency. J Obstet Gynaecol Br Commonw 1971;78:992–1003.
61 Hayman R, Brockelsby J, Kenny L, Baker P: Preeclampsia: the endothelium, circulating factor(s) and vascular endothelial growth factor. J Soc Gynecol Investig 1999;6:3–10.
62 Krieger J, Laks L, Wilcox I, Grunstein RR, Costas LJ, Sullivan CE: Atrial natriuretic peptide release during sleep in patients with obstructive sleep apnoea before and during treatment with nasal continuous positive airway pressure. Clin Sci 1989;77:407–411.
63 Borghi C, Esposti DD, Immordino V, Cassani A, Boschi S, Bovicelli L, Ambrosioni E: Relationship of systemic hemodynamics, left ventricular structure and function, and plasma natriuretic peptide concentrations during pregnancy complicated by preeclampsia. Am J Obstet Gynecol 2000;183:140–147.
64 Lang JD, Figueroa M, Sanders KD, Aslan M, Liu Y, Chumley P, Freeman BA: Hypercapnia via reduced rate and tidal volume contributes to lipopolysaccharide-induced lung injury. [see comments]. Am J Respir Crit Care Med 2005;171:147–157.
65 Krueger JM, Obal F Jr, Fang J: Humoral regulation of physiological sleep: cytokines and GHRH. J Sleep Res 1999;8:53–59.
66 Munari C, Calbucci F: Correlations between intracranial pressure and EEG during coma and sleep. Electroencephalogr Clin Neurophysiol 1981;51:170–176.
67 Laberge L, Petit D, Simard C, Vitaro F, Tremblay RE, Montplaisir J: Development of sleep patterns in early adolescence. J Sleep Res 2001;10:59–67.
68 Mirmiran M, Kok JH, Boer K, Wolf H: Perinatal development of human circadian rhythms: role of the foetal biological clock. Neurosci Biobehav Rev 1992;16:371–378.
69 Farber DM, Giussani DA, Jenkins SL, Mecenas CA, Winter JA, Wentworth RA, Nathanielsz PW: Timing of the switch from myometrial contractures to contractions in late-gestation pregnant rhesus monkeys as recorded by myometrial electromyogram during spontaneous term and androstenedione-induced labor. Biol Reprod 1997;56: 557–562.
70 Stefos T, Sotiriadis A, Tsirkas P, Messinis I, Dimitrios L: Maternal prolactin secretion during labor. The role of dopamine. Acta Obstet Gynecol Scand 2001;80:34–38.
71 Mirmiran M, Maas YG, Ariagno RL: Development of fetal and neonatal sleep and circadian rhythms. Sleep Med Rev 2003;7: 321–334.
72 Barcroft J, Barron D: The genesis of respiratory movements in the foetus of the sheep. J Physiol London 1937;88:56–61.
73 Dawes GS, Fox HE, Leduc BM, Liggins GC, Richards RT: Respiratory movements and rapid eye movement sleep in the foetal lamb. J Physiol London 1972;220:119–143.
74 Dornan J, Ritchie J: Fetal breathing movements and maternal hyperoxia in the growth retarded fetus. Br J Obstet Gynaecol 1983; 90:210–213.
75 Joel-Cohen SJ, Schoenfeld A: Fetal response to periodic sleep apnea: a new syndrome in obstetrics. Eur J Obstet Gynecol Reprod Biol 1978;8:77–81.
76 Barker DJ: The fetal and infant origins of disease. Eur J Clin Invest 1995;25:457–463.
77 Chatelain P: Children born with intra-uterine growth retardation (IUGR) or small for gestational age (SGA): long term growth and metabolic consequences. Endocr Regul 2000;34: 33–36.
78 Blyton DM, Sullivan CE, Edwards N: Lactation is associated with an increase in slow-wave sleep in women. J Sleep Res 2002;11:297–303.
79 Pien GW, Fife D, Pack AI, Nkwuo JE, Schwab RJ: Changes in symptoms of sleep-disordered breathing during pregnancy. Sleep 2005;28:1299–1305.
80 Leung PL, Hui DSC, Leung TN, Yuen PM, Lau TK: Sleep disturbances in Chinese pregnant women. BJOG 2005;112:1568–1571.
81 Izci B, Vennelle M, Liston WA, Dundas KC, Calder AA, Douglas NJ: Sleep-disordered breathing and upper airway size in pregnancy and post-partum. Eur Respir J 2006;27: 321–327.
82 Yinon D, Lowenstein L, Suraya S, Beloosesky R, Zmora O, Malhotra A, Pillar G: Preeclampsia is associated with sleep-disordered breathing and endothelial dysfunction. Eur Respir J 2006;27:328–333.

Prof. Dr. Colin E. Sullivan
David Read Laboratory, Medicine
University of Sydney
Sydney (Australia)
Tel. +61 2 9351 6123, Fax +61 2 9550 3851
E-Mail ces@med.usyd.edu.au

Author Index

Subject Index